# Clinical Nursing Procedures:
# The Art of Nursing Practice

COLLEGE OF NURSING
CHRISTIAN MEDICAL COLLEGE,
LUDHIANA, PUNJAB, INDIA-141008

PRIZE AWARDED
AT 33rd CONVOCATION
HELD ON 21st March, 2009

TO *Sharanjit Kaur*

FOR *securing second highest marks in GNM aggregate*

# Clinical Nursing Procedures: The Art of Nursing Practice

*Editors*

**Annamma Jacob** MSc N
Professor
Bhagwan Mahaveer Jain College of Nursing
Bangalore

*Formerly*
- Professor, St. Philomina's College of Nursing, Mother Teresa Road, Bangalore
- Principal, Graduate School for Nurses, BNE, SIB, CMAI
- Nurse Supervisor, Suburban Medical Center, Paramount, Southern California, USA
- Assistant Director of Nursing, Al-Sabah Hospital, Ministry of Public Health, Kuwait
- Sister Tutor, LT College of Nursing, SNDT Women's University, Mumbai
- Junior Tutor, College of Nursing, CMC Hospital, Vellore, Tamil Nadu

**Rekha R** MSc N
Associate Professor
Bhagwan Mahaveer Jain College of Nursing
Bangalore, Karnataka

*Formerly*
- Lecturer and Asst. Professor, Sree Mookambika College of Nursing, Kanyakumari, Tamil Nadu

**Jadhav Sonali Tarachand** MSc N, PG Diploma in Medical Law & Ethics
Asst. Professor of Nursing
Bhagwan Mahaveer Jain College of Nursing
Bangalore, Karnataka

*Formerly*
- Lecturer in Medical Surgical Nursing, St. Marthas College of Nursing, Bangalore, Karnataka
- Assistant Lecturer, Bharathi Vidyapeeth's College of Nursing, Pune, Maharashtra

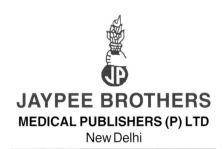

**JAYPEE BROTHERS**
**MEDICAL PUBLISHERS (P) LTD**
New Delhi

*Published by*

Jitendar P Vij
**Jaypee Brothers Medical Publishers (P) Ltd**
EMCA House, 23/23B Ansari Road, Daryaganj
**New Delhi** 110 002, India
Phones: +91-11-23272143, +91-11-23272703, +91-11-23282021, +91-11-23245672
Fax: +91-11-23276490, +91-11-23245683   e-mail: jaypee@jaypeebrothers.com
Visit our website: www.jaypeebrothers.com

*Branches*

- 2/B Akruti Society, Jodhpur Gam Road, Satellite
  **Ahmedabad** 380 015, Phone: +91-079-30988717, +91-079-26926233

- 202 Batavia Chambers, 8 Kumara Krupa Road, Kumara Park East
  **Bangalore** 560 001, Phones: +91-80-22285971, +91-80-22382956, +91-80-30614073
  Tele Fax: +91-80-22281761   e-mail: jaypeemedpubbgl@eth.net

- 282 IIIrd Floor, Khaleel Shirazi Estate, Fountain Plaza, Pantheon Road
  **Chennai** 600 008, Phones: +91-44-28262665, +91-44-28269897
  Fax: +91-44-28262331   e-mail: jpchen@eth.net

- 4-2-1067/1-3, Ist Floor, Balaji Building, Ramkote, Cross Road
  **Hyderabad** 500 095, Phones: +91-40-55610020, +91-40-24758498
  Fax: +91-40-24758499   e-mail: jpmedpub@rediffmail.com

- "KURUVI BUILDING", 1st Floor, Plot/Door No. 41/3098-B &B1, St. Vincent Road
  **Kochi** 682 018, Ph: +91-0484-4036109   e-mail: jaypeekochi@rediffmail.com

- 1A  Indian Mirror Street, Wellington Square
  **Kolkata** 700 013, Phones: +91-33-22456075, +91-33-22451926
  Fax: +91-33-22456075   e-mail: jpbcal@cal.vsnl.net.in

- 106 Amit Industrial Estate, 61 Dr SS Rao Road, Near MGM Hospital, Parel
  **Mumbai** 400 012, Phones: +91-22-24124863, +91-22-24104532, +91-22-30926896
  Fax: +91-22-24160828   e-mail: jpmedpub@bom7.vsnl.net.in

- "KAMALPUSHPA", 38 Reshimbag, Opp. Mohota Science College, Umred Road
  **Nagpur** 440 009, Phones: +91-712-3945220, +91-712-2704275   e-mail: jpnagpur@rediffmail.com

*Clinical Nursing Procedures: The Art of Nursing Practice*

*First Edition:* **2007**

ISBN   81-8061-883-8

*Typeset at* JPBMP typesetting unit
*Printed at* Ajanta Offset & Packagings Ltd., New Delhi

# CONTRIBUTORS

**Jessy Jacob** MSc N
Asst. Professor of Nursing
Bhagwan Mahavir Jain College of Nursing
Bangalore

**Subha Shankari G** BSc N
Asst. Lecturer of Nursing
Bhagwan Mahavir Jain College of Nursing
Bangalore

**Nalini SR** BSc N
Asst. Lecturer of Nursing
Bhagwan Mahavir Jain College of Nursing
Bangalore

**Jain Binny John** BSc N
Asst. Lecturer of Nursing
Bhagwan Mahavir Jain College of Nursing
Bangalore

**Harsha Joy** BSc N
Asst. Lecturer of Nursing
Bhagwan Mahavir Jain College of Nursing
Bangalore

**Anne Dorcas** BSc N
Asst. Lecturer of Nursing
Bhagwan Mahavir Jain College of Nursing
Bangalore

**Mary Daniel** BSc N
Asst. Lecturer of Nursing
Bhagwan Mahavir Jain College of Nursing
Bangalore

**Lakshmi** BSc N
Asst. Lecturer of Nursing
Bhagwan Mahavir Jain College of Nursing
Bangalore

**Anita Grace Daniel** BSc N
Asst. Lecturer of Nursing
Bhagwan Mahavir Jain College of Nursing
Bangalore

**Sindhu Narendran** BSc N
Asst. Lecturer of Nursing
Bhagwan Mahavir Jain College of Nursing
Bangalore

**Naveena J** BSc N
Asst. Lecturer of Nursing
Bhagwan Mahavir Jain College of Nursing
Bangalore

# PREFACE

Today's nursing practice has evolved through many changes influenced by advances in science and technology which has made medical care more complex. As modalities for diagnosing and treating illnesses and managing patients in different stages of health-illness continuum change, several nursing procedures are added and rewritten.

Use of specialized equipments, articles and assisting with advanced procedures have become a necessity in caring for patients. Several nursing procedures taught and practiced in yesteryears have become obsolete as a result of new knowledge of disease pathology and therapy.

The growing body of nursing research further challenges and stimulates nurses to acquire new knowledge and refine their critical thinking skills. Nursing education today aims to provide students a broad knowledge base which would help them provide expert and need-based care to clients with varying health problems. It is, therefore, essential that they master basic theories and skills and become equipped to further develop and refine their abilities to apply analytical thinking in clinical situations.

Nurse educators in India have always been faced with the need to have reference materials suited to present day practice standards. Books which meet the above criteria are written in the context of developed countries where advanced equipments and commercially prepared articles and materials are used for performing most nursing procedures. A procedure manual written in the Indian context, where health care facilities range from most advanced in the tertiary level multi-speciality hospitals in large cities to primary care centers in rural India has been a felt need.

This manual will help in preparing nurses who can demonstrate critical thinking and analytical ability, capable of making adaptations in varying situations. A manual of procedures that is relevant to the present day nursing practice in India has been a need, felt by nurse educators here. The book *Clinical Nursing Procedures: The Art of Nursing Practice* is an all-in-one compilation of nursing procedures.

Basic, Advanced and Community Health Nursing procedures are organized and presented in 15 chapters.

The editors and contributors have taken care to present the material in a concise, straight forward and simplified format in an easy to follow language and most importantly in the Indian context. Scientific rationale of every nursing action is included so as to enable nursing students and practicing nurses to use sound clinical judgement while emphasizing cognitive, interpersonal and psychomotor skills needed to carry out nursing procedures. Special considerations are included wherever additional explanations for deviations and adaptations are required.

The contents of the book include nursing procedures to be performed independently by nurses and interdependently by providing assistance to either health care professionals or clients themselves. Most nursing procedures prescribed for undergraduate education by Apex bodies in India are included.

A special feature of this book authored and contributed by Indian Nurses is the many illustrations and colour photographs which would aid to master and reinforce the skills of nursing students as well as practicing nurses.

The editors are confident that this book will prove to be an useful tool for undergraduate students as well as professional nurses working in different settings all over India.

Annamma Jacob
Rekha R
Jadhav Sonali Tarachand

# ACKNOWLEDGEMENTS

It takes more than great determination and sustained interest to write a book . For completion of the task, encouragement, support and cooperation of many are essential.

For the production of this book, the editors are deeply thankful to the administration of Bhagwan Mahaveer Jain College of Nursing. The President of Bhagwan Mahaveer Memorial Jain Trust, Mr. Sampathraj Gadia always encouraged us and provided the freedom and the facilities needed to the principal and senior faculty of the college to gather knowledge and teach professional nursing of high quality to their students. The members of BMMJ Trust, Mr. Parasmal Bansali and Mr. Phoolchand Jain did an excellent job of providing the library in the college with large collection of books and periodicals for reference. This greatly enhanced preparation of materials for the book.

As the idea of putting together all the nursing procedures taught to nursing students in the college emerged in the minds of the first group of faculty, the Chief Executive Officer of the Hospital and College of Nursing, Dr. Kishore Murthy offered great encouragement and support. The editors are thankful to Dr. Kishore Murthy.

Most of the faculty members who worked in the college of nursing, since its inception in 2003, contributed by way of writing and editing the procedures for the book. The editors thank each one of them for their contribution.

The nursing staff of BMJ Hospital whose practice standards needed updation for providing safe and effective nursing care to patients and the students of BMJ College of Nursing were our inspiration to embark on the task of preparing this manual of nursing procedures.

For the many photographs and illustrations included in the book, college and hospital staffs, their family members, students and patients offered themselves and their efforts, and we record our sincere thanks to everyone of them.

It was Miss Anuradha who in the final stages undertook the job of typing all the material in a professional manner. The preliminary work was done by Mrs. Vachala, Mrs. Sudheshna Mukherjee and Miss Sylvia Eileen. We thankfully acknowledge their contributions.

Finally but importantly, we once again acknowledge the administration of BMJ College of Nursing, the BMMJ Trust in honour of which this book may be published.

# CONTENTS

## 3. SAFETY, BODY MECHANICS AND INFECTION ........................................ 121

## 4. NUTRITION ........................................................................................ 163

## 5. ELIMINATION ..................................................................................... 183

## Contents

## Contents

# Chapter 1

# Health Assessment

1.1      Measuring Body Temperature
1.2      Assessment of Pulse
1.3      Assessing Respiration
1.4      Monitoring Blood Pressure
1.5      Checking Height and Weight of a Patient
1.6      Collecting Urine Specimen for Routine Examination
1.7      Testing Urine for pH
1.8      Testing Urine for Specific Gravity
1.9(a) Testing Urine for Glucose (Benedict's Solution)
1.9(b) Testing Urine for Glucose (Reagent Strip or Tape)
1.10    Testing Urine for Albumin
1.11    Collecting Urine Specimen for Culture
1.12    Collection of 24 hours Urine
1.13    Collecting a Stool Specimen for Routine Examination
1.14    Collecting a Stool Specimen for Culture
1.15    Collecting a Throat Swab for Culture
1.16    Collecting a Wound Swab for Culture
1.17    Protocol for Sample Collection of Blood
1.18    Collecting Blood for Routine Examination
1.19    Measuring Blood for Glucose Level using Glucometer
1.20    Collection of Blood for Culture
1.21    Collecting Blood for Peripheral Smear
1.22    Collection of Sputum for Culture
1.23    Assisting with Obtaining a Papanicolaou Smear
1.24    Measuring Intake and Output
1.25    Teaching Breast Self-examination
1.26    Teaching Testicular Self-examination

## 1.1: MEASURING BODY TEMPERATURE

### DEFINITION

Measuring temperature of the body using a clinical thermometer.

### COMMON METHODS

1. Oral
2. Rectal
3. Axillary
4. Tympanic membrane

### INDICATIONS

1. Routine part of assessment on admission for establishing a base-line data.
2. As per agency policy to monitor any change in patient condition.
3. Before, during and after administration of any drug that affects temperature control function.
4. When general condition of patient changes.
5. Before and after any nursing intervention that affects temperature of the patient.

### PURPOSES

1. To assess the general health status of patient.
2. To assess for any alteration in health status.

### CONTRAINDICATIONS

A. Oral method
   1. Patients who are not able to hold thermometer in their mouth.
   2. Patients who may bite the thermometer like psychiatric patients.
   3. Infants and small children
   4. Surgery/infection in oral cavity
   5. Trauma to face/mouth
   6. Mouth breathers
   7. Patients with history of convulsion
   8. Unconscious/semi conscious/disoriented patients.
   9. Patients having chills
  10. Unco-operative patients.
  11. Patients who cannot follow instructions.
B. Rectal method
   1. Patients after rectal surgery
   2. Any rectal pathology (piles/tumor)
   3. Patients having difficulty in assuming position
   4. Acute cardiac patient
   5. Patients having diarrhea
   6. Reduced platelet count.
C. Axillary method
   1. Any surgery/lesion in axilla.

### ARTICLES

A clean tray containing
1. A bottle with disinfectant solution (dettol 1: 40/savlon 1:20)

2. A bottle with water
3. Thermometer (rectal thermometer in case of rectal method)
4. A small bowl with cotton swabs
5. Paper bag/kidney tray
6. Pens
7. Flow sheet/graphic chart/paper
8. Lubricant (in case of rectal/method)
   If using more than one thermometer, use 3 bottles (2 with antiseptic solution and one with water).

## PROCEDURE

| | Nursing action | Rationale |
|---|---|---|
| 1 | Ascertain method of taking temperature and explain procedure to the patient and instruct him how to co-operate. | |
| | a. In case of oral method, ensure that patient had not taken any hot or cold food and fluids orally or smoked in 15-30 minutes prior to procedure. | Causes alteration in temperature reading. |
| | b. For rectal method, provide privacy and position the patient in a Sim's position. In young children position laterally with knees flexed or prone across lap. | Position ensures easy access to insert thermometer. |
| | c. For axillary method, expose axilla and pat dry with a towel. Avoid vigorous rubbing. | Friction produced by rubbing can cause increase in temperature. |
| 2 | Wash hands | |
| 3 | Prepare equipment | |
| | a. If glass thermometer is in disinfectant solution, transfer it to container with plain water using dominant hand. | Ensures complete removal of disinfectant and reduces irritation to tissues.<br>Using dominant hand reduces chances of accidental breakage. |
| | b. Wipe thermometer dry, using a clean cotton swab using rotatory motion from bulb to stem. | Wiping from an area of least contamination to an area of greatest contamination prevents spread of organisms. |
| | c. Shake down the mercury (if needed) by holding thermometer between thumb and forefinger at the tip of stem. Shake till mercury is below 35 degree centigrade (95 degree Fahrenheit). | Reduces chances of error in reading temperature. |
| 4 | Take temperature | |
| | a. For oral method | |
| |   i. Place bulb of thermometer at base of tongue on the side of frenulum in the posterior sublingual pocket (Figure 1.1(a)). | Blood supply is more in this area and hence reflects the temperature of blood in the larger blood vessels. |

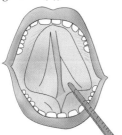

**Figure 1.1(a):** Positioning thermometer for oral temperature (thermometer under tongue)

*Contd...*

*Contd...*

| | |
|---|---|
| ii. Instruct patient to close the lips and not teeth around thermometer. | Clenching teeth can cause the thermometer to break and cause injury. |
| iii. Leave thermometer in place for 2-3 minutes. | Ensures accurate recording |

b. For rectal method
  i. Don disposable gloves
  ii. Apply lubricant on the bulb of thermometer using cotton ball.
  iii. With non-dominant hand, expose the anus raising upper buttocks.(Figure 1.1(b) (i))
  iv. Instruct patient to breathe deeply and insert thermometer into anus. (Figure 1.1(b) (ii))
      3.5 – 4 cm in adults
      1.5 cm in infant
      2.5 cm in child
      Do not force insertion
  v. Hold thermometer in place for 1-2 minutes.

Lubricant facilitates easy insertion without irritating mucous membrane.
Taking deep breathe relaxes external sphincter thereby facilitating easy insertion.
Ensures accurate recording

Prevents thermometer from falling down.
Ensures accurate recording

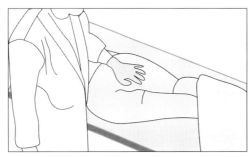 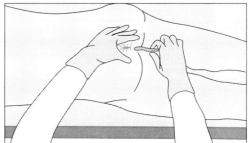

**Figure 1.1(b):** (i) Positioning patient for inserting rectal thermometer, (ii) Inserting rectal thermometer

c. For axillary method
  i. Place bulb in the center of axilla (Figure 1.1(c))
  ii. Place arm tightly across chest to hold thermometer in place.
  iii. Hold thermometer in place for 3-5 minutes.

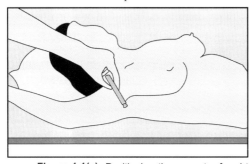 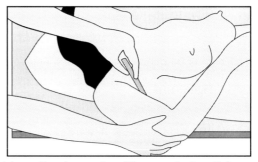

**Figure 1.1(c):** Positioning thermometer for obtaining axillary temperature (Thermometer in axilla)

| | |
|---|---|
| 5  Remove thermometer<br>Wipe using a cotton ball from stem to bulb in a rotatory manner. | Wiping from an area of least contamination to an area of greatest contamination will help in preventing spread of microorganisms. |

*Contd...*

*Contd...*

| | | |
|---|---|---|
| 6 | Read the temperature, holding thermometer at eye level and rotate it till reading is visible and read it accurately. | Holding at eye level prevents error in reading. |
| 7 | Shake down the mercury level | |
| 8 | Clean thermometer using soap and water. | Removes organic material. |
| 9 | Dry it and store it in disinfectant solution. | |
| 10 | Document temperature | |
| 11 | Wash hands | Reduces risk of transmission of microorganisms. |
| 12 | Replace articles. | |

## SPECIAL POINTS

1. It is always best to use individual thermometer for each patient.
2. When individual thermometer is not used in patient care-units (wards), axillary method is recommended.
3. For converting temperature from centigrade to Fahrenheit following conversion formula can be used.
   $C = 5/9 \times F-32$
   [C = degree centigrade]
   [F = degree Fahrenheit]

## 1.2: ASSESSMENT OF PULSE

### DEFINITION

Checking pulse rate, rhythm, volume, etc. for assessing circulatory status.

### PURPOSES

1. To establish baseline data
2. To check abnormalities in rate, rhythm and volume
3. To monitor any change in health status of the patient.
4. To check the peripheral circulation.

**Table 1.2.1:** Common sites for checking pulse (Figure 1.2 (a))

| | Site | Location | Reasons for use |
|---|---|---|---|
| 1 | Radial | Inner aspect of the wrist on thumb side (Figure 1.2(b)). | Easily accessible. |
| 2 | Temporal | Site superior (above) and lateral to (away from the midline) the eye (Figure 1.2(c)). | Used when radial pulse is not accessible. Easily accessible pulse in children. |
| 3 | Carotid | At the side of the trachea where the carotid artery runs between the trachea and the sternocleidomastoid muscle (Figure 1.2(d)). | To assess cerebral perfusion. |
| 4 | Apical | Left side of the chest in the 4th , 5th or 6th intercostal space in the midclavicular line (Figure 1.2(e)). | Used to find out discrepancies with radial pulse. |
| 5 | Brachial | Medially in the antecubital space (Figure 1.2(f)). | Used to monitor blood pressure and assess for lower arm circulation. |
| 6 | Femoral | Below inguinal ligament, midway between symphysis pubis and anterosuperior iliac spine  (Figure 1.2(g)). | To assess circulation to lower hip. |
| 7 | Popliteal | Medial or lateral to the popliteal fossa with knees slightly flexed (Figure 1.2(h)). | Used to determine circulation to the leg. To take blood pressure in the lower limb. |
| 8 | Posterior tibial | On the medial surface of the ankle behind the medial malleolus. | To assess circulation to the foot. |
| 9 | Dorsalis pedis | Along dorsum of foot between extensor tendons of great and first toe (Figure 1.2(i)) | To assess circulation to the foot. |
| 10 | Ulnar pulse | On the little finger side, outer aspect of the wrist. | To assess circulation to ulnar side of hand. To perform Allen's test. |

### ARTICLES

1. Wrist watch with second hand
2. Pen (color as per agency policy)
3. Vital signs chart and flowsheets

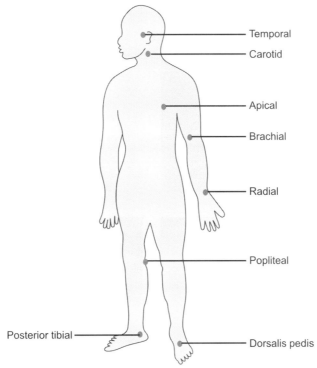

**Figure 1.2(a):** Common sites for checking pulse

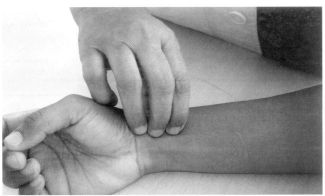

**Figure 1.2(b):** Checking radial pulse

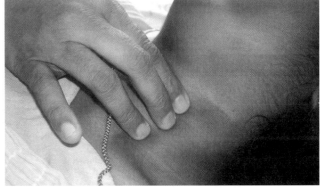

**Figure 1.2(d):** Checking carotid pulse

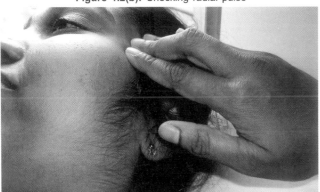

**Figure 1.2(c):** Checking temporal pulse

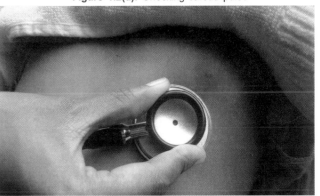

**Figure 1.2(e):** Checking apical pulse

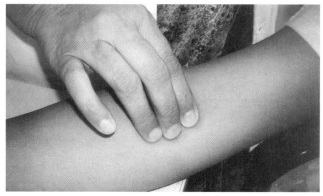

Figure 1.2(f): Checking brachial pulse

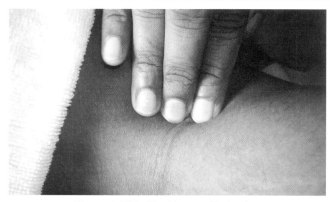

Figure 1.2(h): Checking popliteal pulse

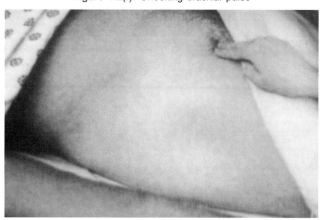

Figure 1.2(g): Checking femoral pulse

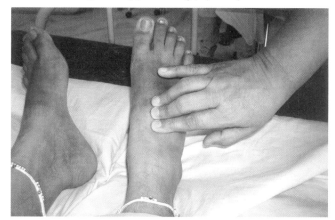

Figure 1.2(i): Checking dorsalis pedis pulse

## PROCEDURE

| | Nursing action | Rationale |
|---|---|---|
| 1 | Explain procedure to patient and check if the patient had been involved in any activity. If so allow the patient to rest for 10 minutes before taking pulse. | Activity can increase the pulse rate. |
| 2 | a. Select the pulse site | Usually radial pulse is selected. If any particular extremity is to be assessed then another pulse site is to be selected. |
| | b. Assist the patient to a comfortable position. For radial pulse, keep the arm, resting over chest or on the side with palm facing downward. In sitting position, keep the arm resting over thigh with palm facing downward. | |
| 3 | Palpate and check pulse | |
| | a. Place tips of 3 fingers other than thumb lightly over pulse site. | Thumb is not used for assessing pulse as it has its own pulse which can be mistaken for patient's pulse. |
| | b. After getting the pulse regularly, count the pulse for one whole minute looking at the second hand on the wrist watch. | Irregularities can be noticed only if pulse is counted for one whole minute. |
| | c. Assess for rate, rhythm and volume of pulse and condition of blood vessel. | |
| 4 | Document and report pertinent data in the appropriate record. | |
| 5 | Wash hands. | |

## SPECIAL POINTS

1.  Never press both carotids at the same time, as this can cause reflex drop in blood pressure/pulse rate.
2.  Carotid pulse is used for victims of shock and cardiac arrest when pulse is not palpable at other sites.
3.  Brachial and femoral sites are used with cardiac arrest in infants.

## 1.3: ASSESSING RESPIRATION

### DEFINITION

Monitoring inspiration and expiration in a patient.

### PURPOSES

1. To assess rate, rhythm and volume of respiration.
2. To assess for any change in condition and health status.
3. To monitor the effectiveness of therapy related to respiratory system.

### ARTICLES

Wrist watch with second hand, graphic record, pen (color according to agency policy).

### PROCEDURE

|   | Nursing action | Rationale |
|---|----------------|-----------|
| 1 | Ensure that patient is relaxed Assess other vital signs such as pulse or temperature prior to counting respirations. | Awareness of the procedure may alter the rate of respiration. Conscious patients when relaxed and unaware of procedure tend to have accurate respiratory rate. |
| 2 | Assess for factors that may alter respiration. | Allows nurse to accurately assess for presence and significance of respiratory alteration. |
| 3 | Wait for 5 –10 minutes before assessing respiration if patient had been active. | Activity may increase rate and depth of respiration. |
| 4 | Position patient in sitting or supine position with head elevated at 45-60 degree. | Ensures proper assessment. |
| 5 | Keep your fingers over the wrist as if checking pulse, and position patient's hand over his lower chest or abdomen. | Makes the patient less aware of his respiration. Keeping hand over chest or abdomen makes the movement of chest more visible. |
| 6 | Observe one complete respiratory cycle-inspiration and expiration. | |
| 7 | Assess rate, depth, rhythm and character of respiration. | Depth of respiration reveals volume of air moving in and out of lungs. Abnormalities of rhythm and character reveals specific disease condition. |
| 8 | Count respiration for one whole minute. | |
| 9 | Wash hands | |
| 10 | Record the findings and report any abnormal findings. | |

## 1.4: MONITORING BLOOD PRESSURE

### DEFINITION

Measuring blood pressure using a sphygmomanometer.

### PURPOSES

1. To determine patient's blood pressure as a baseline for comparing future measurements.
2. To aid in diagnosis.
3. To aid in the assessment of cardiovascular system preoperatively and postoperatively, during and after invasive procedures.
4. To monitor change in condition of the patient.
5. To assess response to medical therapy.
6. To determine patient's hemodynamic status.

### ARTICLES

1. A sphygmomanometer comprising of:
   a. Compression bag/inflatable rubber bladder enclosed in a cloth cuff (appropriate size)
   b. An inflating bulb (by which pressure is raised)
   c. A manometer (mercury) from which pressure is read.
   d. A screw type release valve for inflation and deflation (pressure control.)
2. Stethoscope.
3. Patient chart for recording.
4. Black/blue pen for charting.

### PROCEDURE

|   | Nursing action | Rationale |
|---|---|---|
| 1 | Check physician's order, nursing care plan and progress notes | Obtains any specific instruction/information. |
| 2 | Explain the procedure and reassure the patient. Ensure that patient has not smoked, ingested caffeine or involved in strenuous physical activity within 30 minutes prior to procedure. | Obtains patient consent and co-operation and also relieves anxiety. Smoking, caffeine can increase blood pressure. |
| 3 | Wash and dry hands | Prevents cross-infection |
| 4 | Assist the patient to either sitting or lying down position | Obtains an accurate reading |
| 5 | Collect and check equipment | Ascertains evidence of malfunction |
| 6 | Position the sphygmomanometer at approximately heart level of the patient ensuring that mercury level is at zero. (Figure 1.4(a)) | Helps in obtaining accurate reading. |

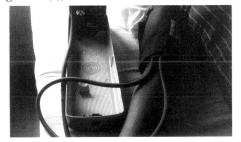

**Figure 1.4(a):** Positioning sphygmomanometer at heart level

*Contd...*

*Contd...*

| 7 | Select a cuff of appropriate size (Figure 1.4(b)) 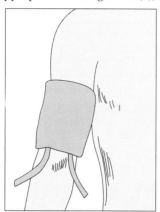 **Figure 1.4(b):** Selecting blood pressure cuff of appropriate size | Ensures that compression bladder width is at least 20% wider than the diameter of the mid-point of the exterimity used. If the bladder is too wide the reading may be erroneously low. If it is too small, the reading may be erroneously high. |
|---|---|---|
| 8 | Expose the arm to make sure that there is no constrictive clothing above the placement of cuff. | Ensures accurate reading. |
| 9 | Apply the cuff approximately 2.5 cm above the point where brachial artery can be palpated. The cuff should be applied smoothly and firmly with the middle of the rubber bladder directly over the artery (Figure 1.4(c)). 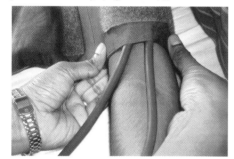 **Figure 1.4(c):** Application of blood pressure cuff over arm | Ensures accurate reading Wrapping the cuff too tightly will impede circulation. Wrapping the cuff very loosely will lead to false elevation of pressure. |
| 10 | Secure the cuff by tucking the end under or by fixing the velcro fastener. | Prevents unwrapping of the cuff. |
| 11 | Place the entire arm at the patient's heart level. | Obtains accurate reading. For every cm that the cuff is above/below heart level. Blood pressure varies by 0.8 mm of mercury. |
| 12 | Keep the arm well rested and supported | Ensures comfort of the patient thereby enabling an accurate reading. Movement of arm can cause noise when auscultating. |
| 13 | Place yourself in a comfortable position. | |
| 14 | Connect the cuff tubing to the manometer tubing and close the valve of the inflation bulb. | |
| 15 | Palpate the radial pulse and inflate the cuff until pulse is obliterated | Estimates systolic pressure in order to determine how high to pump the mercury in order to avoid error related to auscultatory gap. |

*Contd...*

*Contd...*

| 16 | Inflate the compression bag a further 20-30 mm of mercury and then deflate cuff slowly. Note the point at which pulse reappears. Release the valve. | Ensures that mercury column is high enough to minimize error related to auscultatory gap. The point at which pulse reappears is the systolic pressure. |
|----|----|----|
| 17 | Palpate brachial artery and place diaphragm of the stethoscope lightly over the brachial artery. Ensure that ear pieces of the stethoscope are placed correctly (slightly tilted forward and ensure that tubing hangs freely) Raise mercury level 20-30 mm of mercury above the point of systolic pressure obtained by means of palpatory method (Figure 1.4(d)). | Ensures accurate reading. If diaphragm is placed too firmly the artery gets compressed. Sounds are heard better with correct placement of stethoscope. Rubbing of stethoscope against an object can obiliterate Korot-Kov's sounds. |

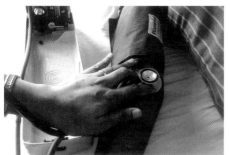

Figure 1.4(d): Auscultatory method of checking blood pressure

| 18 | Release the valve of the inflation bulb, so that mercury column falls at the rate of 2-3 mm of mercury/sec. | Prevents venous congestion and falsely elevated pressure reading due to slower rate of deflation and prevents erroneous reading due to faster rate of deflation. |
|----|----|----|
| 19 | When first sound is heard, the mercury level is noted, this denotes systolic pressure. | First sound is heard when the blood begins to flow through brachial artery . |
| 20 | Continue to deflate the cuff. When the sound disappears note the mercury level. This is diastolic pressure. | |
| 21 | Deflate cuff completely. Disconnect the tubing and remove the cuff from the patient's arm. | Occlusion of artery during the pressure reading causes venous congestion in the forearm. |
| 22 | Repeat the procedure after one minute if there is any doubt about the reading. | Waiting time of one minute allows venous blood to drain completely. |
| 23 | Ensure that patient is comfortable. | |
| 24 | Remove equipment and clean ear piece with a spirit swab. | |
| 25 | Wash and dry hands | Prevents chances of cross-infection. |
| 26 | Document the reading in appropriate observation chart or flow chart. | |
| 27 | Report any abnormal findings. | |

## SPECIAL PRECAUTIONS

1. Do not take blood pressure on a patient's arm if
   a. The arm has an intravenous infusion on it
   b. The arm is injured/diseased.
   c. The arm has a shunt/fistula for renal dialysis.
   d. On the same side if the patient had a radical mastectomy
   e. If the arm is paralysed.

2. Always check supine measurement before checking upright measurement.
3. If blood pressure has to be taken at the same time in two or more positions— Lying, sitting or standing at the same time for comparison, wait for a minimum of 3 minutes after assuming that position before taking the reading.
4. If comparison is needed for blood pressure in lying/standing position, the patient must be in lying/standing position for a minimum of 3 minutes.
5. Appropriate sized cuff should be used.

## 1. 5: CHECKING HEIGHT AND WEIGHT OF A PATIENT

Measuring the height and weight using accurate scales and measuring devices.

## PURPOSES

1. To assess fluid balance in patients with fluid retention, renal problems and cardiac problems.
2. To assess the response to therapy, e.g. diuretics
3. To ascertain the response to physiological changes or prescribed diet, e. g. pregnancy, high calorie diet.
4. To obtain baseline data about patient's health status.

## ARTICLES

1. Weighing machine (electronic weighing scale)
       OR
   Sling scale
2. Measuring tape and stick
3. Ruler.

## PROCEDURE

| | Nursing action | Rationale |
|---|---|---|
| 1 | Assess the patient's ability to stand independently on the weighing machine. | Ensures safety of patient while checking weight and height. |
| **Checking of weight while standing on electronic scale:** | | |
| 2 | Wash hands | Reduces transmission of microorganisms. |
| 3 | Explain the procedure to the patient and ask patient to void. Instruct patient to wear a hospital gown. | Helps to gain cooperation of the patient and voiding will reduce the weight of urine in the bladder. Extra clothing will cause errors in reading of weight. |
| 4 | Place the weighing machine near the patient. | Reduces risk of fall/injury. |
| 5 | Turn on the scale and calibrate it to zero. | Ensures accurate reading. |
| 6 | Instruct patient not to step on the scale until the digital display shows zero. | For accurate reading. |
| 7 | Ask patient to remove shoes and heavy clothing and step on the scale and stand erect and still. | |
| 8 | Read weight after digital numbers have stopped fluctuating. | Reading is not accurate when numbers are still fluctuating. |
| 9 | Ask the patient to step down and assist the patient back to bed or chair. | Reduces risk of injury. |
| 10 | Wash hands | Reduces transmission of microorganisms. |
| **Checking of weight in a sling scale:** | | |
| 11 | A sling is placed under the patient carefully without any folds. | More accurate weight will be obtained by leaving no bedding between sling and the patient. |
| 12 | Put on the scale and calibrate it to zero. | |
| 13 | Lower the arms of the sling scale and slip hooks through the holes of the sling. | This is to attach the sling to the sling scale to measure the weight. |
| 14 | Pump scale until sling rests completely off the bed. | Ensures accurate weight reading. |
| 15 | Read weight after digital numbers have stopped fluctuating. | Reading is not accurate when numbers are fluctuating. |

*Contd...*

*Contd...*

| | | |
|---|---|---|
| 16 | Lower the sling arms and place the patient comfortably on the bed. | Ensures patient comfort. |
| **Measuring height:** | | |
| 17 | Ask the patient to remove the shoes. | Ensures accurate checking of height. |
| 18 | A measuring tape or stick can be held or attached to the wall vertically. | |
| 19 | Instruct the patient to stand erect, with heels together. | Helps in obtaining accurate measurement. |
| 20 | With a stick or ruler placed horizontally on the head at 90 degree angle to the measuring tape, the height is measured in inches/cms. | |
| 21 | Provide the patient a comfortable position in bed. | Ensures patient's comfort. |
| 22 | Replace the articles | |
| 23 | Wash hands | Reduces transmission of microorganism. |
| 24 | Record the procedure with date, time and height and weight. | Documentation helps in continuity of care. |

## SPECIAL CONSIDERATIONS

1. Weigh patient at the same time with same amount of clothing each day to enhance accurate reading.
2. Preferably use the same weighing scale while weighing patients daily.
3. Weighing machine with attached scale for measuring height can be used to measure height and weight.

# 1.6: COLLECTING URINE SPECIMEN FOR ROUTINE EXAMINATION

## DEFINITION

Collection of a small quantity (4 ounce /120 ml) of urine sample in a clean container for testing it in the laboratory.

## PURPOSE

To detect and measure the presence of abnormalities in urine such as red blood cells, white blood cells, casts, pH, sugar, albumin and specific gravity.

## ARTICLES

1. Clean, wide mouthed container.
2. Bed pan or urinal
3. Appropriate laboratory forms
4. Soap and water
5. Laboratory requisition form
6. Gloves.

## PROCEDURE

| | Nursing action | Rationale |
|---|---|---|
| 1. | Check the physician's order and nursing care plan | Obtains specific instructions and information |
| 2. | Identify the patient | Ensures that right procedure is performed for right patient. |
| 3. | Explain procedure to the patient with specific instructions about washing the genital area (skin around the urethral meatus) with soap and water and give the labelled container. Instruct patient not to wet the label on the out side (Figure 1.6(a)) | Washing the genital area prevents contamination of urine specimen. Label on the container must have the patient's full name, ward, register number of the patient, type of test to be done and date. |

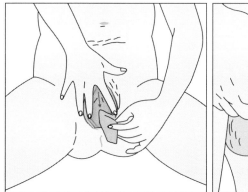 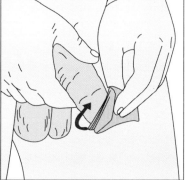

**Figure 1.6(a):** Cleaning genitalia

| | | |
|---|---|---|
| 4. | Ask the patient to direct the first and last part of the urine stream into a urinal or toilet and to collect the middle part of the stream into the specimen container (Figure 1.6(b)). | Collecting the midstream urine avoids contamination of the specimen with organisms normally present on the skin. Four ounces of urine is required for the test. |

*Contd...*

*Contd...*

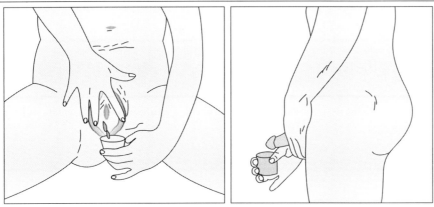

**Figure 1.6(b):** Collecting midstream specimen

| | | |
|---|---|---|
| 5. | Have the patient place the specimen container in proper/designated place | |
| 6. | With gloved hand place the specimen container in polythene bag | Protects health care worker from possible exposure to microorganisms. |
| 7. | Send specimen to the laboratory with completed, signed laboratory form | |
| 8 | Remove gloves and wash hands | |
| 9. | Record the procedure in the nurse's notes and other appropriate forms. | |

## SPECIAL CONSIDERATIONS

1. It is preferable to collect morning specimens whenever possible.
2. A clean – catch midstream urine specimen is collected to detect any urinary tract infection.
3. Specimens collected from menstruating and postpartum patients should have the information included in the requisition form.
4. Always cover specimen to prevent carbon dioxide from air diffusing into urine which will result in urine becoming alkaline and fostering bacterial growth.

# 1.7: TESTING URINE FOR pH

## DEFINITION

Testing urine for pH by dipping litmus paper into it and noting resultant color change.

## PURPOSE

To determine acid-base balance.

## ARTICLES

1. Urine specimen container.
2. Litmus strip
3. Clean gloves
4. Kidney tray.

## PROCEDURE

| | Nursing action | Rationale |
|---|---|---|
| 1. | Explain procedure to the patient and provide specimen container | Obtains co-operation of the patient |
| 2. | Don gloves obtain specimen from patient | Reduces risk of contamination with urine. |
| 3. | Dip litmus strip in urine and keep for one minute and note color change <br> • If blue litmus turns red, urine is acidic. <br> • If red litmus turns blue , urine is alkaline | Shows the reaction of urine |
| 4. | Discard strip into container for infected waste | Proper disposal ensures safety |
| 4. | Discard urine specimen in sluice room/toilet | |
| 5. | Record the procedure in nurse's notes including the result noted | Recording gives information about the result of the procedure. |

Note - The normal pH of urine is 4-8

## 1.8: TESTING URINE FOR SPECIFIC GRAVITY

## DEFINITION

Measuring specific gravity of urine using a caliberated hydrometer/urinometer.

## PURPOSES

1. To determine the level of concentration of urine.
2. To diagnose conditions like diabetes insipidus.

## ARTICLES

1. Container to collect urine
2. Calibrated urinometer
3. Jar for urine
4. Clean gloves.

## PROCEDURE

| | Nursing action | Rationale |
|---|---|---|
| 1. | Explain procedure to the patient and provide container to collect urine | Facilitates co-operation of the patient to collect urine |
| 2. | Don gloves . | Reduces risk of contamination. |
| 3. | Fill three fourths of jar with urine | Permits urinometer to float free in urine |
| 4. | Gently place urinometer into jar | |
| 5. | Make sure that instrument floats freely and does not touch bottom and sides of jar (Figure 1.8(a)) | If urinometer touches the jar reading will be false |

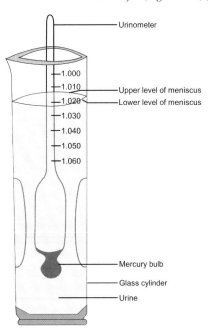

Figure 1.8(a): Measuring specific gravity of urine

*Contd...*

*Contd...*

| | | |
|---|---|---|
| 6. | When urinometer stops bobbing, read specific gravity directly from scale marked on calibrated stem of urinometer. Read scale at lowest point of meniscus to ensure an accurate reading at eye level (Normal specific gravity of urine is 1.010-1.025) | Reduces errors of reading. |
| 7. | Discard urine, and rinse jar and urinometer in running water | Prevents contamination |
| 8. | Remove gloves and wash hands. | Reduces transmission of microorganisms. |
| 9. | Replace articles and record the procedure in Nurse's Record or flowsheet according to policy | Recording gives information about the procedure results to health workers. |

## SPECIAL CONSIDERATION

Presence of faeces, tissue and menstrual blood falsely elevate specific gravity reading.

# 1.9 (A): TESTING URINE FOR GLUCOSE (Benedict's Solution)

## DEFINITION

Testing a specimen of double-voided urine using Benedict's solution for presence of glucose.

## PURPOSE

To estimate the amount of glucose present in urine.

## ARTICLES

1. Spirit lamp
2. Match box
3. Test tube with test tube holder
4. Test tube stand
5. Benedict's solution
6. Dropper
7. Duster
8. Kidney tray
9. Clean, disposable gloves.

## PROCEDURE

| | Nursing action | Rationale |
|---|---|---|
| 1 | Explain about method of collecting a double voided specimen of urine | Proper explanation helps the patient to collect specimen in a correct manner. |
| 2 | Provide labeled container for collecting urine | |
| 3 | Don gloves and collect urine specimen from patient | Reduces risk of contamination |
| 4 | Take test tube and fix in holder. Pour 5 ml of Benedict's solution into test tube. | Benedict's solution is used to find out presence of glucose in urine |
| 5 | Light spirit lamp and heat Benedict's solution till it boils, holding test tube with mouth facing away from the nurse. | On heating if color of solution changes, it indicates that the solution is not suitable for testing. |
| 6 | Add eight drops of urine using dropper, through the sides and allow to boil for another few seconds | |
| 7 | Put off flame and allow it to cool | Cooling completes color change when glucose is present in urine |
| 8 | Watch for color change and compare with standard color code <br> • Blue –nil <br> • Green liquid without deposit <br> • Green liquid with yellow deposit <br> • Colorless liquid with orange deposit <br> • Brick red | Normal urine does not contain sugar <br><br> No sugar <br> +/ 1% sugar <br> ++/2% sugar <br> +++/3% sugar <br> ++++/5% or above |
| 9 | Discard urine in toilet or sluice room and rinse container | |
| 10 | Replace the equipment after washing in proper place | |
| 11 | Discard gloves and wash hands. | Reduces risk of transmission of microorganisms. |
| 12 | Record result in "Diabetic urine chart" and inform doctor for appropriate management/insulin order. | Recording the reaction gives information for further management. |

# 1.9 (B): TESTING URINE FOR GLUCOSE (REAGENT STRIP OR TAPE)

## DEFINITION

Testing urine for glucose using reagent strips such as Diastix or test tape.

## ARTICLES

1. Urine specimen in a container
2. Reagent strips in container
3. Clean disposable gloves
4. Receptacle for used strip.

## PROCEDURE

| | Nursing action | Rationale |
|---|---|---|
| 1 | Provide labeled container for collecting urine | |
| 2 | Explain about method of collection of double voided specimen | Proper explanation helps the patient to collect specimen in a correct manner |
| 3 | Don gloves and and collect urine specimen from patient | |
| 4 | Dip the portion of the strip with reagent in urine | Colour change occurs in the strip according to the amount of glucose present in urine |
| 5 | Compare the color of the strip with the color chart on the reagent strip container or separate chart (Figure 1.9 a) | Colour change indicates the presence and amount of glucose in urine |

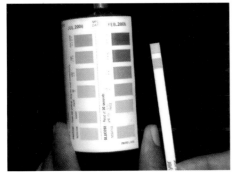

**Figure 1.9(a):** Comparing color of reagent strip with color chart

| | | |
|---|---|---|
| 6 | Discard the used strip and used articles. | |
| 7 | Replace the reusable items and wash hands. | |
| 8 | Record in the patient's chart result of the test. | Conveys information to physician and other staff. |

Note:
Presence of Ketone bodies (acetone) are also tested using reagent tablets (Acetest) or reagent strips (Ketostix). Combined Ketone glucose reagent strips (keto-diastix) are also available for use.

## SPECIAL CONSIDERATION

- The part of the strip with the reagent should not be touched with bare hands. Care should be taken to see that the dipstick should not be exposed to sunlight while storing.

## 1.10: TESTING URINE FOR ALBUMIN

### DEFINITION

Testing urine for presence of albumin using hot test method.

### ARTICLES

1. Spirit lamp.
2. Match box.
3. Test tube and holder.
4. Test tube stand
5. Two percent acetic acid.
6. Dropper
7. Specimen container.
8. Duster
9. Kidney tray.
10. Litmus paper
11. Clean disposable gloves.

### PROCEDURE

| | Nursing action | Rationale |
|---|---|---|
| 1. | Explain to the patient about the test to be done and provide container for collecting urine | Obtains co-operation of patient |
| 2. | Don gloves | |
| 3. | Fill ¾ th of a test tube with urine, secure test tube holder at its top end | |
| 4. | Check the reaction of urine, if found alkaline, add one drop of acetic acid and make it acidic | If the urine is highly alkaline or acidic, it will give false reading. |
| 5. | Heat the upper third of urine over the spirit lamp and allow it to boil. Keep the mouth of the test tube away from your face. | Prevents scalding |
| 6. | A cloud may appear either due to phosphate or albumin. Add 2-3 drops of acetic acid into the test tube. If the urine still remains cloudy, it indicates the presence of albumin.<br>Clear = nil<br>Trace = +<br>Cloudy = ++<br>Thick cloudiness = +++<br>If it becomes clear, it indicates the presence of phosphates | Confirms the presence of albumin<br>Normal urine does not contain albumin |
| 7. | Discard the urine and rinse the test tube. Replace articles | Cleaning the test tube and keeping ready helps for the next use. |
| 8. | Discard gloves and wash hands. | Prevents transmission of microorganisms. |
| 9. | Record the procedure with date and time in nurse's record or flowsheet according to hospital policy | Gives the information about patient's health status. |

# 1.11: COLLECTING URINE SPECIMEN FOR CULTURE

## DEFINITION

Collection of a small sample of urine (30 to 60 ml) for detecting the presence and growth of microorgnisms in the sample.

## PURPOSES

1. To culture pathogenic microorganisms present in the urine.
2. To determine antibiotic sensitivity of the pathogens in the urine.

## ARTICLES

1. Sterile urine container
2. Laboratory form
3. Soap and water
4. Bed pan (for non-ambulatory patient)

## PROCEDURE

| | Nursing action | Rationale |
|---|---|---|
| 1 | Check the physician's order and identify patient. | Helps to understand purpose of procedure for the patient. |
| 2 | Assess the patient's mobility status and activity tolerance to use the toilet facilities | Determines the level of assistance required |
| 3 | Explain procedure to patient including reason for collecting specimen, and how patient can collect an uncontaminated specimen (if patient is able to) | Contaminated urine may result in false results. |
| 4 | Wash hands and don gloves if nurse is to perform procedure | |
| 5 | Provide privacy by closing curtains and/or door. | Privacy allows patient to relax and reduces embarrassment. |
| 6 | Instruct patient to cleanse the perineum (See Figure 1.6(a))<br>*Female:*<br>Wash the urethral meatus and surrounding area with soap and water.<br>*Male:*<br>Hold the penis with one hand and cleanse the end of penis moving from center to outside using soap and water.<br>*For helpless patients:*<br>The nurse should provide hygienic perineal care. | |
| 7 | Assist bedridden patient on to bed pan | |
| 8 | Instruct to open specimen container and place cap with sterile inside surface up and not to touch inside of container and lid. | Contaminated specimen will lead to inaccurate reporting of culture and sensitivity. |
| 9 | Instruct ambulatory patients to:<br>*Female:*<br>• Sit with legs separated on toilet<br>*Male:*<br>• Sit down to control splashing. | Prevents contamination of container from outside |

*Contd...*

*Contd...*

| | | |
|---|---|---|
| 10 | Instruct patient to direct the first and last part of the urine stream into the toilet or bedpan, collect the middle part of the stream into the sterile container. (Midstream sample) | Prevents contamination of the specimen with skin flora |
| 11 | Replace cap securely on specimen container, cleanse any urine from external surface of container and place container in plastic bag or in the designated place. | Prevents transfer of microorganisms to others |
| 12 | Remove bedpan (if applicable) and assist patient to comfortable position | Promotes relaxing enviornment |
| 13 | Label specimen and send to laboratory with completed requisition form. | Prevents inaccurate identification that could lead to errors in diagnosis and therapy. |
| 14 | Remove gloves and dispose in proper receptacle (if used for bed-ridden patient) and wash hands | Reduces transmission of microorganisms. |
| 15 | Transport urine specimen to laboratory within 15 minutes or refrigerate immediately. | Bacteria grow quickly in urine and specimen should be analyzed immediately to obtain correct results. |
| 16 | Record in the nurse's notes the time of urine collection and any other observation. | Documents implementation of physcian's order. |

## SPECIAL CONSIDERATIONS

1. Patients who are catheterized should have the specimen withdrawn using a sterile needle and syringe from the catheter's sampling port. Clamp the collection tube for about 30 minutes before taking sample.
2. Urine specimen must be transported to the laboratory promptly. If not cultured within 30 minutes of collection, urine must be refrigerated and culture done within 24 hours.
3. About 30 minutes prior to collecting the specimen, patient may be encouraged to drink fluids unless contraindicated.

# 1.12: COLLECTION OF 24 HOURS URINE

## DEFINITION

Collection of urine specimen for a period of 24 hours without any spillage or wastage.

## PURPOSES

1. To detect kidney, liver and cardiac conditions.
2. To measure total protein, creatinine, electrolytes, 17 ketogenic steroid, oxylate, porphyrins, drugs, vitamins, VMA, minerals, hormones etc.

## ARTICLES

1. Clean container with preservative, of not less than 3 liters capacity with label, obtained from the laboratory (biochemistry).
2. Urinal or kidney tray to collect urine at each voiding.
3. Appropriate laboratory form, duly filled.

## PROCEDURE

| | Nursing action | Rationale |
|---|---|---|
| 1. | Check the physician's order and nursing care plan | Obtains specific instructions/information |
| 2. | Identify the patient | Ensures that right procedure is performed on the right patient |
| 3. | Explain to the patient, the purpose of procedure and, that all urine for the full 24 hours must be saved | Gains patient's consent and co-operation |
| 4. | Instruct the patient to void at the time set to begin the procedure. E.g: at 6.00 am. Discard this specimen. Record in Nurses Notes, the time when collection began | Ensures that urine collected is produced within the 24 hours of testing |
| 5. | Measure and pour all the subsequent voidings into the container | A 24 hours collection will accommodate all the variables in body chemistry within a representative period |
| 6. | Collect the final specimen at exactly the same time the patient voided 24 hours earlier. E.g: 6.00 am the following day | |
| 7. | Send the container with urine to laboratory when the collection is over, with requisition forms | |
| 8. | Record in the Nurse's notes time of completing the collection and despatching the urine to the lab | |
| 9. | Clean, disinfect and replace the kidney tray or urinal if they are reusable. | |

## 1.13: COLLECTING A STOOL SPECIMEN FOR ROUTINE EXAMINATION

### DEFINITION

Collection of a small quantity of stool sample in a container for testing in the laboratory.

### PURPOSE

To test the stool for normalcy and presence of abnormalities.

### ARTICLES

1. A clean specimen container.
2. A spatula for putting the specimen into the container.
3. Dry bed-pan (for helpless patients). Additional bedpan for rinsing and cleaning.
4. Laboratory requisition form.
5. Clean gloves.
6. Waste paper (for wrapping used spatula).
7. A pitcher of water (for helpless patient).
8. Tissues/towel.

### PROCEDURE

| | Nursing action | Rationale |
|---|---|---|
| 1. | Check the physician's order and 'Nursing Care Plan'. | Obtains specific instruction and information. |
| 2. | Identify the patient. | Helps to perform the right procedure for the right patient. |
| 3. | Explain to patient the procedure and make clear what is expected of him/her. | Aids in proper collection of specimen. |
| 4. | Give the labelled container and spatula to the patient with instructions. i.To defecate into clean dry bedpan ii.Not to contaminate specimen with urine. | |
| 5. | Don gloves | |
| 6. | For helpless patient: assist patient on to the clean bedpan. | |
| 7. | Leave him with instructions | |
| 8. | When done, remove and keep aside the bedpan after placing the second one for cleansing | |
| 9. | Once the specimen is collected sent it to lab with the appropriate requisition forms | |
| 10. | Wash and replace the reusable articles | |
| 11. | Dispose off the used spatula wrapped in waste paper. | Prevents contamination |
| 12. | Wash and dry hands. | Prevents cross contamination. |
| 13. | Record information in the patient's chart. | |

### SPECIAL CONSIDERATIONS

1. Send specimen to be examined for parasites immediately, so that parasites may be observed under microscope while viable, fresh and warm.

2.  Inform if bleeding hemorrhoids or hematuria is present.
3.  Postpone test if woman has menstrual periods, until three days after it has ceased.
4.  Consider that intake of folic acid , anticoagulant , barium, bismuth, mineral oil , vitamin C, and antibiotics may alter the results.
5.  Use two bedpans for helpless patient – one for collecting specimen and the another for cleaning.

# 1.14: COLLECTING A STOOL SPECIMEN FOR CULTURE

## DEFINITION

Collection of a small quantity of stool sample for culture/microbiological examination.

## PURPOSE

To culture the organisms that are not part of the normal bowel flora, e.g.: Salmonella, Shigella, Rotavirus, etc.

## ARTICLES

1. Sterile stool container/specimen container.
2. Sterile spatula/swab stick.
3. Bedpans (two bedpans for helpless patients).
4. Laboratory requisition form.
5. Clean gloves.
6. Tissues.

## PROCEDURE

| | Nursing action | Rationale |
|---|---|---|
| 1. | Check the physician's order and nursing care plan | Obtains specific instructions and information. |
| 2. | Identify the patient | Helps in performing the right procedure for the right patient. |
| 3. | Explain to patient the procedure and make clear what is expected of him/her.<br>i.To defecate into clean dry bedpan .<br>ii.Instruct not to contaminate specimen with urine. | Aids in proper and adequate collection of specimen. |
| 4. | Give labelled container and spatula to the patient with instructions. | |
| 5. | Once the specimen is collected , wear gloves, take the container from patient and send it to the lab with the completed lab requisition | |
| 6. | Wrap spatula in waste paper and discard appropriately. | |
| 7. | Wash and replace the reusable articles | |
| 8. | Wash and dry hands | Prevents cross contamination. |
| 9. | Record the procedure in the patients' record. | |

## SPECIAL CONSIDERATIONS

1. Stool specimen for culture can be obtained directly from the rectum using a sterile swab.
2. If a patient passes blood and mucus, include this information in specimen label.
3. Provide assistance to helpless patients for sitting on pan, cleaning after defecation and collecting specimen.

# 1.15: COLLECTING A THROAT SWAB FOR CULTURE

## DEFINITION

Collecting the exudates from throat or tonsil for laboratory test.

## PURPOSE

To identify the pathogenic organisms.

## ARTICLES

1. Tongue depressor to hold the tongue down.
2. Cotton tipped applicators in sterile packed test tube to collect the specimen for transportation to the lab.
3. Laboratory requisition form.
4. Clean, dry, gauze pieces.
5. Disposable gloves.

## PROCEDURE

| | Nursing action | Rationale |
|---|---|---|
| 1. | Check the physician's order | |
| 2. | Identify the patient | |
| 3. | Explain to patient the procedure and instruct him how he/she must co-operate. | Knowledge of the procedure facilitates patient co-operation |
| 4. | Wash hands and put on gloves | Protects the health care worker from contamination with saliva. |
| 5. | Instruct the patient to open his mouth and hold the tongue down with a tongue depressor. If gag reflex is active in patient, make him to sit upright and if health permits, instruct patient to open mouth, extend tongue and say "Ah". | Sitting position and extension of tongue helps to expose the pharynx. Saying "Ah" relaxes throat muscles. |
| 6. | Carefully yet firmly rub the swab or cotton applicator over areas of exudate or over the tonsil and posterior pharynx, avoiding the cheeks, teeth and gums (Figure 1.15(a)) | Firm rubbing will aid in obtaining an adequate sample. |

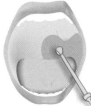

**Figure 1.15(a):** Obtaining a throat swab for culture examination

| | | |
|---|---|---|
| 7. | Insert swab or applicator into the sterile packet, or test tube. | Keeping the applicator directly in the packet will avoid contamination |
| 8. | Send specimen to the laboratory immediately with the requisition form duly filled | |
| 9 | Clean and replace the reusable articles | |
| 10. | Remove gloves and discard wash hands | |
| 11. | Record in appropriate patient record | |

## 1.16: COLLECTING A WOUND SWAB FOR CULTURE

### DEFINITION

Collection of wound exudates/discharge for laboratory examination.

### PURPOSE

To identify aerobic and anaerobic organisms present in the wound.

### ARTICLES

1. Cotton applicators.
2. Culture tube or container for transporting the specimen
3. Laboratory requisition form
4. Disposable gloves

### PROCEDURE

| | Nursing action | Rationale |
|---|---|---|
| 1. | Check the physician's order | |
| 2. | Identify the patient | Ensures that the right procedure is done on right patient. |
| 3. | Explain the procedure to patient | Allays anxiety and promotes patient co-operation |
| 4. | Screen the bed and provide privacy | Reduces anxiety |
| 5. | Wash hands and wear gloves | Reduces risk of transmission of microorganisms. |
| 6. | Expose the wound area | |
| 7. | Using the cotton – tipped applicators, swab and collect as much exudate as possible from the center of the lesion. | Swabbing the surrounding skin will alter the findings |
| 8. | Place the swab immediately in appropriate transport culture tube and send to laboratory labelled clearly, specifying the anatomic part from where the specimen was obtained. | Clear labelling aids in accurate reporting of the test |
| 9. | Record information in the patient's chart | |

## 1.17: PROTOCOL FOR SAMPLE COLLECTION OF BLOOD

| | Test | Sample type | Volume required | Container | Related instruction | Normal values |
|---|---|---|---|---|---|---|
| 1. | Blood glucose | Serum | 3.0 ml clotted | Plain red top | FBS (Fasting) RBS (Random) | 70-110 mg% less than 200 mg/dl |
| 2. | BUN (Blood urea nitrogen) | Serum | 3.0 ml clotted | Plain red top | | 8-25 mg% |
| 3. | Creatinine | Serum | 3.0 ml clotted | Plain red top | | 0.6-1.5 mg% |
| 4. | Total protein | Serum | 3.0 ml clotted | Plain red top | | Albumin 3.5- 5 mg% |
| 5. | AST (Asparatate aminotransferase) | Serum | 3.0 ml clotted | Plain red top | | 10-40 units/ml |
| 6. | Bilirubin | Serum | 3.0 ml clotted | Plain red top | | Total 1.0 mg/100 ml Direct 0.4 mg/100 ml Indirect 0.6 mg/100 ml |
| 7 | Cholesterol | Serum | 3.0 ml clotted | Plain red top | | 120-220 mg/100 ml |
| 8 | Triglycerides | Serum | 3.0 ml clotted | Plain red top | | 40-150 mg/100 ml |
| 9 | Lipid profile Total lipids HDL,LDL,VLDL | Serum (fasting) | 3.0 ml clotted | Red top | | Normal HDL cholesterol – more than 45 mg/dl LDL cholesterol-upto 130 mg/dl VLDL cholestrol-7-33 mg/dl |
| 10 | Triglycerides | Serum | 3.0 ml clotted | Red top | | 35-150 mg/dl |
| 11 | LDH (Lactic dehydrogenase) | Serum | 3.0 ml clotted | Red top | | 50-150 U/L |
| 12 | Blood gases arterial $O_2$ saturation $PO_2$, $PCO_2$, pH | Arterial heparinized blood | 1 ml clotted | Syringe | PCO2 Above 500 mm Hg while on 100% O2 | O2 saturation 96-100% PO2 = 75-100mm Hg PCO2 = 35 –45 mm Hg pH = 7.35 – 7.45 |
| 13 | Electrolytes Na K Mg Cl Urea Uric acid | Serum clotted | 3 ml clotted | Red TOP | | Sodium 135-145 mEq/L Potasium 3.5-5 mEq/L Magnesium 1.5-2mEq/L Chloride 98-110 mEq/L Urea 10-50 mg/dl Uric acid 2-6 mg/dl |
| 14 | P.T. (prothrombin time) | Citrated | | Blue top | Mix well avoid hemolysis send to lab in 30 minutes | Less than 2 seconds deviation from control |
| 15 | PTT (partial thromboplastin time) | Citrated | | Blue top | | 25-37 seconds |
| 16 | Bleeding time | Finger prick | | Capillary tube and blotting paper | | 3-7 minutes |
| 17 | WBC | EDTA | 3.0 ml clotted | Purple top | | Total (4000-11000/100 ml) Differential Neutrophils 60-70% |

*Contd...*

*Contd...*

|  |  |  |  |  |  | Lymphocytes-25-35% <br> Monocytes-5-10% <br> Eosinophils-1-4% <br> Basophils-upto 1% |
|---|---|---|---|---|---|---|
| 18. | RBC | EDTA | 3.0 ml clotted | Purple top |  | Male-4.5-6.5 x $10^6$/μl <br> Female-3.8-4.8 x $10^6$/μl |
| 19. | Hemoglobin | EDTA | 3.0 ml clotted | Purple top |  | Male – 13-18 gm% <br> Female-12-16 gm % |
| 20 | Platelets | EDTA | 3.0 ml clotted | Purple top |  | 150-400 x $10^3$/μl |
| 21 | Hematocrit | EDTA | 2.0 ml | Blue top |  | Male 45-52% <br> Female 37-48% |
| 22 | ESR (Erythocyte sedimentation rate) | EDTA with anticoagulant | 2.0 ml | Blue top |  | Male less than 15 mm/hr <br> Female less than 20 mm/hr |
| 23 | Calcium | Serum clotted | 4-6 ml | Red top | No tourniquet | 8-10 mg/dl |
| 24 | CPK (Cretinine phosphokinase) | Serum | 3.0 ml | Red top |  | Male 15-105 U/L <br> Female 10-80 U/L |
| 25 | Thyroid hormone | Serum | 5.0 ml | Red top |  | TSH—0.3-5.4 μU/ml <br> $T_3$—110-230 ng/dl <br> $T_4$—5-12 μg/dl |
| 26 | PCV (Packed cell volume) | EDTA (with anti-coagulant) | 2 ml | Blue top |  | Male—40-54% <br> Female—37-47% |

## 1.18: COLLECTING BLOOD FOR ROUTINE EXAMINATION

### DEFINITION

Obtaining blood sample by veni puncture for routine lab investigations.

### PURPOSES

1. To determine variations if any in blood composition.
2. To determine any abnormality in order to aid in diagnosis.

### ARTICLES

1. Tourniquet.
2. Small mackintosh.
3. Syringes 5 ml, 10 ml.
4. No.20 gauge needles or vacutainer assembly.
5. Alcohol swabs.
6. Disposable gloves.
7. Specimen container – test tube or bottle.
8. Laboratory requisition form.
9. Sterile gauze pads (2" × 2")
10. Adhesive tapes.

### PROCEDURE

| | Nursing action | Rationale |
|---|---|---|
| 1. | Check the physician's order | |
| 2. | Identify the patient | Ensures performance of procedure on right patient. |
| 3. | Reassure the patient and explain that relatively little blood will be taken | Obtains patient's co-operation and confidence. |
| 4. | Wash hands and put on gloves | Protects health care worker from possible exposure to blood. |
| 5. | Select and examine the vein, visualize the vein, including the antecubital area, wrist, dorsum (back) of the hand and top of foot (if necessary). Palpate the vein | Select a vein that is visible, palpable and fixed to the surrounding tissues so that it does not roll away |
| 6. | Instruct the patient to extend his arm. Hold the arm straight at the elbow with fist clenched | Proper positioning reduces risk of injury |
| 7. | Apply the tourniquet 5 to 15 cm above the selected site with just sufficient pressure to obstruct venous flow | A tourniquet when applied increases venous pressure and makes the vein more prominent and easier to enter. |
| 9. | Cleanse the skin with alcohol swab in a circular motion – center to periphery. Allow to dry | Cleansing the skin reduces the number of micro-organisms |
| 10. | Fix chosen vein with thumb and draw the skin taut immediately below the site before inserting needle to stabilize the vein. | The vein may roll beneath the skin when the needle approaches its outer surface, especially in elderly and extremely thin patients. |

*Contd...*

*Contd...*

11. Hold the syringe between the thumb and last three fingers with the bevel up and directly in line with the course of the vein. Insert the needle quickly and smoothly under the skin and into the vein (Figure 1.18(a))

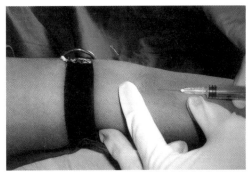

**Figure 1.18(a):** Inserting needle into vein

| | |
|---|---|
| 12. Obtain blood sample by gently pulling back on the plunger (Figure 1.18(b)) | Use minimal suction to prevent hemolysis of blood and collapse of vein. |

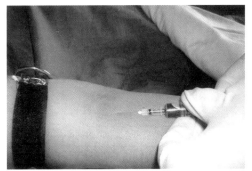

**Figure 1.18(b):** Obtaining blood sample

| | |
|---|---|
| 13. Release the tourniquet as soon as the specimen is obtained and ask the patient to open the fist. | |
| 14. Apply sterile 2′ × 2′ gauze piece to puncture site without applying pressure and withdraw needle slowly along the line of vein | Slow withdrawl of the needle is less painful and reduces trauma |
| 15. Request patient to apply gentle but firm pressure to site for 2 – 4 minutes | Firm pressure over puncture site prevents leakage of blood into surrounding tissues with subsequent hematoma development |
| 16. Remove the needle from the syringe as soon as possible after withdrawing blood, gently eject the blood sample into the appropriate container without forming bubbles in the test tube or bottle (Some tests require container with anticoagulant) | Gentle ejection of blood prevents hemolysis |
| 17. Invert the tube gently several times to mix blood with anticoagulant where applicable. For some tests blood is allowed to coagulate in the test tube | Gentle handling of specimen prevents risk of hemolysis. |
| 18. Label specimen correctly and send to laboratory immediately with completed requisition forms. | Specimen should reach the laboratory with the minimum of delay for optimum reliability. |
| 19. Dispose the needle and syringe in appropriate containers . | Avoids possible spread of blood–borne diseases. |

*Contd...*

*Contd...*

| | |
|---|---|
| 20. Clean all spills with 10% bleach (sodium hypochlorite) solution. Remove gloves and wash hands. | Avoids possible spread of blood–borne diseases. |
| 21. Record in the patient's chart the procedure and the tests for which the sample was sent to the laboratory. | |
| 22. Replace the tray with the reusable articles in proper place | |

## 1.19: MEASURING BLOOD GLUCOSE LEVEL USING GLUCOMETER

### DEFINITION

Measuring the blood glucose level with the help of a portable glucometer.

### ARTICLES REQUIRED

1  Blood glucose meter
2  Testing strips/reagent strips
3  Sterile lancet
4  Cotton balls
5  Alcohol swab
6  Disposable gloves.

### PROCEDURE

| | Nursing action | Rationale |
|---|---|---|
| 1 | Check physician's order | Confirms time for checking blood glucose. |
| 2 | Review manufacturer's instructions for glucometer use. | Helps in doing procedure accurately. |
| 3 | Gather articles at the bedside | Provides an organised approach during the procedure. |
| 4 | Explain the procedure to the patient. | Helps to gain patient's co-operation |
| 5 | Have the patient wash hands with soap and water. Use warm water if available. | Washing hands reduces transmission of microorganisms. |
| 6 | Position the patient comfortably in a semi-fowlers position or upright position | Increases blood flow to puncture site. |
| 7 | Wash hands. Don disposable gloves | Prevents spread of microorganisms. Gloves protects from exposure to blood and body fluids. |
| 8 | Remove test strip from the container and recap container immediately | Immediate recapping protects strips from exposure to light and discoloration. |
| 9 | Turn monitor on and check whether the code number on strip matches with the code number on the monitor screen. | Matching the code numbers on the strip and glucometer ensures that machine is calibrated correctly |
| 10 | Take the lancet without contaminating it. Select appropriate puncture site. | Aseptic technique maintains sterility. |
| 11 | Massage side of finger for adults (heel for children) toward puncture site and wipe with alcohol swab. | Massage increases blood flow to the area. |
| 12 | Hold lancet perpendicular to skin and prick site with lancet. (Figure 1.19(a)) | Holding lancet in proper position facilitates proper skin penetration. |

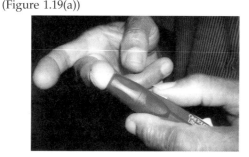

**Figure 1.19(a):** Patient pricking side of his finger

*Contd...*

*Contd...*

| | | |
|---|---|---|
| 13 | Wipe away the 1st drop of blood from the site. | The first drop may impede accurate result because it may contain large amount of serous fluid. |
| 14 | Lightly squeeze or milk the puncture site until a hanging drop of blood has formed. | The blood droplet should be large enough to cover the test pad on the strip and it also facilitates accurate test results. |
| 15 | Gently touch the drop of blood to pad on the test strip without smearing it (Figure 1.19(b)). | Smearing of the blood will alter results. |

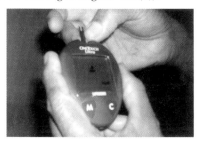

**Figure 1.19(b):** Inserting strip into gloucometer

| | | |
|---|---|---|
| 16 | Insert strip into glucometer according to directions for that specific device. Some devices require that the drop of blood is applied to a test strip that has already been inserted in the monitor. (Figure 1.19(c)) | Correctly inserted strip allows glucometer to read blood glucose level accurately. |

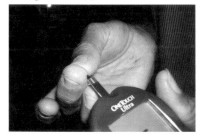

**Figure 1.19(c):** Touching drop of blood to test strip

| | | |
|---|---|---|
| 17 | Apply pressure to puncture site using a dry cotton ball. | This will stop bleeding at the site. |
| 18 | Read blood glucose results displayed on the monitor and inform the patient about results. (Figure 1.19(d)) | |

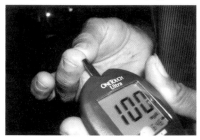

**Figure 1.19(d):** Display of blood glucose level in monitor

| | | |
|---|---|---|
| 19 | Turn off the glucometer | |
| 20 | Dispose supplies appropriately and discard lancet in sharp's container. | Reduces contamination by blood. Sharps must always be handled properly to protect others from accidental injury. |

*Contd...*

*Contd...*

| | | |
|---|---|---|
| 21 | Remove gloves and discard. Wash hands. | |
| 22 | Record blood glucose level in the chart | This facilitates documentation of procedure and provides for comprehensive care. |

## SPECIAL CONSIDERATIONS

1.  In patients who require regular blood-glucose monitoring, shallow penetration should be encouraged to avoid tissue damage.
2.  Rotate or change sites to allow time for the penetrated site to heal.
3.  To reduce pain, choose side of fingertips or side of heel for children. where few nerve endings are present rather than central part of fingertips.
4.  Patients should compare their personal glucometer reading with the laboratory measured blood glucose level, every 6-12 months.

# 1.20: COLLECTION OF BLOOD FOR CULTURE

## DEFINITION

Collection of blood for culture to determine presence of microorganisms in the blood.

## ARTICLES REQUIRED

1 Blood culture bottles (3)
2 Cotton swab
3 Spirit
4 Syringe(10- 20 ml)
5 Needle
6 Povidone – Iodine solution
7 Sterile gloves
8 Tourniquet
9 Laboratory requisition form.

## PROCEDURE

| | Nursing action | Rationale |
|---|---|---|
| 1 | Assess the physician's order for blood culture investigation. | Obtains knowledge of samples to be collected and the reason for doing culture. |
| 2 | Explain procedure to the patient and provide a comfortable position. | Gains co-operation of the patient during the procedure. |
| 3 | Wash hands. Don sterile gloves | Reduces transmission of microorganisms and maintains aseptic technique . |
| 4 | Apply tourniquet above the puncture site and palpate the venipuncture site. | Restricts blood flow and promotes easy visibility of veins. |
| 5 | Wipe the site with 70% alcohol in a circular manner from center to peripheri for approximately 5 cm in diameter and allow to dry. | |
| 6 | Cleanse the site again with povidone —iodine starting from center in even widening circles. Allow the iodine to remain on the skin for at least one minute. | Avoids contamination and maintains a sterile field. |
| 7 | Clean the cover of the culture bottles with povidone iodine followed by spirit. | Maintains sterility of equipment. |
| 8 | Puncture the site and draw 10 ml of blood (Adults 10-20 ml of blood preferred) | |
| 9 | Remove the tourniquet once the blood is collected. | Restores circulation. |
| 10 | Remove the needle and apply pressure to the puncture site with dry cotton simultaneously. | Stops bleeding from the puncture site. |
| 11 | Wipe the site with 70% alcohol. | |
| 12 | Change the needle with a fresh needle before injecting the blood into the bottles. | |
| 13 | Remove the metal cover on the cap of culture bottles and push 10 ml of blood into each of the bottles. While injecting blood into the bottles be careful not to touch the sides of the bottle (Figure 1.20(a)) | Maintains strict aseptic technique |

*Contd...*

*Contd...*

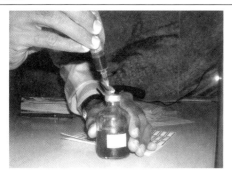

**Figure 1.20(a):** Injecting blood into culture bottle

| 14 | Mix the blood and culture media by shaking the bottle gently. | |
|----|----|----|
| 15 | Discard the contaminated articles. Remove gloves | |
| 16 | Wash hands | Reduces transmission of infection. |
| 17 | Fill the lab requisition form appropriately and label the bottles with patient's name, identification number, date and time of collection | |
| 18 | Transfer the specimen to the lab immediately. | |
| 19 | Record the procedure in the patient's chart with date and time of collection. | Communicates pertinent information to members of health care team. |
| 20 | Repeat the procedure within an interval of 30 minutes to one hour as per the number of samples required from different puncture sites. | |

## SPECIAL CONSIDERATIONS

1   Blood for culture should be taken before antibiotics are administered.
2   If there is regular periodicity of the fever, the advantageous time to draw blood will be just before the anticipated rise in temperature.
3   For children, 2-5 ml and neonates 1-2 ml of blood is required for culture investigation.
4   Blood should never be taken from an IV line or from above an exisiting IV line.
5   For patients with clinical diagnosis of endocarditis, two or three sets of blood cultures (a set consists of one aerobic and one anaerobic culture from one site) should be performed over a 24-hour period to assess for sustained bacteremia.

# 1.21: COLLECTING BLOOD FOR PERIPHERAL SMEAR

## DEFINITION

Obtaining a small sample of blood by skin puncture for peripheral smear.

## PURPOSES

1. To detect malarial parasites.
2. To detect blood cell abnormalities.

## ARTICLES

1. Disposable lancet.
2. Pipette and tubing.
3. Slides.
4. Cotton swabs / Alcohol prep pads.
5. Alcohol.
6. Disposable gloves.
7. Laboratory forms.

## PROCEDURE

| | Nursing action | Rationale |
|---|---|---|
| 1. | Check the physician's order and nursing care plan. | Obtains specific instructions and information. |
| 2. | Identify the patient. | Ensures that right procedure is performed for right patient. |
| 3. | Give explanation to patient about the procedure. | Obtains patient's co-operation and consent. |
| 4. | Wash hands and put on gloves. | Protects health care workers from possible exposure to blood. |
| 5. | Cleanse site (ball of finger) with alcohol and dry with sterile cotton swab. | If any alcohol remains, it will alter red cell morphology. Blood will not collect into a compact drop, but will run down the finger if it is not dry. |
| 6. | Prick the skin sharply and quickly with sterile, disposable lancet. | Pricking the skin sharply and quickly minimizes pain during procedure and helps to obtain a flowing sample. |
| 7. | Release pressure on the finger, wipe off the first drop of blood. | Epithelial and endothelial cells may be found in the first drop of blood and may render the count inadequate. |
| 8. | Allow the blood to flow freely with an adequate puncture. | Pressing out the blood dilutes it with tissue fluid. |
| 9. | Obtain the blood sample, fill the pipette and make blood smears on the slides (Figure 1.21(a)) | |

Figure 1.21(a): Preparing a peripheral smear

*Contd...*

*Contd...*

|   | a. | Thin smear |
|---|---|---|
|   |   | • Put a drop of fresh blood on the middle of the slide. |
|   |   | • Use another slide end to allow the drop of blood to spread along the slide. |
|   |   | • Push the spreader quickly from the center to the left of the slide drawing the blood behind it. |
|   |   | • Leave the film to dry. Do not blow on it. |
|   | b. | Thick smear |
|   |   | • Put three drops of fresh blood on the left hand quarter of the slide |
|   |   | • With the corner of another slide mix the blood and smear it in a round form about 1 cm in diameter. |
|   |   | • Leave the film to dry. Do not blow on it or shake the slide. |
| 10. | Apply pressure over the puncture site, with a dry cotton ball until bleeding stops. | |
| 11 | When the film is dry, label the slide wrap it and dispatch to laboratory. | |
| 12. | Remove gloves, wash hands and dispose off articles in approved containers. | |

# 1.22: COLLECTION OF SPUTUM FOR CULTURE

## DEFINITION

Collection of coughed out sputum for culture to identify respiratory pathogens.

## EQUIPMENTS

1  Sterile specimen container
2  Sputum cup
3  Tissue paper
4  Gloves
5  K-basin
6  Suction catheter (optional)
7  Suction apparatus (optional).

## PROCEDURE

| | Nursing action | Rationale |
|---|---|---|
| 1 | Check the physician's order | |
| 2 | Explain to client that the specimen must be taken from sputum , coughed up from back of the throat or lungs | Promotes patient's co-operation |
| 3 | Ask the patient to sit erect in bed if possible. | Provides easy access for collection of specimen. |
| 4 | Wash hands and put on gloves | Reduces transmission of microorganisms. |
| 5 | Keep a sterile specimen container ready for the sample and take a tissue paper in hand. | |
| 6 | Remove lid of container and place with inner side facing upwards | Prevents contamination. |
| 7 | Instruct the patient to take deep breaths and then cough out deeply. | It helps to loosen the secretions and obtain adequate specimen. |
| 8 | Explain to the patient that he has to expectorate the sputum into sterile labelled container without touching the inside of it. | Prevents contamination of the specimen. |
| 9 | Close the container without touching inside of lid. | |
| 10 | Provide client with tissue paper and a comfortable position. | Promotes patient comfort. |
| 11 | Replace articles | |
| 12 | Wash hands | Reduces transmission of microorganisms. |
| 13 | Provide mouth care if patient needs it or encourage patient to carry out oral hygiene. | Removes unpleasant taste in mouth. |
| 14 | Document obtained specimen, date and time of collection and characteristics of the specimen and send specimen to lab. | Helps in continuity of care. |

## SPECIAL CONSIDERATION

It is preferable to collect an early morning sputum specimen before brushing/rinsing the mouth.

## 1. 23: ASSISTING WITH OBTAINING A PAPANICOLAOU SMEAR

### DEFINITION

It is a cytologic examination of desquamated epithelial tissue to differentiate normal from anaplastic cells and it is also a widely used cancer screening test.

### PURPOSES

1. To detect cervical and vaginal carcinomas.
2. To perform routine screening and for diagnosing disorders of reproductive system.

### METHODS OF OBTAINING PAP (PAPANICOLAOU) SMEAR

1. Slide method
2. Liquid method (Thin Preparation)

### ARTICLES NEEDED

1. A glass slide
2. A sterile Ayre's spatula
3. Cusco's speculum
4. A pipette
5. A sterile cotton swab
6. Sterile gloves
7. Ether/95% alcohol solution (1: 1)
8. Spray fixative
9. A graphite pencil
10. Light source
11. K-Y jelly.

### PROCEDURE

| | Nursing action | Rationale |
|---|---|---|
| 1 | Check the physician's order and progress notes. | Obtains specific instructions/ information. |
| 2 | Identify the patient and check identification against physician's order. | Ensures that the right procedure is performed on the right patient. |
| 3 | Explain the pap cytology test to the patient. Allow questions to be asked. Consider the protocols to be followed in specific cases. | Obtains patient's consent and co-operation. Promotes patient education. In rape cases, vaginal swabs may be used for forensic evidence . |
| 4 | For patients of child bearing age, test should be done 10-20 days after the first day of LMP, and definitely not when the patient is menstruating or bleeding, unless bleeding is a continuous condition. | A smear taken any time other than in the mid menstrual cycle can result in abnormal findings. Heavy menstrual flow and blood may make the interpretation of the results difficult and may obscure atypical cells. |
| 5 | Instruct the patient not to douche for 2 to 3 days before the test. | Douching may remove the exfoliated cells. |
| 6 | Instruct the patient not to use vaginal medications or vaginal contraceptives during the 48 hrs before the examination. Intercourse to be avoided the night before the examination. | Use of contraceptives before examination may result in false test results. |

*Contd...*

*Contd...*

| | | |
|---|---|---|
| 7 | Instruct the patient to empty her bladder and rectum before examination. | Ensures comfort during the procedure. |
| 8 | Ask the patient to give the following information:<br>  a. Age | Identifies if patient is an adolescent, pregnant or post–menopausal woman. |
| |   b. Use of hormone therapy, birth control pills or contraceptive devices. | Hormones and contraceptive devices can alter the findings. |
| |   c. Past vaginal surgical repair or hysterectomy. | |
| |   d. All medications taken, including prescribed, over-the–counter, and herbal medications. | Some medications alter the test results. |
| |   e. Any radiation therapy | |
| |   f. Any other pertinent clinical history (e.g previous abnormal Pap smear, signs of inflammation or bleeding) | |
| 9 | Obtain the requirements of the procedure | |
| 10 | Using the graphite pencil, label the ends of the slide with the patient's name and the collection site. | |
| 11 | Ask the patient to undress from waist down. | |
| 12 | Position the patient in a lithotomy position on an examination table and drape | Ensures good visibility and promotes comfort and provides privacy. |
| 13 | Don sterile gloves, lubricate and insert a sterile Cusco's speculum. | |
| 14 | a. For endocervical smear:<br>Insert a sterile cotton swab into the cervical os (Figure 1.23(a))and rotate it 360°. Leave the swab in place for 10-20 sec. Remove the swab and smear onto a glass slide. Fix it immediately.<br>Note: fixative must be applied to the slide before drying of the specimen occurs. | |

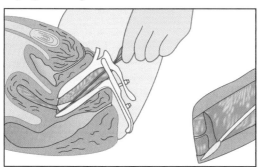

**Figure 1.23(a):** Obtaining a cervical swab for smear

    b. Ectocervical scraping:
       Insert Ayre's spatula into the cervical os, rotate or scrape the entire surface at the squamocolumnar junction (Figure 1.23(b)). Remove the spatula and smear onto a glass slide. Fix it immediately (Figure 1.23(c)).

*Contd...*

*Contd...*

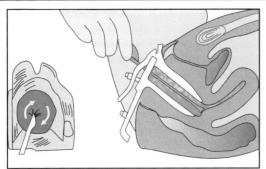

Figure 1.23(b): Ayre's spatula in cervical os

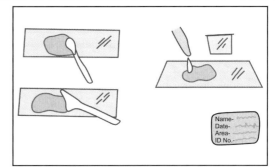

Figure 1.23(c): Preparing slides

c. Cervical scraping:
Insert the pointed edge of a wooden Ayre spatula into the cervical os and rotate the spatula 360 degrees.
Spread the cervical scrapings on a glass slide, fix it with an ether/95% ethyl alcohol solution, and dry the slide. A cervix - brush sampling device may be used, and it is recommended to be rotated a full 180 degree to improve the sampling for abnormal cervical cells.

d. Vaginal pool:
Using the blunt side of a wooden Ayre spatula, scrape the vaginal floor behind the cervix. Spread the vaginal pool secretions on a glass slide, spray or soak them in fixative,and dry the slide. Vaginal fluid is obtained for suspected endometrial cancer or for a hormonal evaluation.

e. Vulval smear:
Using the blunt side of a wooden Ayre spatula, directly scrape the vulvar lesion. Spread the scraping on a glass slide and fix immediately with spray fixative.

| 15 | Give the patient a perineal pad after the procedure to absorb any bleeding or drainage. |
| 16 | Write the patient's age: the reason for the study , the LMP, etc. on the requisition form  and send the slides to the cytology laboratory. |

## SPECIAL CONSIDERATIONS

1. Smears that dry before fixative is applied cannot be properly interpreted.
2. Do not lubricate the speculum as it may distort cells.
3. A smear taken any time other than in the mid menstrual cycle can result in abnormal findings.
4. Tetracycline or digitalis preparations can affect the appearance of squamous epithelium.
5. Blood, mucus or pus on the slide makes interpretation difficult.

# 1.24: MEASURING INTAKE AND OUTPUT

## DEFINITION

It is defined as the measuring and recording of fluid intake and output (I and O) during a 24-hour period which provides important data about a patient's fluid and electrolyte balance.

## PURPOSES

1. To assess patient's general health.
2. To monitor specific disease conditions
3. To assess the fluid and electrolyte balance.

## ARTICLES

1. Intake and output form at bedside
2. Intake and output graphic record in chart
3. Bedpan or urinal or bedside commode
4. Graduated drinking cup/tumbler
5. Graduated container for output
6. Clean gloves
7. Sign at bedside that patient is on intake and output measurement.

## PROCEDURE

| | Nursing action | Rationale |
|---|---|---|
| 1. | Identify the patient | |
| 2. | Explain the methods of maintaining. Intake and output. All fluids taken orally must be recorded on the patient's intake and output form (Input and output flow sheet) | Helps to obtain patient's co-operation and encourages patient's participation. |
| 3. | Wash hands every time prior to giving oral fluids | Reduces transmission of microorganisms |
| 4. | Measure all oral fluids in accordance with institutional policy Example: a. Water glassful = 200 ml b. Cupful = 120 ml Paper cup a. Large = 200 ml b. Small = 120 ml Soup bowl full = 180 ml Water pitcher full = 1000 ml Measure all fluids in the graduated cup/tumbler before giving to patient. | Provides for consistency of measurement |
| 5. | Record time and amount of fluid intake in the designated space on bedside chart. Include all semi solid and liquid food rich in fluids (oral, IV, tube feedings and IV fluids) | Documents the amount of fluids accurately |
| 6. | Transfer eight hours total fluid intake from bedside intake and output chart to 24 hour intake and output record in patient's chart. | Provides for data analysis of the patient's fluid status every 8 hour shift. |
| 7. | Record all fluid intake in the appropriate column of the 24-hour record | Documents intake by type and amount |

*Contd...*

*Contd...*

| | |
|---|---|
| 8. Complete 24-hour intake record by adding all eight hour totals. | Provides consistent data for analysis of the patient's fluid status over a 24 hours. |
| 9. For measuring output include urinary output and other drainage from patient. **(Figure 1.24(a)).** | Documents the amount of output accurately. |

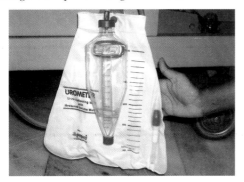

**Figure 1.24(a):** Measuring urine from urometer

10. Urinary output
    • After each voiding measure the urine using a measuring container and record it with the time of voiding on the intake and output form (Figure1.24(b)).

Name:      Room No/Bed No:      Hosp. No.:    I.P. No.:

| Date | Time | Oral | I.V. fluids started infused | Urine | Emesis | Other | Stool | Misc |
|------|------|------|------------------------------|-------|--------|-------|-------|------|
| | | | | | | | | |
| | | | | | | | | |
| | | | | | | | | |
| | | | | | | | | |
| | | | | | | | | |
| | | | | | | | | |
| | | | | | | | | |
| | | | | | | | | |
| | | | | | | | | |
| | | | | | | | | |
| | | | | | | | | |
| | | | | | | | | |
| | | | | | | | | |
| | | | | | | | | |
| | | | | | | | | |
| | | | | | | | | |
| | | | | | | | | |
| | | | | | | | | |

**Figure 1.24(b):** Intake–output chart

*Contd...*

*Contd...*

| | | |
|---|---|---|
| | • For patients with retention catheter empty the drainage bag into a measuring container at the end of the shift or at prescribed times if output is measured more often. Note and record it.<br>• For infants and incontinent patients the output may be measured by first weighing diapers or incontinent pads that are dry and then subtracting this weight from the weight of soiled items | |
| 11. | The amount and type of fluid (urine , drainage from NG tube, drainage tube) are recorded in the intake and output form | Documents output. |
| 12. | Transfer 8 hour output total to 24 hours intake and output record on the patient's chart. | Provides for data analysis of the patient's fluid status. |
| 13. | Complete 24 hours output record by totaling all 8 hours total. | Provides consistent data for analysis of the patient's fluid status over a 24 hours period |

## SPECIAL CONSIDERATIONS

- Proper aseptic technique should be taken while handling patient's body fluid output viz blood, urine etc.
- Remember that fluids taken to swallow pills must be recorded as intake
- Do not have visitors or family members empty bedpan, urinal or catheter bags.

## 1.25: TEACHING BREAST SELF-EXAMINATION (BSE)

### DEFINITION

Breast self–examination is a technique which women use to assess their own breasts to detect breast carcinomas at the earliest.

### ARTICLES

1. Mirror
2. Gloves
3. Small pillow/rolled towel.

### PROCEDURE

| | Nursing action | Rationale |
|---|---|---|
| 1. | Identify the patient and review personal history and family health history. | Identifies risk factors and previous baseline data |
| 2. | Explain procedure to the patient. Ask her to disrobe to the waist and to put on a gown with the opening in the front | Provides easy access while maintaining maximum privacy |
| 3. | Wash hands. Don gloves if required by agency policy | Prevents transfer of microorganisms and possible contact with discharge when palpating nipples |
| 4. | Provide privacy and assist the patient to sitting position facing you and expose chest and breasts. | Allows comparison of breasts bilaterally |
| 5. | Explain and teach breast self–examination as you examine. For inspection, ask the patient to stand before the mirror and check both breasts for anything unusual with patients:<br>• Arms at sides<br>• Arms raised<br>• Hands pressed on hips<br>• Arms extended straight ahead as patient leans forward (Figure 1.25(a)) | • Flesh color, slight inequities in size and symmetry, rounded shape and smooth skin surface is normal.<br>• Redness, blue hue, retraction, dimpling , enlarged pores, edema, lumps , lesions, rashes, ulcers and discharge are abnormal .<br>• Supernumerary nipples along the milk line are a normal variant. |

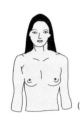 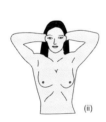 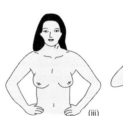 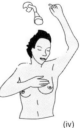 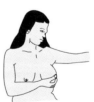 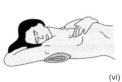

(i)    (ii)    (iii)    (iv)    (v)    (vi)

**Figure 1.25(a):** Breast self-examination

| | | |
|---|---|---|
| 6. | Explain and teach the palpation method. Teach the patient to use the right hand to palpate the left breast and vice versa. During the examination, place the patient's fingers under your fingers | Teaching during examination reinforces the need for and understanding of breast examinations, and enables the patient to identify normal breast tissue and abnormal tissue if present thus increasing confidence in performing BSE |

*Contd...*

*Contd...*

| | |
|---|---|
| 7. Using the pads of the palmar surfaces of the fingertips, palpate the right breast by gently compressing the mammary tissues against the chest wall. Palpation may be performed from the periphery to the nipple, in either concentric circles, wedge sections or vertical strip (Figure 1.25(b)). | Warm temperature, elasticity, tenderness, pain , erythema, masses or nodules are abnormal. |

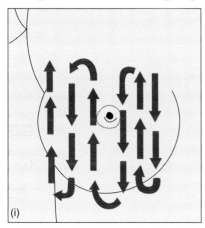 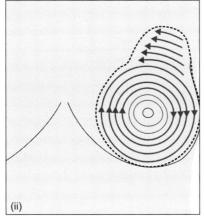 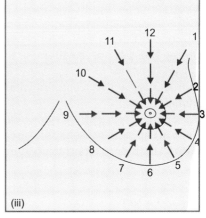

**Figure 1.25(b):** Palpation method. (i) Wedge setion, (ii) Concentric circles pattern for breast palpation, (iii) Hands-of-the-clock pattern of breast palpation

| | |
|---|---|
| 8. Palpate areola and nipple using a similar circular technique as with breast. Pay special attention to subareolar part and gently press the nipple between the fingers | Inflammation, discharge, nodules fissuring and lesions are abnormal. |
| 9. Palpate into axilla starting at anterior axillary line and continuing at an angle to the mid axillary line and up into the axilla (using same circular fingertip motion). Have patient place arm at side and palpate deep into the axilla. Identify posterior axillary, central axillary, anterior axillary and lateral axillary node locations. | Nodes should be less than 1 cm and non tender |
| 10. Repeat steps 7-9 on the left breast , areola, nipple and axilla. Identify normal versus abnormal as with the right breast. Compare breasts bilaterally | |
| 11. Assist the patient to supine position. Place arm on examination side under the head, and place a small pillow under the same side scapula | This position spreads breast tissue over the chest wall maximizing palpation accuracy |
| 12. Assist the patient to palpate the breast, areola and nipple as in steps 7–9 with the other hand and vice versa | Re-evaluate examination findings in second position |
| 13. Assist the patient to a sitting position. Review the steps and ask the patient to demonstrate breast self–examination | Provide more comfort for patient. Evaluate success of the teaching |
| 14. Allow patient to dress | Provide for patient's comfort |
| 15. Remove gloves and wash hands | Reduce transmission of micro-organisms |
| 16. Give the patient written materials to reinforce teaching | Reinforce teaching. Provides a readily available form to patient for reference when at home |
| 17. Record date, time, findings of abnormalities and absence of abnormalities , patient's response to findings and teachings | |

## SPECIAL CONSIDERATIONS

1. Instruct patients not to use creams, lotions or powders and not to shave underarms 48 hours before the scheduled assessment, because these things could alter the breast skin or cause folliculitis and lymph node enlargement.
2. Explain that BSE is best performed after menses (5th -7th day) for pre-menopausal women and first day of the month for postmenopausal women.
3. Educate even men to perform a monthly BSE and obtain a clinical examination every 1 to 3 years because 1% of all breast cancer is found in men.
4. Advise the patient to palpate her breasts during shower, as the fingers will glide easily over soapy skin, so that one can concentrate on feeling for changes in the breasts.
5. During BSE pay special attention to upper outer quadrant area and the tail of Spence, where about 50% of breast cancers develop.
6. Instruct patient that a baseline mammogram is to be obtained at 35 years and followed by annual mammogram after 40 years.
7. Determine if patient is taking oral contraceptives, digitalis, diuretics, steroids or estrogen hormones. These medications may cause nipple discharge and hormones may cause fibrocystic changes in breast.
8. Instruct mother to report if any lumps, tenderness or nipple discharge exists.

# 1.26: TEACHING TESTICULAR SELF–EXAMINATION (TSE)

## DEFINITION

Testicular self-examination is a technique used to examine the testes by self for detecting abnormalities like testicular cancer.

## PROCEDURE

| | Nursing action | Rationale |
|---|---|---|
| 1. | Identify the patient and review personal history, medication, and family health history | Identifies risk factors and previous baseline data |
| 2. | Explain the procedure to patient , provide privacy and ask the patient to disrobe completely and to put on a gown | Obtains patient's co-operation and provides easy access while maintaining maximum privacy |
| 3. | Wash hands, and apply clean gloves | Practices clean technique |
| 4. | Instruct the patient to stand and fold up his gown to expose the genitalia | Provides best exposure for examination |
| 5. | Advise the patient to use both hands to palpate the testes. The normal testicle is smooth and uniform in consistency. Note the size, lie, shape, consistency and tenderness The length of a normal testes should be greater than 4 cm and the volume greater than 20 ml | The left testicle normally sits slightly lower than right testicle. The testicles are rubbery and approximately equal in size Pressure on testes normally produces a deep visceral pain. Twisting or torsion of the testes causes venous obstruction, edema and eventually arterial obstruction. |

6. Advise the patient to palpate each testis one at a time and feel for any evidence of a small, pea size lump or abnormality (Figure 1.26(a))

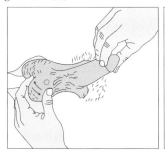 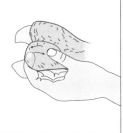

**Figure 1.26(a):** Testicular self–examination

7. Teach the patient to locate and palpate the spermatic cord and vas deferens between the thumb and fingers (from epididymis to the inguinal ring) (Figure 1.26(b))  —  Note any nodules or swelling

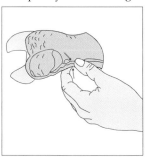

**Figure 1.26(b):** Palpating spermatic cord

*Contd...*

*Contd...*

| | | |
|---|---|---|
| 8. | Explain that it is normal to find that one testis is larger than the other | |
| 9. | Assist the patient to a comfortable position. Review the steps and ask the patient to redemonstrate testicular self–examination | Provides more comfort for patient. Evaluate success of the teaching given. |
| 10. | Remove gloves and wash hands | Reduces risk of transmission of microorganism |
| 11. | Give the patient written materials if available. | Reinforces teaching. Provides a readily available form to patient for reference when at home |
| 12. | Record date, time, findings of palpation and patient's response to findings and teaching. | |

## SPECIAL CONSIDERATIONS

1. Advise patient to perform testicular self–examination on one particular day of each month.
2. It is advisable to perform testicular self–examination after a warm relaxing shower.

# Chapter 2

# Client Care: Hygiene and Comfort

# 2.1: ADMISSION OF A PATIENT IN HOSPITAL

## DEFINITION

Receiving a patient to stay in the hospital for observation, investigation, diagnosis, treatment and care.

## PURPOSES

1. To welcome and establish a positive relationship with patient and close relatives.
2. To offer immediate management and care in acute conditions.
3. To orient patient to immediate environment and services available.
4. To acquire baseline data of a patient through history and physical examination.
5. To collaborate with patient in planning and providing comprehensive care.

## ARTICLES

1. Prepared bed.
2. Thermometer tray.
3. B.P. apparatus.
4. Weighing machine (scale)
5. Admission advisory form (from admitting department)
6. Documents such as:
   i. Doctor's order sheet.
   ii. T.P.R.Sheet.
   iii. Nursing assessment form
   iv. Nurses record.
   v. Progress record.
   vi. Lab master sheet.
   vii. Additional sheets as indicated, such as diabetic urine chart, intake output chart, and specific flow sheets, admission consent form.
7. Kidney tray or emesis basin.
8. Tissue paper.
9. Bedpan and/or urinal
10. Bath towels and wash cloth.

## PROCEDURE

| | Nursing action | Rationale |
|---|---|---|
| 1. | Lower the bed and turn down top sheet and bedspread | Makes it convenient for the patient to get into bed |
| 2. | Arrange room furniture for easy access to bed | Reduces risk of fall |
| 3. | Assemble special equipment such as suction equipment, oxygen supplies, pole for I. V. line etc. and make sure they are in working condition | Prevents delay in case immediate treatment is required. |
| 4. | Receive the patient and family cordially. Identify the patient with the admission slip. Check the details such as advance payment, unit and room assigned. | Reduces anxiety about admission |
| 5. | Introduce yourself and escort the patient and family to the assigned room. | Reduces anxiety |

*Contd...*

*Contd...*

| | | |
|---|---|---|
| 6. | Prepare the patient's record with all the necessary information like name, hospital number, unit, room or bed number, in each record. | |
| 7. | Check for admission consent whether it is duly signed by patient and or relative. Collect the patient's old records if indicated from medical records department. | Provides base line for assessment of condition on admission. |
| 8. | Check the patient's weight, vital signs and record it | Provides base line for assessment of condition on admission |
| 9. | Collect the history and do a simple physical examination and observe the general condition of the patient. | Provides base line for assessment of condition on admission |
| 10. | Orient patient to the physical set up of the ward such as nurse's station, treatment room, toilet and bathroom facilities, drinking water supply, patient's cupboard, call light, kitchen, etc. and also orient the patient to the ward routines. | Reduces the strain of finding the details by himself |
| 11. | Explain about the facilities available such as canteen, dietary, telephone, pharmacy, safety rules related to fire, accident etc. | Reduces the strain of findings the details by himself |
| 12. | Explain the hospital policies regarding visiting hours, gate pass, attendants staying with patients and restrictions in the ward. | |
| 13. | Have family leave patient's room unless they choose to assist patient with undressing. Close door and curtains. | Provides for privacy and prepares patient for care. |
| 14. | Give an admission bath if needed and provide hospital gown. | |
| 15. | Initiate care which do not require physician's order if needed, such as cold compress, tepid sponge etc. | |
| 16. | Obtain detailed nursing history and physicial examination findings as per hospital policy. | Alerts nurses to substances to which the patient is allergic and gains understanding of the patients problems. |
| 17. | Obtain specimens such as urine, blood or any other for tests if not already obtained. | Serves for basic screening |
| 18. | Inform patient about procedures or treatments scheduled for the next shift or day and clarify any related questions. | Provides opportunity for the patients to remain informed |
| 19. | Encourage patient to send the valuables home. If the patient prefers to keep them, list on a paper and have the patient or family member sign it . Place the valuables in safe custody. | Accounts for safe placement of valuables and prevents loss. |
| 20. | Be sure that the call light is within reach, bed is in lowered position and side rails are raised. | Provides for patient safety. |
| 21. | Wash hands | |
| 22. | Record history and assessment findings in appropriate forms. | |
| 23. | Notify physician of patient's arrival, report any unusual findings | Patient's condition may require immediate attention. |
| 24. | Inform dietary department regarding patient's arrival and type of diet ordered. | |
| 25. | Write the admission note including the following details: date, time of patient's arrival to the ward, age, mode of arrival, patient's complaints for which he is hospitalized, variations in vital signs and any other abnormalities observed such as pressure sores, rashes, etc. the orientation given and the full signature of the nurse. | |

## SPECIAL CONSIDERATIONS

1. Information regarding an admission is received from out-patient admitting office or emergency department.
2. In admissions of sick patients or emergency situations, steps of the procedure may be altered, considering the priority of needs.
3. General information regarding facilities available can be provided in written form. e. g. pamphlets.

# 2.2: DISCHARGE OF A PATIENT FROM HOSPITAL

## DEFINITION

Discharge planning is a centralized, co-ordinated, multidisciplinary process that ensures that the patient has a plan for continuing care after leaving the hospital.

## GENERAL PRINCIPLES

1. Patient and family understands the diagnosis, anticipated level of functioning, discharge medications and anticipated medical follow-up.
2. Specialized instructions or training is provided to the patient and family to ensure that proper care after discharge will be provided to the patient.
3. Community support systems are co-ordinated to enable the patient to return home.
4. Relocation of the patient and co-ordination of support system or transfer to another health care facility are performed.

## ARTICLE

1. Wheel chair or stretcher.

## PROCEDURE

| | Nursing action | Rationale |
|---|---|---|
| 1 | Assess patient's health care needs at the time of discharge using nursing history, care plan and ongoing assessment of physical abilities and cognitive function from time of admission | Planning for discharge begins at the time of admission and continues throughout patient's stay in agency. |
| 2 | Assess patient's and family's need for health teaching related to home therapies, restrictions resulting from health alterations and possible complications. | Improves understanding of health care needs and ability to achieve self care at home. |
| 3 | Assess with patient and family any environmental factors within home that might interfere with self care, e.g. size of room, bathroom facilities, stairs etc. | May pose risks to safety as a result of limitations created by illness or certain therapies. |
| 4 | Collaborate with physician and staff in other disciplines, e.g. physical therapist, social worker, etc. | A multidisciplinary assessment ensures a comprehensive discharge plan. |
| 5 | Consult other health team members about needs after discharge, e.g. dietitian, social worker. Make appropriate referrals. | Members of all health care disciplines should collaborate to determine patient's needs and functional abilities. |
| 6 | Preparation before day of discharge<br>a. Suggest ways to change physical arrangement of home to meet patient's needs if required.<br>b. Provide patient and family with information about community health care resources<br>c. Conduct teaching sessions with patient and family as soon as possible during hospitalization in anticipation of preparation for discharge, e.g. signs and symptoms of complications. Use of medical equipment etc. | Patient's level of independence and ability to retain function can be maintained within safe environment. Community resources may offer support to patient and family.<br>Gives opportunities to practice new skills, ask questions and obtain necessary feedback. |

*Contd...*

*Contd...*

| | |
|---|---|
| 7 Day of discharge | |
| a. Allow patient and family to ask questions | Relieves anxiety and ensures that safe care is provided to patients |
| b. Check physician's discharge orders for prescription and change in treatments. | Discharge is authorized only by physician. Early information about discharge permits the nurse to attend to any last minute treatment or procedure well in advance before discharge. |
| c. Determine whether patient or family has arranged for transportation home | Determines method of transport |
| d. Check all closets and drawers for belongings. Obtain copy of valuables list signed by patient. Account for all valuables when required. | Prevents loss of items. Relieves nursing department of liability for losses. |
| e. Provide patient with prescriptions for medications ordered by physician | Review of drug information provides feedback to determine success in learning about medications and its administration. |
| f. Provide information about follow-up visit and home health care facilities available. | Ensures that patient attends regular follow-up in the hospital. |
| g. Provide printed teaching material as per patient's requirement with necessary instructions. | Helps patient review instructions that are provided by the health care team. |
| h. Obtain wheel chair for patients who are unable to ambulate. | Provides for safe transport. |
| 8 Complete documentation of patient's discharge in nurse's notes. | |
| 9 Ensure that the discharge summary from physician is ready. | Discharge summary is essential for documenting patient's status and time patient leaves the hospital. |

## SPECIAL CONSIDERATIONS

1. If patient is getting discharged "against medical advice" inform physician and nurse-in-charge and complete the AMA form as per hospital policy.
2. Patients who may need detailed instructions and follow-up visit to the home after discharge include;
   - Newly diagnosed chronic disease like diabetes mellitus
   - Patients after major and radical surgery
   - Patients who are socially isolated
   - Patients with emotional or mental instability
   - Patients who lack of financial resources
   - Patients who are terminally ill.

# 2.3: TRANSFER OF A PATIENT FROM UNIT TO UNIT/HOSPITAL TO HOSPITAL

## DEFINITION

Transfer of a patient is defined as shifting a patient from one department to another department in the same hospital or between hospitals.

## PURPOSES

1. To receive different forms of therapy and management
2. To have care continued closer to home
3. To have care continued when financial resources prohibit receiving care in the current facility.
4. To provide for more skilled care and close observation in specialised units.

## ARTICLES

1. Wheel chair or stretcher
2. Oxygen tank and tubing
3. I.V. pole
4. Cardiac monitor
5. Requistion forms
6. Records
7. Isolette for care of newborns.

## PROCEDURE

| | Nursing action | Rationale |
|---|---|---|
| 1 | Assess reason for patient's transfer in collaboration with physician (e.g. change in condition, resources available at agency, patient or family preference regarding patient's transfer) | Patient should have access to agency with best resources to meet his health care needs. |
| 2 | Inform the nurse-in-charge of the new ward about the transfer. | Prior information will help the staff in the new unit to receive the patient with adequate preparation |
| 3 | Check the belongings of the patient and keep ready for shifting. | Ensures that patient's belongings are safe. |
| 4 | Complete patient's charts and make it up-to-date. Keep ready the patients record with X-rays, ECG, lab reports and the medicine card. | Provides information about the care and treatment provided. |
| 5 | Assess patient's physical condition and determine the mode of transportation (if patient needs to be shifted to another hospital) | Determines if patient is stable for transfer. Patient's safety is best assured by using a vehicle equipped with life support equipment. |
| 6 | Determine patient's level of understanding regarding purpose of transfer and feelings about the change in care setting. | Transfers are sometimes planned quickly. Patient requires adequate psychological preparation. |
| 7 | Inform patient and his relatives about the purpose of transfer. | Reduces anxiety. |
| 8 | Prepare summary of patient's treatment and condition. Complete the nurse's record and transfer form. | Provides summary of patient's nursing care needs and ensures continuity of care. |
| 9 | Anticipate problems patient may develop just before or during transfer and perform necessary nursing therapies like nebulization, medicine administration etc. | Ensures patient's comfort and safety during transport. |
| 10 | Assist in transferring patient to stretcher or wheel chair using proper body mechanics. | Reduces risk of injury to patient and nurse. |

*Contd...*

*Contd...*

| | | |
|---|---|---|
| 11 | Perform final assessment of patient's physical stability. (check vital signs, airway) | Minimizes risk of patient developing complications during transfer. |
| 12 | Accompany the patient to the receiving unit or hospital. | |
| 13 | Hand over all documents and belongings of patient to the receiving nurse and ensure that the items given are noted. | Ensures completion of transfer procedure. |
| 14 | Complete the needed documentation after transfer according to agency policies. | Nurse is legally responsible for documenting transfer of patient. |

## 2.4: PREPARING AN OPEN BED/UNOCCUPIED BED

### DEFINITION

Preparing a bed that is comfortable and suitable for a hospitalized patient.

### PURPOSES

1. To provide comfort and to promote rest.
2. To maintain a clean environment and neat appearance to the unit.
3. To reduce transmission of microorganisms.
4. To economize time, material and effort.
5. To promote cleanliness
6. To observe patient and to prevent complications.
7. To ambulate the patient.
8. To provide smooth, wrinkle free bed thus minimizing sources of skin irritation.

### ARTICLES

1. A tray containing
   a. Duster - 2
   b. A bowl /basin with disinfectant solution (1:20 savlon)
   c. Kidney tray
2. Chair or stool to keep the clean linen.
3. Hamper or dirty linen basket.
4. Clean bed linen, draw sheets, pillow case, counter pane (optional).
5. Mackintosh.
6. Linen bag/bucket.

### PROCEDURE

| | Nursing action | Rationale |
|---|---|---|
| 1. | Assess patient's general condition | Determines if patient can be made to sit out of bed |
| 2. | Explain to patient the need and purpose for making bed and how he has to cooperate. | Wins the patient's co-operation and confidence |
| 3. | Assess whether there is need for change of linen and collect fresh linen as needed | Ensures an organized approach towards carrying out procedure |
| 4. | Provide privacy | |
| 5. | Move furniture away from the bed | Provides adequate space for nurse to move |
| 6. | Place the tray on bedside locker. Keep hamper/linen basket at the bed side. | Arranging articles at the bed side saves time and energy |
| 7. | Place stool at footend of bed and place fresh linen on it in the reverse order of use | Keeping articles at convenient place and within reach promotes ease of work and saves time |
| 8. | Assist patient to get out of bed (if not contraindicated) and sit comfortably on a stool or chair near the bed. | |
| 9. | Lower head end of bed. Keep bed in flat position and lower side rails | • Working with the bed in lowered position promotes good body mechanics.<br>• Keeping the bed in flat position enables the nurse to make a wrinkle free bed. |

*Contd...*

*Contd...*

| | |
|---|---|
| 10. Remove wrist watch and wash hands | Prevents chances of cross-infection |
| 11. Switch off fan | Prevents spread of dust and microorganisms |
| 12. Remove pillow and place it over the seat of the chair/stool with open end away from the entrance to room | Reduces chance of accumulation of dust. |
| 13. Remove any personal items on the bed, inside the pillow cover, under the pillow, under the mattress etc. | Avoids loss of patient's belonging |
| 14. Stand on the side of the bed | |
| 15. Strip linen from all sides starting from head end to foot end. Move around the bed systematically. | Moving around the bed systematically prevents stretching, reaching, and possible muscle strain |
| 16. Bundle the linen each at a time and discard it into the linen hamper if they are not to be reused. | |
| 17. If reusing linen <br> • Remove blanket from foot end, dust, fold and place on the stool <br> • Remove towels, dust and place neatly on stool <br> • Take pillow, hold free end downwards, dust and place on the stool. If pillowcase is dirty, remove and discard into the hamper. <br> • Fold top sheet on the bed itself into 4 folds. Hold both ends of sheet, shake gently into the hamper and place on the stool <br><br> • Remove drawsheet, dust it and four–fold and place on stool <br> • Clean mackintosh with the damp duster from head end to foot end, roll it and keep on the stool <br> • Fold bottom sheet lengthwise with head end of both sides touching and feet end on both sides touching, into four folds | <br><br><br><br><br><br>Prevents sheet from dragging on the floor. Dusting into hamper avoids spread of dust and micro-organisms. Vigorous shaking of sheets should never be done <br><br><br><br>Folding lengthwise reduce risk of contamination from foot end to head end. |
| 18. Clean top of mattress with a dry duster from head end to foot end and collect into kidney tray. | Damp dusting causes mildew on the mattress |
| 19. Fold mattress from top to bottom and clean under surface of mattress with dry duster | |
| 20. Clean head end and half of body of cot with damp duster | |
| 21. Now fold mattress from bottom to top, clean the under surface of mattress and body of cot from the middle to foot end as described above | |
| 22. Replace duster and keep mattress flat | |
| 23 Place bottom sheet at the center of the bed (Figure 2.4(a)) | |

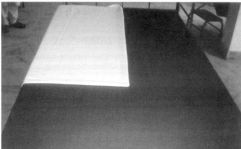

**Figure 2.4(a):** Placing bottom sheet at center of bed

*Contd...*

# Client Care: Hygiene and Comfort

*Contd...*

| | |
|---|---|
| 24. Open up the bottom sheet, make mitered corners, (Figure 2.4(b))first at the head end and then at the foot end and tuck on that side moving from head to foot. Separate the feet slightly apart and flex the knees instead of bending the back when tucking linen under the bed. | Making mitered corners and tucking prevents slipping of sheet and keeps bed firm .<br><br>Maintaining good body mechanics prevents undue strain on nurse's back |

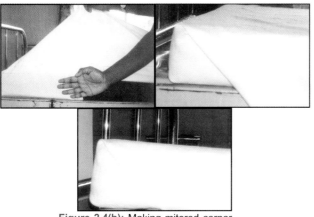

Figure 2.4(b): Making mitered corner

| | |
|---|---|
| 25. Spread mackintosh and place draw sheet over it. Tuck them together on the side you are standing. Tuck the middle portion first, then head end followed by foot end (Figure 2.4(c) | Mackintosh prevents soiling of bottom sheet. Draw sheet avoids direct contact of mackintosh with the skin |

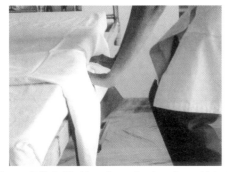

Figure 2.4(c): Tucking draw sheet and mackintosh

| | |
|---|---|
| 26. Move to other side of bed, tighten bottom sheet and make mitered corners at head and foot ends (if sheet is not long enough, make mitered corner at head end only. Leave foot end of sheet even with foot end of bed.) While tucking pull the sheets with both hands. | Pulling and tucking the sheet ensures a wrinkle free bed |
| 27. Tuck the mackintosh and draw sheet together on the side. | While tucking, keep palms downwards in order to get even appearance |
| 28. Place the top sheet in four-fold, with the top end at level with head end of the mattress. Spread the sheet. | |
| 29. Place blanket over the top sheet, 15 to 20 cm below from the top of the mattress. Cuff the top of the sheet over the blanket (Figure 2.4(d)). | Smooth cuff protects patient's skin from irritation caused by the blanket. |

*Contd...*

*Contd...*

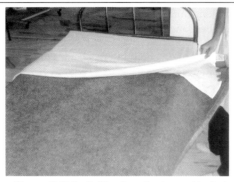

**Figure 2.4(d):** Cuffing top sheet over blanket

| | | |
|---|---|---|
| 30 | Make a toe fold about 15 cm from the bottom of mattress (Figure 2.4(e)) | Ensures adequate space for the toes under the sheet. |

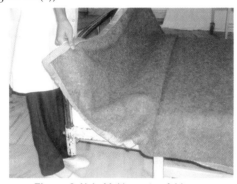

**Figure 2.4(e):** Making a toe fold

| | | |
|---|---|---|
| 31 | Tuck the top sheet and blanket together at the foot end and make a modified mitered corner, allowing the sides to hang free | |
| 32. | Change pillow case and replace pillow with free end facing away from the entrance of room or door (Figure 2.4(f)) | Free end of pillow away from entrance gives neat appearance and prevents collection of dust. |

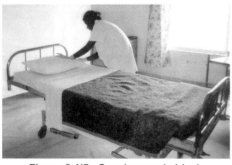

**Figure 2.4(f):** Open/unoccupied bed

| | | |
|---|---|---|
| 33 | Place or tie towels at the head end of bed (bath towel, sponge towel and face towel) | Allows easy access for the patient. |
| 34 | Clean inside and outside of locker and arrange patient's belongings neatly | Promotes a neat appearance. |

*Contd...*

*Contd...*

| 35 | Replace articles | |
|----|----|----|
| 36 | Wash hands | Reduces risk of transmission of microorganisms. |

## SPECIAL CONSIDERATIONS

1. Assess the patient's pulse, respiration and blood pressure before ambulating
2. Any comfort device used by the patient should be replaced.
3. The patient should be assisted back to bed.
4. The whole unit of the patient must be made neat and tidy.
5. Used dusters must be disinfected, washed and dried.
6. If linen is soiled with feces, urine or any other body fluids, segregate such linen for laundry as per the hospital policy.

## 2.5: PREPARING AN OCCUPIED BED

## DEFINITION

Making a comfortable bed with a patient who is confined to the bed in it.

## PURPOSES

1. To provide comfort for patients whose physical condition confines them to bed and for patients on imposed bed rest for therapeutic reasons
2. To change wet/soiled linen for the bed-ridden patients.
3. To maintain neat appearance and clean environment.
4. To provide a smooth wrinkle free bed foundation thus minimizing sources of skin irritation.

## ARTICLES

1. Dusters - 2 (Nos.)
2. Chair/stool
3. Basin with disinfectant solution
4. Hamper or dirty linen basket
5. Bucket
6. Clean bed linen
7. Clean gloves(optional)
8. Kidney tray.

## PROCEDURE

| | Nursing action | Rationale |
|---|---|---|
| 1. | Assess patient's general condition and check for any limitation in physical activity. | Determines level of activity and ensures patient's safety during the procedure. |
| 2. | Explain to patient the need for bed making. | Facilitates patient co-operation. |
| 3. | Wash hands | Prevents spread of microorganisms |
| 4. | Assemble all equipment and arrange on the bed side chair in the order of use. | Organized efforts facilitate ease of performance of task. |
| 5. | Close door/curtain. | Provides privacy. |
| 6. | Adjust the height of the bed. Lower side rails near to you, leaving the opposite side rails up. Release any equipment attached to the bed linen with clips like call light, IV tubes, Foley's catheter, drains etc. | Adjusting height of bed reduces strain on the nurse. Releasing equipment attached to bed linen prevents discomfort and accidental dislodgement of the tubes. |
| 7. | Check bed linen for patient's personal items. Remove extra pillows | Avoids loss of personal items. |
| 8. | Loosen the top bedding from head end to foot end. Remove blanket leaving the top sheet over the patient. | Makes removal of blanket easier. |
| 9. | If blanket and bedspread are to be re-used, fold lengthwise and keep on the chair. | Facilitates replacement and prevents wrinkling. Lengthwise folding prevents contamination of head end of sheet |
| 10. | Position the patient on side on the far side of the bed facing away. Adjust the pillow under the head. Be sure that the farthest side rails are up. | Provides space for placement of fresh bed linen. Side rails ensure safety. |

*Contd...*

*Contd...*

| | | |
|---|---|---|
| 11. | Loosen bottom linen from head end to foot end on both sides. | |
| 12. | Fan–fold the draw sheet towards the patient and push it as close to the patient as possible. (Figure 2.5(a))<br>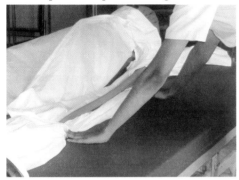<br>**Figure 2.5(a):** Fan folding linen close to patient | |
| 13. | Clean and roll the mackintosh towards the patient | Provides maximum work space for placing clean linen |
| 14. | Fan–fold the bottom sheet towards the patient. | When the patient turns to the other side these soiled linen can be easily removed. |
| 15. | Dust the mattress with dry duster | Dusting minimizes the number of microorganisms |
| 16. | Apply clean bottom linen, which is fan–folded length wise to the exposed half of the bed, keeping the centerfold in center of the bed (Figure 2.5(b)) | Applying linen over bed in successive layers minimizes expenditure of time and energy. |
| | a. Fan/fold the bottom sheet towards the patient. Smoothen the bottom layer over the mattress and bring edge over near side. Allow the sheets to hang about 25 cm over the mattress edge, make mitered corner at the head end of the bed. Tuck the hanging sheets on the sides till the foot end. The lower hem of the bottom should be even with the bottom edge of mattress | Keeping seam edges down eliminates irritation to patients skin. Mitered corners will secure the sheet on the bed. |
| | b. Bring the mackintosh back into place and clean it using dry duster (if soiled replace the mackintosh). Place the clean draw sheet over the mackintosh and tuck both mackintosh and draw sheet under the mattress<br>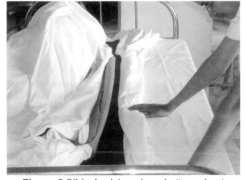<br>**Figure 2.5(b):** Applying clean bottom sheet | Protects bed linen from soiling |
| 17. | Raise the side rails on working side and go to the other side. | Maintains safety. |

*Contd...*

# Clinical Nursing Procedures: The Art of Nursing Practice

*Contd...*

| | |
|---|---|
| 18. Lower the side rails and assist the patient to roll slowly to the other side of bed over the fold of linen. | Exposes opposite side of bed for removal of soiled linen and placement of clean linen. |
| 19. Loosen the edges of the soiled linen from underneath the mattress. | Makes linen easier to remove. |
| 20. Remove the draw sheet by folding it into a bundle and place in the linen bag. Remove the bottom sheet and put it in linen bag. Clean and roll mackintosh towards the patient | |
| 21. Dust the mattress with dry duster and spread the fan–folded clean linen smoothly over the edge of the mattress from head end to foot end. | Dusting minimizes the number of microorganisms. |
| 22. Pull taut and secure the bottom sheet under the head of the mattress. Miter corners. Pull the side of the sheet taut and tuck under the side of the mattress. | Removes wrinkles and creases in linen, which are uncomfortable to lie on. |
| 23. Straighten the mackintosh and draw sheet. | Smooth linen will not irritate patients skin. |
| 24. Assist the patient in rolling back to supine position and reposition the pillow. | Maintains patient's comfort. |
| 25. Tuck the mackintosh and draw sheet in the same manner | Tucking will keep the bed firm. |
| 26. Place top sheet over the patient with center–fold lengthwise down the middle of the bed. Open the sheet from head to foot and unfold it over the patient. | Sheets should be equally distributed over bed by correctly positioning the center–fold. |
| 27. Ask the patient to hold the top linen and tuck around the shoulders. Remove the used top sheet by pulling from down and place it in the linen bag. | Top sheet prevents exposure of body parts. Having patient hold the sheet encourage participation in care. |
| 28. Place the blanket over top sheet as in an open bed (Figure 2.5(c)) | Provides warmth for the patient. |

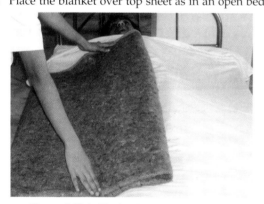

**Figure 2.5(c):** Placing blanket over top sheet

| | |
|---|---|
| 29. Make a horizontal toe pleat and modified mitered corner in the foot end allowing the sides to hang free. | Tucking the linen together gives neat appearance and toe pleat provides adequate room for the legs under the sheet. |
| 30. Place the upper edge of blanket 5-6 inches lower than the top sheet as in open. Fold it over the blanket's upper border to form a cuff. | Provides warmth for the patient. This type of fold, covering the upper edge of blanket avoids irritation from direct contact of patient's skin with blanket. |
| 31. Change the pillow case and replace pillow /pillows with open end facing away from door or entrance to room | Maintains neat appearance |

*Contd...*

*Contd...*

| | |
|---|---|
| 32. Place the call signal and all other tubing back and place the patient in comfortable position. | Ensures safety and comfort. |
| 33. Discard the dirty linen in the linen bag and wash hands. | Prevents transmission of microorganisms |
| 34. Record the observations made on the patient in the nurses notes | Provides accurate documentation of patient. |

## SPECIAL POINTS

Patients with respiratory and cardiac disorders may be unable to tolerate lying flat during bed making. Top to bottom method of occupied bed making can be used for such patients.

# 2.6: PREPARING A POSTOPERATIVE BED

## DEFINITION

Preparing a hospital bed to receive the patient who has undergone surgical procedure.

## PURPOSES

1. To provide a safe, clean and comfortable bed for a postoperative patient.
2. To provide appropriate position to the patient who has undergone an operation.
3. To protect the patient from being hypothermic.
4. To be equipped to meet any possible postoperative emergencies.
5. To protect the mattress and bedding from getting soiled from bleeding, vomiting, drainage/discharges.
6. For quick transfer of patient from trolley to bed.

## ARTICLES

1. All articles needed to make an open bed.
2. Additional articles.
   a. A small mackintosh and towel.
   b. A tray containing (postanesthetic tray)
      - Clean rag pieces or gauze pieces.
      - Artery forceps
      - Mouth gag
      - Airway
      - Tongue depressor
3. Temperature tray.
4. IV stand and other requisites for IV administration
5. Hot water bag
6. Bed blocks – 2 (in case of surgery under spinal anesthesia)
7. Suction apparatus.
8. Articles needed for oxygen administration.
9. Additional articles as per patient requirement (e g. pillows)
10. B P apparatus
11. Kidney tray.

## PROCEDURE

| | Nursing action | Rationale |
|---|---|---|
| 1. | Prepare the foundation of the bed as in open bed | |
| 2. | Place extra mackintosh and towel at the head end | Protects the bed from soiling with vomitus |
| 3. | The foot end of the top linen are left untucked. They are folded back evenly with the mattress | |
| 4. | Fanfold the top linen to the opposite side of the entrance standing on side of the bed (Figure 2.6(a)) | Helps in transferring patient easily from stretcher to bed |

*Contd...*

*Contd...*

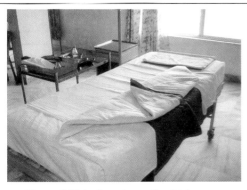

**Figure 2.6(a):** A postoperative bed

| | | |
|---|---|---|
| 5. | Place hot water bags beneath the fan folded top linen and remove it before receiving the patient | Keeps the bed warm |
| 6. | Place articles such as infusion stand, bed blocks and post–anesthetic tray near the bed ready for use | |
| 7. | Pillow is not used but can be kept at the head end | Protects the patient from injury by hitting against the bars at head end |
| 8. | Additional mackintosh and draw sheet can be used according to the site of operation | Protects the bed from getting soiled |
| 9. | Additional pillows if used should be protected with water proof covers | Additional pillows are used to support the operated area |
| 10. | Rinse and replace the dusters and basin | |
| 11 | Wash hands | Reduces risk of transmission of microorganisms. |

# 2.7: PREPARAING A CARDIAC BED

## DEFINITION

A cardiac bed is used to help the patient to assume a sitting position, which can afford him greatest amount of comfort with least strain.

## PURPOSES

1. To relieve dyspnea caused by cardiac diseases
2. To provide comfort with least strain
3. To reduce work load of heart in cardiac diseases.

## ARTICLES

1. Bedsheets
2. Mackintosh
3. Drawsheet
4. Blanket
5. Dusters (2)
6. Basin with disinfectant solution (savlon 1:20)
7. Laundry bag
8. Pillows(Additional)
9. Back rest
10. Cardiac table
11. Foot rest.

## PROCEDURE

| | Nursing action | Rationale |
|---|---|---|
| 1. | Explain to patient what will be done and how it would help him to be comfortable. | |
| 2. | Collect articles, fold and arrange the linen on the stool in the order of use. | Arranging linen in the order of use aids for smooth functioning |
| 3. | Prepare the bed as an open bed | |
| 4. | Place back rest at patient's back and arrange pillows. | Supports the patient's back and provides comfortable position to the patient |
| 5. | Assist patient to assume comfortable position in bed and cover him properly | Provides warmth to the patient |
| 6. | Place a pillow under the knees | Prevents slipping of the patient |
| 7. | Arrange pillows on either side of the patient below both the arms | Supports the arms |
| 8. | Place cardiac table in front of the patient (Figure 2.7(a)) | Helps patient to lean forward. |

*Contd...*

*Contd...*

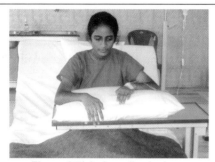

**Figure 2.7(a):** A cardiac bed

| | |
|---|---|
| 9. | Ensure that patient is sitting comfortably in the new position. |
| 10. | Record the observation made on the patient in the Nurse's notes | Promotes communication among staff. |

# 2.8: ASSISTING IN ORAL HYGIENE FOR A CONSCIOUS PATIENT

## DEFINITION

Assisting the weak or debilitated patient for cleansing mouth by mechanical brushing of the teeth and rinsing of the mouth.

## INDICATIONS

1. Mouth breathers.
2. Patients on NPO.
3. Oral surgery patients (sterile special mouth care).
4. Patients on oxygen inhalation.
5. Children under three years.
6. Patients who are unable to maintain adequate oral hygiene.

## PURPOSES

1. To maintain the healthy state of mouth, teeth, gums and lips.
2. To clean the mouth off food particles, plaque and bacteria.
3. To relieve discomfort resulting from unpleasant odors and tastes.
4. To enhance the well- being and comfort and to stimulate appetite.
5. To prevent sordes, caries and infection to oral tissues.

## ARTICLES

A clean "mouth toilet tray" containing:
1. Face towel
2. Tumbler/feeding cup containing water.
3. Soft bristled toothbrush.
4. Tooth paste/Tooth powder/Available dentrifice.
5. Mouth wash solution (according to patient's preference and availability)
    i. Sodium chloride.
    ii. Thymol.
    iii. Diluted solution of potassium permanganate 1: 1000
    iv. Listerine.
    v. Chlorhexidine
6. Cotton applicators/cotton balls
7. Emollient in a container – Glycerin, Liquid paraffin, Vaseline, coconut oil
8. K-basin/Emesis basin – 2 (one could be a paper bag)
9. Small mackintosh.
10. Clean gloves

## PROCEDURE

| | Nursing action | Rationale |
|---|---|---|
| 1. | Assess the condition of the patient, the condition of his mouth and level of consciousness. | Helps to determine the type of oral hygiene, the patient requires. |
| 2. | Inspect the integrity of lips, teeth, buccal mucosa, gums, palate and tongue. | Determines the status of the patients oral cavity and extent of need for oral hygiene. |

*Contd...*

# Client Care: Hygiene and Comfort

*Contd...*

| | | |
|---|---|---|
| 3. | Assess the patient's ability to grasp and manipulate toothbrush. | Determines the level of assistance required. |
| 4. | Explain procedure to patient and encourage him to participate. | Reduces anxiety and promotes patient participation. |
| 5. | Pull the screen. | Provides privacy. |
| 6. | Wash hands and Don gloves. | Prevents spread of infection. |
| 7. | Bring patient to edge of the bed nearest to the nurse. | Promotes correct body mechanics and ease of working |
| 8. | Position patient in high fowlers/semi fowlers position as tolerated | Provides comfortable working position |
| 9. | Place the small mackintosh with the face towel on the chest. | Prevents patient's clothing from soiling. |
| 10. | Place K. basin close to the patient's chin. | Prevents soiling. |
| 11. | Apply toothpaste to brush. Holding brush over K. basin, pour small amount of water over toothpaste (Figure 2.8(a)) | Moisture aids in distribution of toothpaste over tooth surface. |

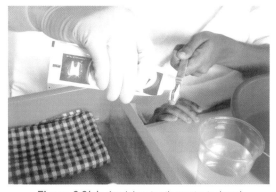

**Figure 2.8(a):** Applying tooth paste to brush

| | | |
|---|---|---|
| 12 | Instruct patient to hold toothbrush bristles at 45 degree angle to gum line. Brush inner and outer surfaces of upper and lower teeth by brushing from gum to crown of each tooth (Figure 2.8(b)) | Angle allows brush to reach all tooth surfaces and to clean under gum line where plaque and tartar accumulate. |

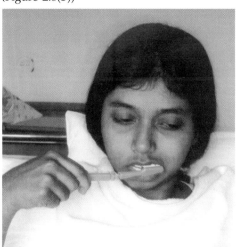

**Figure 2.8(b):** Brushing teeth, holding brush at 45 degree

| | | |
|---|---|---|
| 13 | Clean the biting surface back and forth; farther side first and then nearer side and upper jaw first and then lower jaw. | Back and forth motion dislodges food particles caught between teeth and along chewing surface. |

*Contd...*

*Contd...*

| | |
|---|---|
| 14. Have the patient hold the brush at the same angle (45 degree) over tongue and brush lightly over surface horizontally taking care not to initiate gag reflex. | Microorganisms collect and grow on tongue surface and contribute to bad breath. Gagging may cause aspiration of toothpaste or may induce vomiting. |
| 15. Allow patient to rinse mouth thoroughly by taking mouthful of water and spitting into the K. basin (Figure 2.8(c)) | Vigorous swishing motion helps to remove debris and toothpaste |

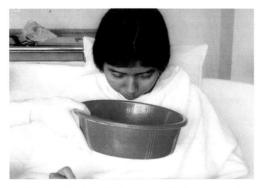

**Figure 2.8(c):** Assisting patient in rinsing mouth

| | |
|---|---|
| 16. Allow patient to rinse mouth with mouthwash as desired. | Mouthwash leaves a pleasant taste in mouth. |
| 17. Assist wiping mouth with face towel. | Promotes sense of comfort. |
| 18. Apply emollient to lips | Prevents cracking and drying of lips |
| 19. Assist patient to comfortable position. | |
| 20. Discard the waste, clean the used articles and replace equipment as appropriate | Leaves the unit clean and articles ready for further use. |
| 21. Wash hands. | |
| 22. Record the procedure including time, solution used and condition of mouth. | |

# 2.9: PERFORMING ORAL CARE FOR AN UNCONSCIOUS PATIENT

## DEFINITION

Performing mechanical cleansing of the teeth and the mouth, for an unconscious patient.

## PURPOSES

1. To maintain integrity of the lips, tongue and mucous membrane of the mouth.
2. To prevent and treat oral infection.
3. To clean and moisturize oral mucous membrane.
4. To stimulate salivation.
5. To prevent dental caries and tooth decay.
6. To prevent halitosis.

## ARTICLES

1. Small mackintosh and face towel
2. Artery forceps
3. Dissecting forceps/thumb forceps
4. Small bowl with mouthwash solution or normal saline
5. Kidney tray
6. Emollient
7. Tongue depressor
8. Disposable gloves
9. Cotton applicator
10. Small jug with plain water
11. Mouth gag
12. Suction apparatus
13. Square gauze piece(2" × 2")

## PROCEDURE

| | Nursing action | Rationale |
|---|---|---|
| 1. | Assess patient's oral hygiene . | Certain conditions such as coated tongue, ulceration / red dry swollen tongue, halitosis, immunosuppressed patients, with diabetes mellitus etc. may require frequent oral care. |
| 2. | Test for presence of gag reflex by placing tongue blade on back half of tongue | Reveals whether the patient is at risk of aspiration |
| 3. | Check the doctor's orders for specific precautions regarding the movement and positioning of patient | Prevents injury to patient. |
| 4. | Explain the procedure to patient and/or relatives | Unconscious patients may retain ability to hear |
| 5. | Pull curtains | Provides privacy |
| 6. | Raise bed to comfortable working level. Arrange articles by bedside | Use of good body mechanics prevents fatigue |
| 7. | Position the patient on side, head turned towards you. | Allows secretions to drain from mouth instead of collecting in back of pharynx and thus preventing aspiration |

*Contd...*

*Contd...*

| | | |
|---|---|---|
| 8. | Place towel and mackintosh under the patients head and spread one towel over chest and an emesis basin under the chin. | Collects saliva that may drool from the mouth and prevents soiling of bed. |
| 9. | Raise side rails of bed on both sides | Prevents the patient from falling |
| 10 | Wash hands and don gloves | Reduces transfer of micro-organisms |
| 11. | Lower the side rails on the working side | Use of good body mechanics prevents fatigue |
| 12. | Do not pour water into the mouth of an unconscious patient | Prevents aspiration of fluid into the lungs because of poor gag reflex |
| 13. | Separate the upper and lower teeth with padded tongue depressor by inserting it quickly and gently if required. | Provides access to oral cavity |
| 14. | Take gauze piece with the dissecting forceps. | |
| 15. | Wrap the gauze piece around the artery forceps covering its tip. Moisten the gauze piece with normal saline or dip in the cleaning agent (Figure 2.9 (a) and Figure 2.9(b)) | Covering tip of forceps prevents injury to the mucous membrane and gums. |

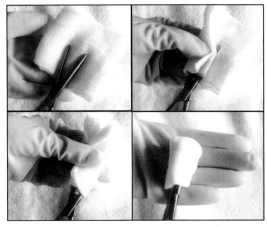

Figure 2.9(a): Wrapping gauze over artery forceps

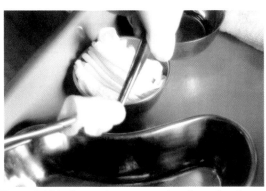

Figure 2.9(b): Squeezing gauze using dissecting forceps

| | | |
|---|---|---|
| 16. | Swab each tooth gently but firmly and clean all the sides of the tooth. Clean chewing surface first and then, inner and outer surface from gum to crown (Figure 2.9(c)) | Ensures thorough cleaning and prevents injury to the oral mucous membrane and gums |

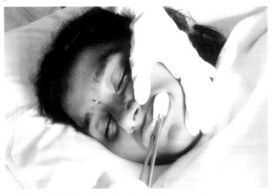

Figure 2.9(c): Cleaning teeth from gum to crown

| | |
|---|---|
| 17. | Clean lower teeth on both sides followed by upper teeth on both sides. |

*Contd...*

# Client Care: Hygiene and Comfort

*Contd...*

| | | |
|---|---|---|
| 18. | Gently swab roof of the mouth, gums and inner side of cheeks | |
| 19. | Clean the tongue from back to front using artery forceps covered with gauze | Ensures thorough cleaning of the tongue |
| 20. | Clean the teeth and tongue in similar way using plain water | Ensures thorough removal of dentrifice or cleaning agent which may cause unpleasant taste |
| 21. | Apply emollient to the lip using cotton applicators. | Lubricates the lips to prevent drying and cracking |
| 22. | Position the patient in comfortable position. Raise side rails, lower bed | |
| 23. | Replace all the articles after discarding the waste, remove gloves, discard it and wash hands. | Prevents transfer of microorganisms |
| 24. | Record date, time, solution used, condition of mouth and any abnormalities, like bleeding/inflammation. | |

# 2.10: BATHING A PATIENT IN BED

## DEFINITION

Cleansing the entire body of a dependent patient in bed.

## PURPOSES

1. To remove transient microorganisms, body secretions, excretions and dead skin cells.
2. To stimulate circulation
3. To produce a feeling of well being
4. To promote relaxation and comfort
5. To improve self–esteem
6. To prevent or eliminate bad odour.

## ARTICLES

1. Bed pan/urinal
2. Basin
3. Jugs with hot water and cold water (water of 110 to 115 degree Fahrenheit (43–45° centigrade) for adults and 100 to 105degree F for children).
4. Table or trolley
5. Bath blanket/sheet
6. Clean gloves
7. Wash clothes (2)
8. Soap
9. Towels (2)
10. Lotions, powders, deodorants (optional)
11. Change of bed linen (1 set)
12. Change of patient's dress (1 set).

## PROCEDURE

| | Nursing action | Rationale |
|---|---|---|
| 1 | Prepare patient and environment | |
| | a. Explain procedure to patient and relative and encourage participation from patient or relative. | Reduces anxiety and encourages co-operation. |
| | b. Close windows and doors to make sure that room is free from drafts and switch off fan/AC | Air currents increase loss of heat from the body. |
| | c. Provide privacy by drawing curtains and closing doors | Reduces patient's embarrassment. |
| | d. Offer bedpan or urinal if he or she requires. | Enhances comfort of the patient. |
| 2 | Prepare bed and position patient appropriately | |
| | a. Place bed in a high position | Reduces strain to nurse's back. |
| | b. Position patient close to right side of the bed or close to nurse. | |
| | c. Raise side rails on both sides. | |
| 3 | Wash hands and put on clean gloves | Reduces transmission of microorganisms. |
| 4 | Lower side rails on the right side. | |
| 5 | Arrange articles within your reach | |
| 6 | Make mitts with the wash cloth. | Mitts conserve heat of water and prevents tip of wash cloth from trailing and dripping over patient's body. |

*Contd...*

*Contd...*

| | | |
|---|---|---|
| 7 | Check temperature of water mixed in the basin by pouring water on the inner aspect of the palm of the patient. | Prevents risk of burns |
| 8 | Remove patient's clothings and cover with a bath blanket or sheet. Expose only that part of the body which is to be washed. | Ensures privacy and prevents chills for the patient. |
| 9 | Wash face<br>a. Place one bath towel under patient's head<br>b. Wet bath mitt, squeeze water from it, so that it is not dribbling<br>c. Wash patient's eyes using separate corners of the bath mitt for each eye and wipe from inner canthus to outer canthus.<br><br><br>d. Ask patient if he prefers using soap for the face (in unconscious patients avoid soap)<br><br><br>e. If using soap, apply soap with the second mitt and then rinse with the first mitt, till soap is removed fully<br>f. Wash, rinse and dry patient's face, neck and ears. | Prevents wetting of pillows and bed linen.<br>Bath mitt retains temperature of water.<br><br>Prevents transmission of organisms from one eye to another, wiping from inner to outer canthus prevents secretions from entering nasolacrimal duct.<br>Soap has a drying effect and face is more exposed to the air than any other body part and hence tends to be more drier<br>Soap if remaining on skin will cause irritation. |
| 10 | Wash arms and hand.<br>a. Place bath towel lengthwise under arm farther to you.<br>b. Wash, apply soap, rinse and dry arms using long strokes from distal to proximal areas.<br>c. Pat dry using the 2nd bath towel. Do not rub.<br>d. Wash axilla well. Exercise precaution, if there is an IV infusion on arm.<br>e. Place folded towel on bed under hands, and place basin on it. Attend to inter-digital spaces. Immerse hand in basin and assist patient in washing hand.<br>f. Repeat entire procedure for other arm. | Protects bed linen from becoming wet.<br>Firm strokes from distal to proximal areas will increase venous return.<br>Rubbing may cause skin injuries. |
| 11 | Wash chest and abdomen<br>a. Fold bath blanket upto pubic area. Place towel over chest and abdomen.<br>b. Wash, rinse and dry chest and abdomen giving special attention to skin folds under breasts.<br>c. Keep chest and abdomen covered all along and use long firm strokes to wash the area.<br>In women, wash chest and abdomen separately. | Prevents unnecessary exposure of patient. |
| 12 | Change water if cold, dirty or soapy. | |
| 13 | Wash back of patient<br>a. Turn patient to side lying or prone position and expose back.<br>b. Place towel lengthwise alongside back of patient.<br>c. Wash, rinse and dry using long, firm strokes from neck to buttocks.<br>d. Give back massage. | |
| 14 | Change bath water | |
| 15 | Turn patient back to supine position. | |
| 16 | Wash legs<br>a. Place towel lengthwise under farther leg away from you. | |

*Contd...*

*Contd...*

| | | |
|---|---|---|
| | b. Bend leg at knee, supporting under leg and ask patient to hold position. If patient is unable to do it ask another nurse/family member to support leg.<br>c. Use long, firm strokes to wash from distal to proximal/ from ankle to knee and knee to thigh. Do not use such long strokes in patients having blood clots in lower extremities. Eg: in DVT as it may dislodge the clot.<br>d. Wash, rinse and dry the extremity<br>e. Fold towel and place beneath foot of the patient. Place basin with water under the foot and clean with mitt.<br>f. Take out the foot and dry the extremity.<br>g. Discard water.<br>h. Repeat entire procedure for the other leg. | Moving from distal to proximal improves venous circulation and removes dirt from skin pores. |
| 17 | Encourage patient to clean perineal area with mitt. Discard it into a kidney tray. | Promotes patient's independence. |
| 18 | Position patient in a comfortable manner. | |
| 19 | Apply moisturizer or body lotion if patient prefers or if skin is dry. | Lotions prevent drying and chapped skin. |
| 20 | Assist patient in dressing. | |
| 21 | Comb hair | |
| 22 | Change bed linen | |
| 23 | Wash hands | |
| 24 | Record procedure | |
| 25 | Replace all articles. | |

## SPECIAL CONSIDERATIONS

1. Obtain assistance if required in case of helpless/unconscious patient.
2. If patient is obese or cannot move in bed, nurse may move from one side of the bed to the other side to ensure good body mechanics.
3. Assess patient's general condition before giving bath. If unstable, refrain from giving bath.
4. Bath should not be given immediately after food because it interferes with the process of digestion.

# 2.11: PERFORMING NAIL AND FOOT CARE

## PURPOSES

1. To keep the feet clean and dry.
2. To teach the patient proper way to inspect all surfaces of feet and hands for lesions, dryness or signs of infection.
3. To trim nails and keep them short to prevent injury.
4. To prevent accumulation of dirt and microorganisms underneath the nails.

## ARTICLES

1. Wash basin.
2. Wash cloth.
3. Bath or face towel.
4. Nail cutter with a nail file
5. Warm water.
6. Soap in soap dish.
7. Body lotion.
8. Clean disposable gloves
9. Paper bag/kidney tray.
10. A bowl with cotton swabs.
11. Bowl with antiseptic solution.
12. Bowl with cotton swabs soaked in antiseptic solution.
    (optional: for diabetic and unconscious patients).

## PROCEDURE

| | Nursing action | Rationale |
|---|---|---|
| 1. | Inspect all surfaces of fingers, toes, feet and nails. Pay particular attention to areas of dryness, inflammation and cracking. Also inspect areas between toes, heels and soles of feet. | Integrity of feet and nails determines frequency and level of hygiene required. Heels, soles and sides of feet are prone to irritation from ill-fitting shoes. |
| 2. | Assess color and temperature of toes, feet and fingers. Assess capillary refill of nails, palpate radial and ulnar pulses of each hand and dorsalis pedis pulse of feet, note character of pulses. | Assess adequacy of blood flow to extremities. Circulatory alterations may change integrity of nails and increase patient's chance of localized infection, when break in skin integrity occurs. |
| 3. | Observe patient's gait. Have patient walk down the hall or walk in straight line (if able) | Painful disorders of feet can cause limping or unnatural gait. |
| 4. | Ask female patients whether they use nail polish and polish remover frequently. | Chemicals in these products can cause excessive dryness. |
| 5. | Assess type of footwear worn by patients. | Types of shoes and footwear may predispose patient to foot and nail problems (e.g.: infection, areas of friction, ulceration) |
| 6. | Identify patients at risk for foot or nail problems<br>a. Older adults | Poor vision, lack of co-ordination or inability to bend may contribute to difficulty in performing foot and nail care. Normal physiological changes and aging also result in nail and foot problems. |
| | b. Diabetes mellitus | Vascular changes associated with diabetes mellitus reduce blood flow to peripheral tissues. Break in skin integrity places diabetic patients at high risk for skin infection. |

*Contd...*

# Clinical Nursing Procedures: The Art of Nursing Practice

*Contd...*

| | |
|---|---|
| c. Heart failure and renal disease | Both conditions can increase tissue edema particularly in dependent areas like legs and feet. Edema reduces blood flow to neighboring tissues |
| d. Cerebrovascular accident or stroke | Presence of residual foot or leg weakness or paralysis results in altered walking patterns. Altered gait pattern causes increased friction and pressure on feet. |
| 7. Assess type of home remedies patient uses for existing foot problems. | |
| a. Over the counter liquid preparations to remove corns | Liquid preparations can cause burns and ulcerations. |
| b. Cutting of corns or calluses with razor blade or scissors | Cutting of corns or calluses may result in infection caused by break in skin integrity. |
| c. Application of adhesive tape | Skin of older adult is thin and delicate and is prone to tearing when adhesive tape is removed. |
| 8. Assess patient's ability to care for nails or feet, visual alteration, fatigue, musculoskeletal weakness etc. | Determines patient's ability to perform self–care and degree of assistance required from nurse. |
| 9. Assess patient's knowledge of foot and nail care practices. | Determines patient's need for health teaching. |
| 10. Explain procedure to patient including the fact that proper soaking requires several minutes. In case of patients who are unconscious, soak nails with wet cotton swabs. In patients with diabetes soak only for a few minutes | Soaking softens the nails and enables easy cutting of the nails. In diabetic patients extended soaking can result in accidental injury at the time of procedure leading to delayed wound healing. |
| 11. Wash hands and arrange equipment on the over- bed table. | Easy access to equipment prevents delay. |
| 12. Pull curtain around bed or close room door. | Maintains patient's privacy. |
| 13. Assist ambulatory patient to sit in bedside chair. Help bed-bound patient to supine position with head of bed elevated. Place towel on mattress | Sitting position facilitates immersing feet in basin. |
| 14. Fill washbasin with warm water. Test water temperature and have it about 43 to 44° C. | Warm water softens nails and thickened epidermal cells, reduces inflammation of skin and promotes local circulation. Proper water temperature prevents burns. |
| 15. Place basin on towel and help patient place feet in basin for soaking toe nails. Place call light within patient's reach. | Patients with muscular weakness or tremors may have difficulty positioning feet. Patient's safety is maintained. |
| 16. Adjust over bed table to low position and place it over patient's lap (patient may sit in chair or lie in bed). | Easy access prevents accidental spills. |
| 17. Fill basin with warm water and place basin on towel on over bed table for soaking finger nails. | Warm water softens nails and thickened epidermal cells. |
| 18. Instruct patient to place fingers in basin and place arms in comfortable position. | Prolonged positioning can cause discomfort unless normal anatomical alignment is maintained. |
| 19. Allow patient's feet and fingernails to soak for 10 to 20 minutes and rewarm the water after 10 minutes if necessary. | Softening of corns, calluses and cuticles ensures easy removal of dead cells. |
| 20. Dry hands with towel | |
| 21. Clip fingernails straight across and even with top of fingers using nail clipper. Shape nails with file. Wipe each finger tip with cotton dipped in antiseptic solution | Cutting straight prevents splitting of nail margins and formation of sharp nail spikes that can irritate lateral margins. |
| 22. Move over bed table away from patient | Provides easier access to feet. |
| 23. Put on disposable gloves and scrub callused areas of feet with washcloth. | Gloves prevent transmission of fungal infection,. Friction removes dried skin layers |
| 24. Remove feet from basin and dry thoroughly | |

*Contd...*

*Contd...*

| | |
|---|---|
| 25. Clean and trim toenails. Do not file corners of toenails. | Shaping corners of toenails may damage tissues. |
| 26. Apply lotion to feet and hands and assist patient back to bed and into comfortable position. | Lotion lubricates dry skin by helping to retain moisture. |
| 27. Remove disposable gloves and place in receptacle. Clean and replace equipment and supplies to proper place. Dispose off soiled linen in hamper . Wash hands. | Reduces transmission of infection |
| 28. Inspect nails and surrounding skin surfaces after soaking and nail trimming. Place nail cutter in a bowl with antiseptic solution for 20-30 minutes then wash, dry and replace | Evaluates condition of skin and nails. Allows nurse to note any remaining rough nail edges. |
| 29. Record procedure and observations (e.g.: breaks in skin, inflammation, ulceration, etc. and patients response). | |
| 30. Report any breaks in skin or ulcerations to nurse in-charge or physician. | These abnormalities can seriously increase patient's risk of infection and must be carefully observed. |

## 2.12: PROVIDING GENITAL CARE/HYGIENIC PERINEAL CARE

### DEFINITION

Genital care involves thorough cleansing of external genitalia and surrounding skin.

### PURPOSES

1. To promote patient's comfort and cleanliness
2. To prevent infection in high risk patients.

### INDICATIONS

1. Patients who are unable to do self–care.
2. Patients with indwelling catheter
3. Patients with incontinence of urine or stool.
4. Patients having excessive vaginal discharge
5. Patients recovering from rectal or genital surgery
6. Following childbirth.

### ARTICLES

1. Wash basin
2. Soap dish with soap
3. Wash cloths (2)
4. Bath towel
5. Bath blanket/bedsheet
6. Bed pan
7. Disposable gloves
8. Cotton swabs
9. Kidney tray
10. Toilet tissues or diaper wipes.

### PROCEDURE

| | Nursing action | Rationale |
|---|---|---|
| 1 | Explain procedure and its purpose to patient | Helps to minimise anxiety and embrassment during procedure. |
| 2 | Wash hands and Don clean gloves | Prevents cross infection |
| 3 | Position patient with legs spread apart | |
| 4 | Assess genitalia for signs of inflammation, skin breakdown, infection or contamination with fecal matter. | Determines the extent of perineal care required by patient |
| 5 | If fecal material is present enclose in a fold of pad or toilet tissue and remove. With disposable wipes or tissue cleanse buttocks and anus, washing from front to back. Cleanse, rinse and dry area thoroughly. Remove and discard underpad and replace with clean one. | Cleansing reduces transmission of microorganisms from anus to urethra or genitalia. |
| 6 | Change gloves if they are soiled | |
| 7 | Help patient to flex knees and spread legs apart. | Provides full exposure of genitalia. |

*Contd...*

# Client Care: Hygiene and Comfort

*Contd...*

| | |
|---|---|
| 8 | Fold top linen down toward foot of bed and fold patient's gown above genital area. | Draping prevents unnecessary exposure of body parts and maintains patient's warmth and comfort during procedure. |
| 9 | Diamond drape patient by placing bath blanket/top sheet with one corner between patient's legs, and another corner over patient's chest. The two side corners should hang over sides of bed. Tuck side corner around patient's legs and under hips. (Figure 2.12(a)) | |

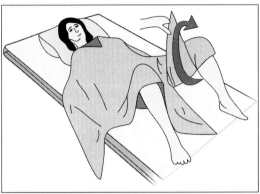

**Figure 2.12(a):** Positioning and draping female patient for genital care

| | |
|---|---|
| 10 | Raise side rails, fill basin with warm water. | Prevents patient from falling. Use of warm water promotes comfort. |
| 11 | Place wash basin and toilet tissue on over bed table, place wash clothes in basin | Articles placed within reach of nurse prevents accidental spills. |
| 12A a. | Female genital care Lower side rails and instruct patient to maintain dorsal recumbent position with knees flexed and legs apart. Note any restriction or limitation in positioning patient. | Provides full exposure of female genitalia. Minimise degree of abduction if position causes pain because of arthritis or reduced joint mobility. |
| b. | Fold lower corner of bath blanket/sheet up between patient's legs onto abdomen. Wash and dry patient's upper thighs (Figure 2.12(b)) | Minimises transmission of microbes. Keeping patient draped until procedure begins minimises anxiety. Accumulated perineal secretions can soil surrounding skin surface. |
| c. | Wash labia majora while using non-dominant hand to retract labia from thigh. With dominant handwash carefully in skin folds and wipe in direction from perineum to rectum. Repeat on opposite side using separate section of wash cloth. Rinse and dry area thoroughly. | Skin folds may contain body secretaions which harbour microorganisms. Wiping from perineum to rectum reduces chances of transmitting fecal organisms to urinary meatus |
| d. | Separate labia with non-dominant hand to expose urethral meatus and vaginal orifice. With dominant handwash downwards from pubic area towards rectum using separate quarters of wash cloth for each stroke. Clean the vulva and labia minora on both sides and inside of labia majora on both sides. | Cleansing method reduces transfer of microorganisms to urinary meatus. (For menstruating women and patients with indwelling urinary catheter, cleanse with cotton balls). |
| e. | If patient can use bedpan, place bedpan and pour water over perineal area. Dry perineal area thoroughly with bath towel from front to back. | Rinsing removes soap and microorganisms more effectively than wiping. Retained moisture harbours microorganisms. |

*Contd...*

*Contd...*

f. Fold lower corner of bath blanket back between patient's legs and over perineum. Ask patient to lower legs and assume comfortable position.

12B Male genital care:

a. Lower side rails and assist patient to supine position. Note restriction in mobility if any.

b. Fold top half of bath blanket/sheet down below the penis. Position gown to cover chest. Wash and dry patient's upper thighs (Figure 2.12(b)). | Minimises transmission of microorganisms. Keeping patient draped until procedure begins minimizes anxiety. Accumulation of perineal secretions can soil surrounding skin surfaces.

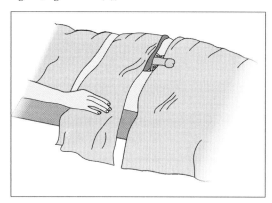

**Figure 2.12(b):** Draping male patient for genital care

c. Gently raise penis and place bath towel underneath. Firmly grasp shaft of penis, if patient is uncircumcized, retract foreskin. If patient has an erection, defer procedure until later. | Towel prevents moisture from collecting in inguinal area. Gentle but firm handling reduces chance of patient having an erection. Secretions capable of harbouring microorganisms collect underneath foreskin.

d. Wash top of penis at urethral meatus first using circular motion. Cleanse from meatus outwards. Discard wash cloth and repeat with clean cloth until penis is clean. Rinse and dry gently. | Direction of cleaning moves from area of least contamination to area of most contamination. This prevents microorganisms from entering urethra. Tightening of foreskin around shaft of penis can cause local edema and discomfort.

e. Return foreskin to its original position. | Vigorous massage of penis can lead to erection, which can embarrass patient and nurse. Underlying surface of penis may have greater accumulation of secretions. Abduction of legs provides easier access to scrotal tissues.

f. Wash shaft of penis with gentle but firm downward strokes. Pay special attention to underlying surface of penis. Rinse and dry penis thoroughly. Instruct patient to spread legs apart slightly. | Pressure on scrotal tissues can cause pain.

g. Gently cleanse scrotum. Lift it and wash underlying skin fold. Rinse and dry.

13 Fold bath blanket over patient's perineum and assist patient in turning to side lying position. | Draping promotes comfort and minimises patient's anxiety. Side lying position provides access to anal area.

14 If patient has urinary or bowel incontinence, apply thin layer of skin barrier containing petroleum jelly over skin. | Protects skin from excess moisture and irritants from urine or stool.

*Contd...*

*Contd...*

| | | |
|---|---|---|
| 15 | Apply underpads if required | Reduces risk of bed linen from getting soiled. |
| 16 | Remove disposable gloves and dispose in proper receptacle | Moisture and body secretions on gloves can harbor microorganisms. |
| 17 | Assist patient to comfortable position and cover him or her with top sheet. | |
| 18 | Remove bath blanket, dispose of all soiled bed linen and return unused articles to storage area. | Reduces chances of transmitting microorganisms. |
| 19 | Record procedure and presence of any abnormal finding. E.g character and amount of discharge and condition of genitalia. | Provides documented evidence and communication among health team members. |
| 20 | Report any abnormality observed to nurse in-charge and physician. | |

## 2.13: PERFORMING A BED SHAMPOO/HAIR WASH

## DEFINITION

Cleaning of hair with shampoo or soap to remove dirt, oil and odour on scalp and hair, for a helpless patient in bed.

## PURPOSES

1. To keep hair clean and healthy.
2. To promote growth of hair.
3. To prevent loss of hair.
4. To prevent itching and infection.
5. To prevent accumulation of dirt, dandruff and oil.
6. To prevent tangles.
7. To stimulate circulation.
8. To clean hair after pediculosis treatment.
9. To enhance personal appearance and self-esteem.
10. To observe the scalp.
11. To provide a sense of well being.

## CONTRAINDICATIONS

1. Head and neck injuries.
2. Spinal cord injuries.
3. Surgeries on back and neck.

## ARTICLES

*A tray containing:*
1. Bath towels – (2 Nos.)
2. Washcloth or face towel
3. Mackintosh – (2 Nos.)
4. Non-absorbent cotton balls
5. Bath blanket/sheet
6. Oil (optional)
7. Shampoo or liquid soap
8. Hair comb.
9. Kidney tray or paper bag
10. Basin
11. Bucket
12. Mug
13. Jugs – (2 Nos.)
14. Low stool
15. Clean linen
16. News paper

# PROCEDURE

| | Nursing action | Rationale |
|---|---|---|
| 1. | Check the physician's order for specific precautions if any for movement and positioning of the patient. | Patient may be at risk for injury while manipulating the head. In some hospitals a physician's order is required for bed shampoo. |
| 2. | Assess the general condition of the patient, the scalp, hair and need for shampoo. | Determines the presence of any condition that may require the use of special shampoo or treatment. |
| 3. | Check the patient's preference for soap/shampoo. | |
| 4. | Explain procedure to the patient | Relieves anxiety and helps the patient to co-operate. |
| 5. | Adjust the bed to comfortable height | Use of good body mechanics prevent injury. |
| 6. | Close windows and put off the fan | Prevents patients from going into hypothermia. |
| 7. | Pull the curtains | Provides privacy for the patient |
| 8. | Fan fold the top linen to the foot-end of the bed leaving a sheet or bath blanket over the patient. | A sheet or bath blanket prevents patient from chilling. |
| 9 | Make a trough with the mackintosh or use a kelly's pad if available. | Allows dirty water to flow into the bucket. |
| 10. | Unless contraindicated, move the patient's head to the edge of the bed, position the patient diagonally with head positioned inside trough (Figure 2.13(a)) | Prevents over stretching and allows use of good body mechanics. |

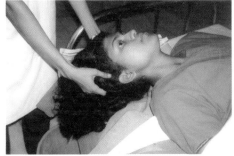

Figure 2.13(a): Positioning patient for bed shampoo

| | | |
|---|---|---|
| 11. | Place pillow under the shoulder so that the head is slightly tilted backwards | Prevents soiling of the bed. |
| 12. | Protect the pillow and bed with a mackintosh and towel | Prevents soiling of bed and pillow. |
| 13. | Place the bucket on a low stool close to the side of bed | Collects the dirty water. |
| 14. | Plug the ears with cotton balls. | Prevents shampoo entering into the ears |
| 15. | Place a wash cloth or a towel over the eyes | Prevents shampoo entering into the eyes. |
| 16. | Wash hands | Prevents spread of microorganisms. |
| 17. | Loosen and remove tangles | |
| 18. | Mix cold and hot water and test the temperature with the back of hand. | Warm water is comfortable and facilitates removal of dirt and sebum. |
| 19. | Start cleaning at hairline and working towards the back of the head symmetrically using shampoo. | Shampoo helps to remove dirt, sebum and dandruff from the scalp. |
| 20. | Rub shampoo and massage the scalp well (Figure 2.14(b)) | Rubbing and massaging of scalp adds to the comfort of the patient and effectiveness of shampoo. |

*Contd...*

*Contd...*

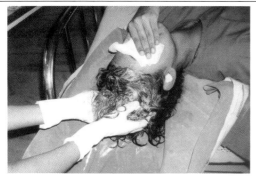

**Figure 2.13(b):** Massaging scalp using shampoo

| 21. | Rinse thoroughly with water | Removes soap and dirt. |
|-----|------------------------------|------------------------|
| 22. | Repeat washing and rinsing until hair is clean, squeeze off water from hair | Prevents chilling |
| 23. | Instruct patient to inform nurse, if any discomfort or pain occurs. | |
| 24. | Dry hair with second towel (Figure 2.13(c)) | |

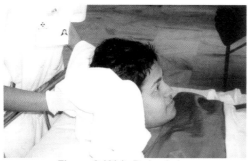

**Figure 2.13(c):** Drying hair

| 25. | Remove the trough and place it in the bucket. Discard the cotton plugs used to plug ears into the paper bag. | |
|-----|---------------------------------------------------------------------------------------------------------------|------------------------|
| 26. | Reposition the patient in proper alignment. | Enhances patient's comfort. |
| 27. | Spread the hair over mackintosh and towel placed on the pillow and allow it to dry. | Enhances patient's comfort |
| 28. | Change linen if wet | Enhances patient's comfort |
| 29. | Offer hot drink | Enhances patient's comfort |
| 30. | Take all articles to the utility room and clean them. Disinfect the towels, mackintosh, basin and bucket. Send soiled linen to laundry. Wash hands. | Reduces risk of transmission of microorganisms. |
| 31. | Return to bedside when the hair is dry. Comb and arrange the hair. Remove mackintosh and towel from the bed. Make the patient comfortable. | Improves self–esteem of patient. |
| 32. | Record the procedure and report any abnormalities if present | Ensures communication between staff members. |

## SPECIAL CONSIDERATIONS

1. Consider cultural, religious and personal preferences of patients.
2. Special precaution should be taken in positioning patient if central venous lines are present.

## 2.14: PERFORMING AN EYE CARE

### DEFINITION

Process of cleaning one/both eyes using prescribed solution for removing secretion and for preventing infection.

### PURPOSES

1. To relieve pain and discomfort
2. To prevent infection
3. To prevent any further injury to the eye
4. To provide instillation of an eyedrop or application of an eye ointment.

### ARTICLES

1. A clean tray containing:
2. Sterile eye dressing pack containing.
   a. Gallipot
   b. Cotton balls
   c. Disposable towel
   d. Sterile swabbing solution, e.g. normal saline.
   e. K-basin
   f. Sterile glove (if eye is infected)
   g. Mackintosh
   h. Pillow.

### PROCEDURE

| | Nursing action | Rationale |
|---|---|---|
| 1 | Check the physician's order, progress notes and nursing care plan | Obtains specific instruction/information. |
| 2 | Identify the patient. | |
| 3 | Explain to patient what will be done and how he may co-operate. Allow patient to ask questions. | Obtains patient's consent and co-operation and promotes patient education. |
| 4 | Ensure privacy | Avoids unnecessary embarassment. |
| 5 | Collect and prepare articles. | |
| 6 | Position the patient comfortably. Preferably in the supine position or seated with head inclined backwards. | |
| 7 | Ensure adequate light source taking care not to dazzle the patient. | Enables maximum observation of the eye without causing the patient harm or discomfort. |
| 8 | Wash and dry hands | Prevents infection. |
| 9 | Always treat the uninfected eye first. | Avoids cross infection. |
| 10 | Always bathe the lids first, with the eyes closed . | Avoids secretion on the lid from entering into eyes. |
| 11 | Lightly moisten swab in the prescribed solution. | If the swab is too wet, the solution will run down the patient's cheek. This increases the risk of cross-infection. |
| 12 | Gently swab from the inner canthus of the eye to the outer canthus using each swab only once until all discharge has been removed. | Avoids the risk of discharge entering into the lacrymal duct. |

*Contd...*

*Contd...*

| 13 | Gently dry the patient's eyelids to remove excess moisture. |
| 14 | Ensure that the patient is comfortable. |
| 15 | Replace the equipment safely. |
| 16 | Wash hands and dry. |
| 17 | Document the procedure appropriately and report any abnormal findings. |

## 2.15: USE OF COMFORT DEVICES

## DEFINITION

Comfort devices are articles which would add to the comfort of the patient when used, by relieving discomfort and helping to maintain correct posture.

## PURPOSES

1. To relieve discomfort
2. To provide and maintain correct body alignment
3. To immobilize a body part
4. To relieve pressure in parts of body
5. To prevent falls and accidents.

### Uses of common comfort devices and their clinical implications

| | Names of comfort devices | Uses | Clinical implications |
|---|---|---|---|
| 1 | **Pillows** | • It is used to support parts of the body like head and neck, arms, legs and parts of back.<br>• Relieves pain on abdominal muscles and tendons beneath the knees.<br>• Used in positioning patients | • It is used to splint incision area in abdominal and thoracic surgeries to reduce post–operative pain during activity or coughing and deep breathing.<br>• Pillows placed directly under popliteal fossa may obliterate blood supply in vessels passing through this area. |
| 2 | **Foot board**<br>A flat panel or board made of plastic or wood which is placed perpendicular to the mattress and parallel to and touching the plantar surfaces of the patient's feet | • Used to prevent plantar flexion of feet. | • The patient's feet should be placed firmly against the board. |
| 3 | **Posey foot guard**<br>Made of foam structures. | • Used to maintain the patient's feet in a dorsiflexed position and prevent food drop. | • It is used to prevent foot drop. |
| 4 | **Trochanter roll**<br>Can be made of thick cotton blankets or towels.<br>A cotton bath blanket is folded lengthwise to a width that extends from the greater trochanter of the femur to the lower border of the popliteal space. | • Used to prevent external rotation of legs when the patient is in supine position. | • The blanket is placed under the buttocks and then rolled counter clockwise until the thigh is in the neutral position or in inward rotation. |
| 5 | **Sand bags**<br>These are sand filled bags which are available in various sizes. | • Used in application of pressure in case of bleeding.<br>• Used to provide support and shape to body contours, and maintains specific body alignment | • Prevents foot drop and external rotation of thighs. |

*Contd...*

*Contd...*

| 6 | **Hand rolls**<br>Can be made by folding a wash cloth, rolling it and securing it in place with tape. | • Used to maintain thumb in slightly adducted position and in apposition to fingers.<br>• Used to maintain fingers in slightly flexed position. | • Helps in maintaining the hand, thumb and fingers in a functional position. |
|---|---|---|---|
| 7 | **Hand wrist splints**<br>These are individually moulded splints for patients to maintain proper alignment of thumb They are slightly adducted in apposition to fingers and maintains wrist in slight dorsiflexion. | • Used to maintain immobility of the fingers and maintains functional position. | • The nurse should ensure that pressure of the splints are not obliterating circulation. |
| 8 | **Trapeze bar**<br>It is a triangular device that is attached to an over bed frame | • Used to enable patient to raise trunk from bed.<br>• Used to enable patient to move from bed to wheel chair.<br>• Used to help the patient in performing exercises that strengthen upper arms. | • Ideal for patients in traction and plaster cast for assisting with changing position in bed and in carrying out nursing procedures. |
| 9 | **Bed boards**<br>Plywood boards placed under the entire mattress. | • Used for increasing back support and vertebral alignment with a soft mattress.<br>• Used in patients with spinal problems<br>• Used in giving CPR in the proper manner. | |
| 10 | **Bed cradle**<br>Vary widely in size and material | • Used to support the weight of the top bed clothing and to prevent them from coming in contact with the patient's body.<br>• Used especially for patients with burns. or when the plaster cast is yet to be dry or for patients after amputation. | • Cradles with electric bulbs provide desired warmth to burns patients. |
| 11 | **Air and water mattresses**<br>Special types of mattresses filled with water or air which moves from one part of the mattress to the other, thus reducing pressure to the same area. | • Used to prevent pressure ulcers in patients at risk. | • All nursing interventions should be carried out to prevent pressure ulcer development even if such mattresses are used. |
| 12 | **Cardiac table** | • Used for patients to lean forward especially when the patient has been in the sitting position for a long time.<br>• Used as a book support to read or write or as a table to take food in bed itself.<br>• Used in positioning patients who are to undergo some diagnostic procedures like thoracentesis. | • Generally used by patients suffering from cardiac and respiratory diseases. |

*Contd...*

*Contd...*

| 13 | **Bed blocks** | | |
|---|---|---|---|
| | Made up of wood or metal used to raise the head or foot end of the bed. | Used for providing Trendelenburg position for patients:<br>• Following spinal anesthesia<br>• For preventing shock<br>• For arresting hemorrhage<br>• For retaining fluids in retention enema. | • Do not raise foot end in case of increased intracranial pressure. |
| 14 | **Backrest** | | |
| | A mechanical device used as a suitable support and rest for the back of the patient in Fowler's position. | • Used to relieve dyspnea as in asthmatic patients by providing Fowler's or high Fowler's position.<br>• Used in positioning cardiac patient to reduce workload on heart. | |

# 2.16: ADMINISTERING A BACK MASSAGE

## DEFINITION

Scientific form of massaging the back using different massaging strokes to provide cutaneous stimulation and thus promote comfort.

## PURPOSES

1. To relieve muscle tension
2. To promote physical and mental relaxation
3. To relieve insomnia
4. To stimulate blood circulation
5. To assess condition of skin.

## CONTRAINDICATIONS

Patients with
a. Rib fracture
b. Burns
c. Immediate postoperative period after coronary artery bypass graft
d. Patient's at risk for developing pressure ulcer
e. Spinal injuries
f. Surgeries on back.

## ARTICLES

1. Lotion or oil
2. Bath towel
3. Bath blanket
4. Soap
5. Washcloth
6. Warm water in basin
7. Mackintosh and draw sheet
   If patient requires hygienic care, it should be provided, followed by massage

## PROCEDURE

| | Nursing action | Rationale |
|---|---|---|
| 1. | Explain procedure and desired position to patient. Determine if patient is comfortable with massage strokes | Helps in promoting relaxation |
| 2. | Adjust bed to comfortable height | Ensures proper body mechanics and prevents strain on back muscles. |
| 3. | Adjust light, temperature and sound within room. | Environmental distractions can prevent patient from relaxing |
| 4. | Close curtains around bed. Lower side rail and help patient assume prone or side – lying (sims) position with back towards you. | Privacy promotes relaxation. Position makes it easier to apply necessary pressure to back muscles. |
| 5. | Expose patient's back, shoulders, upper arms and buttocks. Cover remainder of body with bath blanket/top sheet | Prevents unnecessary exposure of body parts and prevents excess lotion from touching linen |

*Contd...*

*Contd...*

| | | |
|---|---|---|
| 6. | Wash your hands in warm water. | Cold water causes muscle tension |
| 7. | Inform patient that lotion will feel cool and wet | Warning patient of what to expect reduces startle response |
| 8. | Apply hands first sacral area massaging in circular motion. Stroke upward from buttocks to shoulders. Massage over scapulae with smooth, firm strokes. Continue in one smooth stroke from upper back to arm and laterally alongside of back, down to iliac crests (Figure 2.16(a)). Do not take the hands off from patient's back till the end of the procedure. Continue massage pattern for at least 3 minutes (effleurage) (Figure 2.16(b)) | Gentle, firm pressure applied to all muscle groups promotes relaxation. Continuous contact with skin surface is soothing and stimulates circulation to tissues. |

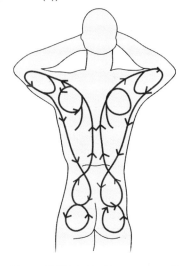

Figure 2.16(a): Back massage pattern

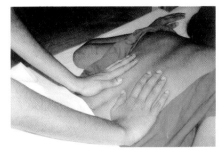

Figure 2.16(b): Effleurage

| | | |
|---|---|---|
| 9. | Knead skin by gently grasping tissue between your thumb and fingers, knead upward along one side of spine from buttocks to shoulders and around nape of the neck, knead downwards towards sacrum, repeat along other side of back (petrissage) (Figure 2.16(c)) | Kneading increases circulation. Kneading motion is soothing and relieving |

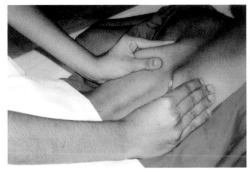

Figure 2.16(c): Petrissage

| | | |
|---|---|---|
| 10. | Perform tapotement (tapping movement with medial aspects of hands on side of spine from sacral region upwards) for 2 minutes (Figure 2.16(d)) | Provides relaxation to back muscle. |

*Contd...*

*Contd...*

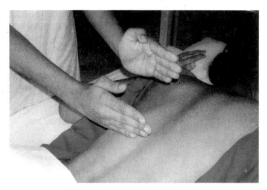

**Figure 2.16(d):** Tapotement

| | | |
|---|---|---|
| 11. | End massage with long, stroking movement for an additional 3 minutes and tell patient you are ending massage. | Long stroking is most soothing |
| 12. | If lying on side, ask patient to turn to opposite side and massage other hip | |
| 13. | Apply oil or lubricant to back as required | Helps to reduce friction |
| 14. | Wipe excess lubricant from patients back with bath towel/tissues. Re-tie gown or assist with pajamas. Help patient to comfortable position. Raise side rails as needed, open curtain and lower bed. | Excess lotion can act as an irritant and soil sheets. Comfortable position enhances back rub's effects. |
| 15. | Dispose off soiled towel and wash hands | Promotes infection control |
| 16. | Record response to massage and condition of skin. | |

## SPECIAL CONSIDERATIONS

- For patients with history of hypertension and dysrhythmias assess pulse and blood pressure as massage may cause stimulation of autonomic nervous system, which increases heart rate, and BP
- Consider cultural preferences of patient. Some cultures may consider it as an invasion of personal space
- Do not give massage if any discoloration of skin is present.

## 2.17: ADMINISTERING A SITZ BATH

### DEFINITION

A procedure whereby patient's perineal area/buttocks are submerged in warm water.

### PURPOSES

1. To aid the healing process of perineal wounds
2. To reduce pain and discomfort
3. To reduce swelling and irritation
4. To increase circulation
5. To promote relaxation.

### INDICATIONS

1. Following surgery in the ano-rectal region
2. Following incision in the perineum, e. g. episiotomy
3. Swollen painful hemorrhoids.

### CONTRAINDICATIONS

1. Diabetes, peripheral vascular diseases
2. Impaired, peripheral sensory function
3. Immediate post hemorrhoidectomy.

### ARTICLES

1. Sitz bath basin
2. Warm water (temp 105-110 degree F./40-43 degree centigrade)
3. Medication if ordered
4. Bath thermometer
5. Clean gloves (optional)
6. Towel
7. Robe or sheet.

### PROCEDURE

| | Nursing action | Rationale |
|---|---|---|
| 1. | Check the physician's order and nursing care plan. | |
| 2. | Identify the patient | |
| 3. | Assess the patient's condition, pain level and ability to ambulate to the bathroom | Patients who have taken pain medication may experience lightheadedness or drowsiness impairing their ability to ambulate and tolerate the procedure. |
| 4. | Wash hands | Reduces transmission of microorganisms. |
| 5. | Add required quantity of ordered medication. E g: betadine into the Sitz bath basin | |
| 6. | Fill the basin with warm water at a temperature of 105 to 110 degree F (40 – 43 degree C) | Warm water is soothing and results in vasodilatation to enhance healing |
| 7. | Keep the basin on a low stool/potty chair/ toilet bowl with toilet seat up. | |

*Contd...*

*Contd...*

| | | |
|---|---|---|
| 8. | Assist patient with removal of any dressing or peripad and position and assist to sit in sitz bath basin (Figure 2.17(a)) | For postpartum patients peripad must be removed from front to back to prevent contamination |

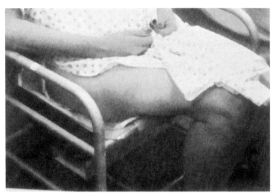

Figure 2.17(a): Positioning patient in sitz bath basin

| | | |
|---|---|---|
| 9. | Place a towel on the patient's thigh and cover the shoulders with a sheet | Promotes warmth and prevents chills. |
| 10. | Do not leave the patient unattended during the procedure. Instruct patient to contract and relax anal sphincter while taking sitz bath. | |
| 11. | Allow patient to sit for 20 minutes, then assist with drying and applying dressing or peripad as required | Beneficial effects of heat are lost after 20 minutes due to vasoconstriction |
| 12. | Discontinue the procedure if any adverse effects like dizziness, weakness, accelerated pulse rate or pallor occurs. | |
| 13. | Assist patient back to bed, and instruct to stay in bed for 20 minutes with hip elevated | Use of warm water and prolonged sitting in one position may result in light headedness on arising. |
| 14. | Clean and replace all the reusable articles. If the basin is to be autoclaved, arrange for it. | |
| 15. | Wash hands | |
| 16. | Document tolerance of procedure, pain and appearances of the perineal area/wound area. | Decreased swelling, redness and drainage and complete healing are the goals. |

## SPECIAL CONSIDERATION

If the patient has received epidural anesthesia, be sure that complete sensation has returned before using a warm sitz bath.

## 2.18: APPLICATION OF HOT WATER BAG

### DEFINITION

Local application of dry heat to a specific body part for a short duration using a rubber bag.

### PURPOSES

1.  To stimulate circulation by dilating blood vessels
2.  To relieve pain and congestion by encouraging flow of blood
3.  To supply warmth and comfort
4.  To promote healing
5.  To relieve retention of urine
6.  To relieve muscle spasm
7.  To reduce tissue swelling
8.  To counteract sudden drop in temperature during cold sponging
9.  To raise body temperature in case of hypothermia

### ARTICLES

1.  Hot water bag with cover
2.  Boiling water
3.  Mug – to pour water into the bag
4.  Duster
5.  Towel
6.  Bath thermomete.
7.  Vaseline or oil in a bottle – to apply if redness develops
8.  Kidney tray

### CONTRAINDICATIONS

1.  Acute inflammation, e g: acute appendicitis, tooth abscess
2.  Very young or very old patien.
3.  Patients who are unconscious or insane
4.  Patients with sensory–neural deficits, e.g. diabetes mellitus, peripheral neuropathy
5.  Patients with high temperature
6.  Open wounds
7.  Malignancy
8.  Blisters/burns

### PROCEDURE

|  | Nursing action | Rationale |
|---|---|---|
| 1. | Identify the patient and check the patient's chart for any special instructions and nursing care plan | |
| 2. | Provide explanation to the patient regarding the procedure and the care to be taken | Knowledge about the care during bag application will help prevent accidental burn injury. |
| 3. | Assess for presence of lotion or oil over skin surface at the site of application | Heat can be retained with the presence of these products and lead to increased risk of heat intolerance and burns. |

*Contd...*

*Contd...*

| | | |
|---|---|---|
| 4 | Wash hands | Prevents chances of cross infection. |
| 5. | Fill the hot water bag with hot water, secure the cap and turn it up side down | Ensures that there are no leaks and pre-warms the bag |
| 6. | Empty the bag and refill with hot water (temp, 105–115°F) to about two – third full. | Filling to 2/3rd level ensures comfort when applied |
| 7. | Place the bag on a flat surface such as a table and expel all air by forcing the water up to the neck of the bag (Figure 2.18(a)) | When air is removed the bag is easier to mold over the body part. |

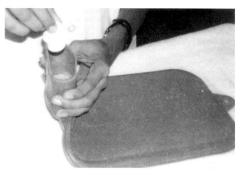

Figure 2.18(a): Expelling air from hot water bag

| | | |
|---|---|---|
| 8. | Screw the cap tightly, dry outside of the bag using duster and check it for leakage. | Prevents chances of scalding |
| 9. | Wipe off any moisture on the outside of the bag. | Moisture on the outside of bag increases risk of burns |
| 10. | Put on the cover and take to the bedside. If cover is not available, use a pillow case or towel (Figure 2.18(b)). | Use of bag directly over the skin can cause burns. Thick covers can reduce effect of hot application |

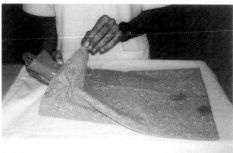

Figure 2.18(b): Placing hot water bag inside cover

| | |
|---|---|
| 11. | Apply to the area as ordered (Figure 2.18(c)) |

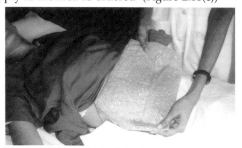

Figure 2.18(c): Applying hot water bag

*Contd...*

# Client Care: Hygiene and Comfort

*Contd...*

| | | |
|---|---|---|
| 12. | Remove the bag after 20 to 30 minutes | Keeping the bag for 20 to 30 minutes avoids chances of burn injury. |
| 13. | Check the site for redness, blisters, etc. If present apply Vaseline/oil | Vaseline/oil soothes the skin |
| 14. | Make patient comfortable in bed | |
| 15. | Record in the patient's chart the time, site, duration of application and effects observed. | |
| 16. | Take all articles to the utility room. Empty the hot water bag, wash outside of the bag with soap and water and hang upside down to dry it. | |

## SPECIAL CONSIDERATIONS

1. Do not leave the patient unattended with hot water bag applied/in place.
2. Never place an extremity on top of hot water bag as it can cause burn injury.

# 2.19: APPLICATION OF AN ICE CAP

## DEFINITION

Application of a rubber bag filled with small pieces of ice and salt to a specific body part.

## PURPOSES

1. To relieve pain of muscle strain.
2. To relieve congestion/edema.
3. To relieve urinary retention
4. To reduce temperature (101 to 102 degree Fahrenheit).

## ARTICLES

1. Ice cap with cover
2. Ice in a bowl (ice chips if available)
3. Water in a bowl
4. Ice pick (if ice need to be broken)
5. Salt
6. Table spoon
7. Duster to wipe ice cap after filling
8. Towel and mackintosh
9. Kidney tray.

## CONTRAINDICATIONS

1. Hypothermia
2. Muscle spasm
3. Peripheral neuropathy.

## PROCEDURE

| | Nursing action | Rationale |
|---|---|---|
| 1. | Identify patient and check the physician's order and nursing care plan | Ensures that right procedure is done on right patient. |
| 2. | Provide explanation to patient | Promotes patient's co-operation and participation |
| 3. | Fill ice cap with tepid water and tilt the ice cap | Checks for presence of leakage |
| 4. | Crack the ice to pieces of required size, if not obtained as small chips | Facilitates filling of the ice cap |
| 5. | Add salt to ice chips | Salt prevents the ice from melting faster |
| 6. | Fill ice cap half-full with ice chips and expel air (Figure 2.19(a)) | Air inside ice cap will make it uncomfortable for patient when applied. |

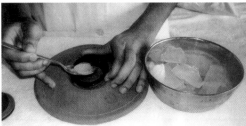

**Figure 2.19(a):** Filling an ice cap

*Contd...*

*Contd...*

| | | |
|---|---|---|
| 7. | Screw on cap tightly and put cover over ice cap | Spilling of water can be prevented by tight screwing of the cap |
| 8. | Apply ice cap to the area for about 30 minutes | Application beyond this time causes secondary effects |
| 9. | Check tolerance of patient periodically Observe for presence of cyanosis/mottling. | Identifies complications at an early stage. |
| 10. | Clean and replace the articles used | |
| 11. | Wash hands | |
| 12. | Record the procedure in the Nurse's Notes including time of application and observation | |

## SPECIAL CONSIDERATION

- Controls localized hematoma or hemorrhage, such as following thyroid surgery, tonsillectomy and dental surgery.
- For application on neck, bags of different shape such as ice collars are used.

## 2.20: APPLICATION OF COLD COMPRESS

## DEFINITION

Application of cloth pieces or gauze wet in cold water to a specific body part.

## PURPOSES

1. To reduce inflammation and edema resulting from strains, contusions, insect bites, etc.
2. To control bleeding and pain in conditions as in sprain, epistaxis and black eye.
3. To reduce body temperature in fever.
4. To inhibit bacterial growth and thus prevent suppuration.

## ARTICLES

A tray containing:
1. Bowl with cold water. (15 degree Centigrade/59 degree Fahrenheit)
2. Folded lint or gauze. – 2 Nos.
3. Small mackintosh and towel.
4. A small bowl with non-absorbent cotton balls (for plugging ears if applying to forehead).
5. Kidney tray.

## PROCEDURE

| | Nursing action | Rationale |
|---|---|---|
| 1. | Identify the patient | Obtains specific instructions and information. |
| 2. | Check the physician's order and care plan | Ensures that right procedure is performed on the right patient. |
| 3. | Explain procedure to patient | Improves understanding of patient regarding procedure and enhances patient co-operation. |
| 4. | Ensure privacy | Avoids embarrassment during the procedure. |
| 5. | Wash and dry hands | Prevents cross contamination. |
| 6. | Expose the area and place mackintosh and towel under the area to be treated | Prevents soiling of bed linen |
| 7. | Plug ears with cotton plugs (if compress is applied to forehead/eyes) | |
| 8. | Soak 3 – 4 gauze/lint in cold water, squeeze gently and apply to the area | When cold is applied to the skin or a part of the body, vasoconstriction of the superficial blood vessels occurs. |
| 9. | After 2-3 minutes remove the compress and apply fresh one | |
| 10. | Squeeze the used compress into K. basin and immerse into bowl of cold water | |
| 11. | Observe skin area every five minutes for any adverse reaction like burning, numbness, bluish discoloration, mottling of skin, erythema or extreme pallor. | Tissue damage can occur from prolonged vasoconstriction |
| 12. | Discontinue procedure if adverse reactions are seen | |

*Contd...*

*Contd...*

| | |
|---|---|
| 13. Continue the procedure for specified length of time that is until desired result is obtained /15 to 20 minutes, and repeat every 2 –3 hours | |
| 14. Remove compresses, dry the area and make the patient comfortable. | |
| 15. Clean and replace articles in its proper place as appropriate | |
| 16. Wash and dry hands | |
| 17. Document the procedure in the nurse's notes. Include time, area to which compress was applied, duration, patient's tolerance and any other pertinent observation.<br>Example: If applied for reducing fever, record the temperature. | Documentation promotes communication among staff. |

## 2.21: GIVING A TEPID SPONGE

### DEFINITION

Sponging of body with tepid (tap) water for reducing body temperature.

### PURPOSE

To reduce body temperature when fever in itself may be deleterious, e.g. temperature between 102 to 103 degree Fahrenheit.

### ARTICLES

1. Bath basin
2. Tepid water (temp 98.6 degree F or 37 degree Celisius) in bucket
3. Bath thermometer
4. Wash cloths – 6
5. Long mackintosh/waterproof pad to protect the bed
6. Bath blanket
7. Thermometer tray
8. Bath towels – 2
9. Linen, e g: bedsheet and gown
10. Articles for cold compress and ice cap.

### PROCEDURE

| | Nursing action | Rationale |
|---|---|---|
| 1. | Assess patient's body temperature and pulse rate. | Provides baseline for evaluating response to therapy. Sudden temperature changes may alter pulse |
| 2. | Explain to patient that the purpose of sponging with tepid water is to cool the body slowly. Briefly describe steps of procedure | Procedure can be uncomfortable because of cold applications. Anxiety over procedure can increase body temperature |
| 3. | Close room door or curtain | Ensures privacy |
| 4. | Wash and dry hands | |
| 5. | Place mackintosh under patient and remove gown | Mackintosh prevents soiling of bed linen. Removing gown provides access to all surfaces. |
| 6. | Keep the bath blanket over body parts not being sponged. Close the windows and door, and put off fan. | Prevents drafts |
| 7. | Check water temperature | Prevents chilling |
| 8. | Immerse wash cloths in water and apply wet clothes in each axilla and over groin | Axilla and groin contain large superficial blood vessels. Application of wet wash cloths promote reduction of temperature by conduction |
| 9. | Cover one extremity with a wet towel | |
| 10. | Wet a wash cloth and wipe down towards fingers/toes from outer aspect of each extremity and move up from the inner aspect | |
| 11. | Follow a clockwise sequence for wiping the extremities, each in turn for 5 minutes and then the back and the abdomen | |

*Contd...*

## Client Care: Hygiene and Comfort

*Contd...*

| | |
|---|---|
| 12. Reassess temperature and pulse every 15 minutes | Prevents sudden temperature fall |
| 13. Change water and reapply sponges to axilla and groin as needed | Water temperature rises as a result of exposure to patient's warm body surface |
| 14. When the body temperature falls to slightly above normal, discontinue procedure | Prevents temperature drift to subnormal level |
| 15. Dry extremities and body parts thoroughly | Prevents chilling |
| 16. Dress patient and cover with sheet. | Promotes patient comfort. Excessively heavy covering increases body temperature |
| 17. Measure patient's body temperature and pulse rate. | Temperature indicates response to therapy. |
| 18. Record time when procedure was started and terminated, vital sign changes and patient's response | Recording communicates care provided in accurate and timely fashion |

## 2.22: GIVING A COLD SPONGE

### DEFINITION

Moist cold application using ice water when patient's temperature is dangerously raised to more than 103 degree Fahrenheit.

### PURPOSE

To reduce body temperature.

### CONTRAINDICATION

Patient with rigors.

### ARTICLES

Tray containing
1. Sponge towels – 6 nos.
2. Bath towels - 2 nos.
3. Basin for bath water
4. Long mackintosh
5. Thermometer tray
6. Linen
7. Hot water bag
8. Bath thermometer
9. Ice chips in a container
10. Clean disposable gloves.

### PROCEDURE

| | Nursing action | Rationale |
|---|---|---|
| 1. | Assess body temperature | Identifies if procedure is required for the patient. |
| 2. | Obtain doctor's written order since procedure involves hot water bag application to counteract secondary effects | Ensures right procedure is done on right patient. |
| 3. | Explain to patient what will be done, the expected result and how he may participate. | Reduces patient's anxiety and promotes co-operation during procedure. |
| 4. | Add ice cubes to basin of water till temperature of water reaches 65 degree Fahrenheit. | Adding ice cubes brings down water temperature to meet requirements. |
| 5. | Provide privacy and spread mackintosh under the patient | Prevents soiling of the bed |
| 6. | Remove dress and cover patient with top sheet | Avoids exposing the patient |
| 7. | Place a bath towel over chest and another over pubic region | Provides privacy |
| 8. | Apply hot water bag at soles of feet | Avoids sudden cooling of the body |
| 9. | Don gloves | |
| 10. | Wet five sponge towels in the basin | |
| 11. | Take a wet sponge towel, dab face and replace at edge of basin | |
| 12. | Take the second sponge towel, wipe distal arm, start from acromion process, proceeding laterally to fingers and reach axilla. Place towel in axilla | Helps in reducing the temperature |

*Contd...*

# Client Care: Hygiene and Comfort

*Contd...*

| | | |
|---|---|---|
| 13. | Repeat same for proximal arm | |
| 14. | Wipe abdomen and back with first sponge towel which was left at edge of basin | |
| 15. | For legs, start from thigh proceed laterally to feet and medially to groin. Keep sponge in groin, wipe face and neck again | |
| 16. | Take sponge from distal axilla, squeeze into bucket and continue procedure as before | |
| 17. | Check patient's temperature every 15 minutes | Gives information about decline of temperature |
| 18. | Stop procedure when temperature reaches 100 degree F. | Prevents secondary effects on the body |
| 19. | Check pulse and observe skin colour | Know about adverse reactions |
| 20. | Continue procedure for maximum of 20 to 30 minutes and then stop, irrespective of reaction or result | |
| 21. | Check temeperature after 15 minutes, half hour and one hour of treatment | Continuous monitoring of vital signs gives information on the patient's response to the procedure |
| 22. | Remove sponge towels, dry patient, cover with top sheet and remove towels | |
| 23. | Replace wet linen, dress and position patient | Makes patient feel comfortable |
| 24. | Clean and replace articles | |
| 25. | If temperature remains same, institute other measures to bring down temperature | |
| 26. | Record time and period of procedure, effect on patient, vital signs at 15 minutes, 30 minutes and one hour after procedure is completed | Continuous monitoring of vital signs gives the patient's response to the procedure and information for further steps to be followed |

# 2.23: CARE OF BODY AFTER DEATH

## DEFINITION

Care of body in 30 to 45 minutes following declaration of death by physician.

## PURPOSES

1. To maintain normal body alignment before rigor mortis sets in.
2. To reduce mental distress of family
3. To facilitate transportation to mortuary/residence.

## ARTICLES

1. Tray lined with towel.
2. Long artery clamp.
3. Bandage.
4. Absorbent and non-absorbent cotton.
5. Hospital gown or patient's clothes.
6. Mackintosh
7. Mortuary cards in transparent plastic cover.
8. Valuables envelope
9. Shroud/body bag/sheet.
10. Clean disposable gloves
11. Articles for cleaning or bathing the body.

## PROCEDURE

| | Nursing action | Rationale |
|---|---|---|
| 1. | Assess for presence of family or significant others and whether they have been informed of the patient's death. Ask if they wish to view the body, observe their response and offer them the opportunity to ask questions | It is the physician's responsibility to notify the family of patient's death. Nurses provide emotional support and prepare body for viewing. |
| 2. | Assess patients religious preference or cultural heritage. Determine if family wishes to have a minister or priest at the bedside | Specific religions dictate ceremonies at time of death |
| 3. | Determine if patient was on isolation precautions for an infectious disease | Precautions must be taken to prevent spread of infection to others |
| 4. | Wash hands | Reduces transmission of microorganisms |
| 5. | Don disposable gloves and gown or protective devices as applicable | Body secretions may harbor infectious micro-organisms |
| 6. | Close room door or draw bedside curtains | Provides privacy for the deceased and family |
| 7. | Identify the body according to agency policy | Ensures proper name use in labelling |
| 8. | Position body supine with arms at side, palms down or arms across the abdomen. Do not place hands one on top of the other because bottom hand will become discolored. | Body appears in natural position |
| 9. | Place small pillow or folded towel under the head or elevate head of bed 10 to 15 degree. | Prevents pooling of blood in the face and subsequent discoloration |

*Contd...*

# Client Care: Hygiene and Comfort

*Contd...*

| 10. | Gently place fingers over the closed eyelids for a few seconds | Holds eyelids in place to create a natural appearance |
|---|---|---|
| 11. | Insert dentures into mouth (if applicable). If mouth fails to close, place a rolled towel under the chin | It is difficult to insert dentures after rigor mortis occurs. Dentures maintain normal facial expression |
| 12. | Remove all bottles, bags or receptacles from urinary catheters, nasogastric tubes, I.V lines or drainage tubes | In case when autopsy is needed these need to be preserved. |
| 13. | For tubes remaining in the body, either remove clamp or cut within one inch of the skin and tape in place | Hospital policy dictates tube care. Specific guidelines apply if an autopsy is to be performed |
| 14. | Remove soiled dressing and replace with clean gauze dressings | Controls odour caused by microorganisms |
| 15. | Wash body parts soiled with blood, urine, faeces or other drainage and put clean gown on | Prepares body for viewing and reduces odours |
| 16. | Apply jaw bandage (four tailed bandage) | Keeps the mouth closed |
| 17 | Plug body orifices such as nose, mouth, vagina and rectum with absorbent cotton followed by nonabsorbent cotton (ears to be plugged only if there is cerebrospinal fluid leakage). Nose to be packed in such a way that cotton is not visible. | Release of sphincter muscles after death may cause release of urine faeces and body fluids. |
| 18. | Close eyes by keeping wet cotton balls on eyelids | Eyelids remain closed with wet cotton on them |
| 19. | Fold hands as in praying position and tie thumbs together | |
| 20. | Straighten legs, bring feet together and tie big toes | |
| 21. | Complete mortuary card and place in plastic cover and tie to the big toes | Use ball point pen to avoid ink from spreading |
| 22. | Place an absorbent pad under the patients buttocks | Relaxation of sphincter muscles after death may cause release of urine or faeces. |
| 23. | Brush and comb patient's hair. Remove any clips hairpins or rubber bands. | During viewing the patient should appear well groomed. Objects such as pins can damage or discolor the face and scalp |
| 24. | Remove all jewellery. Exception: family may request wedding band be left in place. Place a small strip of tape around finger over the ring. | Prevents loss of valuables |
| 25. | Account for all valuables remaining in the patient's room and label each item. Prepare a 'valuables list' to inventory all items. Return valuables to immediate family members when they arrive or store in locked container/cupboard. | Nurse is responsible for safe keeping of personal valuables, such as jewellery, wallet, eye glasses or religious medals |
| 26. | Place patient's clothing and shoes in a labelled bag and return to family members | Keeps items safely secured |
| 27 | Complete identification tags and attach one to the patient's ankle. The remaining tag should be saved in order to attach to the outside of the sheet/shroud after the body is covered. (step 31) | |
| 28. | If the family requests viewing, place a sheet or light blanket over the body with only the head and upper shoulders exposed. Provide soft lighting and offer chairs to the family | Maintains dignity and respect for the patient and family and prevents exposure of body parts |
| 29. | After the family has left, remove all linen and the patient's gown, then place body in body bag or apply the shroud. Be sure that the shroud completely encircles all body parts. | Prevents injury to skin and extremities, avoids unnecessary exposure of body parts. |

*Contd...*

*Contd...*

| 30. | Secure shroud with tape wrapped over the shoulders, waist and legs | Keeps shroud secure, protects body during transfer |
|---|---|---|
| 31. | Attach second completed label to outside of the body bag or shroud | Ensures proper identification of the body |
| 32. | If patient had a transmissible infection, special labelling may be used | Protects health care workers who transport and store the body |
| 33. | Arrange for transportation of the body to the morgue or mortuary | The body should be cooled in the morgue to prevent further tissue damage |
| 34. | Carefully transfer the body to a stretcher keeping the body aligned. Cover with a clean sheet | Prevents damage to body tissues. A false bottom stretcher makes it appear there is no body lying on stretcher |
| 35. | Close other patient's room doors and arrange to transport the body | Appearance of a body can be emotionally upsetting to other patients |
| 36. | Remove remaining items and linen from the patient's room, wash hands | Prevents transfer of micro-organisms |
| 37. | Record date and time of death, time physician was notified, name of physician announcing death, disposition of valuables and belongings, care delivered to family, consent form signed by family, disposition of the body and information provided to family members | Ensures that patient's death is recorded accurately and legally. |
| 38. | Document any marks, bruises or wounds on body before death or those observed during care of the body | Reduces risk of liability for creating such marks in the care of the body after death or in transport to the morgue. Certain markings can identify the body if identification tags are lost or destroyed |
| 39. | Document any infectious process that the patient had when death occurred and document procedure used to identify the risk on body bag | Reduces liability for inadvertent contamination by persons handling the body after transfer from the division or agency |

## RELEASING BODY

1. Check all documents such as:
   - Copies of death certificate
   - Autopsy permit if needed
   - Entries in mortuary register
   - Authorization paper to take body to destination.
2. Hand over body to relatives after the bill has been settled and the body dressed in own clothes.
3. Assist for transporting body into conveyance from mortuary.
4. Replace articles brought back from mortuary after adequate disinfection
5. Document in nurse's record, the date and time of release of the body.

# Chapter 3

# Safety, Body Mechanics and Infection

# 3.1: PRACTICING PRINCIPLES OF BODY MECHANICS

## DEFINITION

Body mechanics is the efficient use of the body as a machine and as a means of locomotion.

## ADVANTAGES/BENEFITS

1. Maintains good body alignment
2. Maintains balance of the body
3. Prevents fatigue and deformities (kyphosis, lordosis, scoliosis)
4. Promotes physiological functions of the body
5. Reduces expenditure of energy
6. Prevents and reduces the risk of musculoskeletal injury.

## PROCEDURE

| | Principle | Rationale | Example |
|---|---|---|---|
| 1 | When planning a transfer or move, free the surrounding area of obstacles. | Appropriate preparation prevents potential falls and injury and safeguards the patient and equipment | Make sure that path is cleared of obstacles whenever planning a transfer or move. |
| 2 | The heavier an object, the greater the force needed to move the object | Using mechanical devices or assistance to move objects reduces muscular effort and prevents injury. | Use cot keys when lowering or elevating up the bed of the patient while lifting or moving. Encourage patients to assist as much as possible by pushing or pulling themselves to reduce the nurse's effort. |
| 3 | Objects that are close to the center of gravity are moved with the least effort | Bringing the center of gravity of the object close to the center of gravity of the person, prevents unnecessary strain on muscles | Adjust the working area to waist level, e.g. lowering side rails while making bed or shifting the patient from bed to wheel chair, prevents stretching, reaching and injury to the lower back. Holding objects close to body when moving or lifting them. |
| 4 | Reduced friction between the object moved and the surface on which it is moved requires less energy | | Provide firm, or smooth surfaces to move an object, e.g. using a pull sheet to move patient in bed. |
| 5 | Effective use of major muscles while carrying heavy objects minimises strain on abdomen and back. | | While carrying the heavy objects, moving the feet towards the direction instead of moving upper body minimizes muscle strain on abdomen and back and avoids twisting. Facing the direction of the movement avoids twisting and helps to maintain body balance |

*Contd...*

*Contd...*

| | | | |
|---|---|---|---|
| 6 | Balance is maintained and muscle strain is avoided as long as the line of gravity passes through the base of support | | Arrange the articles near to the patient's bed before starting the procedure, prevents reaching, stretching and unnecessary wasting of time and energy . Standing as close as possible to the object avoids stretching, reaching and twisting which may place the line of gravity outside the base of support |
| 7 | The wider the base of support and lower the center of gravity the greater the stability. | | Widening your stance by keeping the feet apart, maintains body balance while performing activities like lifting transferring etc. |
| 8 | Using the longest and strongest muscles of the extremities for moving an object requires less energy and reduces the musculo-skeletal injury and strain | | Use your gluteal and leg muscles rather than muscles of your back when lifting heavy objects. |
| 9 | The greater the preparatory con-traction of the muscles before moving an object the lesser will be the energy required to move it and lesser the likeli-hood of strain and injury. | | Before performing a task contract your gluteal, abdominal, leg and arm muscles to prepare them for action. |
| 10 | Moving an object along a level surface requires less energy than lifting it or pushing it up on an incline. | | Push, pull, roll or turn objects instead of lifting them. Lower the head of the bed before moving the patient up in bed. |
| 11 | Balance is maintained with minimal effort when the base of support is enlarged in the direction in which the movement will occur | | When pulling an object, moving the rear leg backward or when pushing the patient in wheel chair, moving the front foot forward |
| 12 | Body weight of the person counteracts the weight of the object and reduces strain to the back. | Reduces the amount of strain on the arms and back | Using the weight of the body as a force for pulling or pushing by rocking the feet or leaning forward or backward. |
| 13 | Continuous muscle exertion can result in muscle strain, injury and fatigue | | Taking rest between activities. Alternate rest periods, prevents fatigue, back injury, strain etc. |

## FACTORS AFFECTING BODY ALIGNMENT AND ACTIVITY

- Growth and development
- Physical health
- Mental health
- Nutrition
- Personal values and attitudes
- External factors
- Prescribed limitations.

# 3.2: MOVING A PATIENT UP IN BED

## DEFINITION

Assisting a patient who has slid down in bed to move up.

## PURPOSES

1. To promote comfort.
2. To maintain proper alignment of the body.

## PROCEDURE

| | Nursing action | Rationale |
|---|---|---|
| 1. | Adjust the bed and the patient's position.<br>Position patient in supine<br>  a. Lower the head of the bed to a flat position or as low as the patient can tolerate<br><br>  b. Raise the bed to the height of your center of gravity<br><br>  c. Lock the wheels of the bed and raise the side rails on the side opposite to you<br>  d. Remove all pillows and place one against head of the bed | <br><br>Moving the patient upward against gravity requires more energy expenditure<br>Ensures good body mechanics and prevents strain on nurse's back<br>Prevents falls and accidents<br><br>Protects from accidental injury by hitting against head end of bed when moving up. |
| 2 | Assess the mobility status and strength of patient. | Assesses the patient's ability to co-operate and participate in the procedure |
| 3. | Explain procedure to patient, the purpose of the procedure and how he can co-operate. | Reduces anxiety and ensures patient co-operation. |
| 4. | Instruct patient on how he can help during the procedure<br>  a. Ask patient to flex hip and knees and position feet flat on the bed. So that they can be used effectively for moving the body up in bed.<br>  b. If patient can pull up holding a trapeze or holding the head of the bed that should be encouraged | Patient participation can lessen nurse's workload<br>Flexing hips and knees keeps entire leg off bed surface, thereby reducing friction<br><br>Utilizing a trapeze when moving patient reduces effort on the part of the nurse |
| 5. | Position 2-3 nurses depending on patient's ability to assist in the lifting and moving efforts<br>  a. Two Nurses: One nurse is positioned at the level of patient's upper body with arm closest to the head of bed, under the neck supporting head and shoulder on the opposite side. The other arm of the nurse is under the trunk of the patient. The second nurse is positioned against the lower part of patient's body with one arm under the waist of the patient and the other arm under the thighs just below the buttocks (Figure 3.2(a)) | Ensures adequate and equal distribution of weight between the two nurses. |

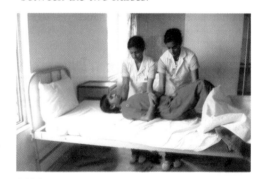

**Figure 3.2(a):** Positioning 2 nurses for moving a patient up in bed

*Contd...*

*Contd...*

| | | |
|---|---|---|
| | b. Three Nurses: If a third nurse is present, she is positioned at the lower extremities, one arm supporting under the thighs and second arm supporting under the legs. (three nurses are needed if patient is unable to help himself) | |
| 6. | Flex at the knees. Support patient's weight on forearms with forearms resting on bed | Supporting weight on forearms bring object closer to your center of gravity reducing the effort required. |
| 7. | Stand with feet apart.The foot near the head of bed, behind the other foot (forward, backward stance) | Standing with feet apart increases stability |
| 8. | Instruct patient to push with heels and elevate trunk if possible, thus moving towards head end of bed, to the count of three | Patient's assistance will help in reducing friction |
| 9. | On count of three shift your weight from front foot to back foot and at the same time shifting patient to the top of bed. Tighten your gluteal, abdominal, leg and arm muscles as you do it. | Shifting your weight counteracts patient's weight and helps in reducing force needed to move the load. Using the gluteal, leg and arm muscles reduces strain on the back. |
| 10 | Realign and position patient as required | Prevents injury to musculoskeletal system |
| 11 | Wash hands | Reduces risk of transmission of microorganisms. |
| 12 | Lower bed | Reduces risk of falls. |
| 13. | Position patient comfortably. | |

## VARIATION : WITH TWO NURSES AND A TURN SHEET

| Nursing action | Rationale |
|---|---|
| Follow steps (1 to 4) | |
| 5. a. Place a draw sheet/Pull sheet folded in half under patient extending from shoulder to thighs. | A draw sheet distributes weight more evenly |
| b. Fan fold the sheet close to the body of patient with two nurses standing on either side of patient | Draws the weight closer to the nurses center of gravity. |
| c. Grasp the sheet at shoulder and buttocks (Figure 3.2(b)) | Increases nurse's balance and stability permitting a smooth movement. |

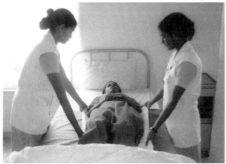

**Figure 3.2(b):** Grasping turn sheet for moving a patient up in bed

| | |
|---|---|
| 6 | Continue with step (7) of above procedure |

# 3.3: TURNING A PATIENT TO LATERAL AND PRONE POSITION

## DEFINITION

Changing position from supine to lateral/prone for repositioning or for doing procedures.

## PURPOSES

1. To ensure comfort of patient.
2. To perform procedures such as changing linen and giving bedpan.
3. To offer relief on pressure points in supine position.

## PROCEDURE

| | Nursing action | Rationale |
|---|---|---|
| 1. | Explain to patient what will be done and how it would help. | Knowledge of what to expect would reduce anxiety. |
| 2. | Position yourself and the patient appropriately, before the procedure | |
| | a. Move the patient to the side of bed opposite the side the patient will face when turned using pull sheet/by shifting gently with help of one or two nurses | This ensures that the patient will be positioned safely in the center of bed when turned. |
| | b. While standing on the side of the bed nearest the patient, place the patient's near arm across chest. Abduct the far arm–flexing at the elbow | Pulling one arm forward facilitates turning motion. Pulling the other arm away from body prevents that arm from being caught beneath the body |
| | c. Flex the knees of the leg near to you/place patient's nearest ankle across the far ankle and foot. | Facilitates turning motion |
| | d. Raise side rails next to patient. Go to the other side of the bed | |
| | e. Position yourself on the side of the bed towards which patient will turn directly in line with the patient's waist line. | |
| | f. Incline your trunk forward from the hips. Flex your hips, knees and ankles. Assume a broad stance with weight placed on the forward foot. | |
| 3. | Pull/roll the patient to a lateral position (Figure 3.3 (a)) | |

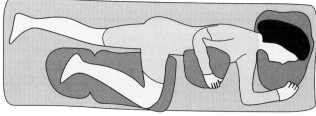

**Figure 3.3(a):** Lateral position with pillows in place

Two-heaviest parts of the body are supported.
a. Place one hand on the patient's far hip and one hand on the patient's far shoulder.
b. Tighten your gluteal muscles, rock back shifting your weight and abdominal muscles from forward to backward foot. Roll patient to side of the bed to face you.

• To roll on to prone position. The arm far to you should be kept along side the body, when turning roll completely

## SPECIAL CONSIDERATION

Never pull the patient across the bed when the patient is in a prone position as it may injure a woman's breast or man's genitals.

## 3.4: LOGROLLING A PATIENT

### DEFINITION

Log rolling is a technique used to turn a patient whose body must at all times be kept in straight alignment, e.g. in spinal injury.

### PURPOSES

1. To turn the patient in straight alignment.
2. To prevent further injury.

### PROCEDURE (THREE NURSES)

| Nursing action | Rationale |
|---|---|
| 1. Inform patient of the position change and provide needed explanation. | Explanation of what will be done reduces anxiety and promotes relaxation. |
| 2. Place pillow between patient's knees | Prevents tension on the spinal column and adduction of the hip |
| 3. Cross patient's arms on chest | Prevents patient's arms from being trapped under the body when turned |
| 4 Position two nurses on side of bed to which the patient will be turned. Position third nurse on the other side of bed (Fig. 3.4(a)) | Distributes weight equally between nurses |

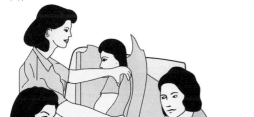
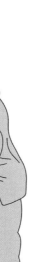

Figure 3.4(a): Logrolling by three nurses

| | |
|---|---|
| 5. Fanfold or roll the draw sheet or pull sheet | Provides strong handles in order to grip the draw sheet or pull sheet without slipping |
| 6. Nurses on either side place their hands under the patient supporting at the shoulder, waist, buttocks and thighs | Ensures equal distribution of weight |

*Contd...*

*Contd...*

| 7. | Move the patient to lateral position unit in a smooth, continuous motion on the count of three | This maintains proper alignment by moving all body parts at the same time preventing tension or twisting of the spinal column. |
|---|---|---|
| 8. | Nurse on the opposite side of the bed places pillows along the length of the patient | Pillows keep patient aligned |
| 9. | Gently lean the patient as a unit back towards the pillow for support | Ensures continued straight alignment of spinal column preventing injury |
| 10. | Put up side rails on either side | Ensures safety |
| 11. | Following each position change. Evalute patient's body alignment and presence of any pressure areas | Provides opportunity to recognize presence of pressure ulcers |
| 12. | Perform handwashing | Reduces transmission of microorganisms. |

## VARIATION: 2 NURSES AND TURN SHEET

1. Both nurses stand on the same side of the bed assuming a broad stance with one foot forward and grasp half of the fan-folded or rolled edge of the turn sheet (Fig. 3.4(bi))

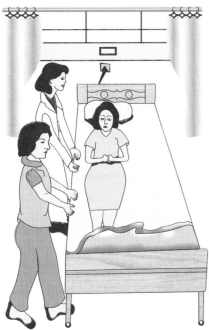

Figure 3.4(bi): Logrolling by two nurses

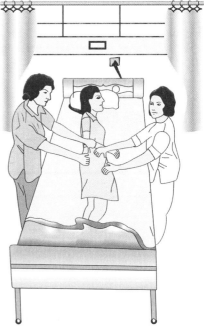

Figure 3.4(bii): Logrolling by two nurses

| 2. | On a signal both nurses pull the patient towards both of them | Bringing the patient to edge of the bed before turning ensures central-positioning of patient after turning |
|---|---|---|
| 3. | One nurse moves to other side of the bed and places supportive devices for the patient when turned<br>• Place a pillow where it will support the patient's head after the turn | The pillow prevents lateral flexion of the neck and ensures elignment of the cervical spine |

*Contd...*

*Contd...*

| | |
|---|---|
| • Place one or two pillows between the patient's legs to support the upper leg when the patient is turned | Prevents adduction of the upper leg and keeps the legs parallel and aligned |
| 4. Reaching over the patient, grasp the far edges of the turn sheet and roll the patient towards you. The second nurse (behind the patient) helps turn the patient and provides pillows for support to ensure good alignment in the lateral position (Fig. 3.4(bii)) | |

# 3.5: ASSISTING A PATIENT TO SITTING POSITION

## DEFINITION

Assisting a patient to move from a lying down position to a sitting position in bed.

## PURPOSES

1. To enable change of position without injury
2. To maintain good body mechanics.

## PROCEDURE

| | Nursing action | Rationale |
|---|---|---|
| 1. | Explain to patient that he will be assisted to sitting position. | Prepares him to accept the new position knowing how it would help. |
| 2. | Place patient in side lying position, facing you on the side of the bed on which patient will be sitting | Prepares patient to move to the sitting position |
| 3. | Raise head of the bed to the highest level possible as patient is able to tolerate | Decreases the amount of work needed by the patient and nurse to raise patient to sitting position |
| 4. | Stand opposite to patient's hip and turn diagonal so that you are facing patient and far corner of foot of the bed | Facing in the direction of work reduces a twisting motion |
| 5. | Place feet apart with one foot close to head of bed in front of other foot (Figure 3.5 (a) (i)) | Increases balance and enables you to transfer weight as you change position of patient |

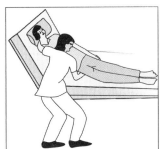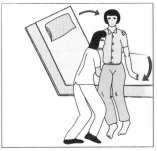

**Figure 3.5(a) (i and ii):** (i) Assisting a patient to sitting position, (ii) Assisting a patient to sit on edge of the bed with feet down

| | Nursing action | Rationale |
|---|---|---|
| 6. | Place arm nearer head of bed under shoulder supporting head and neck of the patient | Maintains good body alignment |
| 7. | Place other hand over patient's thighs | Supports hip and prevents falling |
| 8. | Move patient's lower leg and feet over side of bed | Decreases resistance and friction. |
| 9. | Pivot towards your rear leg allowing patient's upper legs to swing downward (Figure 3.5 (a) (ii)) | Allows you to transfer weight in the direction of motion |
| 10. | At the same time shift your weight to the rear leg and elevate patient | Reduces risk of falling |
| 11. | Remain in front of the patient till balance is regained | Reduces risk of falling |
| 12. | Support feet on the floor or on foot board | This allows patients to sit comfortably |
| 13. | Straighten patient's clothes and bed linen | Allows for neat appearance and improved self-esteem. |
| 14. | Assess patient's position and comfort frequently or as required | |
| 15. | Assess vital signs as indicated by patient's health status. | |

## 3.6: TRANSFERING A PATIENT FROM BED TO CHAIR

### DEFINITION

Assisting patient to a chair from the bed.

### PURPOSES

1. To enable change of position without injury
2. To maintain good body mechanics.

### PROCEDURE

| | Nursing action | Rationale |
|---|---|---|
| 1. | Explain the procedure to patient and instruct him on how he has to co-operate | Reduces anxiety and promotes patient's participation. |
| 2. | Assist the patient to sitting position on the side of the bed. Position a chair at 45 degree angle to the bed or parallel with the bed | Positioning patient in sitting position helps in starting transfer. The chair should be within easy access of the bed. |
| 3. | Spread your feet apart | Ensures a wider base of support |
| 4. | Flex your knees and hip on line with patient's knees | Lowers center of gravity to the object to be raised |
| 5. | Reach under the axilla of patient and place hands on scapula (Figure 3.6(a)) | Reduces pressure on axilla |

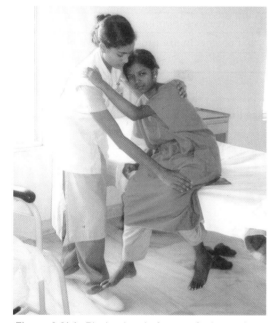

**Figure 3.6(a):** Placing hands for transferring patient

| | | |
|---|---|---|
| 6. | Help patient up to standing position on count of three. While straightening your hips and knees | Reduces effort required |
| 7. | Pivot on foot that is farthest from the chair (Figure 3.6 (b)) | Maintains support of patient while allowing adequate space for patient to move |

*Contd...*

*Contd...*

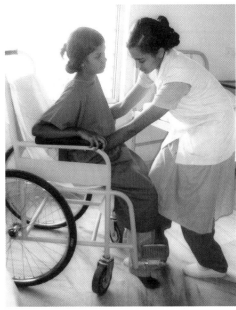

**Figure 3.6(b):** Pivoting on feet

| 8. | Ask patient to sit only after he feels the seat of the chair on the back of his knees | Reduces risk of fall |
|---|---|---|
| 9. | Instruct patient to use arm rest of chair for support, if present | Increases support and stability |
| 10. | Flex your hips and knees and lower patient to chair | Prevents injury caused by poor body mechanics |
| 11. | Align patient properly to sitting position | |

**Note:**
If patient is to be shifted to a wheelchair, ensure that its wheels are locked and that foot plate is raised.

# 3.7: TRANSFERING A PATIENT BETWEEN A BED AND STRETCHER

## DEFINITION

Shifting a helpless patient from bed to stretcher or from stretcher to bed.

## PURPOSES

1. To transfer patient safely.
2. To maintain proper body alignment.

## ARTICLES

1. Stretcher.
2. Roller bar (optional).

## PROCEDURE

Three persons to carry the patient

| | Nursing action | Rationale |
|---|---|---|
| 1 | Explain procedure to patient and how he has to co-operate. | Helps in obtaining patient's participation. |
| 2. | Adjust the patient's bed in preparation for the transfer<br>  a.  Adjust the bed to be in flat position<br>  b.  Raise the bed/stretcher, from where the patient is to be transferred to a slightly higher level<br>  c.  Ensure that the wheels of the bed and stretcher are locked<br>  d.  Untuck the draw sheet out from both sides of the bed pulling along a flat surface. | Facilitates easy transfer.<br>Placing patient in flat position facilitates easy transfer.<br>Facilitates easy transfer of patient by pulling downward with less force<br>Avoids accidental moving of bed or stretcher during procedure |
| 3. | Move patient to the edge of the bed and position the stretcher (Figure 3.7(a))<br>  a.  Roll draw sheet to the patient's side<br>  b.  Position the patient to the edge of the bed and cover patient with a sheet<br>  c.  Place the stretcher parallel to the bed next to the patient, and lock its wheels | |

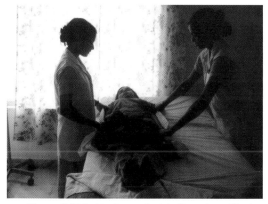

**Figure 3.7(a):** Moving patient to the edge of bed

*Contd...*

*Contd...*

4. Position yourself for the transfer (Figure 3.7(b))
   a. The first nurse should kneel on the bed on the side away from the stretcher.
   b. The other two nurses should reach over the stretcher holding the draw sheet; one nurse at the head and chest areas of the patient, supporting head and neck and the other nurse supporting at the waist and thigh area.

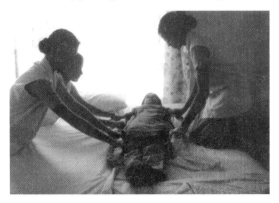

**Figure 3.7(b):** Position of nurses for transferring patient from bed to stretcher

| | |
|---|---|
| 5. Transfer the patient securely to the stretcher. | |
| a. In unison with the other staff members press your body tightly against the stretcher. | Prevents the stretcher from moving. |
| b. Roll the pull sheet tightly against the patient. | Achieves better control over patient movement |
| c. Instruct the patient to flex his neck and head during the move if possible. Place his arms across the chest. | Prevents injury to his body parts. |
| d. Flex your hips, and pull the patient on the pull sheet in unison directly towards and on to the stretcher. | |
| 6. Make the patient comfortable, unlock the stretcher wheels and move the stretcher away from the bed | |
| 7. Raise the stretcher side rails and/or fasten the safety straps across the patient | Avoids danger of patient falling out of stretcher. |

- **Having four nurses for the transfer reduces risk of injury to patient.**

## VARIATION

Using a three – person carry: all standing on same side of bed

| | Nursing action | Rationale |
|---|---|---|
| 1. | Three nurses of equal height stand beside the patient on one side of the bed facing the patient's bed. Stretcher is placed at 90 degree to bed and wheels are locked. | Maintains alignment of patient. |
| 2. | Incline trunk, flex knees. Place forearm on bed and slide hands under, head and shoulders, upper trunk, hips, thighs and lower legs with fingers securely around other side of patient's body | Distributes weight evenly. |
| 3. | Roll patient towards the nurse's chests. | Ensures greater stability. |

*Contd...*

*Contd...*

| | | |
|---|---|---|
| 4. | At the count of three patient is lifted and held against nurses' chests. | |
| 5. | On second count of three nurses step back and pivot towards stretcher. Move forward if required. | Maintains adjustment and uniformity of movement. |
| 6. | At count of three place patient gently on center of stretcher by flexing knees and hips till elbows are level with edge of stretcher. | |
| 7. | Put on side rails/safety straps and position patient. | |

# 3.8: PROVIDING RANGE OF MOTION EXERCISES

## DEFINITION

Isotonic exercises that are performed either by patient himself or by the nurse in case of helpless patients to mobilize all joints through their full range of motion.

## PURPOSES

1. To increase muscle strength and endurance.
2. To maintain normal physiological function.
3. To prevent complications caused by immobility-like contracture.
4. To improve patient participation in activities of daily living.
5. To improve physical activity.
6. To increase joint flexibility.

## GENERAL GUIDELINES

1. Passive ROM exercise should be done only on patients who are unable to do it on their own.
2. Passive ROM exercise should be done to the point of slight resistance.
3. Never do ROM exercise beyond the capacity of the individual, that is to the point of discomfort.
4. Move body parts smoothly, slowly and rhythmically.
5. Expect heart rate and respiratory rate to increase during exercise, which should return to resting levels within 3 minutes, if not, exercises are strenuous for patient.
6. If muscle spasticity occurs during movement, stop the movement temporarily, but continue to apply slow gentle pressure on the part until the muscle relaxes, then proceed with the ROM exercises.

## PROCEDURE

| | Nursing action | Rationale |
|---|---|---|
| 1. | Explain to the patient the purpose of doing exercises. | Ensures co-operation of patient. |
| 2. | Remove rings or other constrictive jewellery if present. | In case of hand swelling, this may impede circulation. |
| 3. | Remove all tight fitting clothes and provide a hospital gown. | Ensures comfort of the patient. |
| 4. | Cover patient with a bath blanket/sheet and assist in assuming a supine position. | Ensures comfort of the patient. |
| 5. | Provide privacy and wash hands. | Reduces patient anxiety and reduces risk of transfer of microorganisms. |
| 6. | Expose only the area that is being exercised. | Reduces embarrassment of patient. |
| 7. | Position bed to an appropriate height. | Ensures proper body mechanics. |
| 8. | Start providing passive ROM exercise from the head downwards (Figure 3.8 (a))<br>a. **Neck:**<br>• Move head through flexion, extension, lateral flexion, rotation and hyperextension of the neck.<br>• Movement of head is contraindicated in spinal surgery, spinal trauma and other central nervous system trauma and for patients having central venous line.<br>b. **Shoulder:**<br>Flexion, extension, hyperextension, abduction, adduction and circumduction, external rotation and internal rotation. Shoulder should be supported proximally and distally. | |

*Contd...*

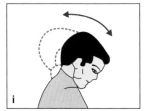

i

Neck flexion, extension, hyperextension

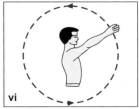

vi

Shoulder–circumduction

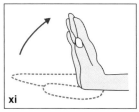

xi

Wrist–hyperextension

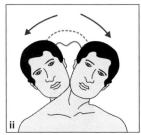

ii

Lateral flexion of neck

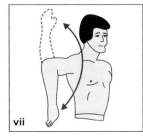

vii

Shoulder–Internal and external rotation

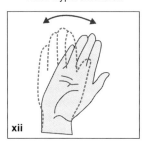

xii

Radial flexion and ulnar flexion

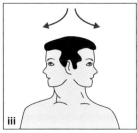

iii

Rotation of neck

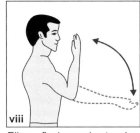

viii

Elbow–flexion and extension

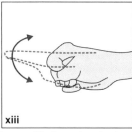

xiii

Hand and fingers–Flexion extension hyperextension

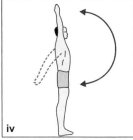

iv

Shoulder–flexion, extension and hyperextension

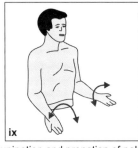

ix

Supination and pronation of palms

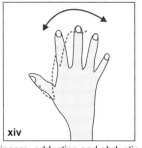

xiv

Fingers–adduction and abduction

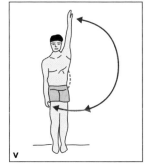

v

Shoulder–abduction and adduction

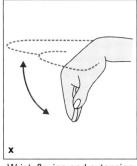

x

Wrist–flexion and extension

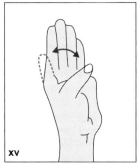

xv

Thumb–flexion extension

**Figure 3.8 (a):** Contd...

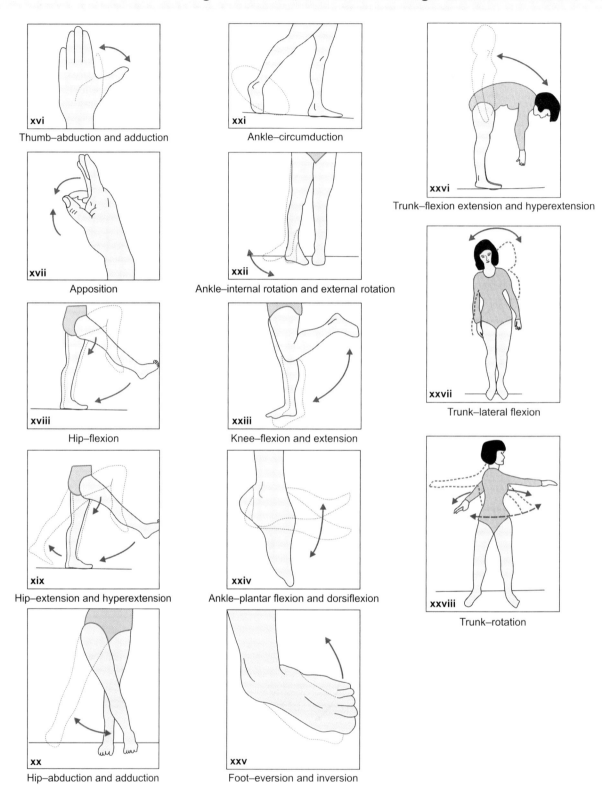

**Figure 3.8 (a):** Range of motion exercises illustrated

*Contd...*

c. **Trunk:**
Flexion, extension, hyperextension
lateral flexion, rotation of the trunk

d. **Elbow:**
Flexion, extension, pronation and supination.
Support elbow joint both proximally and distally.

e. **Forearm:**
Pronation, and supination. Position wrist in functional position.

f. **Wrist:**
Flexion, extension, hyperextension and lateral flexion
(radial and ulnar) Position wrist in functional position.

g. **Hand:**
Move hand through flexion, extension, hyperextension, abduction, adduction, apposition of the thumb and circumduction of thumb.

h. **Hip:**
Move hip through flexion, extension, abduction, adduction, internal rotation and external rotation and circumduction with support above and below joints.

i. **Knee:**
Move knee through flexion and extension

j. **Ankle and foot:**
Extension, plantar flexion, dorsi flexion, eversion and inversion of foot.

k. **Toes:**
Move through flexion, extension, abduction and adduction

9. Wash hands

10. Record procedure

11. Position patient in a comfortable position

## SPECIAL POINTS

- Move each joint through its full ROM exercise three times and follow regular pattern of movement.
- Provide passive ROM exercise two times a day.
- Support measures should be used to prevent muscle strain or injury during ROM exercise (Figure 3.8(b)).

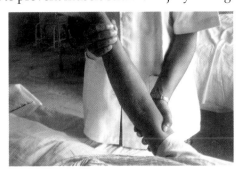

**Figure 3.8(b):** Supporting extremities during
ROM exercises

## 3.9: POSITIONING OF THE PATIENT IN BED

### DEFINITION

Placing the patient in good body alignment as needed therapeutically.

### PURPOSES

1. To promote comfort to the patient.
2. To prevent complications caused by immobility.
3. To stimulate circulation.
4. To promote normal physiological functions.

### ARTICLES

1. Clean, dry, firm bed
2. Different types of mattresses
3. Bed boards
4. Pillows
5. Foot board/foot boot
6. Sand bags
7. Hand rolls
8. Trochanter rolls
9. Bed blocks
10. Over bed table
11. Additional sheets
12. Trapeze bar

{Articles are used as per requirement of each type of position. Additional articles may be used as per availability}

### GENERAL PRINCIPLES IN POSITIONING

1. Maintain good body mechanics.
2. Obtain assistance as required.
3. Ensure that mattress is firm and level of bed is at working height.
4. Ensure that sheets are clean and dry.
5. Avoid placing a body part directly over another to prevent pressure.
6. Plan a regular position change schedule for the patient for 24 hours.
7. Ensure patient comfort.
8. Wash hands before and after procedure.

### A. FOWLER'S POSITION

#### PURPOSES

1. To relieve or minimize dyspnea.
2. To relieve tension on abdominal sutures.

#### PROCEDURE

| | Nursing action | Rationale |
|---|---|---|
| 1. | Inform patient of the position, he will be in and provide needed explanation. | Understanding reduces anxiety and promotes relaxation. |

*Contd...*

*Contd...*

| | | |
|---|---|---|
| 2. | Elevate head of the bed (Fowlers 45 to 90 degree) Semi Fowlers(15 to 45 degree) High Fowlers (90 degree) (Figure 3.9(a)) | Increases comfort and relaxation. |
| 3. | Rest head against mattress or small pillow. | Prevents cervical flexion contractures. |
| 4. | Use pillow to support arm. | Prevents shoulder dislocation, promotes circulation and prevents flexion contractures of arms and wrists. |
| 5. | Place a small pillow at lower back. | Supports lumbar vertebrae and prevents exaggerated flexion of vertebrae. |
| 6. | Place a small pillow/roll under thigh. | Prevents hyperextension of knee and occlusion of popliteal artery from pressure of body weight. |
| 7. | Place small pillow under ankle. | Prevents prolonged pressure on heels. |
| 8. | Place foot board at bottom of patient's feet. | Maintains dorsi- flexion and prevents foot drop. |

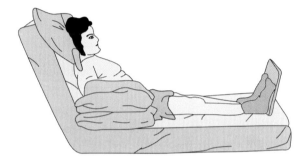

**Figure 3.9(a):** Fowler's position

## PROBLEMS TO BE PREVENTED IN FOWLER'S POSITION

1. Posterior flexion of lumbar curvature.
2. Hyperextension of neck.
3. Edema of hands and arms
4. Possible dislocation of shoulder
5. Flexion contracture of the wrist.
6. Hyperextension of the knees.
7. External rotation of hips (Trochanter roll to be placed)
8. Pressure on heels.
9. Plantar flexion of feet/foot drop.

## B. ORTHOPNEIC POSITION

High Fowler's position with over bed table to be placed across the front of the patient. Patient to rest both hands on over bed table/on pillow placed on it and lean forward. Leaning forward facilitates respiration by allowing maximum chest expansion by reducing pressure of abdominal organs on diaphragm.

### INDICATIONS

1. Patients with severe dyspnea
2. Cardiac patients
3. Position for thoracentesis
4. Patient with chest drainage tubes.

## C. SUPINE POSITION/DORSAL RECUMBENT/BACK LYING

| | Nursing action | Rationale |
|---|---|---|
| 1. | After providing explanation about the procedure, place patient on back with head of the bed flat (Figure 3.9 (b)) | |
| 2. | Place small rolled towel under lumbar area of the back | Provides support for lumbar spine |
| 3. | Place pillow under head, neck and upper shoulders | Maintains correct alignment and prevents flexion contractures of cervical vertebrae and hyperextension of neck |
| 4. | Place Trochanter rolls/sand bags parallel to lateral surface of thighs | Reduces external rotation of hip. |
| 5. | Place small pillow under thighs | Prevents hyperextension of knees. |
| 6. | Place small pillow/roll under ankle to elevate heels | Reduces pressure on heels. |
| 7. | Place foot board under bottom of feet | Prevents plantar flexion/foot drop. |
| 8. | Place pillow under pronated arm maintaining upper arm parallel to body. | Reduces internal rotation of shoulder and extension of elbows. |
| 9. | If patient is paralyzed place hand rolls in hand. | Reduces extension of fingers and abduction of thumb. Maintains thumb in slight adduction and in apposition. |

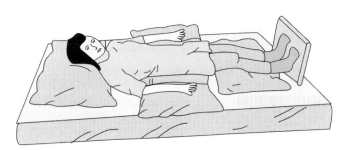

**Figure 3.9(b):** Supine position

### PROBLEMS TO BE PREVENTED IN DORSAL RECUMBENT POSITION

1. Hyperextension of neck.
2. Posterior flexion of lumbar curvature
3. External rotation of legs
4. Hyperextension of knees
5. Plantar flexion
6. Pressure on heels.

## D. PRONE POSITION

### INDICATIONS

1. For patient with pressure sores, burns, injuries and operations on the back.
2. For patients after 24 hours of amputation of lower limbs.
3. Position for renal biopsy

**PROCEDURE**

| | Nursing action | Rationale |
|---|---|---|
| 1. | After providing explanation about the procedure, roll patient over, with arm positioned close to the body with elbows straight, and hands under hips. Position the patient on abdomen in center of bed with bed flat (Figure 3.9(c)) | |
| 2. | Turn patient's head to one side and support with a small pillow. | Reduces flexion or hyperextension of cervical vertebrae. |
| 3. | Place small pillow under abdomen below the diaphragm. | Reduces hyperextension of lumbar vertebrae and strain on lower back. Reduces pressure on breasts for women and on genitals for men. |
| 4. | Support arm in flexed position at level of shoulder. | Reduces risk of shoulder dislocation. |
| 5. | Support lower legs with pillows to elevate toes. | Prevents foot drop and external rotation of legs. Reduces pressure of mattress on toes. |

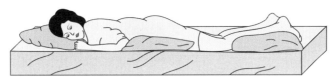

**Figure 3.9(c):** Prone position

**PROBLEMS TO BE PREVENTED IN PRONE POSITION**

1. Flexion/hyperextension of neck.
2. Hyperextension of lumbar curvature.
3. Pressure on breasts, heels and genitals.
4. Foot drop.

## E.  LATERAL/SIDE LYING POSITION

**INDICATIONS**

1. Patients who require periodic position changes, e.g. bed ridden patients.
2. In immediate postoperative patients to prevent the risk of aspiration (except in spinal and epidural anesthesia).

**PROCEDURE**

| | Nursing action | Rationale |
|---|---|---|
| 1. | Provide explanation and prepare patient for the position change. | |
| 2. | Lower head of bed as low as patient can tolerate. | |
| 3. | Position patient to side of bed. | |
| 4. | Turn patient to one side (In helpless patient, flex patient's knee that will be away from mattress, place hand on that side to patient's hip and the other hand at shoulder, then roll patient to side.) (Figure 3.9(d)) | Prevents injury and trauma to tissue. |
| 5. | Place pillow under patient's head and neck. | Maintains alignment, reduces lateral neck flexion and decreases strain on sternocleidomastoid muscle. |

*Contd...*

*Contd...*

| 6. | Bring shoulder blade forward. | Prevents weight from resting directly over shoulder joint. |
|---|---|---|
| 7. | Position both arms in flexed position. Upper most arm is supported by pillow on level with shoulder. | Decreases internal rotation and adduction of shoulder. Ventilation is improved as chest can expand. |
| 8. | Place tuck- back pillow under back (pillow folded lengthwise and smooth area tucked under back). | Provides support to maintain patient on side. |
| 9. | Place pillow under semiflexed upper leg level at hip, from groin to foot. | Prevents hyperextension of leg. Maintains alignment and prevents foot drop. |
| 10. | Place sand bag parallel to plantar surface of dependant foot. | Prevents foot drop. |

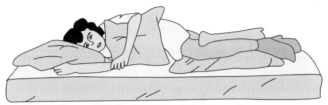

**Figure 3.9(d):** Side lying (lateral) position

## PROBLEMS TO BE PREVENTED

1. Lateral flexion and fatigue of sternocleidomastoid muscle.
2. Internal rotation and adduction of shoulder and limited chest expansion.
3. Internal rotation and adduction of femur and twisting of spine.

## F. SIM'S POSITION/SEMI-PRONE POSITION

### INDICATIONS

1. Vaginal and rectal examination.
2. Administration of enema and suppository.
3. Position for sigmoidoscopy and proctoscopy.

### PROCEDURE

| | Nursing action | Rationale |
|---|---|---|
| 1. | Provide explanation and prepare patient for the position | |
| 2. | Place head of bed flat | |
| 3. | Place patient in supine position | |
| 4. | Turn patient onto lateral position lying partially on abdomen (Figure 3.9(e)) | |
| 5. | Place small pillow under head and neck. | Maintains alignment and prevents lateral neck flexion. |
| 6. | Place pillow under flexed upper arm supporting arm level with shoulder. | Prevents internal rotation of shoulder. |
| 7. | Place pillow under flexed upper leg, supporting leg level with hip | Prevents internal rotation of hip. Maintains proper alignment. |
| 8. | Place sand bags parallel to plantar surface of dependant foot | Prevents plantar flexion. |

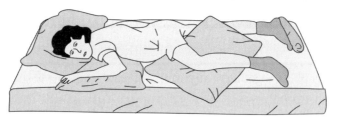

**Figure 3.9(e):** Sim's position

## PROBLEMS TO BE PREVENTED

1. Lateral flexion of neck.
2. Internal rotation of shoulder.
3. Internal rotation and adduction of hip and leg.
4. Foot drop.

# G. LITHOTOMY POSITION

## INDICATIONS

1. For delivery and vaginal examination
2. For rectal surgeries, e.g. Hemorrhoidectomy, fissurotomy.
3. For vaginal hysterectomy.

## PROCEDURE

| | Nursing action | Rationale |
|---|---|---|
| 1. | Place patient in supine position. | |
| 2. | Place pillow under head and neck. | Prevents hyperextension of neck. |
| 3. | Place both legs flexed at hip and knee, at 90 degree with legs supported on stirrups. | |

# H. TRENDLENBURG POSITION

Entire frame of bed tilted with head of bed down.

## INDICATIONS

1. Postural drainage.
2. Management of hypotension and shock.
3. Patients with deep vein thrombosis.

## PROCEDURE

| | |
|---|---|
| 1. | Explain procedure to patient. |
| 2. | Place patient in supine position. |
| 3. | Lower head end of the bed using bed key. If he is not adjustable type, use bed blocke at foot end and tilt entire frame of bed down. |

# 3.10: PERFORMING MEDICAL HANDWASHING

## DEFINITION

Handwashing is a vigorous, brief rubbing together of all surfaces of hands lathered in soap followed by rinsing under a stream of water.

## INDICATIONS

1. Before contact with patients who are susceptible to infection (e.g. newborn infants or immunosuppressed patients).
2. After caring for an infected patient.
3. After touching organic material.
4. Before performing invasive procedures such as administration of injection, catheterization and suctioning.
5. Before and after handling dressing or touching open wounds.
6. After handling contaminated equipment.
7. Between contacts with different patients in high-risk units.

## PURPOSES

1. To remove dirt and transient organisms from the hands and to reduce total microbial counts.
2. To protect nursing personnel from pathogenic organisms.

## ARTICLES

1. Warm running water.
2. Antimicrobial/regular soap.
3. Paper towels/hand drier.

## PROCEDURE

| | Nursing action | Rationale. |
|---|---|---|
| 1. | Inspect surface of hands for breaks/cuts in skin or cuticle. Report and cover lesions before providing patient care. | Open cuts/wounds can harbour high concentrations of micro-organisms. Open wounds serve as a portal for entry of microorganisms. |
| 2. | Inspect hands for heavy soiling. | Requires lengthier handwashing. |
| 3. | Inspect nails for length. | Nails should be short because most microbes on hands come from beneath the fingernails. |
| 4. | Assess patient's risk for infection. | Use of antimicrobial soaps is encouraged when caring for patients who are at risk for infection, e.g. immuno-suppressed patients. |
| 5. | Remove wrist watch and push long uniform sleeves above wristwatch. Remove all jewellery from hands such as ring, watch and bracelet etc. | Provides complete access to fingers, hands and wrist. Wearing of rings increases the number of micro-organisms on hands. |
| 6. | Stand in front of the sink, keeping hands and uniform away from sink surfaces | Inside of sink is a contaminated area. Reaching over sink increases risk of touching edge, which is contaminated. |
| 7. | Turn on water. Avoid splashing water against uniform (Figure 3.10(a)) | Microorganisms travel and grow in moisture. |

*Contd...*

*Contd...*

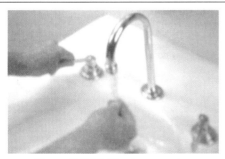

**Figure 3.10(a):** Turning on water

| | | |
|---|---|---|
| 8. | Regulate flow of water and make sure that the water is warm. | Warm water removes less of the protective oils than cold water. |
| 9. | Wet hands and wrists thoroughly under running water. Keep hands and forearms lower than elbows during washing. | Hands are the most contaminated parts to be washed. Water flows from least to most contaminated area, rinsing micro-organisms from the sink. |
| 10. | Apply a small amount of soap or antiseptic, lathering thoroughly. | Use of antiseptic exclusively can be drying to hands and can cause skin irritation. |
| 11. | Wash hands using plenty of lather and friction for at least 10 to 15 seconds. Interlace fingers and rub palms and back of hands with circular motion for at least 5 times each (Figure 3.10(b)) Special attention should be provided to areas such as knuckles and fingernails | Soap cleanses by emulsifying fat and oil thus lowering surface tension. Friction and rubbing mechanically loosen and remove dirt. Interlacing fingers and thumbs ensures that all surfaces are cleansed. Knuckles and fingernails harbour micro-organism. |

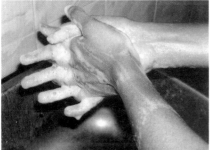

**Figure 3.10(b):** Interlacing fingers and lathering with soap

| | | |
|---|---|---|
| 12. | Area underlying fingernails are often soiled. Clean them with fingernails of other hand and use additional soap if required. (Figure 3.10 (c)) | Area under nails can be highly contaminated which will increase the risk of infection for the nurse or the patient. |

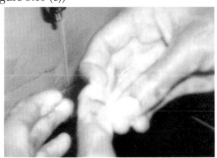

**Figure 3.10(c):** Cleaning underfinger nails

*Contd...*

*Contd...*

| | |
|---|---|
| 13. Rinse hands and wrists thoroughly keeping hands down and elbows up (Figure 3.10(d)) | Rinsing from cleanest to least clean area avoids contamination. |

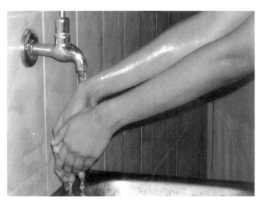

**Figure 3.10(d):** Rinsing hands and wrist

| | |
|---|---|
| 14. Turn off water faucet using paper towel (Figure 3.10(e)) | |

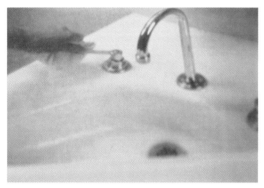

**Figure 3.10(e):** Turning off water using paper towel

| | |
|---|---|
| 15. Dry hands thoroughly from finger to wrist and to forearm with paper towel. | Drying from cleanest to less clean area avoids contamination. |
| 16. Discard used towel | Prevents transfer of micro-organism |

## 3. 11: POLICIES FOR SEGREGATION AND DISPOSAL OF BIOMEDICAL WASTE

Table 3.11.1: Segregation and disposal of biomedical waste

| Option | Waste category | Treatment and disposal |
|---|---|---|
| Category No. 1 | Human anatomical waste (human tissues, organs, body parts). | Incineration/deep burial. |
| Category No. 2 | Animal waste (animal tissues, organs, body parts carcasses, bleeding parts, fluid, blood and experimental animals used in research, waste generated by veterinary hospital colleges, discharge from hospitals, animal houses). | Incineration/deep burial. |
| Category No 3 | Microbiology and biotechnology waste (wastes from laboratory cultures, stocks or specimens of microorganisms, live or attenuated vaccines, human and animal cell culture used in research and infectious agents from research and industrial laboratories, wastes from production of biologicals toxins, dishes and devices used for transfer of cultures). | Local autoclaving/micro waving/ incineration. |
| Category No 4 | Waste sharps (needles, syringes, scalpels, blades, glass etc. that may cause punctures and cuts. This includes both used and unused sharps). | Disinfection (chemical treatment/auto-claving/microwaving and mutilation/ shredding. |
| Category No 5 | Discarded medicines and cytotoxic drugs (wastes comprising of outdated, contaminated and discarded medicines). | Incineration/destruction and drug disposal in secured landfills. |
| Category No 6 | Solid waste (items contaminated with blood and body fluids including cotton, dressings, solied plaster casts, linens, beddings, other material contaminated with blood). | Incineration, autoclaving/ microwaving. |
| Category No 7 | Solid waste (wastes generated from disposable items other than the waste sharps such as tubings, catheters, itravenous sets etc). | Disinfection by chemical treatment, autoclaving/microwaving and mutilation/shredding. |
| Category No 8 | Liquid waste (waste generated from laboratory and washing, cleaning, house-keeping and disinfecting activities). | Disinfection by chemical treatment and discharge into drains. |
| Category No 9 | Incineration ash (ash from incineration of any bio-medical waste). | Disposal in municipal landfill. |
| Category No 10 | Chemical waste (Chemical used in production of biologicals, chemicals used in disinfection, as insecticides etc.). | Chemical treatment and discharge into drains for liquids and secured landfill for solids. |

Chemicals treatment must be done using at least 1% hypochlorite solution or any other equivalent chemical reagent. It must be ensured that chemical treatment ensures disinfection.

Mutilation/shredding must be such so as to prevent unauthorised reuse.

There will be no chemical pretreatment before incineration. Chlorinated plastics are not to be incinerated.

Deep burial shall be an option available only in towns with population less than five lakhs and in rural areas.

**Table 3.11.2:** Color coding and type of container for disposal of bio-medical wastes

| Color coding | Type of container | Waste category | Treatment options as per schedule I |
|---|---|---|---|
| Yellow | Plastic bag | Cat. 1, Cat 2 and Cat 3 Cat 6. | Incineration/deep burial |
| Red | Disinfected container/plastic bag | Cat 3, Cat 6, Cat 7 | Autoclaving/Microwaving/ Chemical treatment |
| Blue/white Translucent | Plastic bag/puncture proof container | Cat 4, Cat 7 | Autoclaving/Microwaving/ Chemical Treatment and destruction/shredding |
| Black | Plastic bag | Cat 5 and Cat 9 and Cat 10 (solid) | Disposal in secured landfill. |

Notes:

1. Color coding of waste categories with multiple treatment options as defined in Schedule 1, shall be selected depending on treatment option chosen, which shall be as specified in schedule 1 (Figures 3.11(a) (i) and (ii))

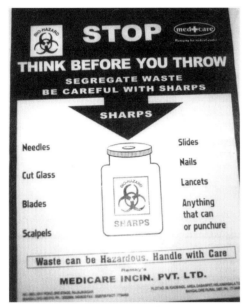
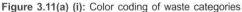

Figure 3.11(a) (i): Color coding of waste categories

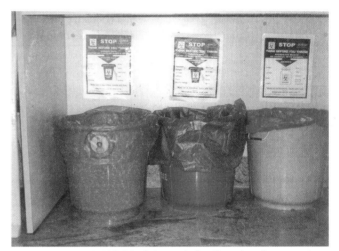

Figure 3.1(a) (ii): Color code for disposing sharps

2. Waste collection bags for waste types needing incineration shall not be made of chlorinated plastics.
3. Categories 8 and 10 (liquid) do not require containers/bags.
4. Category 3 if disinfected locally need not be put in containers/bags.

## 3.12: DISINFECTION OF BLOOD AND BODY FLUIDS SPILLS

### DEFINITION

This process refers to the immediate disinfection of all contaminated articles and bodily discharges in the patient care area/unit.

### PURPOSES

1. To keep the ward or unit clean or free from microorganisms.
2. To prevent spread of infection.
3. To dispose off the spills safely.

### ARTICLES

1. Clean gloves
2. Disinfectants-Sodium hypochlorite, hydrogen peroxide, lysol, Dettol, savlon, formalin
3. Towels
4. Scrubbing brush
5. Soap and water
6. Sterile water.

### PROCEDURE

| | Nursing action | Rationale |
|---|---|---|
| | **Step 1: Cleaning of spills** | |
| 1 | Wash hands and don gloves | Prevents exposure to infective material. |
| 2 | Rinse the article first with cold water. If required, soak them in cold water. | Removes fresh blood, pus and secretions etc. |
| | a. Clean them in cold soapy water until the stains disappear. | Hot water coagulates protien material. |
| | b. If the blood stains are old or infected, soak them in a mixture of hydrogen peroxide and ammonia for several hours, then clean them in cold water and then with soap and warm water. | Emulsifying action of soap reduces surface tension and facilitates the removal of dirt. |
| | c. If the blood stains are fresh, soak in sodium hypochlorite solution for 20-30 minutes. For thick blood stains on the mattress, apply a thick paste of starch and water and allow to stand in the sun, when the paste is dry and discolored, brush off the paste. | |
| 3 | Apply soap | |
| 4 | Use an abrasive (stiff bristled) brush to clean the grooves and corners. | Friction helps to dislodge foreign materials. |
| 5 | Rinse the article well with warm to hot water. | Removes soap thoroughly. |
| 6 | Dry the articles under sunlight. | Moisture allows, growth of microorganisms. |
| 7 | Clean the brush and sink with disinfectant. | Maintains cleanliness. |
| | **Step 2: Disinfection of articles; furniture and floors** | |
| 1 | Identify the causative organisms of disease. | Helps to choose appropriate disinfectant, its concentration, duration of contact etc. |
| 2 | Check the room temperature. | Most disinfectants are intended for use at room temperature. |

*Contd...*

*Contd...*

| 3 | Rinse the article once again with soap and water before disinfecting and remove soap thoroughly. | Presence of soap may inhibit the action of disinfectant. |
|---|---|---|
| 4 | Soak in sterile water | |
| 5 | Check for the presence of any pus, saliva, blood or any secretions before disinfecting. | Presence of saliva, pus, blood may inactivate the disinfectant. |
| 6 | Prepare the disinfectant solution in the correct concentration. | |
| 7 | Soak the articles in disinfectant solution, immersing them completely for about 20 to 30 minutes. | Enables thorough disinfection. |
| 8 | Articles which are not disinfected properly should be sent for autoclaving. | |
| 9 | Disinfect the floors, walls, doors, windows and furnitures by mopping or cleaning with antiseptic (savlon, dettol, sodium hypochlorite, sulphur, formalin and potassium permanganate solutions. | |
| 10 | Take out the articles which are soaked in disinfectant solution and rinse with normal saline/sterile water before use. | |

**Step 3: Fumigation (Terminal disinfection)**

| 1 | Fumigation with sulphur:<br>• Place required quantity of sulphur (220 gm for a 100 square feet room) in an earthern ware pot allow it to stand in a large vessel containing water and boil it until fumes fill the room<br>• Pour methylated spirit over sulphur and light fire to the sulphur and close the door with proper sealing. Open the room after 24 hours. | Sulphur fumes acts better on a damp surfaces. The room should be filled with sulphur fumes by boiling a kettle of water in the room.<br><br>Ensures burning of sulphur completely. For fumigating the room. |
|---|---|---|
| 2 | Fumigation with formalin:<br>Take 140 gram of pottasium permanganate crystals and 250 ml of formalin for a 100 square feet room and mix it well and place them in a metal bowl.<br>The room should be sealed for 12 to 24 hours. | The heat produced by the chemical action evaporates the formaldehyde. |
| 3 | Spray method:<br>Bacillosis sprays can be used to fumigate entire room. | |

**Table 3.12.1:** Commonly used antiseptics and disinfectants, effectiveness and use.

| Agent | Bacteria | Tuberculosis | Fungi | Viruses | Spores | Use on |
|---|---|---|---|---|---|---|
| Iso propyl and ethyl alcohol | X | X | X | X | | Hands, thermometers, vial stoppers. |
| Chlorine (bleach) | X | X | X | X | X | Blood spills |
| Hydrogen peroxide | X | X | X | X | X | Surfaces |
| Iodophors | X | X | X | X | X | Equipment, intact skin and tissues in diluted form. |
| Phenol | X | X | X | X | | Surfaces |
| Chlorhexidine Gluconate (hibiclens) | X | | | X | | Hands |
| Triclosan (bactistat) | X | | | | | Hands, intact skin. |

## POINTS TO BE REMEMBERED WHEN SELECTING THE DISINFECTANT

1. The disinfectant chosen should be efficient to destroy pathogens.
2. They should be used in correct strength.
3. The article should be fully immersed in it.
4. The article should be soaked for about 20 to 30 minutes in disinfectant.
5. The disinfectant should not be injurious to the skin and articles.
6. The article should be thoroughly cleansed prior to immersing in germicide to remove the organic material which will protect the bacteria against the action of disinfectants.
7. The disinfectant should be inexpensive.
8. Instrument soaked in germicides must be adequately rinsed with sterile water or normal saline before being used.

## 3.13: PREVENTION OF NOSOCOMIAL INFECTIONS

## DEFINITION

Infection acquired by patients as a result of medical care received from a health care facility, which was not present or incubating at the time of admission to the hospital.

**Common sites of infection and preventive measures**

| Sites of nosocomial infection | Cause | Preventive measures |
|---|---|---|
| Urinary tract | • Insertion of catheter into urethra | • Catheterize only for accepted indication.<br>• Remove catheter as soon as possible.<br>• Train personnel in proper technique of catheterization.<br>• Use smallest size to promote urine flow(14-16Fr)<br>• Consider silicone catheters for long-term use.<br>• Choose smallest balloon possible. |
| | • Accidental and frequent opening of drainage system | • Maintain closed system throughout.<br>• Follow strict aseptic technique. when connecting or disconnecting system.<br>• Prevent accidental opening of system.<br>• Train personnel, patient and relatives on hazards of open system. |
| | • Improper position of drainage bags, kinking and reflux | • Position bag below level of bladder.<br>• No contact should be there with wall, floor or furniture.<br>• Avoiding kinking or looping of tube.<br>• Clamp tube when lifting above bladder level.<br>• Avoid over filling of bag. |
| | • Lack of aseptic practices in caring for catheter | • Perform proper handwashing and use of gloves before contact with patient, catheter, bag or urinal.<br>• Improve general hygienic practices<br>• Perform catheter and perineal care with soap and water daily. |
| | • Frequent flushing and irrigation | Avoid frequent flushing and irrigation unless absolutely necessary. |
| Respiratory tract | • Contaminated respiratory therapy equipment. | • Disinfect and clean equipment after each use.<br>• Use sterile water to fill in critical and semi critical equipment like humidifiers.<br>• Wash hand before and after each procedure.<br>• Single use equipment should be used for single use only. |
| | • Failure to use aseptic technique during suctioning and other respiratory procedures.<br>• Failure in segregating patients who are infected | • Follow strict aseptic technique when doing procedures.<br>• Use gloves, gown and mask whenever needed.<br>• Restrict staff with respiratory infection to care for the patient.<br>• Use separate rooms for infected and non–infected patients.<br>• In case of pneumonia, tuberculosis etc., admit patients to negative air pressure rooms with independent air supply and exhaust.<br>• Use barrier nursing technique in caring for immuno–compromised patient. |
| | • Improper disposal of secretions and contaminated linen. | • Educate patients regarding disposal of secretions.<br>• Disinfect all collecting equipment after use.<br>• Use appropriate antiseptic solution for disinfection. |

*Contd...*

*Contd...*

| Surgical wound | Improper skin preparation before surgery. | • Clean skin using antiseptic soap and shampoo on the day of surgery.<br>• Report presence of any skin lesions at operative site.<br>• Remove hair by using safe technique (if physician prefers) without traumatizing skin.<br>• Hair should be removed as close to the time of surgery as possible.<br>• Use a broad spectrum antimicrobial agent to disinfect skin.<br>• Permit only trained personnel to perform skin preparation in surgery. |
|---|---|---|
| | • Poor handwashing and aseptic technique before and after surgical wound dressing. | • Educate personnel on handwashing and proper aseptic techniques before handling surgical wound.<br>• Permit only trained personnel to perform surgical wound dressing.<br>• Wear sterile gloves for handling surgical wounds.<br>• Change dressings whenever required.<br>• Use sterile antiseptic solution for cleaning surgical wound. |
| Bloodstream | Use of contaminated catheters, intravenous fluids, tubings etc., and wrong techniques. | • Select catheter type and gauge based on length of use, solution being infused and vein being used.<br>• Plastic catheters are less likely to introduce infection when compared to steel needles.<br>• Discontinue catheters in peripheral vein every 48-72 hours to minimize phlebitis risk.<br>• Discontinue IV devices when signs of phlebitis starts.<br>• Use proper handwashing practices. Don sterile gloves whenever handling IV devices. |
| | Contamination of infusions when adding medications and contaminated heparin locks. | • Use sterile technique when adding medications<br>• Maintain closed system of intravenous infusion.<br>• Administer medications only through medication ports in the set.<br>• Clean ports before inserting syringes or needles into it.<br>• Aseptic technique to be used in passing of IV lines. Replace heparin locks every 96 hours. |
| | • Contamination and improper care of insertion site of intravenous device | • Encourage good skin hygiene.<br>• Use clean linen in contact with patient.<br>• Prevent soiling of dressing site.<br>• Change soiled dressing immediately.<br>• Change dressing every 48-72 hours<br>• When cleaning insertion site, clean from inner to outer area to prevent infection.<br>• Use sterile techniques whenever changing dressing.<br>• Do not retain IV device for longer than required period. |

## MEASURES TO PREVENT NOSOCOMIAL INFECTIONS

1. Universal precautions
2. Body substance isolation
3. Prevention of infection in susceptible patients
4. Specific isolation practices.

## UNIVERSAL PRECAUTIONS

Centers for disease control and prevention (CDC) recommended universal precautions to decrease risk of transmission of unidentified pathogens in 1987.

Universal precautions apply to blood and to other body fluids containing visible blood.

Precautions also apply to semen, vaginal secretions, tissues and fluids such as cerebrospinal, synovial, pleural, peritoneal, pericardial and amniotic fluids.

Universal precautions do not apply to feces, nasal secretions, sputum, sweat, tears, urine and vomitus unless they contain visible blood.

a. Gloves should be worn while contacting with blood and body fluids, mucous membranes, non-intact skin, surfaces soiled with blood or body fluids and for performing venipuncture and other vascular access procedures.
b. Gloves should be changed after contact with each patient.
c. Masks and protective eye wear or face shields should be worn during procedures that are likely to generate droplets of blood or other body fluids.
d. Gowns should be worn during procedures that are likely to generate flashes of blood or other body fluids containing blood.
e. Hands and other skin surfaces should be washed immediately and thoroughly, if contaminated with blood or other body fluids containing blood.
f. To prevent needle stick injuries, needles should not be recapped, purposely bent, broken or removed from disposable syringes. Used needles are to be placed in puncture resistant containers near the work area.
g. To reduce the need for mouth to mouth resuscitation, mouthpieces, resuscitator bags or other ventilation devices should be used.
h. Health care workers who have exudative lesions should refrain from all direct patient care activities and from handling patient care equipment.

## BODY SUBSTANCE ISOLATION (B.S.I)

Body substance isolation are isolation precautions that consider all body substances potentially infectious regardless of a person's diagnosis. BSI precautions should be followed whenever coming in contact with moist body substances, mucous membranes, and non–intact skin. This includes blood, blood tinged fluids, feces, urine, wound drainage, oral secretion, vomitus and any other substances.

BSI was first implemented by CDC in 1996 and the basic premises are:
1 All individuals are prone for infections from microorganisms placed on their non–intact skin and mucous membrane.
2. All people have potentially infectious microorganisms in all of their moist body sites or substances.
3. An unknown portion of patients and health care workers will always be colonised or infected with potentially infectious microorganisms in their blood and other moist body sites and substances.

Body substance isolation requires the following to be done by health care personnel.
1. Wear clean, disposable gloves before contact with mucous membranes, non-intact skin and insertion sites for indwelling devices.
2. Change gloves between patients and between activities with the same patient when gloves become excessively soiled.
3. Wash hands for at least 10 seconds when the hands are soiled, before contact with new patient and after gloves are removed.
4. Use additional barriers such as gowns or plastic aprons, masks, goggles or glasses. Hair covers or shoe covers as needed to keep moist body substances off clothing, skin and mucous membranes.
5. Discard sharp instruments and needles uncapped in a rigid puncture proof container located in the patient's room or treatment area.
6. Handle all laboratory specimens as if they are infectious.
7. Transport all soiled and reusable articles in plastic bags or rigid containers.
8. Secure soiled linen in bags before transport.
9. Isolate patients with communicable diseases and follow appropriate isolation precautions.

## PREVENTION OF INFECTION IN SUSCEPTIBLE PATIENT

The actions for protecting susceptible host includes the following:
1. Promoting basic hygiene practices like bathing, regular oral hygiene which can reduce the numbers of microorganisms that may enter the body.
2. Ensuring ambulation of patient within limitation and deep breathing and coughing exercises to clear respiratory tract.
3. Immunizations of susceptible hosts, both children and adults based on current and accepted schedules.
4. Encouraging a healthy well balanced diet and adequate fluid intake for improving general health status and for ensuring an adequate outflow of urine.
5. Promoting adequate rest and sleep and reducing stress.
6. Encouraging appropriate exercise to meet physiological requirements.
7. Preventing contact of susceptible host with potential source of infection.

## SPECIFIC ISOLATION PRACTICES

A. Strict Isolation
   - Purpose: Prevents spread of highly contagious or virulent infections spread by air and contact.
   - Disease conditions: Chickenpox, diphtheria, etc.
   - Room: Private/separate room
   - Protective devices:
     - Gown
     - Gloves
     - Mask
   - Precautions: Discard or bag all soiled articles, contaminated with infective materials. Reusable articles to be disinfected and sterilized appropriately.
B. Contact Isolation
   - Purpose: Prevents transmission of highly transmissible infections spread by close or direct contact.
   - Disease conditions: Acute respiratory infections in infants and young children, impetigo, herpes simplex and infections by resistant bacteria.
   - Room: Separate room. Patients infected with same organisms may share the room.
   - Protective devices: Gown required if soiling is expected. Gloves required when touching infected material is expected. Mask required when coming in close contact with the patient.
   - Precautions: Discard or bag and label articles contaminated with infective material. Reusable articles to be disinfected and sterilized as appropriate.
C. Respiratory isolation:
   - Purpose: Prevents transmission of infection through air droplets.
   - Disease conditions: Measles, meningitis, mumps, pneumonia, haemophilus influenza in children.
   - Room: Separate room. patient infected with same organism may share room.
   - Protective devices:
     - Gown—Not required
     - Gloves—Not required
     - Mask—Required when coming close to the patient.
   - Precautions: Discard or bag and label articles contaminated with infective material. Reusable items to be disinfected and sterilized. Patients should not use same bathroom.
D. Enteric precautions:
   - Purpose—Prevents infections transmitted by direct or indirect contact with feces.
   - Disease conditions—Cholera, Hepatitis, Gastroenteritis caused by infectious organisms.
   - Room—Separate room if patient's hygiene is poor. Patients with same organsims may share room.
   - Protective devices—
     - Gown—Indicated if soiling is likely.

- Gloves—Indicated when touching infective material.
- Mask—required if patient coughs and does not cover mouth.
- Precautions—Articles to be thoroughly cleansed and disinfected or discarded.

E. Drainage and secretion precautions:
- Purposes—Prevents transmission of organism by contact with purulent material or drainage from infected body site.
- Disease conditions—Abscess, burn infection, infected wounds
- Room—Separate room not indicated
- Protective devices—
  - Gown—required if soiling with infective material is likely.
  - Gloves—Indicated when touching infective material
  - Mask—Not indicated
  - Goggles when there is high risk of exposure to splash.
- Precautions—Discard or bag and label articles contaminated with infective material. Reusable articles to be disinfected and sterilized.

F. Universal blood and body fluid precautions:
- Purpose—Prevents contact with infected blood or body fluids containing blood.
- Disease condition—HIV, hepatitis B, syphilis.
- Room—Separate room if patient's hygiene is poor.
- Protective devices—
  - Gown—Indicated during procedures likely to generate splashes of blood or body fluids.
  - Gloves—Indicated when touching blood or body fluids containing visible blood, mucous membranes or non-intact skin of all patients.
  - Mask—Indicated during procedures likely to generate droplets of blood.
  - Goggles—Indicated if splashes/spurts are expected.
- Precautions
  - Discard or bag and label articles contaminated with blood or body fluids.
  - Disinfect and sterilize articles.
  - Avoid needle sticks
  - Dispose of used needles in puncture—resistant container.
  - Clean blood spills promptly with solution of sodium hypochlorite or bleach.

G. Care of severely immunocompromised patients.
- Purpose—Protects patients with lowered immunity and resistance from acquiring infectious organisms.
- Disease conditions——Leukemia, lymphoma, aplastic anemia
- Room—Separate room
- Protective devices
  - Gown—required
  - Gloves—required
  - Mask—required for all persons coming in contact with patient
- Precautions—Use sterile gloves for open wound or burns.

## 3.14: APPLYING RESTRAINTS

## DEFINITION

Mechanical devices used to immobilize and protect patient from injury or to facilitate examination, treatment and care.
Purposes:
1. To provide safety
2. To facilitate examination
3. To carry out diagnostic and therapeutic procedures.
4. To keep the child in desired position.

## ARTICLES

1. Draw sheet or baby blanket for babies (newborn).
2. Elbow restraint-cloth with 5-6 pockets in which spatulas are kept(children).
3. Clove hitch knot-4"bandage, cottonpads, knitted bandage.
4. Padding to protect bony prominences.

## PROCEDURE

| | Nursing action | Rationale |
|---|---|---|
| 1 | Identify patient in need of restraints, e.g. confused or disoriented patients, patients requiring immobilization of extremity, and children requiring immobilization of elbow joint to prevent dislodgment of therapeutic equipment. | Restraints are used to reduce risk of patient falling from /out of bed, chair or wheel chair. Prevents interruption of therapy such as traction and IV infusion. |
| 2 | Check physician's order and assess type of restraint needed. | Nursing assessment and institutional policies aids in determining what type of restraints are used. Physician's order is necessary to apply restraints. |
| 3 | Explain to patient and family about the importance of restraint, type of restraint selected and anticipated duration of use. | Restraint can increase confusion or combativeness in patient. Family may express anger about restraint. Explanation and reinforcement can reduce or prevent negative perceptions. |
| 4 | Wash hands | Reduces transmission of microorganisms. |
| 5 | Apply selected restraints<br>a. Jacket restraint:Vest like garment that usually crosses in front of patient (Figure 3.14(a)) | a. Restrains patient while lying or reclining in bed and while sitting in chair or wheelchair. |

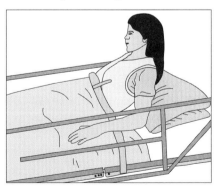 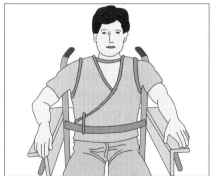

**Figure 3.14(a):** Jacket restraints

*Contd...*

*Contd...*

b. Belt restraint: Device that secures patient on stretcher or chair. Avoid placing belt too tightly across patient's chest or abdomen

b. Restraints prevent patient from falling out of chair or stretcher

c. Extremity restraints (ankle or wrist restraints) (Figure 3.14(b))
Restraints designed to immobilize one or all extremities. Commercially available limb restraints are composed of sheep's skin and foam pads that come in contact with skin. Modification of commercial restraints can be devised by making clove-hitch restraints (Strips of cloth that does not tighten if patient pulls against it.) Make figure of eight with the strip of cloth and then pick up loops before attaching restraints to patient's limbs. Place gauze or padding around extremity to be restrained and then place loops of clove hitch directly over padded surface (Figure 3.14(c))

c. Maintains immobilization of extremity to protect patient from injury or accidental removal of therapeutic device (e.g. IV tube or Foley catheter)

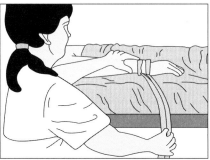 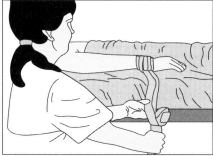

**Figure 3.14(b):** Wrist restraints

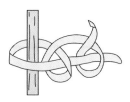 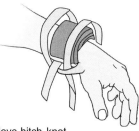

**Figure 3.14(c):** Clove-hitch knot

d. Mitten restraint: Thumb less mitten devices to restrain patient's hand (Figure 3.14 (d))

d. Prevents patient from dislodging, invasive equipment, removing dressing or scratching.

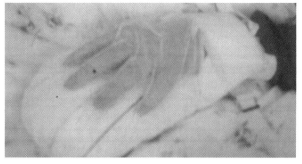

**Figure 3.14(d):** Mitten restraint

*Contd...*

*Contd...*

e. Elbow restraint: Piece of fabric with slots in which wooden spatula are placed so that elbow joints remain rigid (Figure 3.14(e))

e. Used for infants and children to prevent elbow flexion. Maintains short term restraint of small child or infant for examination or treatment involving head and neck.

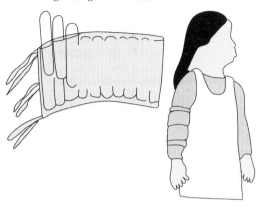

**Figure 3.14(e):** Elbow restraints

f. Swaddle wrap: Blanket or sheet opened on bed or crib, with one corner folded toward center. Baby is placed on blanket with shoulders at fold and feet towards opposite corner.
With baby's right arm straight down against the body, right side of the blanket is pulled firmly across the right shoulder and chest and secured beneath left side of the body. Left arm is placed straight against side and left side of the blanket is brought across shoulder and chest and locked beneath baby's body and tucked or fastened securely with safety pins (Figure 3.14(f)).

f. Swaddle wrapping device effectively controls movement of baby's torso and extremities.

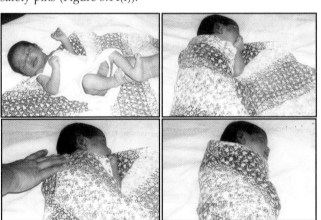

**Figure 3.14(f):** Swaddle wrapping

| 6 | Bony prominences should be padded before applying restraint | Padding decrease injury to underlying skin. |
| 7 | Restraints should be completely removed at least every 2 hours for 30 mins. Patient should not be left unattended. | Provides opportunity to assess skin integrity and provides skin care. Areas on which restraints were applied are often massaged. |

*Contd...*

*Contd...*

| 8 | Restraints should be secured so that they cannot be undone by patient. | When patient is able to undo restraints, purpose of restraint is negated. |
|---|---|---|
| 9 | Restraints applied to patient in bed or on stretcher should be attached to bed frame, not side rails. | Release of side rails while restraint remains attached can result in injury to patient's musculoskeletal system |
| 10 | Wash hands | Reduces transmission of microorganisms. |
| 11 | Assess adequacy of restraints and presence of any potential injury to musculoskeletal system every 2 hours | Timely assessment enables nurse to routinely observe musculoskeletal system and prevents any complication from restraint device. |
| 12 | Observe for correct application of restraints every 2 hours | Incorrect application of restraints can result in injury to patient's musculoskeletal system from fall or muscle strains. |
| 13 | Inspect skin for adequate color change, check capillary refill and palpate pulses distal to restraints every 30 minutes | Timely identification of impaired circulation related to the restraint device reduces risk of damage to extremities. |
| 14 | Perform passive ROM exercises every 2 hours for restrained extremities. | Reduces risk of injury from restricted mobility of extremity. |
| 15 | Record in "nurses" notes nursing assessment before and after restraints were used focussing on patient's safety, patient's level of orientation, type of restraints selected, patient's response to the restraint, skin integrity and status of musculoskeletal system. Notes should also include documentation that the restraints are loosened, ROM is performed and skin integrity is assessed every 2 hours | • Documents that patient's physical safety was at risk and specific restraint was warranted.<br>• Documents presence or absence of any break in skin integrity and status of musculoskeletal system before and after application of restraints. |

## SPECIAL CONSIDERATION

1. If patient is violent and noncompliant, remove one restraint at a time or have staff assistance while removing restraints.
2. Special attention should be given towards safety of patients who are immobilized, emaciated, and for patients with fever, chronic illness and impaired skin integrity since they are at risk of developing musculoskeletal injury

# Chapter 4

# Nutrition

## 4.1: SERVING A NORMAL DIET

### DEFINITION

Meeting the nutritional needs of a patient by serving normal/regular diet.

### PURPOSES

1. To maintain adequate nutrition of the individual.
2. To promote optimal nutrition.
3. To restore the individual to a satisfactory nutritional status, if his nutritional balance has been disturbed.

### ARTICLES

1. A tray containing prepared diet (solid/fluid)
2. Face towel
3. Water

### PROCEDURE

|  | Nursing action | Rationale |
|---|---|---|
| 1 | Wash hands. | Reduces risk of transmission of microorganisms. |
| 2 | Help the patient to wash hands and face, in preparation for eating. | This promotes patient's comfort and helps patient to prepare mentally for a pleasant experience. |
| 3 | Remove any unpleasant visual stimuli such as commodes, bedpans and urinals from the unit. | Unpleasant sights and smell can decrease a patient's appetite. |
| 4 | If possible, raise the head of the patient's bed or have the patient sit in a chair | The upright position reduces the risk of aspiration and reflux. |
| 5 | Check to be sure that the food corresponds to what the patient has ordered | Promotes increased intake of food. |
| 6 | Be sure the food is in a form the patient can eat. Check for presence of any specialised utensils the patient may require, like spoons, forks etc. | Promotes increased intake of food. |
| 7 | Check for tubes, braces or dressings that may make eating more difficult. | |
| 8 | Place a napkin or protective cover over the patient if needed | Promotes cleanliness and improves patient's esteem. |
| 9 | Arrange food in a tray and place on the over-bed table or in a manner convenient for the patient to eat. | |
| 10 | Cut food into large pieces, open cartons and pour fluids. Open straws if present and place them in glasses. | |
| 11 | Allow patient to make choices regarding the order in which food is eaten, the speed at which patient eats, and the amount patient will eat | This promotes patient's independence and self esteem. |
| 12 | Do not hurry the patient through the meal | If hurried, a patient may aspirate. |
| 13 | Use this time as an opportunity to converse with the patient. | Improves interpersonal relationship. |
| 14 | Do not discuss stressful events with the patient | Stressful topics at mealtime can decrease appetite and delay digestion. |

*Contd...*

*Contd...*

| | | |
|---|---|---|
| 15 | When the patient decides she or he is finished with the meal, remove the tray. | |
| 16 | Encourage the patient to remain in sitting position for at least 15 min following the meal | This decreases the risk of reflux and aspiration. |
| 17 | Help the patient to clean up following the meal. Allow patient to wash hands and face and clean dentures if needed | Helps to promote patient's comfort. |
| 18 | Wash hands | Reduces the transmission of microorganisms. |
| 19 | Record the time, type and amount of food taken and tolerance to food. | |

## SPECIAL CONSIDERATIONS

1. Note any food preferences, allergies or restrictions of diet.
2. Note the diet the patient is on and indicate any special preparation or utensils the patient needs while eating.
3. Note any eating difficulties or how well the patient tolerated the meal.
4. Check for medications to be administered before, after and along with the meal, e. g. insulin.

## 4.2: FEEDING A HELPLESS PATIENT

### DEFINITION

Assisting a helpless patient to take food and fluids..

### PURPOSE

1. To assist patient to meet his nutritional needs

### ARTICLES

1. Tray containing prepared diet.
2. Face towel and water.
3. Kidney tray
4. Backrest and cardiac table
5. Fork and spoon
6. Feeding cup with water.

### PROCEDURE

| | Nursing action | Rationale |
|---|---|---|
| 1. | Explain procedure to the patient and assess how he can participate. | Gains confidence and co-operation of patient. |
| 2. | Position the patient comfortably, preferably in Fowler's position. | Fowler's position reduces risk of aspiration. |
| 3. | Assist the patient to wash his hands and face | Prepares patient for taking food. |
| 4. | Place towel over chest and around the neck | Protects garments from soiling. |
| 5. | Make sure that therapeutic restrictions are considered. Check the diet and ensure that it is the one that was ordered. | Ensures that patient takes the right type of diet. |
| 6. | Create a pleasant environment. | Increases appetite. |
| 7. | Wash your hands. | Prevents cross infection. |
| 8. | Sit or stand at the side of patient | |
| 9. | Consider the patient' preferences while feeding and encourage his participation to the extent possible. | Enhances patient co-operation and self esteem. |
| 10. | Feed the patient in small spoonfuls waiting for him to chew and swallow one mouthful before next (Figure 4.2(a)) | Taking small mouthful of food at a time helps in effective chewing and reduces risk of aspiration. |

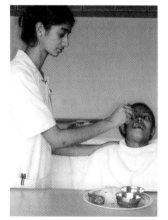

**Figure 4.2(a):** Feeding helpless patient

*Contd...*

*Contd...*

| 11. | Encourage the patient to take all the food served to him, but do not force. | Forcing food causes vomiting. |
|---|---|---|
| 12. | Give water in between if patient prefers water. | Relieves obstruction if any and helps in swallowing. |
| 13. | When the patient has eaten food and he feels satisfied, stop feeding and give him a glass of water if he prefers. | |
| 14. | Provide articles for rinsing mouth and encourage patient to do so. | Rinsing helps in removing food particles from between teeth. |
| 15. | Dry lips and face with towel | Ensures comfort |
| 16. | Replace articles and wash hands | |
| 17 | Record in Nurse's record the type of diet, time of feeding, amount taken and tolerance. | Gives information about patient's response after feeding. |
| 18 | Record fluid taken, in intake – output record | Ensures accurate documentation. |

## SPECIAL CONSIDERATIONS

1. Patient should be undisturbed by treatments, dressing, visitors, doctor's rounds, unpleasant sounds and odour during meal time.
2. Room should be well ventilated, quiet and comfortable and remove all unappetizing objects like bedpan, urinal, etc. from the premises.
3. Encourage patient to eat by himself if possible and to the extent possible.
4. When blind patients are fed, they should be told what feed they are being given as patients have the right to know what they are eating.

# 4.3: INSERTION OF A NASOGASTRIC TUBE

## DEFINITION

Insertion of a small-bore tube to the stomach through the nasopharynx.

## PURPOSES

1. Decompression of stomach (to remove fluids and gas)
2. To prevent or relieve nausea and vomiting after surgery or traumatic events by decompressing the stomach.
3. To determine the amount of pressure and motor activity of GI tract (diagnostic studies).
4. To give gastric lavage (To irrigate the stomach in case of active bleeding or poisoning).
5. To obtain specimen (gastric contents) for laboratory studies.
6. To administer medication.
7. To give gastric gavage (feed directly into the stomach).

## ARTICLES

A tray containing:
1. Kidney trays – 2
2. Mackintosh and towel
3. Cotton tipped applicators
4. Saline
5. Levine's tube or Ryles tube size 8-12 Fr.
6. Water soluble lubricant such as glycerine or liquid paraffin.
7. Adhesive plaster and scissors.
8. Gauze pieces.
9. Clean syringe, size 10-20 ml
10. Measuring cup or marked drinking cup.
11. Bowl with water
12. Clamp
13. Suction apparatus (optional)
14. Pen light/flash light
15. Tongue blade
16. Glass of water

## PROCEDURE

| | Nursing action | Rationale |
|---|---|---|
| 1. | Identify the patient. | Helps in determining the appropriate size of the nasogastric tube for patient. |
| 2. | Check the physician's order for any precautions such as for positioning or movement. | |
| 3. | Ascertain the level of consciousness and ability to follow instructions. | Avoids the risk of aspiration of fluid. |
| 4. | Ascertain the ability of patient to maintain desired position during insertion. | Facilitates insertion of the tube. |
| 5. | Review the patient's medical history for any nasal lesions, bleeding polyps or deviated nasal septum. | May require change in the route of nutritional support, e.g. orogastric insertion. |

*Contd...*

# Nutrition

| 6. | Wash hands | Prevents infection. |
|---|---|---|
| 7. | Explain procedure to patient | Reduces anxiety and helps patient to assist in insertion of the tube. |
| 8. | Place the patient in a high – Fowler's position (comatose patients in semi Fowler's position). | Facilitates insertion of the tube and reduces risk of aspiration. |
| 9. | Place mackintosh and towel across the chest. | Prevents soiling of patient's dress. |
| 10. | Measure the length of the tube, i.e. from tip of nose to tip of the ear lobe and to the tip of xiphoid process and mark with tape.<br>For oro-gastric intubation, the tube is measured from the lips to the tip of xiphoid process of sternum (Figure 4.3(a)). | The measured length approximates the distance from the nose to the stomach. (for duodenal or jejunal placement an additional 20 to 30 cm is required). |

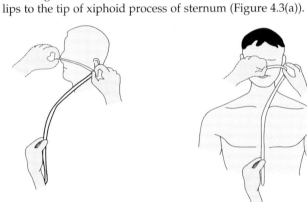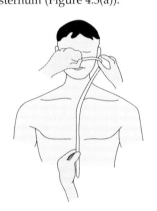

**Figure 4.3(a):** Measuring length of nasogastric tube

| 11. | Cut the adhesive tape 10 cm long. | For easy accessibility. |
|---|---|---|
| 12. | Put on clean gloves | Prevents contamination from secretions. |
| 13. | Lubricate the tip of the tube about 6-8 inches with water soluble lubricant, using a gauze piece. | Lubrication reduces friction between mucus membrane and the tube. Water soluble lubricant easily dissolves if it accidentally enter the lungs. |
| 14. | Insert the tube through the left nostril to the back of the throat, aiming back and down towards the ear (Figure 4.3(b)). | Natural contours facilitate the passage of the tube. |

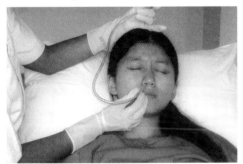

**Figure 4.3(b):** Inserting nasogastric tube

| 15. | Flex the patient's head towards the chest after the tube has passed the nasopharynx. | Reduces the risk of tube entering the trachea. |

*Contd...*

*Contd...*

| | |
|---|---|
| 16. Encourage patient to swallow by giving sips of water when possible. | Facilitates passage of tube. Swallowing closes the epiglottis over the trachea and facilitates passage of tube into esophagus. |
| 17. Advance tube 3-4 inches each time patient swallows until desired length has been passed.<br>Do not force tube. When resistance is met or patient starts to gag, cough, choke or become cyanosed, stop advancing tube and pull tube back. Check for position of tube in back of throat with tongue blade. | Reduces discomfort and trauma.<br><br>Tube may be coiled or kinked or in oro-pharynx or trachea. |
| 18. If there are signs of distress such as gasping, coughing or cyanosis pull back the tube for some length and check if patient's distress is relieved. If it is relieved reinsert after few seconds. If patient develops respiratory distress again, immediately remove the tube. | The tube may have entered the trachea. |
| 19. Perform one of the following measures to check for the placement of the tube:<br>  a. Aspirate gastric contents and check pH using litmus paper if available.<br>  b. Place the end of the tube in a bowl of water to check for continuous air bubbles in water.<br>  c. Ask the patient to speak<br>  d. X-ray may be done | a. Aspirated contents indicates that the tube is in the stomach.<br>b. Continuous air bubbles indicate that tube is in the respiratory tract.<br>c. Patient will not be able to speak if tube is in the trachea |
| 20. Examine the patient's mouth using a tongue blade and flash light/pen light. | The tube may be coiled in the mouth. |
| 21. Secure tube with tape and avoid pressure on nares<br>  a. Use a 10 cm (4 inch) piece of tape, split at one end. (Place intact end of tape over bridge of nose. Carefully wrap two ends around tube) (Figure 4.3(c)).<br><br>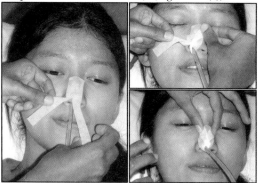<br>**Figure 4.3(c):** Securing tube with tape | |
| 22. Fasten end of tube to gown. | Reduces friction on nares when patient moves. |
| 23. Make patient comfortable in bed and provide oral hygiene every 4-6 hours. | Promotes comfort and integrity of oral mucous membrane. |
| 24. Remove gloves, dispose of articles and wash hands. | Reduces transmission of microorganisms. |
| 25. Record type of tube placed, aspirate returned, and patient tolerance. | Documents exact procedure. |

## SPECIAL CONSIDERATION

Insufflation of air into tube followed by auscultation is no longer considered reliable in determining tube placement, because sounds transmitted by insufflation may be transmitted from the pleural space into upper abdomen, thus giving false impression of tube placement.

## 4.4: ADMINISTRATION OF A TUBE FEEDING

### DEFINITION

Administration of feed directly into the stomach through a tube passed into the stomach through the nose (nasogastric) or mouth (orogastric).

### PURPOSES

1. To provide adequate nourishment to patients who cannot feed themselves.
2. To administer medication.
3. To provide nourishment to patients who cannot be feed through mouth, e.g. surgery in oral cavity, unconscious or comatosed state.

### INDICATIONS

1. Head and neck injury.
2. Coma.
3. Obstruction of esophagus or oropharynx.
4. Severe anorexia nervosa.
5. Recurrent episodes of aspiration.
6. Increased metabolic needs – burns, cancer, etc.
7. Poor oral intake.

### ARTICLES

1. Formula feed
2. Graduated container
3. Large syringe (30 to 60 ml)
4. Water in a container
5. Stethoscope
6. Kidney tray
7. Towel
8. Clean gloves

### PROCEDURE

| | Nursing action | Rationale |
|---|---|---|
| 1. | Identify patient and explain procedure to patient and that feeding will take around 10-20 minutes to complete. Also explain that patient will experience a feeling of fullness after feeding. | Proper explanation allays anxiety and ensures co-operation<br>Explanation to be given to patients who are comatosed or unconscious as they may hear and perceive the instructions. |
| 2 | Assess for food allergies, time of last feed, bowel sounds and lab values. | Proper assessment will prevent risk of complication. |
| 3 | Place container with feed in warm water. | High temperature may damage the tube and cold feeds may cause discomfort to patient. |
| 4 | Assist patient to Fowler's position (35-45 degree) at least | Fowler's position enhances gravitational flow of feed through tube and prevents risk of aspiration. |
| 5 | Wash hands | Reduces risk of transmission of microorganisms. |

*Contd...*

*Contd...*

| | | |
|---|---|---|
| 6 | Spread towel and mackintosh over patient's chest. | Protects patient and bed linen from soiling. |
| 7 | Don gloves and attach syringe to nasogastric tube. | |
| 8 | Aspirate stomach contents. If there is doubt about tube placement (Figure 4.4(a)) inform physician and obtain an order for X-ray. | If residual gastric contents exceed 100 ml for intermittent tube feedings or greater than 1.5 times the hourly rate for continuous feeding, withhold feed and notify physician. |

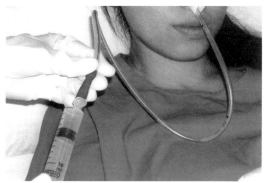

Figure 4.4 (a): Checking placement by aspirating nasogastric tube

| | | |
|---|---|---|
| 9 | If residual contents are within normal limits and placement of the tube has been confirmed, return gastric contents to stomach through syringe using gravity to regulate flow. | Returning gastric contents to stomach prevents fluid and electrolyte imbalance. |
| 10 | If tube placement is confirmed in stomach, pinch the feeding tube and attach barrel of feeding syringe to tube. | Pinching of feeding tube prevents air from entering the stomach and causing distension. |
| 11 | Fill syringe barrel with water and allow fluid to flow in by gravity, by raising barrel above level of patient's head. | Water clears the tube and the rate of flow is regulated by raising or lowering the syringe. |
| 12 | Pour feed into syringe barrel and allow it to flow by gravity. Keep on pouring feed/formula to barrel when it is three quarters empty. Pinch tube whenever necessary to stop when pouring.(Figure 4.4 (b)). | Prevents air from entering tube. |

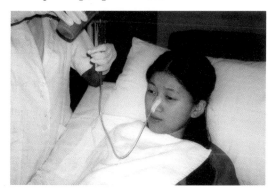

Figure 4.4 (b): Pouring feed into syringe barrel

| | | |
|---|---|---|
| 13 | After feeding is completed, flush tube with at least 30 cc of plain water. | Prevents clogging of feeding tube. |
| 14 | After tube is cleared close end of feeding tube. | Prevents leakage. |

*Contd...*

*Contd...*

| 15 | Rinse equipment with warm water and dry. Replace every 24 hrs as per policy. | Prevents bacterial concentration. |
| --- | --- | --- |
| 16 | Keep head of bed elevated for 30-60 minutes after feeding | Prevents aspiration. |
| 17 | Wash hands. | Reduces risk of transmission of microorganisms. |
| 18 | Document type and amount of feeding, amount of water given and tolerance of feed. | |
| 19 | Monitor for breath sounds, bowel sounds, gastric distension, diarrhoea, constipation and intake and output. | Evaluates for aspiration effects on gastro-intestinal system and therapeutic effect of feeding. |
| 20 | Instruct patient to notify nurse if he experiences sensation of fullness, nausea or vomiting. | May indicate intolerance of feeding. |

## SPECIAL CONSIDERATIONS

1. Intermittent/continuous feeding of solution from, an intravenous pole and adjusting rate of administration by flow regulators are done in some situations (Figure 4.4(c))
2. Siphon method can be used to administer clear fluids. This is done by immersing tip of tube in feed, taking care to avoid air entering into it and then raising container 12 inches above patient's head and observing flow of fluids.

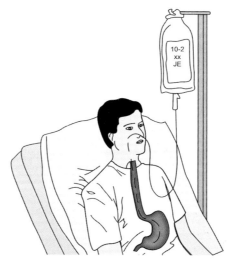

**Figure 4.4(c):** Continuous nasogastric feeding

## 4.5: FEEDING THROUGH A GASTROSTOMY/JEJUNOSTOMY TUBE

### DEFINITION

Administration of food in fluid form through a gastrostomy or jejunostomy tube which is placed through a surgical opening into the stomach or jejunum.

### PURPOSE

To maintain nutritional status of a patient whose upper gastrointestinal tract is bypassed.

### ARTICLES

1. Disposable gavage bag and tubing.
2. 60 ml syringe
3. Stethoscope
4. Feed
5. IV stand
6. Administration set.

### PROCEDURE

| | Nursing action | Rationale |
|---|---|---|
| 1. | Identify patient's need. | The type and timings of feed needs to be planned. |
| 2. | Assess patient for allergies. | Prevents patient from developing localized or systemic allergic responses. |
| 3. | Auscultate for bowel sounds before feeding. | Bowel sounds indicate presence of peristalsis and ability of gastrointestinal tract to digest nutrients. |
| 4. | Verify physician's order for formula, rate and frequency. | Reduces errors in the feeding process. |
| 5. | Assess gastrostomy site for skin breakdown, irritation or drainage. | Infection, pressure from gastrostomy tube, or drainage of gastric secretions can cause skin breakdown. |
| 6. | Obtain baseline weight and laboratory values. | Tube feedings must be ordered by physician. |
| 7. | Wash hands | Prevents cross infection. |
| 8. | Prepare bag and tubing to administer feed<br>a. Connect tubing and bag<br>b. Fill bag and tubing with feed. | Administering of feed through tubing prevents excess air entering gastrointestinal tract |
| 9. | Explain procedure to patient. | Proper explanation enables patient to be informed. Informed patient is more cooperative and feels more at ease. |
| 10. | Place patient in Fowler's position or elevate head of bed 30 degrees. | Elevating patients head helps prevent chances of aspiration. |
| 11. | Check placement of gastric tube<br>a. Aspirate gastric secretions and check gastric residual contents.<br><br>b. Auscultate over left upper quadrant with stethoscope and inject 10-20 ml of air into the tube using a syringe. | Presence of gastric contents indicates that end of tube is in stomach. Gastric residual contents determines if gastric emptying is delayed.<br>A gurgling sound can be heard as air enters stomach. |

*Contd...*

*Contd...*

12. **Initiate feeding:**
    a. *Bolus or intermittent feeding*
    - Pinch proximal end of gastrostomy tube
    - Attach syringe to end of tube and elevate to 18 inches above the patient's abdomen
    - Fill syringe with formula . Allow syringe to empty gradually and refill it until prescribed amount has been delivered to the patient (Figure 4.5(a))

Prevents air from entering the patient's stomach
Gradual emptying of tube feeding by gravity from a syringe or gavage bag reduces the risk of diarrhea induced by bolus tube feedings.

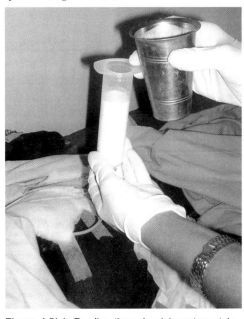

**Figure 4.5(a):** Feeding through a jejunostomy tube

    - If gavage bag is used, attach bag to the end of the feeding tube and raise, bag 18 inches above patient's abdomen. Fill bag with prescribed amount of feed, allow bag to empty gradually over 30 minutes
    b. *Continuous drip method*
    - Hang gavage bag to IV pole.
    - Connect end of bag to the proximal end of the gastrostomy tube
    - Connect infusion pump and set rate

Continuous feeding method is designed to deliver a prescribed hourly feeding. This method reduces the risk of diarrhea. Patients who receive continuous drip feedings should have residual gastric contents checked every 4 hours

13. When tube feedings are not being administered, clamp the proximal end of the feeding tube.

Prevents air from entering the stomach between feedings.

14. Administer water via feeding tube as ordered with or between feedings.

Provides patient with source of water to help maintain fluid and electrolyte balance.

15. Rinse bag and tubing with warm water after all bolus feedings are given.

16. Change gastrostomy exit site dressing as needed. Inspect exit site every shift. Clean ostomy site daily with warm water and mild soap. A small gauze dressing may be applied to exit site.

Leakage of gastric drainage may cause irritation and excoriation of skin around feeding tube.

*Contd...*

*Contd...*

| | |
|---|---|
| 17. Dispose of supplies and wash hands. | Reduces transmission of microorganisms. |
| 18. Evaluate patient's tolerance of tube feeding. | Tolerance of tube feeding is evaluated by checking the amount of aspirate every 4 hours. |
| 19. Monitor blood glucose every 6 hours if hospital policy requires it. | Alerts nurse to patient's intolerance of glucose. |
| 20. Monitor intake and output every shift. | Intake and output are indications of fluid balance. |
| 21. Weigh patient daily. | Weight gain is an indicator of nutritional status. |
| 22. Observe return of normal laboratory values. | Improving laboratory values or electrolytes, indicate return to normal nutritional status. |
| 23. Observe stoma site for skin integrity. | Gastric secretion can cause injury and necrosis at stoma site. |
| 24. Record amount and type of feeding, patency of tube and any untoward effects. | Documents patient's reaction to therapy and identifies presence of any adverse reactions. |
| 25. Report to on coming nursing staff, type of feeding, status of gastrostomy tube, patient's tolerance and adverse effects. | Provides new nursing personnel with status of gastric feeding. Allows new nursing staff to plan for next feeding. |

## SPECIAL CONSIDERATIONS

1. In case of aspiration of feed, suction patient, notify physician and obtain chest X-ray film. Risk of aspiration, may be lessened if head of bed is elevated to 30 to 45 degrees during feeding and for 1 hour after feeding.
2. In case of diarrhea, decrease feeding, review medication and notify physician.
3. In case of nausea and vomiting, notify physician and withhold feeding.
4. If bowel sounds are absent, notify physician before initiating feeding.
5. Gastrostomy tube is appropriate for long-term use.
6. Intermittent feeding is preferred in infants because of possible perforation of stomach and irritation to mucous membrane.
   Tube feeding should be gradually advanced to prevent diarrhea and gastric intolerance of formula.

# 4.6: ADMINISTRATION OF TOTAL PARENTERAL NUTRITION

## DEFINITION

Intravenous administration of varying combinations of hypertonic or isotonic glucose, lipids, amino acid, electrolytes, vitamins and trace elements through a venous access device (VAD) directly into the intravascular fluid to provide nutrients for patients who are unable to receive adequate nutrition through gastrointestinal tract.

## PURPOSES

1. To provide nutrients required for the normal metabolism, tissue maintenance, repair and energy demands.
2. To bypass the GI tract for patients who are unable to take food orally.

## INDICATIONS

1. Patients who cannot tolerate enteral nutrition because of:
   - Paralytic ileus
   - Intestinal obstruction
   - Acute pancreatitis
   - Short bowel syndrome
   - Inflammatory bowel disease
   - Gastrointestinal fistula
   - Severe diarrhea
   - Persistent vomiting
   - Malabsorption.
2. Hypermetabolic states for which enteral therapy is either not possible or inadequate
   - Severe burns
   - Trauma/surgery
   - Sepsis
   - Multiple fractures
   - Tumor in GI tract.
3. Patient at risk for malnutrition because of
   - Gross under weight (more than 80% below the standard)
   - Gross over weight (more than 120% above the standard)
   - Alcoholism
   - NPO for more than 5 days.

## METHODS OF PARENTERAL NUTRITION

1. Total nutrient admixture into a central vein (TNA).
   This parenteral formula combines carbohydrates in the form of a concentrated (20 to 70%) dextrose solution, proteins in the form of amino acids; lipids in the form of an emulsion (10 to 20%), including triglycerides, phospholipids, glycerol and water; vitamins and minerals.
   It is indicated for patients requiring parenteral feeding for seven or more days. Given through a central vein. Often into the superior vena cava.
2. Peripheral parenteral nutrition (PPN)
   This parenteral formula combines carbohydrates a lesser concentrated glucose solution with amino acids, vitamins, minerals and lipids.
   Given through a peripheral vein and it is indicated for patients requring parenteral nutrition for fewer than 7 days.

3. Total parenteral nutrition (TPN)
   This parenteral formula combines glucose, amino acids, vitamins and minerals
   Given through a central IV line. If lipids are needed, they are given
   Intermittently mixed with the TPN.
4. Fat emulsion (lipids)
   It is composed of triglycerides (10-20%), egg, phospholipids, glycerol and water. May be given centrally or peripherally.

## ARTICLES

1. Central venous access devices: Long-term VADs such as Hickman, Broviac or Groshung catheters or peripherally inserted central catheter (PICC line) or peripheral IV access.
2. Volume control infuser.
3. Filters: 0.22 micron for TPN (without fat emulsion).
   3.2 micron filter for TNA or fat emulsion.
4. Bag of parenteral nutrition.
5. Administration tubing with Luer-Lock connections.
6. Hypoallergic tape.
7. Face mask (optional).
8. Sterile gloves.

## PROCEDURE

| | Nursing action | Rationale |
|---|---|---|
| 1 | Assess the need for parenteral nutrition by performing nutritional assessment. | Provides baseline data to compare changes after parenteral nutrition is started. |
| 2 | Check physician's order for method of parenteral nutrition (TNA, TPN, PPN or lipids) and flow rate. | Parenteral therapy must be ordered by physician. |
| 3 | Explain the procedure in detail to the patient and relatives | |
| 4 | Obtain informed consent | |
| 5 | Collect needed equipment for the procedure | |
| 6 | Remove the bag of parenteral nutrition from refrigerator at least 1 hour before procedure (if refrigerated) | Decreases incidence of hypothermia, pain and vasospasm |
| 7 | Inspect fluid for presence of cracking or creaming or any change in constitution. If present, discard and check for expiry date. Confirm with order. | Indicates fluid separation. TPN solution should be clear without clouding. |
| 8 | Wash hands, don cap, mask, gown and sterile gloves | Follows very strict aseptic precautions. |
| 9 | Using strict aseptic technique, attach tubing (with filter) to TNA bag and purge out air. | Prevents chances of developing air embolus. |
| 10 | Close all clamps on new tubing and insert tubing into volume control infuser. | |
| 11 | Place the patient in supine position and turn head away from VAD insertion site. | Supine position opens the angle between clavicle and first rib and turning head away from site will decrease possible microbial contamination of site. |
| 12 | Clean the insertion site with alcohol and povidone iodine solution. | |
| 13 | Assist physician while inserting VAD. | |

*Contd...*

*Contd...*

| 14 | After insertion of VAD, connect tubing to hub of VAD using sterile technique and make sure that the connection is secured using Luer-Lock connection. |
| 15 | Open all clamps and regulate flow through volume control infuser. |
| 16 | Monitor administration hourly, assessing for integrity of fluid and administration system and patient tolerance. |
| 17 | Record the procedure. |

**Table 4.6.1:** Complication of peripheral parenteral nutrition

## COMPLICATIONS

| | Complication | Causes | Interventions |
|---|---|---|---|
| 1 | Sepsis | • High glucose content of fluid.<br>• Venous access device contamination | • Monitor temperature, WBC count and insertion site for signs and symptoms of infection.<br>• Maintain strict surgical asepsis when changing dressing and tubing.<br>• Consider decreasing glucose content of fluid.<br>• Consider removal of venous access device with replacement in alternate site.<br>• If blood culture is positive consider institution of antibiotic therapy. |
| 2 | Electrolyte imblance | • Iatrogenic<br>• Effect of underlying diseases, i.e. fistula, diarrhea, vomiting. | • Monitor for signs and symptoms of electrolyte imbalances.<br>• Treat underlying cause<br>• Change concentration of electrolytes in TNA as necessary. |
| 3 | Hyperglycemia | • High glucose content of fluid<br>• Insufficient insulin secretion | • Monitor blood glucose frequently<br>• Decrease glucose content of fluid if possible.<br>• Administer exogenous insulin. |
| 4 | Hypoglycemia | • Abrupt discontinuation of TNA administration through a central vein | • After discontinuation of centrally administered TNA, start 10% dextrose at the same rate. |
| 5 | Hypervolemia | • Iatrogenic<br>• Underlying disease such as congestive heart failure and renal failure (CHF) | • Monitor intake and output, daily weight, CVP, breath sounds and peripheral edema<br>• Consider administering more concentrated TNA solution. |
| 6 | Hyperosmolar diuresis | • High osmolarity of parenteral nutritional fluid | • Consider decreasing the concentration or amount of fluid administered. |
| 7 | Hepatic dysfunction | • High concentration of carbohydrates/ Fats relative to protein. | • Monitor liver function tests, triglyceride levels and presence of jaundice.<br>• Consider alteration in formula. |
| 8 | Hypercarbia | • High carbohydrate content of fluid | • Consider changing formula to increase the proportion of fat relative to carbohydrate. |
| 9 | Lipids intolerance | • Low birth weight or premature infant<br>• History of liver disease<br>• History of elevated triglycerides | • Monitor for bleeding<br>• Monitor oxygen levels for impaired oxygenation<br>• Monitor fat overload syndrome |

*Contd...*

*Contd...*

| | | | • Monitor triglyceride levels and liver function test, hepatosplenomegaly, decreased coagulation, cyanosis, dyspnea.<br>• Monitor allergic reactions such as nausea, vomiting, headache, chest pain, back pain and fever.<br>• Administer lipid containing solution slowly. |
|---|---|---|---|
| 10 | Lipid particulate aggregation | • Unstable mixture of dextrose solution with lipid emulsion | • Observe for cracking or creaming of fluid and avoid use of fluid with these characteristics. |

## SPECIAL CONSIDERATIONS

1. Strict surgical asepsis is mandatory throughout the insertion of the catheter, when handling the solution and tubes and when caring for the site of insertion. The parenteral line can serve as an excellent culture medium since it directly leads to blood, bacterial invasion leads to septicemia
2. Psychological support is necessary, as the patient is not taking anything orally, for a long time.
3. As nothing enters the GI tract, bowel elimination will decrease and it should be explained to the patient.
4. To prevent hypoglycemia, while discontinuing parenteral nutrition, the solution should be reduced gradually over 48 hours.

# 4.7: PERFORMING A TEST FEED

## DEFINITION

Providing clear oral fluids to a postoperative patient to assess for return of bowel function.

## PURPOSES

1. To evaluate return of bowel function.
2. To aid in decision regarding initiating oral feeds after surgery.

## ARTICLES

A clean tray containing
1. Towel
2. Ounce glass
3. Glass with water
4. Kidney tray
5. Syringe – 20 ml

## GENERAL INSTRUCTION

Number of feeds, quantity of each feed and time of aspiration may differ according to surgeon's order.

## PROCEDURE

| | Nursing action | Rationale |
|---|---|---|
| 1. | Check physician's order | Determines the type of feed. |
| 2. | Explain to the patient regarding purpose of test feed and how it will be performed. | Helps in obtaining cooperation of patient. |
| 3. | Aspirate nasogastric tube. | Determines the amount of gastric contents present. |
| 4. | Measure amount of water to be given, as per doctor's order. | |
| 5. | Offer measured quantity of water every hour for four hours. | |
| 6. | Before giving fifth feed aspirate stomach contents, note the quantity. | Assesses patient's tolerance for feed. |
| 7. | If patient develops vomiting, discontinue test feeds and inform physician. | |
| 8. | Record in nurse's record and intake and output chart | Recording aids in communication among health team members. |

# Chapter **5**

# Elimination

# 5.1: ASSISTING WITH THE USE OF AN URINAL

## DEFINITION

Meeting urinary elimination need of bed-ridden male patients using an urinal.

## ARTICLES

1. Urinal.
2. Disposable gloves.
3. Specimen container if specimen needs to be collected.

## PROCEDURE

| | Nursing action | Rationale |
|---|---|---|
| 1. | Assess patient's normal urinary elimination habits. | Identifies normal pattern of urination. |
| 2. | Palpate for distended bladder. | Identifies if bladder is full and patient needs to void. |
| 3. | Assess patient's knowledge regarding urinal use. | Reveals need for patient instruction. |
| 4. | Wash hands and don gloves. | Reduces transmission of microorganisms. |
| 5. | Provide privacy. | Promotes relaxation. |
| 6. | Assist patient into appropriate position. | Men find it easier to void and empty bladder while standing. |
| 7. | Patient should hold urinal and position penis in urinal. If patient can stand by himself leave patient till he has completed voiding. If patient needs assistance, position penis completely within urinal and hold urinal in place or assist patient to hold urinal. If patient prefers a family member to help him allow it. | Placing penis completely within urinal avoids spillage of urine on bed linen. |
| 8. | Once patient has finished voiding, remove urinal. | Avoids spilling and reduces odors. Prevents growth of microorganisms. |
| 9. | Collect urine in container if required and empty the urinal into toilet and flush it down. | |
| 10. | Cleanse urinal and return it to patient for further use. | |
| 11. | Allow patients to wash hands after voiding/handling urinal. | Reduces spread of microorganisms. |
| 12. | Remove gloves and wash hands. | |
| 13. | Record and report patient's ability to use urinal, output and characteristics of urine. Record amount of urine passed if that information is important. | Communicates patient information to all health care personnel. |

## SPECIAL CONSIDERATION

In incontinent patients, offer urina, more frequently.
a. Place urinal near patient.
b. Provide frequent skin care.

## 5.2: APPLYING A CONDOM CATHETER

### DEFINITION

Applying a thin condom sheath to penis for drainage of urine without inserting a catheter into urethra.

### PURPOSES

1. To drain urine in case of an incontinent patient.
2. To permit patient's normal physical activity without fear of embarrassment caused by incontinence.

### INDICATION

Incontinent men who still have complete and spontaneous bladder emptying.

### ARTICLES

1. Rubber condom sheath (Proper size) (Figure 5.2(a))

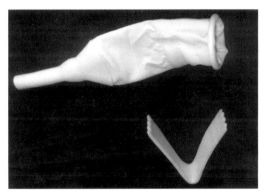

**Figure 5.2(a):** Rubber condom sheath

2. Strip of elastic tape and skin preparation (e.g. Tincture of benzion).
3. Urinary collection bag with drainage tubing.
4. Basin with warm water and soap.
5. Towel and wash cloths.
6. Disposable gloves.
7. Sheets.
8. Razor (optional).

### PROCEDURE

| | Nursing action | Rationale |
|---|---|---|
| 1. | Explain procedure to patient and assess status of patient. | Reduces anxiety and promotes co-operation. |
| 2. | Wash hands. | Reduces transmission of infection. |
| 3. | Provide privacy. | Maintains patient's self-esteem. |
| 4. | Assist patient to supine position. Place bath blanket over upper torso. Fold sheets so that lower extremities are covered. Only genitalia should be exposed. | Promotes patient comfort and prevents unnecessary exposure of body parts. |

*Contd...*

# Clinical Nursing Procedures: The Art of Nursing Practice

*Contd...*

| 5. | Assess condition of penis for skin irritation, excoriation, swelling or discoloration. | Provides baseline to compare changes in condition of skin after condom application. The patient may require an indwelling catheter if there is significant amount of skin breakdown. |
|---|---|---|
| 6. | Apply disposable gloves. Provide perineal care and dry throughly. Clip hair at the base of penis if required. | Removes irritating secretions.Rubber sheath rolls onto dry skin more easily. Hair adheres to condom and pulls during adhesive tape removal causing discomfort. |
| 7. | Prepare urinary collection bag and tubing or prepare leg bag for connection to condom if necessary. Clamp off drainage exit ports. Secure collection bag to bed frame or patient's legs. Bring drainage tubing up through side rails on to bed. | Provides easy access to drainage equipment after condom is in place. |
| 8. | Apply skin preparation to penis and allow to dry for 30 to 60 seconds. | |
| 9. | With non-dominant hand, grasp penis along shaft and with dominant hand roll condom sheath onto penis. | Prepares penis for easy condom placement. |
| 10. | Allow 2.5 to 5 cm (1 to 2 inchs)of space between root of penis and end of condom catheter.This space prevents a irritation of the tip of the penis. | Allows free passage of urine into collecting tubing when patient passes urine. |
| 11. | Encircle penile shaft with a strip of elastic adhesive. Strip should touch only condom sheath. The strip should be applied one inch from the proximal end of penis and do not completely encircle or tighten the penis (Figure 5.2(b)). | Condom must be secured so that it fits snugly and will stay on but not too tight to cause vasoconstriction. |

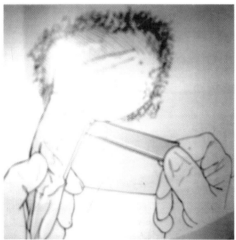

**Figure 5.2(b):** Fixing condom sheath with tape

| 12. | Connect drainage tubing to end of condom catheter. Be sure that condom is not twisted. | Allows urine to be collected and measured. Keeps patient dry. Twisted condom obstructs urine flow. |
|---|---|---|
| 13. | Coil the excess tubing on bed and secure to bottom sheet. | Prevents looping of tubing and promotes free drainage of urine. |
| 14. | Place the patient in safe and comfortable position (lying down/sitting). | Promotes patient's comfort. |
| 15. | Remove gloves. Dispose off contaminated supplies and wash hands. | Prevents spread of infection. |

*Contd...*

# Elimination

*Contd...*

| | | |
|---|---|---|
| 16. | Return in 30 to 60 minutes to observe for urinary drainage | Determines whether normal voiding is occurring. |
| 17. | Regularly inspect skin on penile shaft for signs of breakdown/irritation | Indicates whether condom or urine is causing irritation or whether adhesive is too restrictive. |
| 18. | Record and report, time of condom application, condition of skin and voiding pattern. | Provides data to determine change in elimination status. |

## SPECIAL CONSIDERATIONS

1. Remove the condom once a day to clean the area and assess the skin for signs of impaired skin integrity. This will promote hygiene and reduce the possibility of skin breakdown.
2. Do not reattach the condom catheter if it falls off. It will not stick any better in second try. Apply a new catheter and strip.
3. Clients may have latex allergy and may require latex-free condoms.

# 5.3: PERFORMING AN URINARY CATHETERIZATION

## DEFINITION

Introducing a catheter into the urinary bladder through urethra using aseptic technique for the purpose of emptying the bladder.

## TYPES

1. Intermittent catheterization.
2. Indwelling catheterization.

### INTERMITTENT CATHETERIZATION

*Purposes*

1. To relieve bladder distention
2. To assess for residual urine after voiding
3. To obtain a sterile specimen
4. To empty bladder prior to delivery or abdominal surgery.

### INDWELLING CATHETERIZATION

*Purposes*

1. To facilitate urinary elimination in incontinent patients.
2. To facilitate continuous bladder drainage after injury/surgery on urinary tract or other major surgeries.
3. To splint urethra to promote healing after urological surgery
4. To relieve acute or chronic urinary retention
5. To prevent urine from contacting an incision after perineal surgery.

## ARTICLES

A clean tray containing:
1. Flash light/Drop light
2. Basin with warm water, soap, wash cloth, bedpan, towel, etc.
3. Disposable gloves
4. Kidney tray
5. Antiseptic solution
6. Sterile saline
7. Adhesive tape and scissors (in case of retention catheter)
8. Specimen container
9. Water soluble lubricant.

A sterile tray with:
1. Sterile gloves
2. Sterile drape/fenestrated towel
3. Small bowl
4. Cotton swabs
5. Catheter (indwelling/straight of appropriate size) (Figure 5.3 (a))
6. Kidney tray
7. Artery forceps
8. Dissecting forceps
9. Sterile syringe – 20 ml and distilled water (in case of retention catheter)

# Elimination

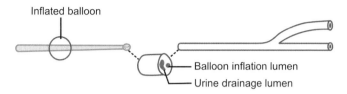

**Figure 5.3(a):** Double lumen indwelling urinary catheter

## PROCEDURE

| | Nursing action | Rationale |
|---|---|---|
| 1. | Review physician's order and nursing care plan | Helps in identifying the reason for catheterization. |
| 2. | Identify patient and assess patient for time of last voiding, level of awareness, mobility, physical limitation, and pathological condition, e.g. prostate enlargement, bladder distention etc. | Proper assessment helps in identifying patient's ability to co-operate during procedure and any possible obstruction in passing catheter. |
| 3. | Explain procedure to patient emphasizing how he/she has to co-operate. | Reduces anxiety and promotes co-operation which ensures smooth insertion of the catheter. |
| 4. | Arrange for help if needed for maintaining position of patient. | Promotes safety and proper body mechanics. |
| 5. | Provide privacy. | Reduces embarrassment to patient. |
| 6. | Wash hands. | Reduces risk of transmission of microorganisms. |
| 7. | Raise bed to appropriate working level. Stand on right side of patient and shift patient closer to you. | Promotes use of correct body mechanics. |
| 8. | Position patient<br>**a. Female:** Dorsal recumbent with knees flexed, and thighs externally rotated<br>**b. Male:** Supine position with thighs slightly abducted | Provides good view of perineal structures<br><br>Prevents tension of abdominal and pelvic muscles. |
| 9. | Wash perineal area/genitalia with soap and water | Cleaning reduces the number of microorganisms around urinary meatus and possibility of introducing microorganisms with the catheter. |
| 10. | Adjust drop light/flashlight to view urinary meatus clearly | |
| 11. | Open the sterile tray, pour antiseptic solution into bowl, open outer cover of catheter and place in tray if prepackaged | Keeping all articles ready for use helps in saving time and prevents chance of contamination. |
| 12. | Open lubricant, squeeze and discard first drop and after that drop some on a sterile gauze in the tray. | First drop of lubricant may be contaminated. |
| 13. | Don sterile gloves | Helps in preventing spread of microorganisms |
| 14. | Drape perineal area (See Figures 2.12(a) and (b)) | |
| 15. | Place sterile tray on drape between patient's thighs | Provides easy access to supplies. |
| 16. | If doing retention catheterization, fill the syringe with sterile water, if not already pre-filled and test balloon of catheter by inflating it (Figure 5.3(b)).<br>Deflate it and keep catheter aside with syringe attached to it | Provides easy access to supplies, checking balloon helps in identifying leaks in the balloon. |
| 17. | Open sterile specimen bottle and sterile urine receiver ready for use in the sterile tray. | |
| 18. | Lubricate tip of catheter liberally and place it in the sterile tray ready for use. | Lubrication aids in easy insertion of catheter by reducing friction. |

*Contd...*

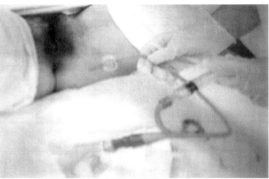

**Figure 5.3(b):** Testing balloon of catheter

19. Clean meatus with antiseptic solution if recommended by agency

    **Female:**

    a. With non-dominant hand, carefully retract labia fully and expose urethral meatus. Maintain position of hand through out the procedure

        Labia coming over meatus before catheter is in situ will cause contamination.

    b. Using dominant, hand take sterile cotton swabs dipped in antiseptic solution and clean perineal area from clitoris towards anus in the following sequence—meatus, labia minora and than labia majora. Use one swab for each wipe (Figure 5.3 (c))

        Disinfectant can be irritating to skin and mucous membrane.

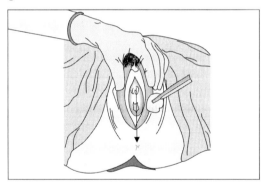

**Figure 5.3(c):** Cleansing female genitalia

    c. Repeat cleaning with cotton swabs dipped in sterile normal saline in same sequence.

    **Male:**

    a. Grasp penis firmly below glans with non-dominant hand . Retract the foreskin and hold it retracted till end of procedure

        Foreskin coming back into position before catheter is in situ will cause contamination

    b. With dominant hand, use sterile swabs dipped in antiseptic solution to clean meatus and moving out in circular motion. (Figure 5.3(d))

    c. Use one swab for each wipe

    d. Repeat the cleaning using sterile saline in same sequence.

        Disinfectant can be irritating to skin and mucous membrane.

20. Insert catheter for 15 to 25 cm in male patients and 2.5 to 5 cm in female, until urine begins to flow, do not force catheter. If met with resistance, twist catheter and wait for some time to

        Male urethra is very narrow and flexing catheter can traumatize sphincter and urethra. Deep breathing can aid in muscle relaxation.

*Contd...*

# Elimination

*Contd..*

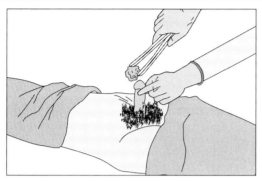

**Figure 5.3(d):** Cleansing male genitalia

allow sphincter to relax. Encourage patients to take deep breaths while inserting (Figure 5.3(e))

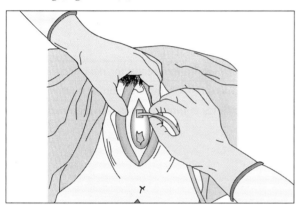

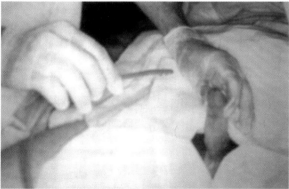

**Figure 5.3(e):** Inserting urinary catheter

| | |
|---|---|
| 21. Collect all urine in the sterile kidney tray. If needed, collect urine specimen in the specimen container. | Collecting urine helps in assessing volume of urine drained. |
| 22. Remove catheter if intermittent catheterization is done. | |
| 23. If retention, catheterization is performed introduce sterile distilled water to inflate balloon. | Inflated balloon helps in retaining catheter inside bladder |
| 24. Pull catheter outward lightly to ascertain stability. | |

*Contd...*

*Contd...*

| 25. | Connect catheter to urosac tied to bed below level of bladder | Urosac above level of bladder will lead to back flow of urine and cause risk of infection. |
| 26. | Fix catheter to thigh using adhesive tapes. Ensure adequate length to avoid traction (Figure 5.3(f)) | Traction on catheter can lead to injury to urinary meatus. |

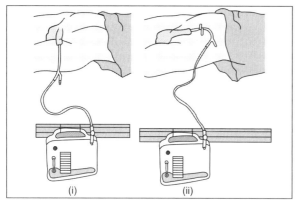

(i)          (ii)

**Figure 5.3(f):** An indwelling catheter in place

| 27. | clean and replace equipment and remove gloves | Keeps equipment ready for next use. |
| 28. | Wash hands | Reduces risk of transmission of microorganisms. |
| 29. | Record procedure and observation in patient's chart. | Promotes communication between staff members. |

# 5.4: PERFORMING CATHETER CARE

## DEFINITION

Cleansing the urethral meatus, the skin surrounding the catheter insertion site and perineum for patients with retention catheter who are bed ridden.

## PURPOSES

1. To promote patient comfort.
2. To reduce chances of developing urinary tract infection.

## ARTICLES

1. A sterile "catheter care kit" containing
   a. Artery forceps
   b. Thumb forceps
   c. Cotton balls/swabs
   d. Bowls for antiseptic lotion and sterile water
2. A clean tray containing
   a. Clean washcloth or towel – 2 Nos.
   b. Warm water and soap
   c. Antiseptic lotion
   d. Normal saline
   e. Mackintosh/waterproof pads and draw sheets
   f. Antibiotic ointment
   g. Clean gloves
   h. Sterile gloves
   i. Drapes
   j. Kidney tray
   k. Adhesive tape and scissors.

## PROCEDURE

| | Nursing action | Rationale |
|---|---|---|
| 1. | Prepare necessary equipment and supplies | Ensures efficiency and smooth functioning. |
| 2. | Explain procedure to patient, offer opportunity for self–care if possible | Reduces anxiety and promotes co-operation. |
| 3. | Provide privacy | Maintains patient's self-esteem. |
| 4. | Wash hands | Reduces transmission of microorganisms. |
| 5. | Position patient **Female:** Dorsal recumbent position with legs flexed **Male:** Supine position | Ensures easy access to perineal area. |
| 6. | Place waterproof pad/mackintosh and drawsheet under patient | Protects bed linen from soiling. |
| 7. | Drape sheet over patient exposing only perineal area | Prevents unnecessary exposure of body parts. |
| 8. | Don clean gloves. | |
| 9. | Remove anchor tapes to free catheter tubing. | |

*Contd...*

*Contd...*

| | |
|---|---|
| 10. Expose the uretheral meatus (with non-dominant hand)<br>**Female:** Gently retract labia to fully expose urethral meatus and catheter insertion site. Maintain position of hand throughout procedure. | Provides full visualization of urethral meatus. |
| **Male:** Retract foreskin if patient is not circumcised and hold penis at shaft just below glans. Maintaining position of hand throughout procedure | Retraction prevents foreskin contaminating the meatus, during cleansing. Accidentally letting go of penis requires that process be repeated. |
| 11. Assess urethral meatus and surrounding tissue for inflammation, swelling and discharge. Note amount, color, odour and consistency of discharge. Ask patient if burning or discomfort is felt. | Determines presence of local infection and hygiene status. |
| 12. Cleanse perineal tissue<br>**Female:** Use clean cloth, soap and water and clean towards anus. Cleanse catheter first and then meatus, labia minora and majora. Be sure to cleanse each side and dry area well.<br>**Male:** Cleanse catheter first and then clean from urethral meatus till glans penis in circular motion. | Cleansing reduces number of microorganisms at urethral meatus. Use of clean cloth prevents transfer of microorganisms. Moving from the most clean area decreases risk of recontamination. |
| 13. Reassess urethral meatus for any discharge | Determines whether cleaning is complete |
| 14. Remove clean gloves and wash hands | |
| 15. Don sterile gloves. | |
| 16. Clean the perineal area with disinfectant<br>**Females:** Retract labia and wipe using sterile cotton swabs dipped in antiseptic solution from center to peripheri in straight strokes from front to back, using one cotton ball for each stroke.<br>**Male:** Retract foreskin and wipe using swabs from center to peripheri in circular stokes. | Moving from an area where there is less number of organisms to an area where there is more number of organisms will help in preventing spread of infection. |
| 17. Repeat step (16) using cotton swabs soaked in sterile water/normal saline | Antiseptic solution may act as an irritant to skin |
| 18. Apply antiseptic ointment at urethral meatus and along 2.5 cm (inch) of catheter. Anchor catheter. | Reduces further growth of microorganisms at insertion site. |
| 19. Place patient in safe and comfortable position | Promotes comfort |
| 20 Remove gloves, dispose of contaminated supplies and wash hands. | Prevents spread of infection. |
| 21. Record and report condition of perineal tissue, the time procedure was performed, patient's response and abnormalities noted. | Provides data to document procedure and informs concerned others of patients condition. |

## SPECIAL CONSIDERATION

Catheter has to be changed periodically as per agency policy.

# 5.5: REMOVING AN INDWELLING URINARY CATHETER

## PURPOSES

1. To promote normal bladder function.
2. To prevent trauma to the urethra.
3. To prevent infection.

## ARTICLES

1. Syringe without needle (10 ml)
2. Clean gloves
3. Protective pad
4. Soap, towel and washcloth
5. Container for waste disposal
6. Urinal or bedpan
7. Kidney tray.

## PROCEDURE

| | Nursing action | Rationale |
|---|---|---|
| 1 | Wash hands and don gloves | Reduces transmission of microorganisms. |
| 2 | If bladder conditioning is to be performed:<br>a. 10 hours before removal, clamp indwelling catheter for 3 hrs.<br><br>b. Unclamp and drain urine for 5 minutes.<br>c. Repeat clamping for 3 hours and draining for 5 minutes two more times. | Volume of urine stretches bladder wall to stimulate muscle tone.<br>Unclamping the catheter simulates voiding.<br>Patients who receive bladder conditioning are able to feel urge to void sooner than those who have no conditioning. |
| 3 | Wash hands. | Decreases the transmission of microorganisms. |
| 4 | Check the doctor's order. | Ensures correct patient and treatment |
| 5 | Identify the patient and explain procedure. | Elicits patient's co-operation |
| 6 | Provide privacy and position patient on back. | Providing privacy demonstrates respect for patient's dignity. |
| 7 | Remove covers and drape so as to expose catheter but do not overly expose perineal area. | Protects patient's privacy and reduces embarrassment. |
| 8 | Place protective pad under patient's thighs. | Prevents bed from becoming soiled. |
| 9 | Empty urine in tubing into urobag. | Prevents leakage from catheter onto patient, when the catheter is removed. |
| 10 | Remove any tape that may be holding the catheter to the leg. | Allows for easy removal of catheter. |
| 11 | Insert syringe end into balloon port and remove all the air or fluid from the balloon, generally 5-10cc. Do not cut the port. | Removal of fluid from balloon prevents damage to urethra, while removing the catheter. |
| 12 | Ask the patient to take a deep breath if able and gently and smoothly remove the catheter on expiration. Stop if you meet resistance and recheck the balloon port. | Damage to the urethra may occur if the balloon is not fully deflated. |
| 13 | Note any sediment, mucus or blood that may be on the catheter. If needed, culture the tip of catheter by cutting it off with sterile scissors and placing in appropriate container. | Assesses for any indications of infection or trauma related to the catheter. |

*Contd...*

*Contd...*

| 14 | Cleanse the patient's perineal area or provide a warm, moist cloth with instructions for self-cleaning. | Provides comfort and reduces transmission of micro-organisms. |
|---|---|---|
| 15 | Remove gloves and wash hands. | Reduces transmission of microorganisms. |
| 16 | Cover patient and position comfortably. | Provides for privacy and comfort. |
| 17 | Instruct the patient to drink oral fluids as tolerated and to call when he/she needs to void. | Determines that patient has returned to usual voiding pattern. |
| 18 | Record time and amount of first voiding. Offer bedpan/urinal every 2-4 hours. | Allows assessment of the patient's voiding pattern. |
| 19 | If the patient is unable to void within 8 hours, report to the physician. | Allows assessment and intervention to determine the cause of the patient's inability to void after catheter is removed. |

## SPECIAL CONSIDERATIONS

1. Instruct patient to inform the nurse, if experiencing any pain, or symptoms of bladder infection, after the catheter is removed.
2. Check if physician has ordered bladder conditioning before removal of catheter.
3. Keep track of intake and output for at least 24 hours after removal of catheter.
4. If patient has not voided within 8 hours after catheter removal, the catheter (intermittent or indwelling, depending on order of physician) may have to be reinserted.

# 5.6: PERFORMING A BLADDER IRRIGATION

## DEFINITION

Flushing out/washing out the urinary bladder with specified solution.

## PURPOSES

1. To flush clots and debris out of the catheter and bladder
2. To instill medication to bladder lining
3. To restore patency of the catheter.

## ARTICLES

1. Disposable gloves
2. Disposable, water resistant, sterile towel/mackintosh
3. Three way retention catheter *in situ*
4. Sterile drainage tubing and bag in place
5. Sterile antiseptic swab
6. Sterile receptacle
7. Sterile irrigating solution warmed or at room temperature
   - Normal saline
   - Distilled water
   - Solution as prescribed by physician
8. Infusion tubing
9. IV pole
10. Kidney basin.

## PROCEDURE

| | Nursing action | Rationale |
|---|---|---|
| 1. | Check physician's order and nursing care plan for type, amount and strength of irrigating fluid and reason for irrigation. | |
| 2. | Prepare the patient <br> a. Explain the procedure and its purpose to the patient <br> b. Provide for privacy and drape the patient <br> c. Empty, measure and record the amount and appearance of urine present in the urine bag. | Clear explanation reduces anxiety <br><br> Emptying the bag allows for more accurate measurement of urinary output after irrigation. Assessment of character of urine helps in obtaining a baseline assessment data for later comparison. |
| 3. | Prepare the equipment <br> a. Wash hands <br> b. Connect the irrigation infusion tubing to the irrigating solution and flush the tubing with solution <br> c. Connect the irrigation tubing to the input port of the 3-way catheter. Connect the drainage bag and tubing to the urinary drainage port if not already in place (Figure 5.6(a)) | Reduces transmission of micro-organisms <br> Flushing the tubing removes air and prevents it from being instilled into the bladder |

*Contd...*

*Contd...*

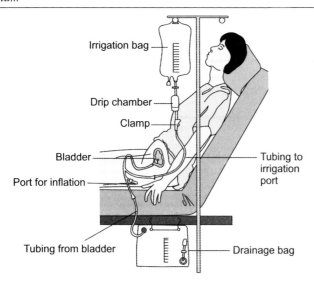

**Figure 5.6(a):** Continuous bladder irrigation

4. *Irrigate the bladder*
   a. Continuous irrigation
   - Open the flow clamp on the urinary drainage tubing (if present)
   - Open the regulating clamp on the irrigating tubing and adjust the flow rate as prescribed by the physician or to 40 – 60 drops/minute if not specified
   - Assess the drainage for amount, color and clarity.

   b. *Intermittent irrigation*
   i. Determine whether the solution is to remain in the bladder for a specified time
   - If solution is to remain in the bladder during a bladder irrigation or instillation close the flow clamp on the urinary drainage tubing
   - Open the flow clamp on the irrigating tubing, allowing the specified amount of solution (75-100 ml) to infuse and then clamp the tubing.
   - After retaining the solution for specified period of time, open the drainage tubing flow clamp and allow the bladder to empty.
   ii. If the solution being instilled is to irrigate the catheter, open the flow clamp on the urinary drainage tubing

| | |
|---|---|
| Open the flow clamp on the urinary drainage tubing (if present) | This allows irrigating solution to flow out continuously. |
| Assess the drainage for amount, color and clarity. | The amount of drainage should equal the amount of irrigant entering the bladder plus expected urine output. |
| If solution is to remain in the bladder... close the flow clamp on the urinary drainage tubing | Closing the flow clamp allows the solution to be retained in the bladder and in contact with bladder walls. |
| Open the flow clamp on the irrigating tubing... | Retains the fluid in the bladder for specified time. |
| If the solution being instilled is to irrigate the catheter... | Irrigating solution will flow through the urinary drainage port and tubing, removing mucous shreds or clots. |

5. Assess the patient 's condition, urinary output, color, odour and clarity of drainage — Proper assessment helps in identifying effectiveness of procedure

6. Discard all used disposable articles, clean and replace reusable articles.

7. Wash hands — Prevents spread of microorganisms

8. Record procedure in nurse's record'

# 5.7: ASSISTING WITH THE USE OF BEDPAN

## DEFINITION

Offering a bedpan to meet the eliminational need of a bed-ridden patient.

## TYPES (FIGURE 5.7(A))

1. Regular bedpan
2. Fracture bedpan.

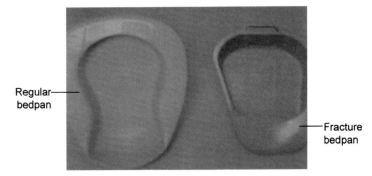

Figure 5.7(a): Types of bedpans

## PURPOSES

1. To facilitate bowel and bladder elimination in a bedridden patient.
2. To collect specimen
3. To give perineal wash
4. To perform bowel and bladder training.

## ARTICLES

1. Disposable gloves (clean)
2. Clean bedpan with lid (2 bedpans may be needed in case of specimen collection).
3. Toilet tissues
4. Specimen container (optional)
5. Wash clothes
6. Towels
7. Draw sheets
8. Soap
9. Warm water in a jug
10. Mackintosh.

## PROCEDURE

| Nursing action | Rationale |
|---|---|
| 1   Assess patient's normal bowel elimination habits, routine pattern, effect of certain foods on bowel elimination and normal fluid intake. | |

*Contd...*

*Contd...*

| | | |
|---|---|---|
| 2 | Assess patient's level of mobility, amount of assistance required and positions that the patient can assume. | Determines the type of bedpan to be used and helps in identifying the level of assistance required from the nurse. |
| 3 | Assess for abdominal pain, hemorrhoids or irritation of skin surrounding anus. | Pain can reduce ability of the patient to bear down during defecation. |
| 4 | Wash hands and don gloves. | Reduces transmission of microorganisms. |
| 5 | Provide privacy. Remove top sheet just enough, so they are out of the way but do not unduly expose patient. | Reduces embarrassment and promotes normal bowel movement. |
| 6 | Warm bedpan under warm running water for few seconds and dry and keep it within reach. | Warm pan helps to relax anal sphincter. |
| 7 | Position bed to convenient height. | Ensures use of good body mechanics and prevents strain on back. |
| 8 | Elevate side rails on opposites side. | Reduces risk of accidental falls. |
| 9 | In patients who can move lower limbs, ask patient to flex knees, resting the weight on back or legs, and then raising the buttocks (with the help of a trapeze if available). | These movements will allow patient to support some of his weight himself. |
| 10 | Place a regular bedpan under patient with the smooth rounded rim under the patient's buttocks. If a fracture bedpan is used, place it with flat low end under the patient's buttocks. (Alteration for placement of bedpan) If patient is not able to move, obtain assistance from another nurse to lift the patient onto the bedpan. Or Position patient to side lying position, place bedpan against buttocks and roll patient onto the bedpan, back to supine position. | |
| 11 | Elevate patient's bed to semi Fowlers position (if permitted) or support patient's back with pillows. | Elevating head end allows for a more normal position. Placing pillows at lumbar curvature prevents hyperextension of the back. |
| 12 | Cover patient with bed linen and permit patient to be alone with call bell within reach. Elevate side rails. | Promotes the dignity of the patient. |
| 13 | When removing bedpan return bed to the position used when giving bedpan. Hold bedpan steady, remove it, cover it and place it away. | |
| 14 | If patient can help by himself, provide tissues to wipe or alternatively place a second bedpan and pour water. So that patient can clean himself. | |
| 15 | If patient is totally helpless, provide perineal and anal care. | |
| 16 | Provide soap and water for the patient to clean his hands and dry hands thoroughly. | |
| 17 | Send bedpan to sluice room. | |
| 18 | Remove gloves and wash hands. | |
| 19 | Position patient comfortably, change linen if wet. | |
| 20 | Record the procedure. | |

# 5.8: ADMINISTERING AN ENEMA

## CLEANSING/EVACUANT ENEMA

### DEFINITION

Introduction of solution into the large intestine for removing feces and cleansing the bowel.

### PURPOSES

1. To relieve constipation or fecal impaction.
2. To prevent involuntary escape of fecal matter during surgical procedure and delivery
3. To promote visualization of the intestinal tract during radiographic or instrumental examination.
4. To help establish regular bowel function during a bowel training program.
5. Pre-operative preparation for bowel surgeries.
6. To relieve retention of urine by reflex stimulation of bladder.

### SOLUTIONS USED

1. Hypertonic – Sodium phosphate, Fleet enema
2. Hypotonic – Tap water
3. Isotonic – Physiological saline (one tsp of table salt in 500 ml of tap water.
4. Others: 3 to 5 ml of concentrated soap solutions in 1000 ml of water.

### CONTRAINDICATIONS

1. Acute renal failure
2. Acute myocardial infarction and cardiac problems.
3. Appendicitis
4. Obstetrical contraindications like antepartum hemorrhage, leaking membranes
5. Recent surgical procedures involving lower intestinal tract.
6. Intestinal obstruction.
7. Inflammation and infection of abdomen.

### ARTICLES

I. **Enema can and tubing method.**

A tray containing:

1. Disposable gloves
2. Water soluble lubricant.(Vaseline)
3. Bath thermometer
4. Soap and water
5. Toilet tissues
6. Enema can (graduated)
7. Tubing and clamp
8. Appropriate size rectal tube
    i. Adult size: 22-30 Fr.
    ii. Child size: 12-18 Fr.
9. IV stand
10. K. Basin - 2 Nos
11. Solution as ordered.
12. Mackintosh/Waterproof under pad
13. Bedpan (for helpless patients)

## TEMPERATURE OF SOLUTION

    i. Adult: 105 – 110 degree F (40 –43 degree Celsius)

    ii. Child:100 degree F (37.1.degree Celsius)

## AMOUNT OF SOLUTION FOR DIFFERENT AGE GROUPS

1. Adult              : 750-1000 ml
2. Adolescent    : 500-750 ml
3. School age     : 300-500 ml
4. Toddler         : 250-300 ml
5. Infant           : 150-250 ml

## PROCEDURE

| | Nursing action | Rationale |
|---|---|---|
| 1. | Assess status of patient (last bowel movement, normal bowel pattern, hemorrhoids, mobility, external sphincter control, abdominal pain and peri-anal lesions | Determines factors indicating need for enema. |
| 2. | Determine the level of consciousness and understanding of patient. | Helps in planning for the procedure. |
| 3. | Provide privacy. | Reduces embarrassment for the patient. |
| 4. | Check the medical record to clarify the rationale for enema and review physician's order. | Determines the purpose of enema administration. |
| 5. | Explain to patient the purpose of enema, what he can expect and how he can participate. | Promotes patient co-operation and reduces anxiety. |
| 6. | Assemble articles. | |
| 7. | Wash hands and don gloves. | Reduces transmission of microorganisms. |
| 8. | Raise the bed to appropriate working height for the nurse. | Promotes good body mechanics. |
| 9. | Assist patient to left side lying position (Sim's position) | Provides easy access to anus. Allows enema fluid to flow downward by gravity along natural curve of sigmoid colon and rectum. |
| 10. | Place waterproof pad or mackintosh under hips and buttocks. | Prevents soiling of linen. |
| 11. | Cover the patient exposing only anal area, clearly visualizing anus. | Decreases exposure of body parts. |
| 12. | Place bedpan or commode in easily accessible position | For use in case the patient is unable to retain enema solution. |
| 13. | Check temperature of the solution on inner wrist or using a bath thermometer. | Hot water burns intestinal mucosa and cold water can cause cramps and is difficult to retain. |
| 14. | Raise container, release clamp and allow solution to flow long enough to fill tubing. | Removes air from tubing. |
| 15. | Clamp the tubing. | Prevents further loss of solution. |
| 16. | Lubricate 6 to 8 cm of tip of rectal tube with jelly. | Allows smooth insertion of rectal tube. |
| 17. | Separate the buttocks and locate anus. Instruct patient to relax by breathing out slowly through mouth. | Promotes relaxation of external anal sphincter. |
| 18. | Insert tip of rectal tube gently by pointing the tip in the direction of patient's umbilicus. Length of insertion varies (Figure 5.8(a)) | Careful insertion prevents trauma to rectal mucosa. The angle follows normal contour of rectum. |

*Contd...*

*Contd...*

Adult: 7.5 cm - 10 cm.
Child: 5.0 cm - 7.5 cm.
Infant: 2.5 cm - 3.7 cm.

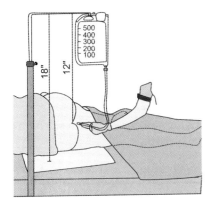

**Figure 5.8(a):** Inserting a rectal tube

| | | |
|---|---|---|
| 19. | Hold the tubing in place with one hand (non-dominant hand) | Bowel contraction can cause expulsion of rectal tube. |
| 20. | Open regulatory clamp and allow solution to enter slowly with the container at the patient's hip level. | Rapid instillation can stimulate evacuation of rectal tube. |
| 21. | Raise the enema can slowly to appropriate level above the anus.<br>Example:<br>   i. 30 cm for regular enema.<br>   ii. 35 – 45 cm for high enema.<br>   iii. 7.5 cm for low enema. | Allows for continuous slow instillation of solution. Raising the container too high causes rapid instillation and possible painful distention of colon |
| 22. | Lower container or clamp tubing for 30 seconds if patient complains of cramping or if fluid escapes around rectal tube. | Administration of enema slowly and stopping the flow momentarily decreases likelihood of intestinal spasm and premature ejection of the solution. |
| 23. | Clamp tubing after all solution is instilled. | Prevents entrance of air into rectum. |
| 24. | Inform patient, that fluid instillation is over and the tube will be removed. | Patient will be prepared for tube withdrawal. |
| 25. | Place layers of toilet tissue around tube at anus and gently withdraw rectal tube. | Provides comfort and cleanliness. |
| 26. | Explain to patient that feeling of distention is normal and ask patient to retain solution as long as possible (5 to 10 minutes) while lying quietly in bed. | Solution distends the bowel. Period of distention varies with type of enema and patient's ability to contract rectal sphincter. |
| 27. | Discard the disposable, used items in proper receptacle. If enema can needs to be reused, rinse out thoroughly with soap and warm water. | Reduces growth of microorganisms. |
| 28. | Assist patient to toilet or help to position on bedpan. | Squatting position promotes defecation. |
| 29. | Observe the fecal matter and expelled solution. (when enema is ordered "until clear", observe contents of solution passed. Return is clear when no solid fecal material is present, but solution may be colored) | Identifies abnormalities such as presence of blood or mucus. |
| 30. | Assist as needed to wash anal area with soap and water. | Hygiene promotes patient's comfort. |
| 31. | Remove and discard gloves, and wash hands. | Reduces transmission of microorganisms. |

*Contd...*

*Contd...*

| | | |
|---|---|---|
| 32. | Assess condition of patient's abdomen. Cramping, rigidity or distention may indicate serious problems. | Excess volume can distend or perforate the bowel. |
| 33. | Record type and volume of enema given and characteristics of return flow. | Communicates with other nurses and members of health team. |
| 34. | Report failure to defecate to the physician. | |
| 35. | Clean and replace the reusable articles. | |
| 36. | Discard any waste and disposable items. | |

## SPECIAL PRECAUTION

Patients with hemorrhoids may experience discomfort/bleeding when enema is administered. Warm sitz bath can be given to relieve discomfort after the procedure. Be observant for persistent rectal bleeding.

## ADMINISTRATION OF EVACUANT ENEMA USING PRE-PACKAGED DISPOSABLE PREPARATIONS

### ARTICLES

A tray containing:
1. Disposable gloves.
2. Packet of enema.
3. Toilet tissues.
4. Soap and water
5. Kidney tray
6. Mackintosh
7. Lubricant jelly
8. Bedpan /commode in case of helpless patient.

## PROCEDURE

| | Nursing action | Rationale |
|---|---|---|
| 1. | Assess status of patient (last bowel movement, normal bowel pattern, hemorrhoids, mobility, external sphincter control, abdominal pain and perineal lesions.) | Determines factors indicating need for enema. |
| 2. | Determine the level of consciousness and understanding of the patient. | Helps in planning for the procedure. |
| 3. | Provide privacy. | Reduces embarrassment for the patient. |
| 4. | Check the medical record to clarify the rationale for enema and review physician's order. | Determines the purpose of enema administration. |
| 5. | Explain to patient the purpose of enema, what he can expect and how he can participate. | Promotes patient co-operation and reduces anxiety. |
| 6. | Assemble articles. | |
| 7. | Wash hands and don gloves. | Reduces transmission of microorganisms. |
| 8. | Raise the bed to appropriate working height for the nurse. | Promotes good body mechanics. |
| 9. | Assist patient to left side lying position (Sim's position). | Provides easy access to anus. Allows enema fluid to flow downward by gravity along natural curve of sigmoid colon and rectum. |

*Contd...*

*Contd...*

| | | |
|---|---|---|
| 10. | Place waterproof pad or mackintosh under hips and buttocks. | Prevents soiling of linen. |
| 11. | Cover the patient exposing only anal area, clearly visualizing anus. | Decreases exposure of body parts. |
| 12. | Place bedpan or commode in an easily accessible place. | For use in case the patient is unable to retain enema solution. |
| 13. | Remove plastic cap from rectal tip (tip is already lubricated. More lubricant may be used if needed). | Lubrication provides for smooth insertion of rectal tube without rectal irritation. |
| 14. | Gently separate the buttocks and locate the anus. Instruct patient to relax by breathing through mouth. | Breathing out through mouth promotes relaxation of anal sphincter. |
| 15. | Insert tip of the tube gently into rectum. (Figure 5.8 (b)) Adult: 7.5 to 10 cm (3 to 4 inch) Child: 5.0 to 7.5 cm (2 to 3 inch) Infant: 2.5 to 3.7 cm (1 to 1½inch) | |

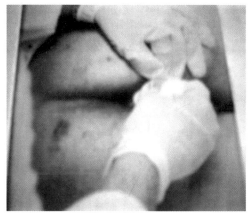

**Figure 5.8(b):** Administering a pre-packaged enema

| | | |
|---|---|---|
| 16. | Squeeze the container until all the solution has entered rectum and sigmoid colon. While squeezing the container roll it up as fluid is instilled. Instruct patient to retain solution until an urge to defecate occurs (2 to 5 minutes) | Prevents subsequent suctioning of the solution. |
| 17. | Place toilet tissue around the tube at anus and withdraw the tube. | Provides comfort and cleanliness. |
| 18. | Discard the disposable items in proper receptacle. | |
| 19. | Assist patient to toilet or help to position on bedpan. | Squatting position promotes defecation. |
| 20. | Observe the fecal matter and expelled solution. | Aids in observing presence of abnormalities. |
| 21. | Remove gloves and discard. Wash hands. | Reduces transmission of microorganisms. |
| 22 | Assess condition of patient's abdomen, cramping or rigidity which can indicate problems. | |
| 23. | Record the enema given and characteristics of results. | |
| 24. | Report any problem if noticed. | |

# 5.9: PERFORMING A BOWEL WASH/COLONIC LAVAGE

## DEFINITION

Washing out colon with large quantities of solution, to clear colon of faeces.

## PURPOSES

1. To prepare colon for specific surgical or diagnostic procedures.
2. To dilute and remove toxic agents that may be present in large intestine, e g. Hepatic encephalopathy
3. To reduce temperature in hyperpyrexia and heat stroke.
4. To supply fluid and electrolytes that are absorbed from intestines.
5. To stimulate peristalsis.
6. To relieve inflammation.
7. To keep the individual clean in case of faecal incontinence.

## CONTRAINDICATIONS

1. Bleeding hemorrhoids
2. Chronic diarrhoea
3. Rectal surgeries, infection
4. Intestinal obstruction
5. Rectal polyps
6. Massive colon carcinoma
7. Loose anal sphincter
8. Debilitation
9. Anal fistula
10. Intestinal diverticulum
11. Painful skin lesions around anus.

## SOLUTIONS USED

1. Plain water
2. Cold water
3. Normal saline
4. Sodium carbonate solution 1 to 2 percent
5. Antiseptic solution such as silver nitrate - 1:5000
6. Potassium permanganate - 1:5000
7. Thymol - 1:100
8. Alum - 1:100
9. Boric solution - 1-2%
10. Tannic acid - 1:100

Amount of solutions used: 2-3 liters or till the return flow is clear.

## TEMPERATURE OF THE SOLUTION

1. For cleansing purpose 104 degree F
2. For reducing temperature 80 – 90 degree F

# ARTICLES

Tray containing:
1. Colonic lavage set with tubing and glass connection
2. Rectal tube
   Adult – 22- 30 Fr
   Children 12-18 Fr
3. Vaseline
4. Rag pieces/Tissue papers
5. Mackintosh
6. Jugs with hot and cold water
7. Kidney tray
8. Bucket
9. Solutions
10. Lotion thermometer
11. Bedpan with lid
12. Duster
13. Perineal toilet tray
14. Clean disposable gloves
15. Plastic apron

# PROCEDURE

| | Nursing action | Rationale |
|---|---|---|
| 1 | Check the patient's chart for physician's order and any specific instructions. | |
| 2 | Explain to the patient about procedure and how he has to co-operate. | Encourages co-operation of patient and reduces anxiety. |
| 3. | Wash hands and don gloves. | Prevents cross infection. |
| 4. | Prepare solution at the required temperature. Test the temperature on the inner aspect of the wrist. | Ensures that it will not cause discomfort to the patient |
| 5. | Attach the tubing and the rectal tube with the funnel. Pour the solution in it and check for leakage. | Ensures that the articles to be used are in good working condition. |
| 6. | Lubricate the tip of rectal tube about 4 inches. | For easy insertion of the tube and to prevent friction. |
| 7. | Fill the funnel with the solution and expel air from the tubing by allowing a small amount of fluid to run into the kidney tray. Pinch the tube or close it with a clamp. | Expelling air from the funnel and tubing prevents air from entering into the colon. |
| 8. | Maintain left lateral position and bring the patient close to the edge of bed. Separate the patient's buttocks to visualize the anus clearly and insert the tip of tube about 4 inches while the patient exhales a deep breath. | The rectum is relaxed when the patient breaths out and makes the insertion of the tube easier. |
| 9. | Lower the funnel below the level of the rectum | Allows flatus if any to escape from the rectum. It will be seen bubbling through the fluid in the funnel. |
| 10. | Raise the funnel and allow the fluid to run in, continue to pour more fluid into funnel before the funnel is empty. | Pouring the solution before the funnel is empty prevents entry of air into rectum. |
| 11. | When 200 – 300 ml of fluid has gone inside, pinch the tube before the funnel is completely empty and invert it into the bucket and siphon off the fluid. | The fluid which has gone in should be drained out before introducing more fluid. |

*Contd...*

*Contd...*

| | | |
|---|---|---|
| 12. | When the return flow ceases, turn the funnel upright and pour more solution, lower the funnel until air from the tube has been expelled. Then raise the funnel and repeat the procedure. | Care is taken to expel air from the tubing as well as from the rectum. |
| 13 | Temporarily stop the procedure if the patient develops any discomfort. | Entry of fluid into the rectum stimulates peristalsis, stopping the procedure for few moments will relax the bowels as the peristaltic movement is passed off. |
| 14. | Continue the procedure until all the fluid ordered has been given or until the return flow is clear. | It helps to know if the entire bowel is cleansed well |
| 15. | Gently remove the rectal tube by pulling it through 3 – 4 layers of rag pieces/tissue papers. | Pulling through the rag pieces removes the faeces on the tube. |
| 16. | Discard the tissue papers in the paper bag. Place the funnel with tubing in the kidney tray | Avoids contamination of the articles and environment with the soiled articles. |
| 17. | Assist patient to the toilet, commode or bedpan | Drains out any fluid left in the rectum |
| 18. | Bring the toilet tray and assist for the perineal care if required | Maintains hygiene of the perineum |
| 19. | Change the bed linen if soiled and assist patient to lie down in comfortable position. | Promotes neat appearance of the bed and comfort of patient. |
| 20. | Take all the articles to utility room. Disinfect the funnel, tubing, catheter and bucket . Clean dry and replace them in their proper place. | Helps in preparing for next use. |
| 21. | Remove gloves and wash hands | Prevents cross infection |
| 21. | Record the type of procedure and the result with date and time in nurse's record. | Gives information about patient's response to the procedure. |

## SPECIAL CONSIDERATION

Colonic irrigation may be given using a Y connector and rectal tube also.

# 5.10: PERFORMING COLOSTOMY CARE

## DEFINITION

Maintenance of hygiene by regular emptying of colostomy bag and cleaning colostomy site.

## PURPOSES

1. To prevent leakage
2. To prevent excoriation of skin and stoma
3. To observe stoma and surrounding skin.
4. To teach patient and relatives about care of colostomy and collection bag.

## ARTICLES

Tray containing:
1. Rubber sheet
2. Long sheet
3. Towel
4. Clean gloves
5. Cotton swabs and gauze pieces
6. Wash cloth
7. Water in basin
8. Soap in dish
9. Disposable colostomy bag with clamp
10. Stoma measuring guide
11. Zinc oxide ointment
12. Skin barrier
13. Bedpan with cover

## PROCEDURE

| | Nursing action | Rationale |
|---|---|---|
| 1 | Explain procedure to the patient and explain to him how he has to cooperate. | Helps in obtaining cooperation of the patient. |
| 2 | Assemble the necessary equipments near by. | Organisation facilitates performance of the task. |
| 3 | Wash hands and don gloves | Prevents spread of microorganisms |
| 4 | Provide privacy and assist patient to a comfortable position (Fowlers, semifowlers, standing or sitting position in bathroom). | Positioning allows patient to view the procedure in preparation for learning. |
| 5 | Empty the partially filled appliance into the bedpan if it is a drainable pouch. | Emptying the contents before removal of the pouch prevents accidental spillage of faecal material. Pouches that are full can detach and leak. |
| 6 | Remove the appliance slowly beginning at the top while keeping the abdominal skin taut. If any resistance is felt, use warm water or adhesive solvent to facilitate removal. | Careful removal protects the underlying skin from damage and minimises discomfort for the patient. |
| 7 | Use tissue paper to remove any excess stool from the stoma. Cover stoma with a gauze pad. | Gauze absorbs any drainage from the stoma while the skin is being prepared. |
| 8 | Gently wash and pat dry the peristomal skin. Mild soap and cleansing agent may be used according to agency policy. | |

*Contd...*

*Contd...*

| | | |
|---|---|---|
| 9 | Assess the appearance of peristomal skin and stoma. A moist-reddish-pink stoma is considered normal. | Change in normal appearance may indicate anemia, altered circulation, and it should be informed to physician. |
| 10 | Apply paste type skin barrier (Zinc oxide) if required and allow the paste to dry for 1- 2 minutes. | Establishes a smooth surface for application of skin barrier and pouch. |
| 11 | Apply the skin barrier and appliance together.<br>• Select size of stoma opening by using the measurement guide.<br>• Trace same size circle on the back at the center of the skin barrier.<br>• Use scissors to cut an opening 1/4 or 1/8 inch larger than stoma.<br>• Remove the backing to expose sticky side.<br>• Remove gauze pad covering stoma.<br>• Ease barrier and pouch over the stoma and gently press onto skin while smoothing out creases or wrinkles. Hold the pouch in place for 5 minutes (Figure 5.10(a)). | Placing both the skin barrier and appliance together over the stoma makes application easier for the patient Smooth application of pouch prevents escape of odour and feces. |

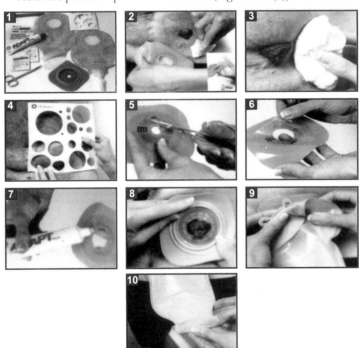

**Figure 5.10(a):** Steps of changing a colostomy bag (2-piece system)

| | | |
|---|---|---|
| 12 | Instill deodrant in bag if required | |
| 13 | Close the pouch if it is drainable by folding the end upward and using a clamp or clip according to manufacturer's direction. | A tightly sealed appliance will not leak and cause embarrasment and discomfort for the patient. |
| 14 | Dispose of used equipment discard gloves and wash hands. | Prevents spread of microorganisms. |
| 15 | Document appearance of stoma, condition of peristomal skin, and patient's reaction to procedure. | Facilitates continuity of care. |

# Elimination

## EMPTYING COLOSTOMY BAG WITHOUT CHANGING

| | | |
|---|---|---|
| 1 | Empty contents into bedpan or toilet. Rinse pouch with tepid water. | Rinsing provides clean appearance and minimises odour. |
| 2 | Wipe the lower 2 inches of the pouch with toilet tissue. | Drying the lower section of the pouch removes additional fecal material. |
| 3 | Instill deodrant in bag and uncuff the edge of the pouch and apply the clamp. | Prevents bad odour. Clamp secures closure of the appliance. |
| 4 | Dispose of used equipment, discard gloves and wash hands. | Prevents spread of microorganisms. |
| 5 | Document procedure and patient's reaction to procedure. | Ensures communication between staff members. |

## SPECIAL CONSIDERATIONS

1. Flatus may cause a pouch to balloon out. This requires immediate attention because if flatus is not released the pouch may separate from the skin barrier causing seepage of fecal contents or release of fecal odour. Open the clamp and release the flatus (never puncture a hole in the appliance).
2. Measure the patient's fluid intake and output. Check the stoma appliance for quality and quantity of discharge. Record intake and output every 4 hours for the first 3 days following surgery.
3. Stoma site should be always dry. Presence of moisture increases chance for candida or yeast infection.
4. Return of peristalsis causes an increase in flatus. Advice patients that this is indicative of bowel functioning. Also tell them to avoid gas containing food since there is no way to voluntarily control passing of flatus.

# 5.11: PERFORMING A COLOSTOMY IRRIGATION

## DEFINITION

An enema given through a colostomy to cleanse lower colon.

## PURPOSES

1. To clean colon.
2. To establish regular pattern of evacuation.
3. To prevent excoriation of skin around stoma.
4. To observe stoma and surrounding skin.
5. To teach patient and family about care of colostomy especially if colostomy is permanent.

## ARTICLES

Tray containing
1. Irrigation can with tubing and clamp
2. Rectal catheter and funnel
3. Irrigation sleeve
4. Jug with solution at body temperature
5. Lubricant
6. Clean cotton swabs
7. Rag pieces/paper tissues
8. Dressing articles
9. Protective ointments such as zinc oxide
10. Protective sheet/mackintosh
11. Clean gloves and colostomy bag
12. Wash cloth
13. Soap
14. Towel and clean linen
15. Kidney tray and paper bag
16. Receptacle with disinfecting lotion for soiled linen
17. Bedpan/bucket for return flow

## PROCEDURE

| | Nursing action | Rationale |
|---|---|---|
| 1. | Assess frequency of defecation, character of stool and placement of stoma, as well as nutritional pattern | Indicates need to irrigate and stimulate elimination function. |
| 2. | Assess time when patient normally irrigates colostomy. In case of new colostomy, confer with physician about when irrigation can begin. Obtain written order. Confer with patient for best time to irrigate | Maintains established routine for bowel emptying. Bowel must be totally healed so irrigation fluid will not cause perforation. Irrigation will initiate attempt to establish regular bowel emptying. This usually occurs 3-7 days after surgery. |
| 3. | Review orders for diagnostic or surgical procedures involving the bowel. | Procedures may indicate need to cleanse bowel of fecal contents or delay in starting irrigation procedure. |
| 4. | Explain procedure to the patient. | Helps in obtaining co-operation of patient. |
| 5. | Assemble equipment and close curtains or door. | Optimizes use of time and conserves patient's and nurse's energy. Provides privacy. |

# Elimination

*Contd...*

*Contd...*

| 6. | Position patient<br>  a.  On toilet, or in chair in front of toilet, if ambulatory<br>  b.  On side of bed with head slightly elevated, if unable to be out of bed. | Allows for placement of irrigation sleeve into toilet or bedpan. |
|---|---|---|
| 7. | Don gloves | Reduces risk of transmission of micro-organisms |
| 8. | Remove used pouch by gently pushing skin from adhesive and barrier. Properly dispose off used pouch. Remove gloves and wash hands. | Prevents skin irritation and controls odor in room. |
| 9. | Apply irrigation sleeve over stoma. Distal end of sleeve should rest in water in toilet or in bedpan. | Directs flow of stool into toilet or bedpan and also controls odor and splashing |
| 10. | Fill irrigation bag with 1000 ml warm tap water, clear tubing of air, hang bag no higher than patient's shoulder height or 18 to 20 inches above stoma. | 500 to 1000 ml are sufficient to distend the colon and effect evacuation. Start with 500 ml. Cold water could trigger syncope, hot water could damage stoma and intestinal mucousa. Air entering the colon may trigger cramping. Raising the bag to 18-20 inches above stoma allows water to slowly enter colon and avoids cramping. |
| 11. | Apply gloves, lubricate cone tip and hold snugly against stomal opening (Figure 5.11(a)). Do not force the cone into stoma. Start inflow of water. Adjust direction of cone to facilitate inflow of water.<br><br><br>**Figure 5.11(a):** Inserting a cone into stoma | • Lubricating tip prevents trauma to stoma<br>• Gentle flow of water avoids perforation of bowel.<br>• Aiming flow of water towards direction of bowel aids in flow |
| 12. | Allow water to flow in over 5 to 10 minutes period. | Avoids rapid distention of bowel, which triggers cramping. If cramping or nausea occurs, stop the inflow of water until it subsides and have patient take a few slow deep breaths. |
| 13. | After the desired amount of water has entered the colon., clamp the tubing and wait 15 seconds before removing the cone. | Avoids sudden back flow of water from the stoma. |
| 14. | Allow 15 to 20 minutes for initial evacuation, dry tip of sleeve and clamp bottom. Fold the sleeve up and leave the top cover in place for 30 to 45 minutes. Discard gloves patient may walk around. | Clamping the sleeve prevents leakage and optimizes evacuation of stool. |
| 15. | Don gloves, unclamp sleeve (Figure 5.11(b)), empty any fecal contents, remove sleeve, rinse with liquid cleanser and cool water. Hang sleeve to dry. | Maintains sleeve in clean condition for future use. |

*Contd...*

*Contd...*

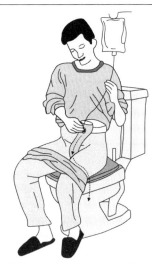

**Figure 5.11(b):** Irrigating colostomy with sleeve in place

| | |
|---|---|
| 16. Apply new colostomy pouch or stoma covering as per procedure | Avoids accidental leakage, soiling of clothes, skin irritation, etc. |
| 17. Remove gloves and wash hands | Reduces risk of transmission of micro-organisms |
| 18. Inspect volume and character of fecal material and fluid that returns after irrigation | Determines if water is retained. If patient is dehydrated, bowel may absorb irrigation solution. Character and amount of stool reveals success in evacuation. |
| 19. Note patient's response during irrigation. Ask if cramping or abdominal pain is felt | Reveals tolerance of irrigation |
| 20. Record procedure, time of irrigation, volume and type of solution if water is used, amount and type of return, patients tolerance | Documents procedure and results, data used for comparison for future irrigation. |
| 21. Record reapplication of pouch and condition of stoma and skin | Enables communication between staff members. |
| 22. Report symptoms of extreme discomfort, onset of severe diarrhea, poor results or excessive bleeding to nurse in charge or physician | Indicates need for additional therapy |

## SPECIAL CONSIDERATIONS

1. Debilitated confused or unconscious patients are at risk for constipation or impaction. Irrigate only with physician's order if obstruction is suspected.
2. Only patients with stoma in the lower descending or sigmoid colon are candidates for colostomy irrigation for routine bowel evacuation.
3. Use of tube without a cone tip carries higher risk of perforation of colon.
4. Patients who develop diarrhea should discontinue irrigation until stool thickens. Diet, medication, radiation, chemotherapy bacterial infection and other factors can cause diarrhea.

# Chapter 6

# Oxygenation

# 6.1(A): OXYGEN THERAPY –CANNULA METHOD

## DEFINITION

A method by which oxygen is administered in low concentration through a cannula which is a disposable plastic device with two protruding prongs for insertion into the nostrils.

## PURPOSES

1. To relieve dyspnea.
2. To administer low concentration of oxygen to patients.
3. To allow uninterrupted supply of oxygen during activities like eating, drinking etc.

## ARTICLES

1. Oxygen source
2. Nasal cannula with connecting tubes
3. Humidifier with distilled water
4. Flowmeter
5. Gauze pads
6. "No smoking" signs.

## PROCEDURE

| | Nursing action | Rationale |
|---|---|---|
| 1 | Determine need for oxygen therapy in patient. Check physician's order for rate, device used concentration etc. | Reduces risk of error in administration. |
| 2 | Perform an assessment of vital signs, level of consciousness, lab values, etc. and record. | Provides a baseline for future assessment. |
| 3 | Assess risk factors of oxygen therapy in patient and environment such as patients with hypoxia drive, faulty electrical connection etc. | Reduces risk of danger to the patient |
| 4 | Explain procedure to patient and relatives and inform them how to cooperate. | Reduces anxiety and ensures cooperation |
| 5 | Post " no smoking" sign on the patients door in view of patient and visitors and explain to them the dangers of smoking when oxygen is on flow | Oxygen supports combustion, smoking in oxygen area can lead to fire hazards. |
| 6 | Wash hands | Reduces risk of transmission of microorganisms. |
| 7 | Set up oxygen equipment and humidifier | |
| | a. Fill humidifier upto the level marked on it with sterile water | Filling beyond this point will cause water to enter tubing. |
| | b. Attach flowmeter to source, set flowmeter in 'off' position | Flow meter helps in monitoring and regulating oxygen flow to patient. |
| | c. Attach humidifier to base of flowmeter | Humidification helps in preventing drying of mucous membranes and promotes comfort of patient. |
| | d. Attach tubing and nasal cannula to humidifier | |
| | e. Regulate flowmeter to prescribed level (Figure 6.1(a)) | Oxygen is a drug and is dangerous to administer at flow rates greater or lesser than prescribed level. |
| | f. Ensure proper functioning by checking for bubbles in humidifier or feeling oxygen at the outlet. | Kinks in the tubing will obstruct flow of oxygen through tube. |

*Contd...*

*Contd...*

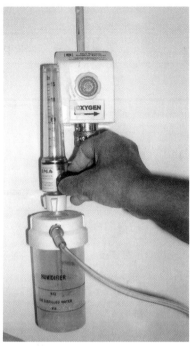

**Figure 6.1(a):** Regulating flowmeter

| | | |
|---|---|---|
| 8 | Place tips of cannula to patients nares and adjust straps around ear for snug fit. The elastic band may be fixed behind head or under chin (Figure 6.1(b)). | Proper fixing ensures comfort and prevents chances of cannula slipping from nostrils. |

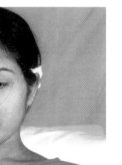

**Figure 6.1(b):** Oxygen delivered through nasal cannula

| | | |
|---|---|---|
| 9 | Pad tubing with gauze pads over ear and inspect skin behind ear periodically for irritation/breakdown | Constant pressure may cause skin breakdown |
| 10 | Inspect patient and equipment frequently for flow rate, clinical condition, level of water in humidifier etc. | Helps in identifying any complications that may arise. |
| 11 | Ensure that safety precautions are followed. | |
| 12 | Wash hands | |
| 13 | Document time, flow rate and observations made on patient. | |

*Contd...*

*Contd...*

| 14 | Encourage patient to breath through his/her nose with mouth closed | Provides for optimal delivery of oxygen to patient |
|----|----|----|
| 15 | Remove and clean the cannula with soap and water, dry and replace every 8 hours. Assess nares at least every 8 hours | Presence of cannula causes irritation and dryness of the mucous membrane. |

## SPECIAL PRECAUTIONS

1. Never deliver more than 2-3 liters of oxygen to patients with chronic lung disease, e.g. COPD.
2. Check frequently that both prongs are in patient's nares.

* Oxygen concentration will vary on many factors like patient's tidal volume and ventilatory pattern.

**Table 6.1.1**: Oxygen concentration with flow rates

| Flow rate | Oxygen concentration |
|----|----|
| 1 Liter | 24 to 25% |
| 2 Liters | 27 to 29% |
| 3 Liters | 30 to 33% |
| 4 Liters | 33 to 37% |
| 5 Liters | 36 to 41% |
| 6 Liters | 39 to 45% |

# 6.1(B): ADMINISTERING OXYGEN BY MASK METHOD

## DEFINITION

Administering oxygen to the patient by means of a mask (simple/venturi) according to requirement of patient.

## PURPOSES

1. To relieve dyspnea.
2. To administer higher concentration of oxygen.

## ARTICLES

1. Oxygen source
2. Mask (simple/or with venturi adaptor of appropriate size)
3. Humidifier with distilled water
4. Flowmeter
5. Gauze pieces
6. "No smoking "sign.

## PROCEDURE

| | Nursing action | Rationale |
|---|---|---|
| 1 | Determine need for oxygen therapy, check physician's order for rate, device to be used and concentration. | Reduces risk of error in administration. |
| 2 | Perform an assessment of vital signs, level of consciousness, lab values, etc. and record. | Provides a baseline for future assessment. |
| 3 | Assess risk factors for oxygen administration in patient and enviornment-like hypoxia drive in patient and faulty electrical connection. | Reduces risk of danger caused to patient. Oxygen is a combustible gas. Hypoxia drive in patients is essential for maintaining respiration. |
| 4 | Explain procedure to patient and relatives and emphasize how he has to cooperate. | Reduces anxiety and enhances cooperation. |
| 5 | Post " no smoking" signals on patient's door in view of patient and visitors and explain to them the dangers of smoking when oxygen is on flow. | Oxygen supports combustion. Smoking in oxygen area can lead to fire hazards. |
| 6 | Wash hands | Reduces risk of transmission of microorganisms. |
| 7 | Set up oxygen equipment and humidifier.<br>a. Fill humidifer upto the mark on it. | Filling humidifier above this level will cause water to enter into tubing. |
| | b. Attach flow meter to source. Set flow meter in "off" position. | Flowmeter will help in monitoring and regulating oxygen flow to patient. |
| | c. Attach humidifer bottle to base of the flowmeter | Humidification helps prevent drying of mucous membrane and promotes comfort of patient. |
| | d. Attach tubing and face mask to humidifier (If venturi device is used attach the color coded venturi adapter to mask s as appropriate) (Figure 6.1(c)) | |
| | e. Regulate flowmeter to prescribed level | Oxygen is a drug and it is dangerous to administer at flow rates greater or lesser than prescribed level. |

*Contd...*

*Contd...*

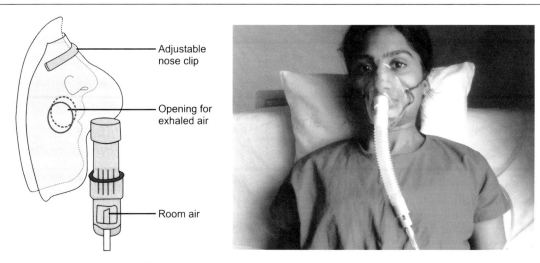

**Figure 6.1(c):** Oxygen delivered through venturi mask

| 8 | Guide mask to patient's face and apply it from nose downward. Fit the metal piece of mask to conform to shape of nose. | The mask should mould to face so that very little oxygen escapes into eyes or around cheeks or chin |
|---|---|---|
| 9 | Secure elastic band around patient's head. | Ensures comfort of patient |
| 10 | Apply padding behind ears as well as scalp where elastic band passes. | Padding prevents irritation to skin around area. |
| 11 | Ensure that safety precautions are followed | |
| 12 | Inspect patient and equipment frequently for flow rate, clinical condition, level of water in humidifier etc. | Identifies complications if they develop. |
| 13 | Wash hands | Reduces risk of transmission of microorganisms. |
| 14 | Remove the mask and dry the skin every 2-3 hours if oxygen is administered continuously. Do not put powder around the mask. | The tight fitting mask and moisture from condensation can irritate the skin on the face. There is danger of inhaling powder if it is placed around mask. |
| 15 | Document relevant data in patient's record. | |

# 6.1(C): ADMINISTERING OXYGEN USING OXYGEN TENT

## DEFINITION

Process of administering oxygen by means of a tent, usually for infants which gives maximum comfort and most satisfactory results.

## DESCRIPTION

An oxygen tent consists of a canopy over the baby's bed that may cover the baby fully or partially and is connected to a supply of oxygen. The canopies are transparent and enables the nurse to observe the sick baby.

## ADVANTAGES

1. Provides an environment for the patient with controlled oxygen concentration, temperature regulation and humidity control.
2. It allows freedom of movement in bed.

## DISADVANTAGES

1. It creates a feeling of isolation.
2. It requires high level of oxygen (10-12 liters per minute)
3. Loss of desired concentration occurs each time the tent is opened to provide care for the infant.
4. There is an increased chance of hazards due to fire.
5. It requires much time and effort to clean and maintain a tent.

## ARTICLES

Oxygen tent and oxygen source, humidifier.

## PROCEDURE

|   | Nursing action | Rationale |
|---|---|---|
| 1 | Explain and reassure the parents and child. | Helps in obtaining cooperation. |
| 2 | Select the smallest tent and canopy that will achieve the desired concentration of oxygen and maintain patient comfort. | Increases the efficiency of the unit. |
| 3 | Tuck the edges of the tent under the mattress securely. This is especially important if the child is restless and can dislodge the tent by pulling the covers loose. | Dislodgement of tent leads to oxygen leakage. |
| 4 | Pad the metal frame that supports the canopy. | Protects the child from injury. |
| 5 | Flush the tent with oxygen (increase the flowrate) after it has been opened for a period of time, to increase the concentration of the gas, then reset the flowmeter to the original level. | Oxygen is circulated in the tent to adjust the concentration. |
| 6 | Analyze and record the tent atmosphere every 1-2 hours. Concentrations of 30 to 50% can be achieved in well maintained tents. | Concentration varies with the efficiency of the tent., the rate of flow of oxygen, and the frequency with which tent is opened to the outside environment. |
| 7 | Maintain a tight fitting canopy whenever possible, provide nursing care through the sleeves or pockets of the tent. | Prevents oxygen leakage and disruption of the tent atmosphere. |

*Contd...*

*Contd...*

| | | |
|---|---|---|
| 8 | Check child's temperature routinely. | Moisture accumulation may result in hypothermia. |
| 9 | 'No smoking' sign should be pasted in the unit. | Oxygen helps in combustion. |
| 10 | Record the flowrate of oxygen, alteration in flowrate and child's reaction. | Serves as a communication between staff members. |

## SPECIAL CONSIDERATIONS

1. Mist is prescribed with oxygen therapy to liquefy secretions.
2. Humidified air may condense into water droplets on the inside walls of the tent, it is important to examine the child's clothing and bedding and change them as necessary to prevent chilling.
3. Electrical equipments used within or near the tent should be grounded properly.
4. It is preferable to monitor $SpO_2$ of patient continuously.
5. Avoid the use of volatile, inflammable materials such as oils, grease, alcohol, ether and acetone near the tent.
6. Nurses should be knowledgeable about the location and technique for using a fire extinguisher.
7. For the baby in oxygen tent toys selected should be such that they retard absorption are washable and will not produce static electricity, e.g. woolen and stuffed toys. This ensures baby's safety.

# 6.2: ADMINISTERING STEAM INHALATION

## DEFINITION

Deep breathing of warm and moist air (vapor) into the lungs for local effect on the air passages or for a systemic effect.

## PURPOSES

1. To relieve the inflammation and congestion of the mucous membranes of the respiratory tract and paranasal sinuses thus to produce symptomatic relief in acute and chronic sinusitis.
2. To soften thick tenacious mucus which helps in its expulsion from the respiratory tract.
3. To provide moisture and heat and to prevent dryness of the mucous membranes of the lungs and upper respiratory passages following operation such as tracheostomy.
4. To aid in absorption of oxygen.
5. To relieve spastic conditions of the larynx and bronchi.
6. To provide antiseptic action on the respiratory tract (e.g.) by using menthol, eucalyptus and tincture benzoin.

## ARTICLES

1. Tray containing
   a. Towel
   b. Nelson's inhaler in a bowl
   c. Sputum cup with antiseptic solution
   d. Inhaler mouthpiece
   e. Gauze piece
   f. Cotton ball
   g. Ounce glass
   h. Face towel
   i. Kidney tray or paper bag
2. Cardiac table
3. Pillows
4. Medication like tincture benzoin if ordered
5. Boiling water (160° F)

## PROCEDURE

| | Nursing action | Rationale |
|---|---|---|
| 1. | Check the physician's order and nursing care plan. | |
| 2. | Explain the procedure to patient and ensure that patient has emptied his bowel and bladder | Helps in promoting relaxation. Patient will have to remain in bed for 1 hour. |
| 3. | Warm the inhaler by pouring a little hot water into the inhaler and emptying it after one minute. | Reduces loss of heat from inhaler during procedure. |
| 4. | Pour the required amount of inhalant into the inhaler and fill to a level below the spout with boiling water. The water should remain just below the spout | If the inhaler is filled up to the level of spout there is possibility of drawing water into the mouth when inhaling and cause scalds. If the spout is filled with water it will not act as an air inlet. |
| 5. | Place sterile mouthpiece and close the inhaler tightly. See that the mouthpiece is in the opposite direction to the spout. | This arrangement keeps the spout away from the patient when inhalations are taken in. |

*Contd...*

*Contd...*

| | | |
|---|---|---|
| 6. | Cover the mouth piece with a gauze piece and plug the spout with a cotton ball. | Covering the mouthpiece with a gauze piece will prevent burns of the lips. Cotton ball in the spout will prevent escape of steam. |
| 7. | Place a towel around the inhaler and position it in the bowl. | Insulates the inhaler and prevents heat loss. |
| 8. | Take it to the patient without losing time. | |
| 9. | Switch off fan/AC or close windows and doors. | |
| 10. | Position the patient in high fowlers or sitting position. | |
| 11. | Place the apparatus conveniently in front of the patient on cardiac table with spout opposite to the patient. Remove the cotton plug and discard it into the paper bag (Figure 6.2(a)). | Keeping the spout opposite to the patient reduces the chances of burns. Removing the cotton plug helps to open spout, so that it can act as an inlet for air. |

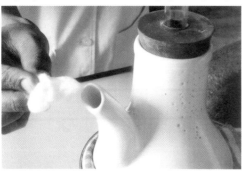

Figure 6.2(a): Removing cotton plug from the spout

| | | |
|---|---|---|
| 12. | Instruct the patient to place lips on the mouthpiece and take deep breath. After removing the lips from the mouthpiece, breathe out air through nose (Figure 6.2(b)). | Directing the steam out through the nostril relieves the congestion of the mucous membranes of the nostril |

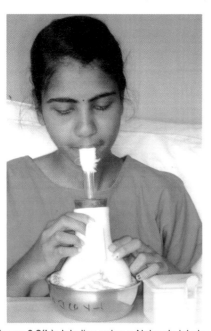

Figure 6.2(b): Inhaling using a Nelson's inhaler

*Contd...*

*Contd...*

| | | |
|---|---|---|
| 13. | Continue the treatment for 15 to 20 minutes as long as patient gets the vapours. Observe the patient during procedure | Helps in effectiveness of the procedure. |
| 14. | Remove inhaler from the patient after the stated time, wipe off perspiration from the patient's face | Enhances comfort of patient. |
| 15. | Give chest physiotherapy and encourage patient to bring out sputum by coughing | |
| 16. | Instruct the patient to remain in the bed for 1 to 2 hours | Reduces chances of dizziness and effects of sudden temperature variation. |
| 17. | Take articles to the utility room, empty the inhaler, clean the inside with alcohol to remove Tr. benzoin. Wash it with warm soapy water and then rinse with clean water. Clean the ounce glass with alcohol swab followed by soapy water. Remove the gauze covering the mouthpiece and wash the mouthpiece with soap and water and send for autoclaving .Dry the articles and replace them. Wash hands. | Cleaning of articles avoids contamination and cross-infection. |
| 18. | Record the procedure in nurse's record with date, time, purpose and patient's response to the procedure. | Communicates to staff about effectiveness and reinforcement of the procedure. |

## SPECIAL POINTS

- Steam inhalation can be given using a kettle or electric inhaler.
- When a wide-mouthed vessel is used for inhalation, patient's head and inhaler may be covered using a sheet or blanket to help increase the concentration of steam.
- During inhalation if patient stops for a while for coughing or expectorating sputum, the spout may be closed with cotton ball to prevent escape of steam.

# 6.3: ASSESSMENT OF OXYGEN SATURATION USING PULSE OXIMETER

## DESCRIPTION

A pulse oximeter is a non-invasive device which has selected wavelength of light passed through a vascular bed to estimate arterial oxyhemoglobin saturation. The pulse oximeter uses infrared light and a process known as spectrophotometry to measure the amount of oxygenated hemoglobin in arterial blood.

**The oximeter unit display indicates:**
Capillary $O_2$ saturation and pulse rate.
The oximeter unit also has provision for setting alarms (High and Low) for pulse rate and $O_2$ saturation.

## PURPOSES

1. To measure the capillary blood oxygen saturation.
2. To detect the presence of hypoxemia before visible signs develop.
3. To assess the response to therapy.
4. To assess the need to decrease the number of arterial blood gas specimens drawn.

## INDICATIONS

1. Patients who may experience sudden change in blood oxygen level (unstable conditions)
2. Patients who will need evaluation for home oxygen therapy.
3. Patients who need supplemental oxygen at rest and with exercise.

## PROCEDURE

|   | Nursing Action | Rationale |
|---|---|---|
| 1 | Explain procedure to patient | Explanation relieves anxiety and facilitates patient's cooperation. |
| 2 | Perform hand hygiene | Prevents spread of microorganisms. |
| 3 | Select an appropriate site for application of the sensor.<br>a. Use the patient's index, middle or ringfinger.<br><br>b. Check the proximal pulse and capillary refill of the pulse closest to the site.<br>c. If circulation at site is inadequate, the earlobe or bridge of nose may be considered.<br>d. Use a toe only if lower extremity circulation is not compromised. | Inadequate circulation can interfere with the $SaO_2$ reading.<br>Brisk capillary refill and a strong pulse indicate that circulation to the site is adequate.<br>These sites are highly vascular alternatives.<br><br>Peripheral vascular disease is common in lower extremities. |
| 4 | Use the proper equipment:<br>a. If one finger is too large for the probe, use a smaller one. A pediatric probe may be used for a small adult.<br>b. Use probes appropriate for patient's age and size.<br>c. Check if patient is allergic to adhesive. A non-adhesive finger clip or reflectance sensor is available. | Inaccurate readings can result if probe or sensor is not attached correctly.<br>Probes come in adult, pediatric and infant sizes.<br>A reaction may occur if patient is allergic to adhesive substance. |
| 5 | Prepare the monitoring site:<br>a. Cleanse the selected area and allow it to dry. | Skin oils, dirt or grime on site, polish and artificial nails can interfere with the passage of light waves. |

*Contd...*

*Contd...*

b. Remove nail polish and artificial nails

| | | |
|---|---|---|
| 6 | Apply the probe securely to the skin, make sure that light emitting sensor and the light receiving sensor are aligned opposite to each other (not necessary to check if placed on the forehead or bridge of the nose). (Figure 6.3(a)) | Ensures accurate recording of $SaO_2$. |

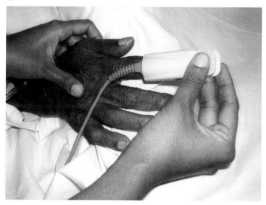

**Figure 6.3(a):** Applying pulse oximeter probe

| | | |
|---|---|---|
| 7 | Connect the sensor probe to the pulse oximeter and check operation of the equipment like presence of audible beep and fluctuation of bar of light or waveform on the monitor of the oximeter. | Audible beep represents the arterial pulse and fluctuating waveform indicates strength of the pulse. A weak signal will produce an inaccurate recording of $SaO_2$. Tone of beep reflects $SaO_2$ reading. If $SaO_2$ drops, tone becomes low pitched. |
| 8 | Set the alarms on the pulse oximeter. Check manufacturer's alarm limits for high and low pulse rate settings. | Alarm provides additional safeguard for patient and signals when high or low limits have been surpassed. |
| 9 | Check oxygen saturation at regular intervals as ordered by physician and necessitated by alarms. Monitor patient's hemoglobin level. | Monitoring $SaO_2$ provides ongoing assessment of patient's condition. A low hemoglobin level may be satisfactorily saturated yet not be adequate to meet a patient's oxygen needs. |
| 10 | Remove sensor on a regular basis and check for skin irritation or signs of pressure. | Prolonged pressure may lead to tissue necrosis and adhesive sensor may cause skin irritation. |
| 11 | Evaluate any malfunctions or problems with equipment.<br>a. For absent or weak signal, check the patient's vital signs and condition. If satisfactory, check connections and circulation to site. | Hypotension makes an accurate recording difficult. Restraint and B.P. cuff may compromise circulation to site and cause venous blood to pulsate, giving an inaccurate reading. If extremity is cold, cover with warm blanket. |
| | b. If reading is inaccurate check prescribed medications and history of circulatory disorders. Try device on a healthy person to see if problem is equipment-related or patient related. | Drugs that cause vasoconstriction interfere with accurate recording of oxygen saturation. |
| | c. If bright light (Sunlight or fluorescent light) is suspected of causing equipment malfunction, cover probe with a dry wash cloth. | Bright light can interfere with operation of light sensors and cause report unreliable. |
| 12 | Record the application of pulse oximeter, its type and size and all nursing assessments. | Documentation ensures continuity of care and ongoing assessment record. |

## SPECIAL CONSIDERATIONS

1. Do not use oximeter if light indicates low battery.
2. The patient with diabetes, peripheral vascular disease or hypothyroidism may have thickened or discolored nailbeds. Assess the patient and move the sensor to an alternate site if required.
3. Finger sensors are generally not sized appropriately for children and are not intended for neonatal or pediatric use. Adhesive sensors can be used on the hand or feet of children or on the hand of the neonate.

# 6.4: ASSISTING THE PATIENT WITH THE USE OF AN INCENTIVE SPIROMETER

## DEFINITION

Assisting the patient for voluntary deep breathing by providing visual feedback about inspiratory volume by using a specially designed apparatus called spirometer.

## PURPOSES

1. To improve pulmonary ventilation.
2. To counteract the effects of anesthesia or hypoventilation.
3. To loosen respiratory secretions.
4. To facilitate respiratory gaseous exchange.
5. To expand collapsed alveoli.
6. To prevent postoperative respiratory complications.

## INDICATIONS

1. Patients on long-term bed rest.
2. Patients with chronic and restrictive lung diseases.
3. Patients on medications that depress respiration.
4. Postoperative patients.

## TYPES

1. Volume-oriented: The tidal volume of the spirometer is set according to the manufacturer's instructions. Purposes: To ensure that the volume of air initiated is increased gradually as the patient takes deeper and deeper breaths.
2. Flow spirometer: There is no preset volume. The spirometer contains a number of movable balls that are pushed up by the force of the breath and held suspended in the air while the patient inhales. The amount of air inhaled and the flow of the air are estimated by how long and how high the balls are suspended.

## ARTICLES

1. Stethoscope
2. Incentive spirometer with appropriate mouthpiece (Figure 6.4(a)).
   a. Flow-oriented or
   b. Volume-oriented
3. Tissue paper
4. Emesis basin
5. Pillow if needed.

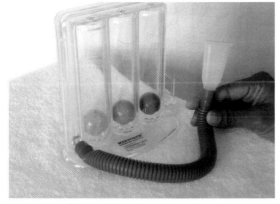

**Figure 6.4(a):** Incentive spirometer

## PROCEDURE

| | Nursing Action | Rationale |
|---|---|---|
| 1 | Explain the reason and objective for the therapy that the inspired air helps to inflate the lungs. The ball or weight in the spirometer will rise in response to the intensity of the intake of air. The higher the ball rises, the deeper the breath. | Helps in obtaining cooperation of patient. |
| 2 | Assess the patient's respiratory status by general observation, auscultation of breathsounds and percussion of thorax. | Helps in comparison after procedure. |
| 3 | Review medical record for recent arterial blood gas. | Determines need for using incentive spirometer. |
| 4 | Remove dentures | Dentures interfere with performance of procedure. |
| 5 | Wash hands | Reduces the transmission of microorganisms. |
| 6 | Instruct patient to assume a semi Fowler's or high Fowler's position. | Promotes optimal lung expansion. |
| 7 | Set pointer on incentive spirometer at appropriate level or point to level where disk or ball should reach. | Encourage patient to reach appropriate goal. |
| 8 | For the postoperative patient try as much as possible to avoid discomfort with the treatment.<br>Co-ordinate treatment with administration of pain relief medications.<br>Instruct and assist the patient with splinting of incision. | More likely to have best results in using incentive spirometry when patient has as little pain as possible. |
| 9 | Demonstrate the technique to the patient<br>a. Hold or place the spirometer in an upright position. A tilted flow-oriented device requires less effort to raise the balls or disks. A volume oriented device will not function correctly unless upright (Figure 6.4(b)). | |

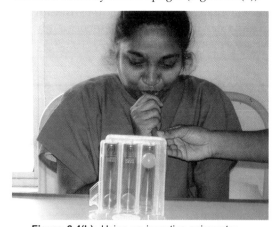

**Figure 6.4(b):** Using an incentive spirometer

    b. Demonstrate how to steady device with one hand and hold mouthpiece with the other hand.

    c. Instruct the patient to exhale normally and then place lips securely around mouthpiece.

    d. Instruct to take a slow, deep breath to elevate the balls or cylinder and then hold the breath for 2 seconds initially increasing to 6 seconds to keep the balls or cylinder elevated if possible.

*Contd...*

*Contd...*

| | | |
|---|---|---|
| | e. Instruct patient not to breath through his or her nose. Use a noseclip if necessary.<br>f. Tell patient to remove lips from mouthpiece and exhale normally. | |
| 10 | Instruct patient to relax and repeat the procedure several times and then four or five times hourly. | Practice increases inspiratory volume, maintains alveolar ventilation and prevents atelectasis. |
| 11 | Instruct patient to cough after the procedure. | Deep ventilation can loosen secretions and coughing can facilitate their removal. |
| 12 | Clean the mouthpiece with water and shake it dry. Change disposable mouthpieces every 24 hours. | |
| 13 | Record lung volume in cubic centimeters. Respiratory assessment (rate and depth of respiration, the amount of secretions expectorated.) | Acts as a communication between staff members. |

## SPECIAL CONSIDERATIONS

1. Patient should take several normal breaths before attempting another one with the incentive spirometer. Usually one incentive breath per minute minimises patient fatigue. No more than four or five maneuvers should be performed per minute to minimise hypocarbia.
2. Assess for tactile fremitus and voice sounds to note the development of consolidation.

# 6.5: PERFORMING POSTURAL DRAINAGE

## DEFINITION

Postural drainage is the gravitational clearance of secretions from specific bronchial segments by using one or more of ten different positions.

Each position drains a specific corresponding section of the tracheobronchial tree, either from the upper, middle or lower lung field into the trachea. Coughing or suctioning can then remove secretions from the trachea.

Areas are selected for drainage based on:
1. Knowledge of patient's condition, and disease process.
2. Physical assessment of the chest.
3. Chest X-ray examination results.

## CONTRAINDICATIONS

1. Increased intracranial pressure (ICP)
2. Unstable head or neck injury
3. Active hemorrhage with hemodynamic instability
4. Recent spinal surgery or injury
5. Empyema
6. Bronchopleural fistula
7. Rib fractures or flail chest
8. Lung tumor
9. Diseases of chest wall
10. Hemorrhage in respiratory tract
11. Painful chest conditions
12. Tuberculosis
13. Osteoporosis.

## ARTICLES

1. A comfortable surface, that can be slanted such as hospital beds in Trendelenburg's position or tilt table and chair if draining upper lobe areas.
2. One to four pillows, depending on patient's posture and comfort.
3. A glass with water.
4. Tissues and paper bag.
5. Sputum cup.

## POSITIONS FOR DRAINING DIFFERENT AREAS OF LUNGS (Figure 6.5(a))

1. *Left and right upper lobe anterior apical bronchi*: Have patient sit in chair leaning back. Percuss with cupped hands and vibrate with heels of hands at shoulders and with fingers over collarbone. Both sides can be done at the same time. Note body posture and arm position of nurse. Nurse's back is kept straight and elbows and knees are slightly flexed.
2. *Left and right upper lobes posterior apical bronchi*: Have patient sit in chair leaning forward on pillow or cardiac table. Percuss and vibrate with hands on either side of the upper spine, can do both sides at the same time.
3. *Right and left anterior upper lobe bronchi*: Have patient lie flat on back with small pillow under knees. Percuss and vibrate just below clavicle on either side of sternum.
4. *Left upper lobe lingular bronchus*: Have patient lie on right side with arm over head in Trendelenburg position with foot of bed raised 30 cm. Place pillow behind back and roll patient one-fourth on to pillow Percuss and vibrate lateral to left nipple below axilla.

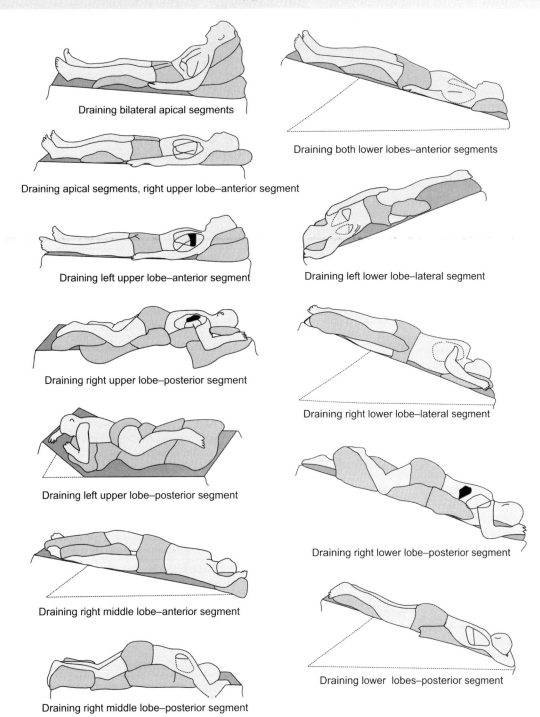

Draining bilateral apical segments

Draining apical segments, right upper lobe—anterior segment

Draining left upper lobe—anterior segment

Draining right upper lobe—posterior segment

Draining left upper lobe—posterior segment

Draining right middle lobe—anterior segment

Draining right middle lobe—posterior segment

Draining both lower lobes—anterior segments

Draining left lower lobe—lateral segment

Draining right lower lobe—lateral segment

Draining right lower lobe—posterior segment

Draining lower lobes—posterior segment

**Figure 6.5(a):** Positions for postural drainage

# Clinical Nursing Procedures: The Art of Nursing Practice

5. *Right middle lobe bronchus*: Have patient lie on left side, raise foot of bed 30 cm. Place pillow behind back and roll patient one-fourth turned on to pillow. Percuss and vibrate area of right nipple below axilla.
6. *Left and right anterior lower lobe bronchi*: Have patient lie on back in Trendelenburg position, with foot of bed elevated 45 – 50 cm. Have knees bent on pillow. Percuss and vibrate over lower anterior ribs on both sides.
7. *Right lower lobe lateral bronchus:* Have patient lie on left side in Trendelenburg position with foot of bed raised to 45 to 50 cm. Percuss and vibrate right side of the chest below scapula posterior to mid axillary line.
8. *Left lower lateral bronchus*: Have patient lie on right side in Trendelenburg position with foot of bed raised to 45 to 50 cm. Percuss and vibrate left side of the chest below scapula posterior to mid axillary line.
9. *Right and left lower lobe superior bronchi:* Have patient lie flat on stomach with pillow under stomach. Percuss and vibrate below scapulae on either side of spine.
10. *Left and right posterior basal bronchi*: Have patient lie on stomach in Trendelenburg position with foot of bed elevated 40 to 50 cm. Percuss and vibrate over posterior ribs on either side of spine.

## PROCEDURE

| | Nursing action | Rationale |
|---|---|---|
| 1. | Identify patient and check physician's order for specific instructions for postural drainage. | Performs correct procedure for the right patient. |
| 2. | Assess for possible impairment of airway clearance. | Certain circumstances, disease process, and conditions place patient at risk for impaired airway clearance. |
| 3. | Identify signs and symptoms that indicate need to perform postural drainage such as changes in X-ray film consistent with atelectasis, pneumonia, bronchiectasis, ineffective coughing with thick sticky tenacious sputum and abnormal breath sounds such as wheezing, crackling and gurgling | X-ray film data and signs and symptoms indicate accumulation of pulmonary secretions. |
| 4. | Identify which bronchial segments needs to be drained by reviewing chest X-ray reports. Auscultate over all lung fields for wheezes, crackles and gurgles, palpate over all lung fields for crepitus, fremitus and chest expansion | Area of lung congestion and postures for drainage will vary depending on disease process, patient condition and patient problem. Areas most in need of and responsive to postural drainage usually can be easily identified by presence of early inspiratory crackles and gurgles. |
| 5. | Determine patient's understanding of and ability to perform home postural drainage | Allows nurse to identify potential need for instruction. |
| 6. | Wash hands | Reduces transmission of microorganisms. |
| 7. | Select congested areas to be drained based on assessment of all lung fields, clinical data and chest X-ray data | To be effective, treatment must be individualized to treat specific areas involved. |
| 8. | Place patient in position to drain congested areas. Area selected may vary from patient to patient. Help patient assume position as needed. Teach patient correct posture and arm and leg positioning, place pillows for support and comfort. | Specific positions are selected to drain each area involved. |
| 9. | Have patient maintain posture for 10 to 15 minutes | In adults, draining each area takes time. |
| 10. | During 10 to 15 minutes of drainage in each posture, perform chest percussion and vibration over areas being drained. | These maneuvers provide mechanical forces that aid in mobilization of airway secretions. |
| 11. | After 10 to 15 minutes of drainage in first posture, have patient sit up and cough. Save expectorated secretions in clear container. If patient cannot cough suctioning to be performed. | Secretions mobilized into central airways should be removed by coughing or suctioning before placing patient into next drainage position. Coughing is most effective when patient is sitting up and leaning forward. |

*Contd...*

*Contd...*

| | |
|---|---|
| 12. Have patient rest briefly if necessary. | Short rest periods between postures can prevent fatigue and help patient for better tolerance to therapy |
| 13. Have patient take sips of water | Keeping mouth moist aids in expectoration of secretions. |
| 14. Repeat procedure until all congested areas selected have been drained. Each treatment should not exceed 30 to 60 minutes. | Postural drainage is used only to drain areas involved and is based on individual assessment. |
| 15. Wash hands | Reduces transmission of microorganisms. |
| 16. Record in nurse's notes baseline and post therapy assessment of chest, frequency and duration of treatment, postures used and bronchial segments drained, cough effectiveness, need for suctioning, color, amount and consistency of sputum, hemoptysis or other unexpected outcome, patient's tolerance and reactions. | Helps to evaluate outcomes and need for changes in therapy. |

## SPECIAL CONSIDERATIONS

1. Provide inhalation using bronchodilators 20 minutes before postural drainage for patients at risk of bronchospasm
2. In severe hemaptysis, stop therapy, remain calm, and stay with patient. Request assistance and keep patient comfortable, warm and quiet.
3. Best times for treatment are:
   • In the morning before breakfast, when patient can clear secretions that accumulate overnight
   • One hour before bed time, so lungs are clear before sleeping and patient has time after treatment to cough up any mobilized secretions.
4. If patient's condition is acute, frequent treatments are tolerated best.
5. If patient is receiving-inhaled bronchodilators or aerosol therapy, postural drainage should be done after 20 minutes.
6. The procedure should be discontinued if tachycardia, palpitation, dyspnea or chest pain occur. These symptoms may indicate hypoxemia.
7. Do not perform postral drainage immediately after taking food.

# 6.6: PERFORMING CHEST PHYSIOTHERAPY

## DEFINITION

Method of facilitating respiratory function by removing thick, tenacious secretions from the respiratory system using techniques of percussion, vibration and postural drainage.

## PURPOSE

To remove tenacious secretions from bronchial walls in conditions like bronchiectasis and chronic bronchitis.

## INDICATIONS

1. Patients who bring out more than 30 ml of sputum in a day.
2. Patients who are at risk of atelectasis.

## ARTICLES

1. Pillows
2. Sputum cup with disinfectant
3. Paper tissues
4. Adjustable bed
5. Kidney tray
6. Stethoscope.

## CONTRAINDICATIONS

1. Undrained lung abscess
2. Lung tumor
3. Pneumothorax
4. Diseases of chest wall
5. Lung hemorrhage/hemoptysis
6. Painful chest condition, e.g. pleural effusion
7. Tuberculosis
8. Osteoporosis
9. Increased intracranial pressure
10. Spinal injuries.

## PROCEDURE

| | Nursing action | Rationale |
|---|---|---|
| 1. | Identify patient and check instruction of physician and nursing care plan. | Ensures that right procedure is done on the right patient. |
| 2. | Explain procedure to patient and check when meals were last taken. | Reassures patient and promotes co-operation. Postural drainage should be avoided immediately after meal times as it can induce vomiting. |
| 3. | Wash hands and dry. | Reduces transmission of microorganisms. |
| 4. | Instruct patient to perform diaphragmatic breathing. | This method of breathing helps patient to relax and widens airways. |
| 5. | Position patient in prescribed postural drainage position, after consulting with physician (refer postural drainage procedure). | Position should be selected according to the area of lung that is to be drained. |

*Contd...*

*Contd...*

| | | |
|---|---|---|
| 6. | Cover area with towel | Reduces discomfort to patient. |
| 7. | Percussion<br>Clap with cupped hands over chest wall for 1to 2 minutes in each lung area. Percuss from<br>• Lower ribs to shoulder in the back<br>• Lower ribs to top of chest in front<br>Avoid clapping over spine, liver, kidney, spleen, breast, clavicle or sternum (Figure 6.6(a)). | Percussion helps in dislodging mucous plugs and mobilizes secretions into main stem bronchi and trachea. The air trapped under cupped hand sets up vibration through chest wall freeing secretions. Percussion over these areas may cause injuries |

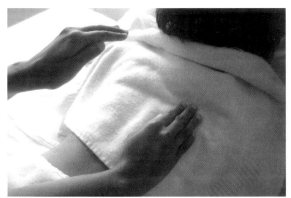

**Figure 6.6(a):** Percussion using cupped hands

| | | |
|---|---|---|
| 8. | Vibration<br>Remove towel and place hand, palm down on chest area to be drained with one hand over the other and fingers together or place hands side by side (Figure 6.6(b)). | |

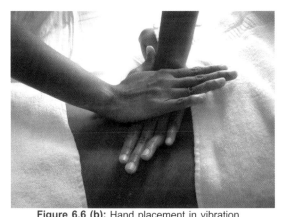

**Figure 6.6 (b):** Hand placement in vibration

| | | |
|---|---|---|
| 9. | Instruct patient to inhale deeply and exhale slowly through pursed lips and perform abdominal breathing. | |
| 10. | Tense all the muscles of hand and arm and vibrate the hand especially heels with moderate pressure during exhalation. | Vibration frees the mucus from bronchial walls. |
| 11. | Stop vibration and relieve pressure on inspiration. | Pressure applied to chest wall inhibits chest expansion during inspiration. |

*Contd...*

*Contd...*

| | | |
|---|---|---|
| 12. | Vibrate for 5 exhalations over each lung area which is affected. After 3 – 4 vibrations, encourage patient to cough/huff and expectorate sputum into sputum cup. | Coughing or huffing aids in the movement and expulsion of secretion from the respiratory tract. |
| 13. | Allow patient to rest for several minutes. | |
| 14. | Auscultate with stethoscope for change in breath sounds. | Presence of crackles/ronchi indicates mucous present in bronchi. |
| 15. | Repeat percussion and vibration cycles according to patient's tolerance and clinical condition, usually for 10-15 minutes. | |
| 16. | Wash hands. | Reduces risk of transfer of microorganisms. |
| 17. | Assist patient to comfortable position. | |
| 18. | Assist with oral hygiene. | Promotes comfort by removing the bad taste of sputum in the mouth. |
| 19. | Record procedure and patient's response in nurse's record. | Enables communication between staff members. |

## SPECIAL CONSIDERATIONS

- Perform chest physiotherapy one hour before meals or 1-3 hours after meals.
- Administer bronchodialator/Metered dose inhaler if ordered or nebulize 15 minutes before procedure.
- Observe patient during treatment for tolerance—like breathing pattern cyanosis, etc.
- Splint incision area, so that pain is tolerable. Administer pain medications if ordered, 15 to 20 minutes before procedure.
- Stop procedure if there is tachycardia, fall in BP, palpitation, dyspnea or chest pain which indicates hypoxemia.

# 6.7: PERFORMING NEBULIZATION THERAPY

## DEFINITION

Process of dispersing liquid medication into microscopic particles (aerosol) and delivering into lungs as patient inhales.

## PURPOSES

1. To administer medications directly into respiratory tract for sputum expectoration.
2. To reduce difficulty in bringing out thick tenacious respiratory secretions.
3. To increase vital capacity.
4. To relieve dyspnea.

## ARTICLES

1. Air compressor
2. Connecting tube
3. Nebulizer
4. Medication and saline solution
5. Sterile water
6. Cotton balls
7. Face mask
8. Sputum cup with disinfectant
9. Disposable tissues
10. Kidney tray.

## PROCEDURE

| | Nursing action | Rationale |
|---|---|---|
| 1. | Identify patient and check physician's instructions and nursing care plan. | Ensures that right procedure is done for right patient. |
| 2. | Monitor heart rate before and after the treatment for patients using bronchodilator drugs. | Bronchodilators may cause tachycardia palpitation, dizziness, nausea or nervousness. |
| 3. | Explain the procedure to the patient. This therapy depends on patient's effort. | Proper explanation of the procedure helps to ensure patient's cooperation and effectiveness of the treatment. |
| 4. | Place the patient in a comfortable sitting or a semifowler's position. | Diaphragmatic excursion and lung compliance are greater in this position. This ensures maximal distribution and deposition of aerosolized particles to base of lungs. |
| 5. | Add the prescribed amount of medication and saline or sterile water to the nebulizer. Connect the tubing to the compressor. A fine mist from the device should be visible. | Aerosol particles enable deep penetration into tracheobronchial tree. |
| 6. | Place mask on patient's face to cover his mouth and nose and instruct him to inhale deeply and slowly through mouth, hold breath and then exhale several times. | This encourages optimal dispersion of the medication. |
| 7. | Observe expansion of chest to ascertain that patient is taking deep breaths. | This will ensure that medication is deposited below the level of oropharynx. |

*Contd...*

*Contd...*

| | |
|---|---|
| 8. Instruct the patient to breath slowly and deeply until all the medication is nebulized. | Medication will usually be nebulized within 15 minutes. |
| 9. On completion of the treatment encourage the patient to cough after several deep breaths. | The medication may dilate airways facilitating expectoration of secretions. |
| 10. Observe patient for any adverse reaction to the treatment | Patient may develop bronchospasms due to inhalation of aerosol. The fluid may also cause dried and retained secretion in airways, leading to narrowing of airway. |
| 11. Record medication used and description of secretions expectorated. | |
| 12. Disassemble and clear nebuliser after each use. Keep the equipment in patient's room. The tubing is changed every 24 hours. | Proper cleaning, sterilization and storage of equipment prevents organisms from entering the lungs. |
| 14. Wash hands. | |

## SPECIAL CONSIDERATION

* If indicated provide nebulization using oxygen source.

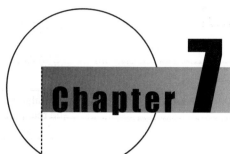

# Chapter 7

# Circulation and Fluid Electrolyte Balance

# 7.1: PERFORMING A VENIPUNCTURE

## DEFINITION

The process of puncturing a vein, with a needle, using aseptic technique.

## PURPOSES

1. To administer fluids intravenously.
2. To administer bolus medication for investigations or treatment.
3. To draw blood specimen.
4. To administer total parenteral nutrition.
5. To administer blood and blood products.

## CONTRAINDICATIONS

1. An arteriovenous fistula in the extremity.
2. Mastectomy on the same side of the arm/ a surgically compromised extremity.
3. Presence of phlebitis, infiltration or sclerosis.

## ARTICLES USED

### A CLEAN TRAY CONTAINING

1. Sterile needle/angiocath/butterfly needle of appropriate size.
2. Sterile cotton swabs in a bowl with antiseptic/alcohol pads.
3. Tourniquet.
4. Tapes for fixing catheter/needle.
5. Syringe of required size for blood draws (optional).
6. Specimen bottle (optional).
7. Syringe loaded with medicine (optional).
8. Infusion made ready for administration.
9. Towel /mackintosh for protecting linen.
10. Gloves.
11. IV pole.
12. K tray/ paper bag.

## PROCEDURE

|    | Nursing action | Rationale |
|----|----------------|-----------|
| 1. | Check physician's order and nursing care plan | Ensures that right procedure is being done for right patient. |
| 2. | Identify client | |
| 3. | Explain procedure to patient that there will be a slight discomfort initially. If required, demonstrate procedure on a doll for children. | Reduces anxiety and ensures client cooperation. |
| 4. | Make sure that clothing can be removed over IV tubing if needed. Provide client with a gown if necessary. | Prevents dislodgment of needle. |
| 5. | Wash hands | Prevents transfer of microorganisms. |

*Contd...*

*Contd...*

6. Select venipuncture site (Figure 7.1(a))
   Unless contraindicated select the non-dominant arm of the client.
   Look for veins that are relatively straight. Consider catheter length so that the wrist/elbow will be away from the catheter tip.

Sclerotic veins are difficult in initiating and maintaining IV. Joint flexion increases risk of irritation of vein walls by the catheter.

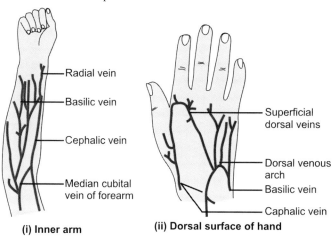

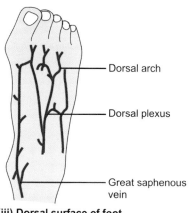

(i) **Inner arm**
- Radial vein
- Basilic vein
- Cephalic vein
- Median cubital vein of forearm

(ii) **Dorsal surface of hand**
- Superficial dorsal veins
- Dorsal venous arch
- Basilic vein
- Caphalic vein

(iii) **Dorsal surface of foot**
- Dorsal arch
- Dorsal plexus
- Great saphenous vein

**Figure 7.1(a):** Common sites used for venipuncture

7. Dilate the vein
   a. Place extremity in a dependant position (lower than heart)

   b. Apply a tourniquet firmly about 15 to 20 cm (6 to 8 inches) above the vein puncture site, explain that tourniquet will feel tight. The tourniquet must be tight enough to obstruct venous flow but not tight enough to obstruct arterial supply.

   c. If the vein is not sufficiently dilated, massage/stroke the vein distal to the site in the direction of venous flow towards the heart.

   d. Encourage the client to clench and unclench the fist.

   e. Lightly tap the vein
   f. If all the above steps fail, remove the tourniquet and apply heat to the entire extremity for 10 to 15 minutes.

Gravity slows venous return and distends the vein. Distending the vein makes insertion of needle easy. Obstructing arterial flow inhibits venous filling. If a radial pulse is felt, arterial flow is not obstructed.

This action helps in filling the vein.

Contracting the muscle compresses the distal veins, forcing blood along the veins and distending them
Tapping the vein may distend it.
Heat dilates superficial blood vessels causing them to fill.

8. Don clean gloves

Prevents nurses from exposure to contaminated blood.

9. Clean venipuncture site (Figure 7.1(b))
   a. Clean with antiseptic swab from center out-ward in circular motion for several inches.
   b. Permit solution to dry on the skin

This movement carries microorganisms away from site of entry.
Povidone iodine should be in contact with skin for at least one minute to be effective.

10. Insert the needle/catheter.
    a. Use non-dominant hand to pull the skin taut below the entry site.
    b. Hold catheter/needle at a 15 to 30 degree angle with bevel up, insert the catheter through the skin and into

This stabilizes the vein and makes skin taut for needle entry
Holding the needle out 15 to 30 degree reduces the risk of counter puncture.

*Contd...*

*Contd...*

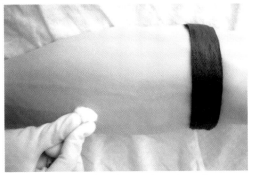

**Figure 7.1(b):** Cleaning venipuncture site

vein in one thrust (Figure 7.1(c)). A sudden lack of resistance is felt as needle enters the vein.

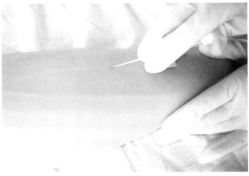

**Figure 7.1(c):** Inserting an IV catheter

c. Once blood is seen in the lumen or when a lack of resistance is felt, reduce the angle of catheter till it is almost parallel to the skin and advance the needle and catheter approximately 0.5 to 2 cm (Figure 7.1(d))
Remove the needle slowly while inserting the catheter inside the vein. When fully inside, loosen tourniquet.

d. Remove needle from inside the angiocath completely and attach syringe with medication/ Syringe for blood draws/ IV infusion tube as required.

Reducing the angle of catheter lower the risk of counter puncture.

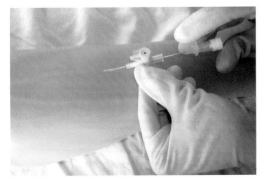

**Figure 7.1(d):** Removing needle from inside the catheter

*Contd...*

*Contd...*

| | |
|---|---|
| 11. Tape the catheter using 3 strips of adhesive tapes.<br>  a. Place one strip with sticky side up under the catheter hub.<br>  b. Fold over each side so that sticky sides are against the skin.<br>  c. Place second strip sticky side down over catheter hub.<br>  d. Place 3rd strip sticky side down over catheter hub/infusion tubing. | Prevents dislodgement of needle. |
| 12 Dress and label the venipuncture site as per agency policy.<br>  a. Place a sterile gauze piece with povidone iodine over the venipuncture site. Apply pad over the site. Apply occlusive dressing over site.<br>  b. Label the dressing with date, time of insertion, size of needle used, catheter used and initials. | Reduces risk of infection. |
| 13. Remove gloves and wash hands. | |
| 14 Discard all soiled equipment appropriately. | |
| 15 Document all relevant data and report any observation. | |

# 7.2: ADMINISTERING OF AN INTRAVENOUS INFUSION

## DEFINITION

Administration of fluid into the bloodstream through an intravenous catheter or butterfly needle inserted into a peripheral vein to replace fluid losses, supply caloric intake or as carrying solution for medications.

## PURPOSES

1. To administer fluid and electrolytes to maintain the balance within the body.
2. To provide glucose necessary for metabolism.
3. To provide water-soluble vitamins and minerals.
4. To establish a lifeline in case of emergency.
5. To administer medications.
6. To administer blood and blood products.

## ARTICLES REQUIRED

### A CLEAN TRAY CONTAINING

1. Infusion set.
2. Sterile solution in container.
3. Adhesive tape.
4. Clean gloves.
5. Tourniquet.
6. Antiseptic swab.
7. Antiseptic ointment (optional).
8. IV catheter (angiocath/butterfly needle).
9. Sterile gauze dressing or transparent occlusive dressing.
10. Arm splint (optional)
11. Towel/pad.
12. Mackintosh/waterproof pad.
13. Kidney tray.

### OTHER ARTICLES

1. IV Pole.
2. Electronic infusion pump (optional).

## PROCEDURE

|   | Nursing action | Rationale |
|---|---|---|
| 1 | Check physician's order indicating type of solution, amount to be administered, rate of flow, etc. | Ensures that right procedure is done for right patient. |
| 2 | Identify the patient. Assess vital signs, skin turgor, allergy to tape or povidone iodine, bleeding tendencies, disease/injury to extremities, status of vein. | Obtains baseline data on patient condition. |
| 3 | Check for any contraindication for venipuncture like arterio-venous fistula, arm on side of mastectomy, phlebitis, infiltration, sclerosis. | Prevents occurrence of any complication. |

*Contd...*

*Contd...*

| | |
|---|---|
| 4. Prepare patient | |
| a. Explain procedure to the patient and that the Venipuncture will cause discomfort for few seconds, but once solution is initiated, there will not be any discomfort. Explain to patient how long the infusion will take to complete. | Reduces anxiety and helps in obtaining co-operation of patient. |
| b. Explain to the patient that movement of the extremity should be minimal (In case of children apply splints) | Movement of the limb can cause needle to be dislodged. |
| c. Make sure that patients clothing can be removed over IV line if needed or provide with a gown. | |
| 5. Wash hands and don gloves. | Prevents infection |
| 6. Open and prepare infusion set. | |
| a. Check infusion container for sediments, turbidity, change in color and expiry date. | Reduces risk of complication caused by solution. |
| b. Remove tubing from the packet and straighten it out | |
| c. Slide the roller clamp along tubing to just below the drip chamber. Close the clamp. | |
| d. Leave the ends of tubing covered with plastic caps until infusion is started. | This will maintain sterility of the ends of tubing. |
| 7. Spike the solution container (Figure 7.2(a)). | |
| a. Remove protective cover from entry point of the container | |
| b. Add any medications if required using syringe and needle. | |
| c. Remove cap from the insertion spike and insertion site of the bag/bottle. | |
| d. Spike the solution container. | |

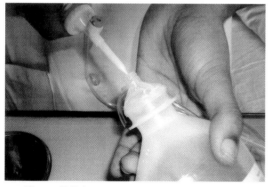

**Figure 7.2(a):** Spiking the solution container

| | |
|---|---|
| 8. Apply a medication label to the solution container if a medication was added. Mix the solution. Apply label upside down. | Applying label upside down will help in easy reading when container is hanging. Mixing ensures uniform distribution of the medication. |
| 9. Apply a timing label on the solution container with the time when infusion was started and flow rate. | Helps in confirming if flow rate is correct or not. |
| 10. Hang solution container on the pole. The pole should be adjusted so that solution container is 3 feet above patient's head. | This height is needed to enable gravity to overcome venous pressure and facilitate flow of solution into the vein. |

*Contd...*

| | |
|---|---|
| 11. Partially fill the drip chamber by squeezing it till half full (Figure 7.2(b)) | Prevents air from moving down the tubing. |

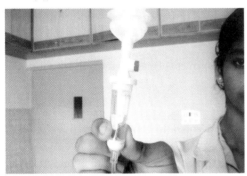

**Figure 7.2(b):** Partially filling the drip chamber

| | |
|---|---|
| 12. Prime the tubing (Figure 7.2(c)) | |
| a. Release the clamp, and let solution run through the tubing till all air bubbles are removed. Tap tubing if necessary with finger to remove air bubbles sticking on sides of tubing. | Prevents introduction of air into the vein. |

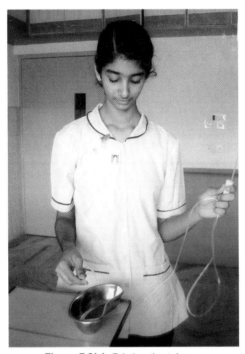

**Figure 7.2(c):** Priming the tube

| | |
|---|---|
| b. Reclamp the tubing and replace tubing cap. | Maintains sterility. |
| c. If an infusion pump is used, set it according to the rate prescribed. Follow manufacturers instructions for setting pump (Figure 7.2(d)). | |

*Contd...*

*Contd...*

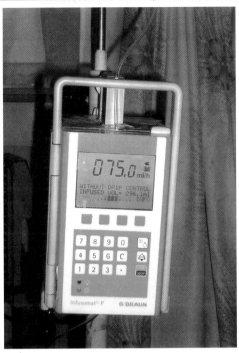

**Figure 7.2(d):** Setting the infusion pump

**Follow steps II to XII of Venipuncture procedure**

| | |
|---|---|
| 13. Label IV tubing with date and time of attachment and signature. | Labelling ensures that tubing is changed every 72 hours. |
| 14. Ensure appropriate infusion flow through pump or by adjusting roller clamp and note patient's response. | |
| 15. Discard all disposable items, clean and replace reusable items. | |
| 16. Wash hands. | |
| 17. Document relevant data-like date and time of starting IV fluids, amount and type of solution used including medication, flow-rate, type and gauge of needle and patient's response. | |
| 18. Position patient comfortably. | |
| 19. Assess frequently for swelling, pain, blanching, coolness of surrounding skin, leaking or bleeding from site and change inflow-rate, etc. | |

# 7.3: CHANGING AN INTRAVENOUS CONTAINER, TUBING AND DRESSING

## PURPOSES

1. To prevent infections.
2. To maintain patency of tubing.

## ARTICLES

1. Container with correct solution in required amount.
2. IV drip set-sterile.
3. Labels for applying to tubing, container and IV cannula .
4. Kidney tray/paper bag.
5. Sterile gauze piece.

### A TRAY CONTAINING

*For dressing:*
1. Clean disposable gloves.
2. Sterile gauze piece.
3. Antiseptic swab.
4. Adhesive tape.
5. Dressing gauze.
6. Towel.

## PROCEDURE

| | Nursing action | Rationale |
|---|---|---|
| 1. | Obtain the correct solution<br>i. Verify with physician order<br>ii. Read label of new container<br>iii. Check name of solution, expiry date, constituents and volume present. Check for any sediments turbidity and color change. | Reduces risk of error. |
| 2. | Wash hands. | Reduces risk of transmission of microorganisms. |
| 3. | Set up intravenous equipment by inserting insertion spike of tubing into container (as in previous procedure)<br>Optional: Add medication to IV solution if required.<br>• Apply label to container – including medication added and timing.<br>• Prime the tubing with solution.<br>• Label the tubing with date and time of changing the tubing. | Communicates the details of medications added and change of tubing. |
| 4. | Prepare dressing equipment.<br>• Prepare strips of tape as needed for the type of catheter or cannula used and hang them from the edges of tray/table.<br>• Open all equipment, swabs, dressing, ointment etc.<br>• Place towel under extremity.<br>• Don gloves | This facilitates access after gloves are worn.<br>Prevents soiling of bed linen.<br>Prevents contamination. |

*Contd...*

*Contd...*

| | | |
|---|---|---|
| 5. | Remove the soiled dressing and all tapes except the one which holds catheter/IV cannula/needle in place. | |
| | • Remove tapes and gauze one layer at a time. | Prevents dislodgment of cannula in case it becomes entangled between layers of dressing. |
| | • Remove adhesive tapes in the line of patient's hair growth. | Reduces discomfort. |
| | • Discard the dressing in appropriate container. | Prevents contamination. |
| 6. | Assess IV site for infiltration/inflammation. If present remove needle from the site. In this case, a new intravenous line should be started. | Reduces chance for further trauma to tissues. |
| 7 | Disconnect the used tubing. | |
| | • Place a sterile swab under the hub of the catheter. | This absorbs any leakage that might occur when tubing is disconnected. |
| | • Clamp the tubing | |
| | • Hold the hub of catheter with non-dominant hand and loosen the tubing with dominant hand using a twisting motion. | Holding the catheter firmly and gently maintains its position in the vein. |
| | • Remove the used IV tubing and place its end in the kidney tray. | |
| 8. | Connect the new tubing | |
| | • Grasp the new tubing with dominant hand. | |
| | • Remove the protective cap at tip and secure it to the hub of cannula or catheter and fix it. | |
| | • Open the clamp to start free flow of solution. | |
| 9. | Remove the tape securing the cannula while holding hub of the needle with one hand. | Prevents inadvertent dislodgment of cannula or catheter. |
| 10 | Clean the IV site with adhesive remover if residues of adhesive tapes are present. Then use alcohol swabs or povidone iodine swabs. Clean the site from center to periphery to a 2-inch diameter, starting from site where catheter enters the skin. | Facilitates new dressing to stick properly. Cleaning in this manner prevents contamination of IV site from bacteria on the peripheral skin areas. Antiseptic reduces the number of microorganisms present thus reducing the risk of infection. |
| 11. | Recap the needle/catheter (as in procedure given before) | Reduces chances of displacement of needle. |
| 12 | Apply antiseptic ointment and apply dressing (sterile gauze over site and fix it with adhesive strips. | Reduces risk of infection. |
| 13 | Label dressing and secure IV tubing with additional tapes if required. | Communicates to all staff members about change of dressing and tubing. |
| 14 | Discard all used articles. | Reduces risk of transmission of infection. |
| 15 | Remove gloves and wash hands. | Reduces risk of transmission of infection. |
| 16 | Document all relevant information. | Enables communication between staff members. |

# 7.4: DISCONTINUING AN INTRAVENOUS INFUSION

## ARTICLES

1. Clean gloves.
2. Dry antiseptic swab.
3. Small sterile gauze piece.
4. Adhesive strip.
5. Kidney tray.

## PROCEDURE

| | Nursing action | Rationale |
|---|---|---|
| 1 | Explain procedure to patient. | Reduces anxiety and helps in obtaining co-operation. |
| 2 | Wash hands and assemble equipment. | Reduces risk of transmission of microorganisms. Assembling equipment saves time and energy. |
| 3 | Clamp infusion tubing. | Clamping prevents fluid from flowing out of the needle onto the patient or bed when removing. |
| 4 | Loosen tape at the venipuncture site while holding the cannula firmly and applying counter traction to skin. | Movement of the cannula can injure the vein and cause discomfort to the patient. Counter traction prevents pulling of skin and causing discomfort. |
| 5 | Don clean gloves and hold sterile gauze over venipuncture site. | |
| 6 | Withdraw IV cannula/catheter from vein by pulling it along the line of vein. | Pulling along the line of vein will avoid vein injury. |
| 7 | Apply firm pressure for 2 to 3 minutes. Hold extremity above level of heart if bleeding persists. | Prevents bleeding and hematoma formation. Raising limb reduces blood flow to the area. |
| 8 | Examine the catheter, removed from patient to see if it is intact. If broken or any part is missing, report it at once to the nurse in charge and physician. If broken piece can be palpated inside the vein, apply a tourniquet above the level of the palpated piece. | If a piece of tubing remains in vein it can travel centrally to heart or lung. Application of tourniquet reduces possibility of the broken piece moving to the heart till physician comes. |
| 9 | Apply sterile gauze piece over venipuncture site with an adhesive tape over it. | Dressing continues to apply pressure over the site. |
| 10 | Discard all disposable articles. | |
| 11 | Wash hands and remove gloves. | Reduces risk of transmission of microorganisms. |
| 12 | Document all relevant information, i.e. time of discontinuing solution, amount of solution left in the old container if any. | |

# 7.5(A): ADMINISTRATION OF BLOOD (BLOOD TRANSFUSION)

## DEFINITION

Blood transfusion consists of administration of compatible donor's whole blood or any of its components to correct/ treat any clinical condition.

## PURPOSES

1. To restore circulating blood volume.
2. To correct platelet and coagulation factor deficiencies.
3. To correct anemia.

## ARTICLES

1. Blood Transfusion set.
2. Normal saline.
3. Blood/blood components – sterile in appropriate container.
4. Cannula No:18/19 (adult).
5. Alcohol/Iodine swabs (disinfectant).
6. Sterile gauze.
7. Tourniquet.
8. Adhesive tape.
9. Scissors.
10. Roller bandage and splint (optional).
11. Infusion stand.
12. Disposal bag/ kidney tray.
13. Disposable gloves.
14. Pressure bag (optional in case of severe bleeding).
15. Specimen container.

## PROCEDURE

| | Nursing action | Rationale |
|---|---|---|
| 1 | Check physician's orders, patient's condition, and history of transfusion /transfusion reaction, reason for present transfusion etc. | Obtains specific data and initiates patient education if required. |
| 2. | Identify patient | Prevents errors and thus eliminates possibility of transfusion reactions. |
| 3. | Check availability of blood with the blood bank | |
| 4. | Explain the procedure to the patient, need for transfusion, blood product to be given, approximate length of time, desired outcome etc. | Provides reassurance and facilitates co-operation. |
| | Emphasize the need for patient to report unusual symptoms immediately. | Early identification of transfusion reactions aids in instituting prompt corrective measures. |
| | Obtain informed consent from patient. | |
| 5. | Obtain blood from blood bank in accordance with agency policy. If transfusion cannot begin immediately, return product to blood bank. Blood out of refrigerator for more than 30 minutes, above | Faulty techniques in storing blood products can cause hemolysis. |

*Contd...*

*Contd...*

| | | |
|---|---|---|
| | 10 degree centigrade cannot be re-issued Never store blood in unauthorized area-like ward refrigerator. Blood must be stored in refrigerated unit at carefully controlled temp. (4° C). | |
| 6. | Encourage patient to empty bowel and bladder and assist to a comfortable position. Collect urine specimen. | Ensures comfort of the patient. Urine specimen collected before transfusion will serve as base line data to identify transfusion reaction, if it occurs. |
| 7. | Ensure privacy. | |
| 8. | Wash and dry hands | Prevents cross infection. |
| 9. | Check vital signs and record. | Obtains baseline data to compare with changes post transfusion. Delay transfusion if temperature is more than 101.8° F. |
| 10. | Don disposable gloves | Reduces risk of contracting infection. |
| 11. | Insert IV cannula (18G /19G), if not already present in a large peripheral vein and initiate infusion of normal saline solution using blood transfusion set. | Normal saline is the only crystalloid that is compatible with blood and priming of the blood set helps in reducing risk of hemolysis of blood in contact with tubing. Large bore cannula permits infusion of whole blood, reducing chances of hemolysis. |
| 12. | Inspect the blood product (By 2 Nurses) for (Figure 7.5(a))<br> I. Identification number<br> II. Blood group and type<br> III. Expiry date<br> IV. Compatibility<br> V. Patient's name<br> VI. Abnormal color, clots, excess air etc. | Safe storage of blood is limited to 35 days before erythrocytes are damaged.<br>Verifies that ABO group, Rh type, unit number, patient's name, etc. matches. This reduces chances of mismatched transfusion and transfusion reaction. |

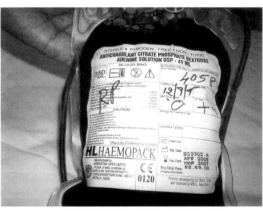

**Figure 7.5(a):** Checking label on blood bag

| | | |
|---|---|---|
| 13. | Warm blood if needed using special blood warmer or immerse partially in tepid water. | Cold blood can cause hypothermia and cardiac arrhythmias. |
| 14. | If blood product is found to be correct, Stop the saline solution by closing roller clamp. Remove insertion spike from saline container and insert spike into blood container | Priming of tubing is essential for preventing hemolysis. |
| 15. | Start infusion of blood product slowly, at the rate of 25 to 50 ml per hour for the first 15 minutes. Stay with patient for first 15 minutes. Check vital signs every 15 minutes for first 30 minutes, or as per agency policy. | Transfusion reaction typically occurs during this period. A slow volume can minimize the volume of RBCs transfused. Checking vital signs frequently helps in early identification of complications. |

*Contd...*

*Contd...*

| | | |
|---|---|---|
| 16. | Increase infusion rate if no adverse reactions are noticed. The flow rate should be within safe limits. | Flow rate is determined by physician's instruction and patient's condition. |
| 17. | Assess the condition of patient every 30 minutes and if any adverse effect is observed stop transfusion and start saline. Send urine sample, blood sample and remaining blood product in container with transfusion set, back to the blood bank. | Helps in identifying early transfusion reaction. Taking urine samples and blood samples helps in confirming transfusion reactions. |
| 18. | Complete transfusion and administer saline (as per physician's order), if no adverse reaction is observed. | |
| 19. | Dispose blood product container and set in appropriate receptacle. | |
| 20. | Wash hands. | |
| 21. | Record the following: product and volume transfused, number and blood group: Time of administration. Started and completed. Name and signature of nursing staff carrying out procedure and Patient's condition. If agency policy requires remove label from blood bag and paste it on patient's record. | |
| 22. | Assist patient to comfortable position. | |

## SPECIAL CONSIDERATIONS

- Do not administer medication through the same line, where blood product is transfused. Start another IV line if medications are to be infused, because of possible incompatibility and bacterial contamination. Blood transfusion should be completed over a period of 4 hours from the time of initiation.
- Cover the blood bag with a towel when it hangs on the IV pole.
- Gently rotate the blood bag periodically to prevent clumping of cells.
- When rewarming the blood by immersing in tap water, do not immerse the blood bag fully into the water as it may cause hemolysis.

# 7.5(B): BLOOD TRANSFUSION REACTIONS AND NURSING MANAGEMENT

Table 7.5.1: Transfusion reactions and nursing management

| | Reaction | Signs and symptoms | Nursing management |
|---|---|---|---|
| 1 | Allergic reaction | Hives, itching, anaphylaxis | • Stop transfusion immediately and keep vein patent with normal saline.<br>• Notify physician stat<br>• Administer antihistamine parenterally as necessary. |
| 2 | Febrile reaction: fever developing during infusion | • Fever and chills<br>• Headache<br>• Malaise | • Stop transfusion immediately and keep vein patent with normal saline.<br>• Notify physician<br>• Treat symptoms. |
| 3 | Hemolytic transfusion reaction: Incompatibility of blood product | • Immediate onset<br>• Facial flushing<br>• Fever, chills<br>• Headache<br>• Lowback pain<br>• Shock | • Stop infusion immediately and keep vein open with normal saline<br>• Notify physician stat<br>• Obtain blood samples from site.<br>• Obtain first voided urine<br>• Treat shock if present.<br>• Send remaining blood in bag, tubing and filter to lab.<br>• Draw blood sample for serologic testing and send urine specimen to lab. |
| 4 | Circulatory overload: | • Dyspnea<br>• Dry cough<br>• Pulmonary edema | • Slow/stop infusion.<br>• Monitor vital signs<br>• Notify physician<br>• Place patient in upright position with feet dependent. |
| 5 | Bacterial reaction: Bacteria present in blood | • Fever<br>a. Hypertension<br><br>b. Dry, flushed skin<br>c. Abdominal pain | • Stop transfusion immediately<br>• Obtain culture of patient's blood and return blood bag to lab.<br>• Monitor vital signs<br>• Notify physician<br>• Administer antibiotics stat. |

## PROCEDURE

| | Nursing action | Rationale |
|---|---|---|
| 1 | Immediately stop the transfusion | Reduces risk of further reaction. |
| 2 | Using gloved hands, remove tubing with blood and replace with new tubing | Prevents blood in the tubing from being infused. |
| 3 | Maintain the IV line patent with normal saline. Do not use any solutions containing dextrose. | Ensures that fluids/medications can be given in the event of anaphylaxis. Dextrose is incompatible with blood. |
| 4 | Obtain vital signs including oxygen saturation. | Assess patient's hemodynamic stability. |
| 5 | Remove gloves and wash hands | Maintains aseptic techniques. |
| 6 | Notify physician of patient's transfusion reaction, including vital signs and specific symptoms with severity of reaction and time frame. Administer oxygen and place in Trendelenburg position if shock occurs. | Transfusion reaction needs prompt medical attention with efficient and accurate communication of the event. |

*Contd...*

*Contd...*

| 7 | Monitor patients vital signs at least every 15 min | Assess patients cardiopulmonary status. |
|---|---|---|
| 8 | Read the blood component bag to ensure that correct unit was given to the correct patient. | Patient may have received incompatible blood intended for another patient. |
| 9 | Administer medications as prescribed: | |
| | • Diphenhydramine | • Antihistamine given IV, counteracts some allergic responses. |
| | • Epinephrine | • Epinephrine stimulates alpha receptors and beta receptors in the sympathetic nervous system and decreases respiratory distress in anaphylactic reactions. |
| | • Broad spectrum antibiotics | • Given when bacterial sepsis is suspected. |
| | • Intravenous fluids | • Counteracts symptoms of septic shock. |
| 10 | Start cardiopulmonary resuscitation if indicated | Prompt resuscitation may reverse cardiopulmonary arrest. |
| 11 | Obtain two blood samples from the other arm. | First sample is for cross match to ensure that the correct ABO matched blood was given. In the second sample the serum is tested for free hemoglobin which indicates hemolysis. |
| 12 | Return the remaining blood and tubing to blood bank. | A sample of blood will be cross-matched with the patient's samples before and after the transfusion to check for any error in cross-matching. |
| 13 | Obtain first voided urine (within one hour of reaction) | Hemoglobinuria occurs with hemolysis so the urine may be red/black. Renal damage requires prompt treatment to promote diuresis and to prevent renal tubular damage. |

**Table 7.5.2:** ABO compatibility chart

| RECIPIENT'S BLOOD | | REACTIONS WITH DONOR'S BLOOD | | | |
|---|---|---|---|---|---|
| RBC antigens | Plasma antibodies | Donor type O | Donor type A | Donor type B | Donor type AB |
| None (Type O) | Anti A Anti B | Normal | Agglutination | Agglutination | Agglutination |
| A (Type A) | Anti B | Normal | Normal | Agglutination | Agglutination |
| B (Type B) | Anti A | Normal | Agglutination | Normal | Agglutination |
| AB (Type AB) | None | Normal | Normal | Normal | Normal |

## ABO BLOOD TYPES

1. Type A—Antigen A on RBCs
2. Type B—Antigen B on RBCs
3. Type AB—Both antigen A and antigen B on RBCs
4. Type O—Neither antigen A nor antigen B on RBCs

**Table 7.5.3:** Adult transfusion flow rates

| Red blood cells | Initial rate no more than 25 ml in 1st 15 min Usual transfusion time is 2 hours and maximum time is 4 hours. |
|---|---|
| Platelets | 10 ml/min |
| Plasma | 10 ml/min |
| Cryoprecipitate | 10 ml/min |

**Table 7.5.4:** Quantity of blood products in one unit

|   | Type of blood product | Amount |
|---|---|---|
| 1 | Fresh blood | 350-450 ml |
| 2 | Plasma (different types) | 130-160 ml |
| 3 | Packed cell | 220 ml |
| 4 | Cryoprecipitate | 15 ml |

## 7.6: MONITORING CENTRAL VENOUS PRESSURE

### DEFINITION

Central venous pressure monitoring refers to the measurement of right atrial pressure or pressure in the great vein within the thorax.

### PURPOSES

1. To obtain pressure in great vessels which reflects right atrial pressure.
2. To provide an estimate of fluid balance and to aid in correction of fluid imbalance.
3. To evaluate blood volume and pumping action of heart.

### ARTICLES

1. Central venous pressure manometer with vented top and gradations (in centimeter of water).
2. Three way stopcock with Luer adapters.
3. Sterile caps.
4. Intravenous fluids with tubing (normal saline).
5. Clean gloves.
6. Scale for ascertaining level of manometer.

### PROCEDURE

| | Nursing action | Rationale |
|---|---|---|
| 1. | Identify patient who is at potential risk for fluid imbalance or hypotension and may require central venous pressure measurement. | Patient at risk for hypotension or fluid imbalance include those with cardiac decompensation, infections leading to sepsis, hemorrhage, any form of shock and other conditions where rapid fluid shift occurs. |
| 2. | Observe for signs and symptoms indicating need for central venous pressure measurement. | Central venous pressure measurement will help in diagnosing hypotension and thus initiating the appropriate treatment. |
| | • Blood pressure low or labile. | Indicates fluid imbalance that cause hypotension |
| | • Intake and output widely diverse. | |
| | • Fluid administration at a rapid rate | Rapid fluid administration can cause congestive heart failure. |
| 3. | Review patient's medical record for physician's order to measure central venous pressure and the frequency that is ordered. | Central venous pressure measurement must be ordered by a physician. |
| 4. | Wash hands. | Reduces transmission of microorganisms. |
| 5. | Explain procedure to the patient | Promotes understanding and reduces the anxiety. |
| 6. | Position the patient supine without any pillows at head end | Lateral positions produce significantly higher central venous pressure reading. Maintaining the same position for each reading provides for more consistent and comparable results. |
| 7. | Mark an "X" with an indelible pen at the level of the right atrium (fourth intercostal space, midaxillary line) (Figure 7.6(a)). | The zero mark on the central venous pressure manometer should always be on level with this "X"(Zero point) to minimize variations in measurement. |

*Contd...*

*Contd...*

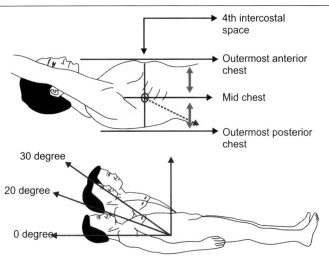

4th intercostal space

Outermost anterior chest

Mid chest

Outermost posterior chest

30 degree

20 degree

0 degree

**Figure 7.6(a):** Identifying phlebostatic axis for monitoring CVP

| | | |
|---|---|---|
| 8. | Connect IV fluid to the three way stopcock and flush the other parts of the stopcock with the fluid. | Flushing IV tubing forces air out of the stopcock. |
| 9. | Connect the central venous pressure manometer to the upper part of the stopcock. | Avoid touching the tips of manometer. |
| 10. | Connect the central venous pressure tubing from the patient to the second side port of the stopcock (Figure 7.6(b)). | Establishes IV line from fluid to central venous pressure catheter. |

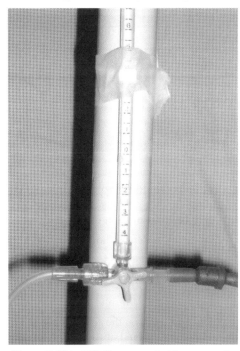

**Figure 7.6(b):** CVP line connected to manometer using 3-way stopcock

*Contd...*

# Circulation and Fluid Electrolyte Balance

*Contd...*

| | |
|---|---|
| 11. Allow intravenous fluid to drip rapidly into patient for several seconds with stop cock closed to manometer. | This assures patency of the central venous pressure line. If intravenous fluids do not flow freely central venous pressure reading will be dampened. |
| 12. Turn stopcock off to patient and fill manometer with intravenous fluid. | Manometer must be vented to air on top for fluid to fill tubing. |
| 13. Level manometer with the "X" on thorax and note the level on the manometer. Turn stopcock off to intravenous fluids, so system is now patent from manometer to patient. | Fluid in manometer will fall rapidly to a level equal to the amount of pressure in the central veins. |
| 14. Take reading when fluid level stabilizes. Read at end of expiration if level fluctuates. | End expiration is associated with constant intravascular pressure. Central venous pressure is decreased with negative pressure breathing and shock and increased by positive pressure breathing, straining, increased blood volume and heart failure. Normal central venous pressure is 2-8 cm of water. |
| 15. Close stopcock to manometer leaving intravenous fluids in place at ordered fluid rate | |
| 16. Wash hands. | Reduces transmission of microorganisms. |
| 17. Compare present readings with any previous readings. | Identifies physiologic changes occurring in relation to fluid volume and BP. |
| 18 Record in nurse's notes the central venous pressure reading. Report any abnormal values to the physician. | Abnormal values often require immediate treatment. |

## SPECIAL CONSIDERATIONS

1. IV fluids without medication if already was being infused into the central venous pressure line, a stopcock may be carefully inserted at the connector site and used for CVP measurement without adding another bottle of fluids.
2. Special flow sheets should be placed in the chart for recording readings when patients require frequent measurement
3. For frequent, repeated measurements, the manometer may be left in place . If the manometer is moved each time, care must be taken that the cap does not become contaminated in which case it should be disposed off and a new one obtained.

# Chapter 8

# Medication Administration

# 8.1: POLICIES ON DRUG ADMINISTRATION

1. Check physician's prescription as it provides information and specific instructions for mediation administration.
2. Remember to check it is right patient, right drug, right dose, right route and right time for administering a medication.
3. To minimize chances of contamination and infection use clean/sterile technique in preparing medications and handling equipments.
4. Ensure that the patient has no history of drug allergy.
5. Ensure that the drug has not already been administered because such errors could result in lethal dosage.
6. To avoid errors check the name of the drug, dosage and expiry date against drug prescription and drug label.
7. Check the label of drug container with the order form of medicine three times.
   1. Before removing medicine from the cupboard
   2. As the amount of drug ordered is being removed from the container
   3. As the medicine is reviewed with the patient before being taken or before disposing off the medication packet.
8. Calculate drug dosage accurately. Standard measuring receptacles should be used in preparing liquid medications.
9. Administer only those medications which are personally prepared. Do not administer a drug prepared by another person.
10. Institute necessary observations and measures before drug administration, e.g. Assessing BP, before giving an antihypertensive medication.
11. Check for specific timings prescribed by physician for administration of medication such as before food or after food, because medication action can be altered by food.
12. Do not leave medications at patient's bedside, this prevents chances of patient hoarding medications, not taking it or taking at inappropriate time.
13. Do not save parts of tablets or capsules to be used later.
14. Check decimal points. Some medications come in quantities that are multiples of one another (e.g. Coumadin in 2.5 mg and 25 mg tablets).
15. Do not administer medication ordered by nickname or unofficial abbreviations.
16. Record the procedure with patient's response, including any undesired effects. This serves as a communication between staff members.
17. Monitor after-effects and report abnormal findingcs to the physician.
18. In case if an error is made report to nursein-charge and physician as this, could help to minimize the effect of error.

## CURRENT PRACTICE

Nurse's six rights for safe medication administration:
1. The right to a complete and clearly written order.
2. The right to have the correct drug route and dose dispensed.
3. The right to have access to information.
4. The right to have policies on medication administration.
5. The right to administer medications safely and to identify problems in the system.
6. The right to stop, think and be vigilant when administering medications.

## PATIENT'S RIGHTS

1. To be informed of the medication's name, purpose, action and potential undesired effects.
2. To refuse a medication regardless of the consequences.
3. To have qualified nurses or physicians assess a medication history including allergies.
4. To be properly advised of the experimental nature of medication therapy and to give written consent for its use.
5. To receive appropriate supportive therapy in relation to medication therapy.

# 8.2: ADMINISTERING ORAL MEDICATION

## DEFINITION

Administration of medication by mouth. Oral medication administration includes buccal (cheek) and sublingual (under tongue).

## PURPOSE

To provide a medication that has systemic or local effect on gastrointestinal tract.

## CONTRAINDICATIONS

1. Alteration in gastrointestinal tract like vomiting
2. Reduced gastrointestinal motility (after general anesthesia, bowel inflammation, etc)
3. Surgical resection of a portion of gastrointestinal tract
4. Inability to swallow (e.g. patients with neuromuscular disorders, esophageal strictures, mouth lesions)
5. Patients with gastric suction/aspiration.
6. Prior to certain tests/surgery.
7. Unconscious/confused patients.
8. Patients on NPO status.
9. Patients with poor gag reflex.

## ARTICLES REQUIRED

1. Medication card/patient's files
2. Medication tray
3. Small plastic cups/paper cups/bottle caps
4. Glass of water
5. Mortar and pestle (optional)
6. Scissors
7. Paper bag
8. Paper towel/tissue paper (for liquid medication).

## PROCEDURE

| | Nursing action | Rationale |
|---|---|---|
| 1 | Assess for any contraindication (see text above). | Proper assessment will help in determining route of administration. |
| 2 | Determine patient's preferences and physician's order for fluid restriction, if any. | Patients on restricted fluids such as those with renal, heart, lung and liver diseases need to be given measured quantity within the prescribed total amount. |
| 3 | Prepare needed supplies and articles. | |
| 4 | Check medication card/form with physician's written order for accuracy, completeness etc. Check patient's name, name of drug, dose, route and time of administration. Clarify any doubt. Report any discrepancy to charge nurse and physician (Figure 8.2(a)). | Physician's order is the most legal and reliable source of information. |

*Contd...*

*Contd...*

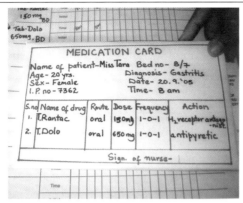

**Figure 8.2(a):** Checking medication card
with physician's order

5   Prepare drug

a.   Wash hands

Reduces transfer of microorganisms to medication and equipment.

b.   Arrange medication tray in nurse's station (optional) (Figure 8.2(b))

Saves time and reduces error.

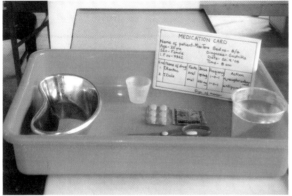

**Figure 8.2(b):** Medication tray

c.   Prepare medicine of one patient at a time, keeping medication card and forms together.

Reduces chance of error.

Select correct drug-container from stock while checking label with name of drug in medication card and expiry date (first check)

Hastiness will increase error

d.   Calculate correct drug dose. Take time and double check calculation

Provides accuracy and maintains cleanliness.

e.   For tablets/capsules, pour required number from bottle into bottle cap and transfer to medication cup. Do not touch with fingers. Extra tablets/capsules may be returned to bottle. For packaged tablet/ capsule, place packaged tablet/capsule directly over cup and remove without touching it (retain strip) check medication before removing from bottle or strip (second check) (Figure 8.2(c))

Retaining strips will help in identifying medication till the last tablet and thus reducing error.

*Contd...*

*Contd...*

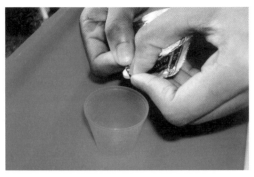

**Figure 8.2 (c):** Removing medication from strip

f.  Place all tablets to be given at the same time in one cup (except those requiring pre-administration assessment), e.g. vital signs

Keeping such drug separately will help in withholding drug if necessary.

g.  If patient has difficulty in swallowing, grind tablets in a mortar with pestle. Crush it to a fine powder and mix it with small amount of semisolid food. (DO NOT CRUSH ENTERIC COATED TABLET/ SUSTAINED ACTION TABLET)

Large tablets are difficult to swallow. When mixed with soft food, ground tablets are easy to swallow. Enteric coated medication willnot be absorbed in stomach.

h.  Prepare liquids
• Shake bottle
• Hold bottle with label against palm of hand when pouring
• Hold medication cup to eye level and fill it to desired level
• Discard if there is excess liquid in cup into sink, wipe mouth of bottle with paper towel. Excess medication should not be returned to medication container.
• For volume less than 5 ml/10 ml a syringe without needle can also be used to measure the quantity of medication.
j.  Do not leave drug unattended.
k.  Return drug container back to cupboard after checking label. (third check)

• Label will not be soiled with spilled liquid
• Ensures accuracy
• Prevents contamination of bottle contents and prevents cap from sticking

Third check of label reduces errors.

6   Administer drug
a.  Take medication to patient at correct time
b.  Identify patient by comparing name on card with the name patient gives when asked
c.  Perform necessary pre-administration assessment for specific medication (e.g. blood pressure, pulse, etc.)
d.  Explain to patient the medications to be given and allow patient to clarify doubts.
e.  Assist patient to sitting or side lying position
f.  Administer drug properly
• Ask if patient wishes to hold medication in cup/hand before placing in mouth.
• Administer only one drug at a time.
• Offer a glass of water with the drug to be administered (Figure 8.2(d)).
• Place medication under tongue and allow it to dissolve completely in case of sublingually administered medication. Caution patient against swallowing.

This gives information as to whether medications should be given at that time.
Patient has the right to be informed and understanding of medications increases compliance to therapy.
Prevents aspiration

• Certain drugs when swallowed are destroyed by the gastric juices or rapidly detoxified by liver and thus therapeutic levels are not attained.

*Contd...*

*Contd...*

- Instruct patient to place the medication in mouth against cheeks until it dissolves completely in case of buccal administration.
- Prepare powdered medication at bed side and give to client for drinking.
- Caution patient against chewing or swallowing lozenges
- Give effervescent tablets immediately after dissolving.
- If patient is unable to hold medication in hand place cup to the lip and introduce each drug into mouth one at a time using a spoon. Do not rush.

• Promotes local activity on mucus membrane.

When prepared in advance, powdered medication becomes more solid and difficult to swallow.

Such drugs acts through slow absorption through oral mucosa and not gastric mucosa.

Effervescence helps to improve taste of drug and is good for gastrointestinal tract problems.

Prevents contamination of medication. Administering single tablet or capsule avoids difficulty in swallowing and aspiration.

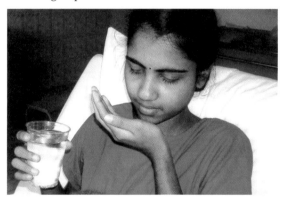
**Figure 8.2 (d):** Patient taking oral medication

g. If tablet/capsule falls to the floor, discard it and repeat tablet preparation

h. Stay with patient until each tablet is swallowed. Ascertain that all tablets are swallowed.

i. Assist patient to comfortable position.
j. Dispose off soiled supplies and wash hands
k. Return medication cards, forms/print outs to appropriate files for next administration.
l. Replenish items in medicine tray and return for next use.
m. Clean work area
n. Record the medication administration with date, time and signature.
o. Return within 30 minutes to evaluate effectiveness of medication.

Drug is contaminated if it falls to the floor.

Nurses assume responsibility for ensuring that patient receives ordered medication. If left unattended, patient may not take medication or may hoard medication.

Maintains comfort
Reduces transmission of microorganisms
Loss of record can lead to errors in administration.

This leads to greater efficiency

Prompt documentation prevents errors such as repeated doses. Signature establishes accountability for administration
Useful in detecting therapeutic effects and also detecting side effect or adverse effect.

## SPECIAL CONSIDERATIONS

1. Administer medications which can irritate the stomach mucosa with a light snack or following a meal, e.g. aspirin, brufen.
2. Administer medication with a light snack or following a meal if required (e.g. aspirin).
3. Administer medication with water and avoid fruit juice, milk, etc. with medications.
4. Do not administer water after giving cough syrup.

# 8.3: WITHDRAWING OR PREPARING MEDICATIONS FROM VIAL AND AMPOULE

## DESCRIPTION

### AMPOULE

Ampoule is a glass container usually designed to hold a single dose of a drug. It is made of clear glass and has a distinctive shape with a constrictive neck.

Ampoules vary in size ranging from 1 to 10 ml or more. Most ampoule necks have colored marks around it indicating where they are prescored for easy opening.

### VIAL

A vial is a small glass bottle with a sealed rubber cap. Vials come in different sizes from single to multi dose vials. They usually have a metal or plastic cap that protects the rubber seal.

## ARTICLES

1. Medication in an ampoule or vial
2. Syringe, needle
3. Small gauze piece
4. File
5. Medication chart
6. Kidney tray.

## PROCEDURE

| | Nursing action | Rationale |
|---|---|---|
| 1 | Check patient's name and medication order, including medication name, dose, route of administration. | Ensures correct administration of medication. |
| 2 | Perform handwashing and assemble equipments. | Reduces transmission of microorganisms. |
| 3 | Check medication order and check label for the name of medication, dose and date of expiry. | Medication potency may increase or decrease when outdated. |
| 4 | Prepare medication. | |

### AMPOULE PREPARATION

| | Nursing action | Rationale |
|---|---|---|
| 1 | Tap top of ampoule lightly and quickly with finger until fluid moves from neck of ampoule. | Drains any fluid that collects above neck of ampoule into lower chamber. |
| 2 | Place small gauze piece or cotton swab around neck of ampoule | Placing gauze piece around neck of ampoule protects nurse's fingers from trauma as glass tip is broken off. |
| 3 | Partially file the neck of the ampoule if necessary, for a clean break (Figure 8.3(a)). | |
| 4 | Snap neck of ampoule quickly and firmly away from hands (Figure 8.3(b)). | Protects nurse's fingers and face from shattering glass. |
| 5 | Place the ampoule on a flat surface. Insert needle into center of ampoule opening. Do not allow needle tip or shaft to touch rim of ampoule (Figure 8.3(c)). | Broken rim of ampoule is considered contaminated. When ampoule is inverted solution dribbles out if needle tip or shaft touches rim of ampoule. |

*Contd...*

*Contd...*

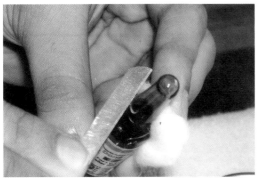

**Figure 8.3(a):** Filling neck of ampoule

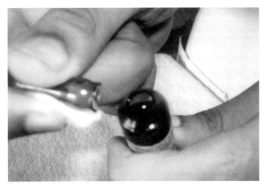

**Figure 8.3(b):** Snapping neck of ampoule

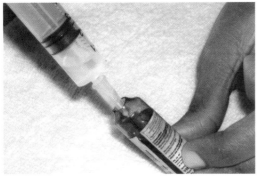

**Figure 8.3(c):** Withdrawing medication from ampoule

| | | |
|---|---|---|
| 6 | Aspirate medication into syringe by gently pulling back on plunger. | Withdrawal of plunger creates negative pressure within syringe barrel, which pulls fluid into syringe. |
| 7 | Keep needle tip under surface of liquid. Tilt ampoule to bring all fluid within reach of the needle. | Prevents aspiration of air bubbles. |
| 8 | If air bubbles are aspirated, do not expel air into ampoule. | Air pressure may force fluid out of ampoule and medication will be lost. |
| 9 | Expel excess air bubbles. Remove needle from ampoule. Hold syringe with needle pointing up. Tap side of syringe to cause | Withdrawing plunger too far will remove it from barrel. Holding syringe vertically allows fluid to settle |

*Contd...*

bubbles to rise toward needle. Draw back slightly on plunger and then push plunger upward to eject air. Do not eject fluid (Figure 8.3(d)).

in bottom of barrel. Pulling back on plunger allows fluid within needle to enter barrel so fluid is not expelled.

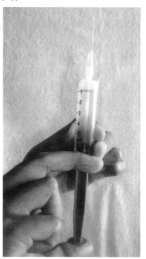

**Figure 8.3(d):** Expelling air from syringe

| | | |
|---|---|---|
| 10 | If syringe contains excess fluid, use kidney tray for disposal. Hold syringe vertically with needle tip up and slanted slightly toward kidney tray. Slowly eject excess fluid into kidney tray. Recheck fluid level in syringe by holding it vertically at eye level. | Medication is safely dispersed into kidney tray. Position of needle allows medication to be expelled without flowing down needle shaft. Rechecking fluid level ensures proper dose. |
| 11 | Cover needle with its safety sheath or cap. Replace the needle with another needle for injection. | Prevents contamination of needle. The outer surface of the needle may be coated with medication which may cause tissue irritation, if used for injection. |

## PREPARATION FROM VIAL

| | | |
|---|---|---|
| 1 | Prepare the medication vial for drug withdrawal:<br>• Mix the solution, if necessary by rotating the vial between the palms of the hands, not by shaking. | Some vials contain aqueous suspensions, which settle when they stand. In some instances shaking is contra-indicated because it may cause the mixture to foam. |
| 2 | Remove cap covering top of unused vial to expose sterile rubber seal.<br>In a multidose vial which has been used before, cap is already removed. Firmly and briskly wipe surface of rubber seal in a circular motion with alcohol swab and allow it to dry (Figure 8.3(e)). | Seals must be swabbed with alcohol before preparing medication. Allowing alcohol to dry, prevents needle from being coated with alcohol and mixing with medication. |

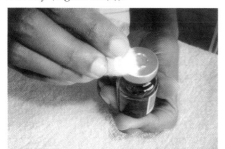

**Figure 8.3(e):** Cleaning rubber seal with alcohol swab

*Contd...*

| | | |
|---|---|---|
| 3 | Pick up syringe and remove needle cap. Pull back on plunger to draw amount of air into syringe equivalent to volume of medication to be aspirated from vial. | Air must be injected into vial to prevent build up of negative pressure in vial when aspirating medication. |
| 4 | With vial on flat surface, insert tip of needle with beveled tip entering first through center of rubber seal. Apply pressure to tip of needle during insertion. | Center of seal is thinner and easier to penetrate. Injecting beveled tip first and using firm pressure prevents curing of rubber seal which could enter vial or needle. |
| 5 | Inject air into the vial keeping the bevel of the needle above the surface of the medication (Figure 8.3(f)). 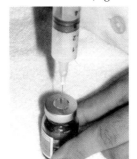 **Figure 8.3(f):** Injecting air into vial | • The air will allow the medication to be drawn out easily because negative pressure will not be created inside the vial. <br> • Avoids creating bubbles in the medication. |
| 6 | Invert vial while keeping firm hold on syringe and plunger. Hold vial between thumb and middle fingers of non-dominant hand. Grasp end of syringe barrel and plunger with thumb and forefinger of dominant hand to counter act pressure in vial. | Inverting vial allows fluid to settle in lower half of container. Position of hands prevents forceful movement of plunger and permits easy manipulation of syringe. |
| 7 | Keep tip of needle below fluid level. | Prevents aspiration of air. |
| 8 | Allow air pressure from the vial to fill syringe gradually with medication. If necessary, pull back slightly on plunger to obtain correct amount of solution (Figure 8.3(g)). 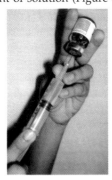 **Figure 8.3(g):** Withdrawing medication from vial | Positive pressure within vial forces fluid into syringe |
| 9 | When desired volume has been obtained, position needle into vial's air space, tap sides of syringe barrel carefully to dislodge any air bubbles. | Forcefully striking barrel while needle is inserted in vial may bend needle. |
| 10 | Remove needle from vial by pulling back on barrel of syringe taking care not to pull the plunger. | Accidentally pulling plunger rather than barrel causes plunger to separate from barrel, resulting in loss of medication. |

*Contd...*

*Contd...*

| | | |
|---|---|---|
| 11 | Hold syringe at eye level at 90 degree angle to ensure correct volume and absence of air bubbles. Remove any air bubbles if present. Draw back slightly on plunger then push plunger upward to eject air. Do not eject fluid. Recheck volume of medication. | Holding syringe vertically allows fluid to settle in bottom of barrel. Pulling back on plunger allows fluid within needle to enter barrel so fluid is not expelled. Air at top of barrel and within needle is then expelled. |
| 12 | Change needle to appropriate gauge and length according to route of medication. | Inserting needle through a rubber stopper may dull bevelled tip. New needles are sharper and will not track medication through tissues. |
| 13 | For multidose vial, make label that includes date of mixing, concentration of medication per milliliter, and nurse's initials. | Ensures that future doses will be prepared correctly. |

## VIAL CONTAINING A POWDER (RECONSTITUTING MEDICATIONS)

| | | |
|---|---|---|
| 1 | Remove cap covering vial of powdered medication and cap covering vial/ampoule of proper diluent. Firmly swab both seals with alcohol swab and allow it to dry. | Maintains sterility and allows alcohol to dry. |
| 2 | Withdraw an equivalent amount of air from the vial before adding the solvent unless otherwise indicated by the directions by the manufacturers. | Reduces pressure inside the vial when injecting the diluent. |
| 3 | Draw up diluent into syringe from vial or ampoule. | Prepares diluent for injection into vial containing powdered medication. |
| 4 | Insert tip of needle through center of rubber seal of vial containing powdered medication. Inject diluent into vial. Remove needle. | Diluent begins to dissolve and reconstitutes medication. |
| 5 | Mix medication thoroughly by rolling in palms. Do not shake. | Ensures proper dispersal of medication throughout solution. Shaking produces bubbles. |
| 6 | Reconstituted medication in vial is ready to be drawn into new syringe. Read label carefully to determine dose after reconstitution. | Once diluent has been added, concentration of medication determines dose to be given. |
| 7 | Clean work area and perform handwashing. | Controls transmission of infection. |

## MIXING INSULINS

If the patient is to receive 10 units of regular insulin and 30 units of NPH insulin follow this procedure (Figure 8.3(h)).
a. Inject 30 units of air into the NPH vial and withdraw the needle (there should be no insulin in the needle). The needle should not touch the insulin.
b. Inject 10 units of air into the regular insulin vial and immediately withdraw 10 units of regular insulin.
c. Reinsert the needle into the NPH insulin vial and withdraw 30 units of NPH insulin.
   By using this method, you avoid mixing NPH insulin with the regular insulin.

## SPECIAL CONSIDERATIONS

Some medications and some institutions require that a filter needle be used when preparing medications from a vial. Check agency policy to determine if use of filter needle is indicated.

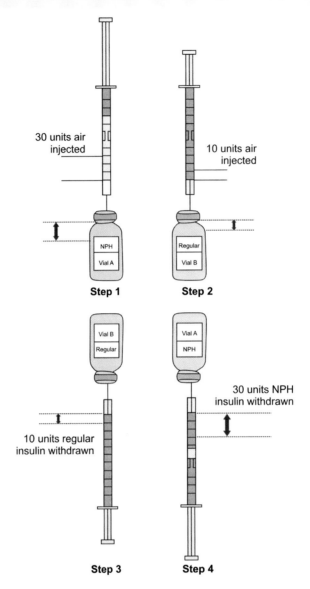

Figure 8.3(h): Mixing insulin in syringe

# 8.4: ADMINISTERING A SUBCUTANEOUS INJECTION

## DEFINITION

Administering medication into subcutaneous tissue.

## ARTICLES

1. Medication card
2. Sterile syringes and needles
3. The prescribed medication in ampoules or vials
4. Alcohol swabs
5. Disposable gloves
6. Kidney tray.

## PROCEDURE

| | Nursing action | Rationale |
|---|---|---|
| 1 | Assemble, equipment and check physician's order. | Avoids medication error from occurring. |
| 2 | Identify patient carefully | Ensures that right procedure is done on right patient. |
| 3 | Explain procedure to patient, the drug that is to be administered, site, and how he has to cooperate. | Encourages cooperation and allays anxiety. |
| 4 | Wash hands. | Reduces spread of microorganisms. |
| 5 | Withdraw medication from an ampoule/vial as prescribed (refer procedure 8.3) | |
| 6 | Assemble all equipment including loaded medication in syringe near the patient's bed side. | |
| 7 | Pull curtains. | Provides privacy. |
| 8 | Help patient assume position depending on site selected (Figure 8.4(a)). | Ensures free access to injection site. |

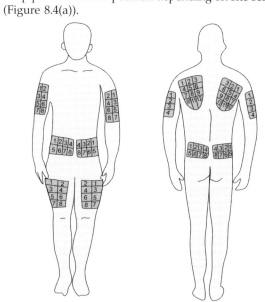

Figure 8.4(a): Common sites for subcutaneous injection

*Contd...*

- Outer aspect of upper arm—arm relaxed and at the sides of the body.
- Anterior thigh-sitting or lying down with muscles relaxed.
- Abdomen –patient in semirecumbent position.

| | | |
|---|---|---|
| 9 | Assess the area. Check for lumps, nodules, tenderness, hardness, swelling, scarring, itching, burning sensation and localised inflammation in the area. | Good visualization helps in establishing the correct location of site and avoids damage to tissues. Nodules and lumps indicate that there is inadequate absorption at previous injection site. |
| 10 | Don gloves | Reduces spread of microorganisms. |
| 11 | Clean the area around injection site with an alcohol swab. Use firm circular motion, while moving outward (5 cm diameter). Allow antiseptic to dry. Keep alcohol swab in the tray for reuse, when withdrawing needle. | Friction helps to clean the skin. |
| 12 | Remove needle cap with non-dominant hand, pulling straight off. | Lessens risk of an accidental needle prick. |
| 13 | Grasp and pinch the area surrounding the injection site or spread skin at site. | Provides for easy and less painful entry into subcutaneous tissue. |
| 14 | Hold the syringe in dominant hand between thumb and forefinger. Inject needle quickly at an angle of 45-90 degree, depending on amount of tissue, turgor of tissue and length of needle. For thin people an angle of 45 degree is preferred. When using an insulin syringe with a 26G needle an angle of 90 degree can be used in normal and obese people (Figure 8.4(b)). | Subcutaneous tissue is abundant in well nourished, well hydrated people and sparse in emaciated, dehydrated or very thin people. |

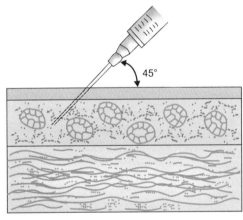

Figure 8.4(b): Angle of needle insertion for subcutaneous injection

| | | |
|---|---|---|
| 15 | After insertion, release the tissue and immediately move your non-dominant hand to steady lower end of syringe. Slide your dominant hand to top of the barrel. | Injecting solution into compressed tissue results in pressure against nerve fibers and creates discomfort. The non-dominant hand secures the needle and allows for smooth aspiration. |
| 16 | Aspirate if recommended, by pulling back gently on the plunger to determine whether needle is in a blood vessel. If blood appears, withdraw needle and discard. Prepare medication again. | Discomfort and serious reactions may occur if a drug intended for subcutaneous administration enters into the bloodstream. |

*Contd...*

*Contd...*

| | | |
|---|---|---|
| | Do not aspirate for heparin/insulin | Heparin is an anticoagulant and can cause bruising on aspiration. Insulin needle is very small and hence aspiration will not give relevant information regarding placement of needle. |
| 17 | Inject medication slowly if no blood appears. | Rapid injection of the medication creates pressure in the tissues and results in discomfort |
| 18 | Withdraw needle quickly at the same angle as it was inserted, while applying counter traction around the injection site with non-dominant hand. | Slow withdrawal of the needle pulls tissue and causes discomfort. Applying counter traction around the injection site helps in preventing pulling of tissues when needle is withdrawn. Removing needle at the same angle minimizes trauma to tissues and discomfort to the patient. |
| 19 | Massage the area gently with alcohol swab.<br><br>Do not massage a heparin/Insulin injection site. | Massaging helps to distribute the medication and hastens its absorption.<br>Massaging a heparin site can lead to bruising massaging after insulin injection will contribute to unpsedictable absorption. |
| 20 | Do not recap needle. Discard syringe and needle in appropriate receptacle. | Proper disposal prevents accidental needle stick injury. |
| 21 | Assist patient to a comfortable position. | |
| 22 | Wash hands after removing gloves | |
| 23 | Document medication administration with date, time, dosage, route, site and nurse's signature. | |
| 24 | Evaluate response of the patient to medication. | |

# 8.5: ADMINISTERING AN INTRADERMAL INJECTION

## DEFINITION

Intradermal injection is administration of medication into the dermal layer of skin.

## PURPOSES

1. To perform sensitivity test.
2. To perform tuberculin test.
3. To administer vaccination.

## ARTICLES

1. Medication card.
2. Medication in vial/ampoule.
3. Disposable gloves.
4. Sterile syringes and needles (Tuberculine syringe or 1 ml syringe).
5. Alcohol swab.
6. Kidney tray.

## PROCEDURE

| | Nursing action | Rationale |
|---|---|---|
| 1 | Check physician's order for medication administration and identify patient. | Eliminates medication error. |
| 2 | Explain procedure to patient, the purpose, the site of injection and how he has to cooperate. | Explanation encourages cooperation and reduces apprehension. |
| 3 | Wash hands | Reduces spread of microorganisms. |
| 4 | Prepare medication from ampoule/vial (refer procedure 8.3) | |
| 5 | Wash hands and don gloves | Reduces spread of microorganisms. |
| 6 | Assemble equipment at the bed side | |
| 7 | Position patient and locate site for intradermal injection (inner aspect of forearm, upper chest or upper back beneath scapulae) | Forearm is the most convenient and easily located and hence the commonly used site |
| 8 | Cleanse the site with alcohol swab in circular motion moving outward. Allow skin to dry. Keep cotton in the clean tray for reuse when taking out the needle. | Pathogens in the skin can be introduced into tissues. Alcohol if enters tissues can cause irritation. |
| 9 | Remove needle cap with the non-dominant hand by pulling it straight off. | Reduces chances of contamination of needle. |
| 10 | Use non-dominant hand to spread skin taut over injection site | Taut skin provides an easy entrance into skin. |
| 11 | Place needle almost flat against patient's skin (Figure 8.5(a)) (15°) and insert the needle into the skin so that the point of the needle can be seen through the skin. Insert needle only about 1/8 inch. | Action facilitates insertion into intradermal tissue. |
| 12 | Slowly inject the drug (0.01-0.1ml). watching for a bleb/blister to develop. If not present, withdraw needle slightly and inject medication (Figure 8.5(b)) | Appearance of a bleb/wheal indicates that needle is in intradermal tissue. |

*Contd...*

*Contd...*

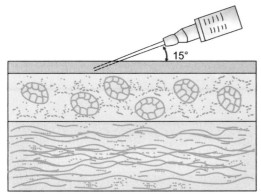

**Figure 8.5(a):** Angle of needle insertion for intradermal injection

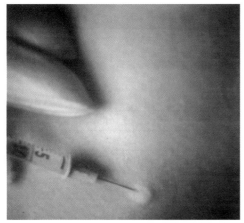

**Figure 8.5(b):** Administration of intradermal injection

| | | |
|---|---|---|
| 13 | Withdraw needle quickly in the same angle as it was inserted | Reduces tissue damage and discomfort of patient. |
| 14 | Do not massage the area | Massaging the area will lead to spread of medication to subcutaneous tissue and false results may occur. |
| 15 | Do not recap the needle. Discard syringe and needle into appropriate receptacle. | Reduces risk of accidental puncture with needles. |
| 16 | Assist patient to comfortable position | |
| 17 | Remove gloves and wash hands | Reduces spread of microorganisms. |
| 18 | Record medication administration—the medication administered, amount, dose, site and patient's response. | Reduces chances of medication errors |
| 19 | Draw a circle using blue/black pen around injection site. Write date and time of administration of medication and medication name on a piece of adhesive tape and stick near to the site. Check reaction within specified time period. | Helps in identifying exact site for checking reaction to medication. |

# 8.6: ADMINISTERING AN INTRAMUSCULAR INJECTION

## DEFINITION

A form of parenteral administration of medication, where a drug is injected into a deep muscle tissue.

## ARTICLES

A tray containing:
1. Medication card
2. Sterile medication (in ampoule/vial)
3. Syringes and needles of appropriate size
4. Antiseptic swab
5. Disposable gloves
6. Kidney tray.

## PROCEDURE

| | Nursing action | Rationale |
|---|---|---|
| 1 | Check physician's order and identify patient. | Prevents errors in medication administration |
| 2 | Explain procedure to patient, the purpose of medication, the site of injection, expected effect and how he has to cooperate. | Reduces anxiety and encourages co-operation. |
| 3 | Wash hands. | Reduces spread of microorganisms. |
| 4 | Prepare medication from ampoule/vial (refer procedure 8.3) | |
| 5 | Wash hands and don gloves. | Reduces spread of microorganisms. |
| 6 | Position patient:<br>• Assist patient to a supine, lateral or prone position depending on site chosen. If ventrogluteal, have patient in supine position with knees flexed or lateral position with upper leg flexed or prone with " toe in "position. | Proper positioning ensures muscle relaxation of patient. |
| 7 | Select, locate and clean site (Figure 8.6(a))<br>• Select a site free of skin lesions, tenderness, swelling, hardness, localized inflammation and one that has not been frequently used.<br>• Determine whether size of muscle is adequate for amount of medication to be injected.<br>• Locate exact site for injection.<br>• Don gloves.<br>• Clean with antiseptic swab in circular motion moving from center to periphery – moving outward upto 5 cm.<br>• Transfer and hold swab between 3rd and 4th finger of non-dominant hand or place in tray. Allow site to dry. | An average adult's deltoid muscle can absorb 0.5 – 1 ml and gluteal muscle can absorb 1-4 ml<br><br><br><br>Cotton swab is kept in readiness for removal of needle. |
| 8 | Remove needle cover without contaminating the needle by pulling straight off. | Reduces risk of accidental needle prik. |
| 9 | Confirm that medication and dosage are correct. | |
| 10 | Ensure that medication is not dripping on needle prior to injection. If it is dripping change needle. | Medication on outside of needle can cause pain and irritation of subcutaneous tissue when it passes into the muscle. |

*Contd...*

*Contd...*

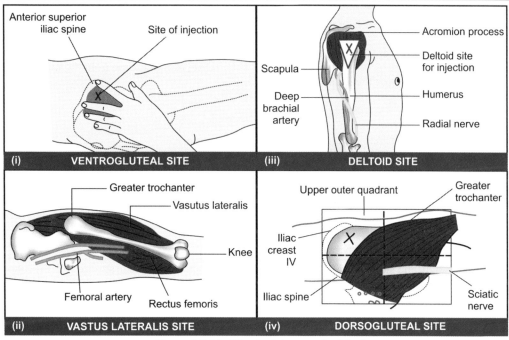

**Figure 8.6 (a):** Sites for intramuscular injection

11  Inject the medication
   - Grasp and pinch the area surrounding the injection site or spread skin at site as appropriate.
   - Hold the syringe between the thumb and forefinger in a pen-holding manner and pierce skin at site at a 90 degree angle and insert the needle (Figure 8.6(b))
   - Aspirate by holding the barrel steady with non-dominant hand and pulling back the plunger with your dominant hand
   - Withdraw needle if blood appears in the syringe, discard and prepare new injection.
   - Inject the medication slowly and steadily if blood does not appear in the syringe on aspiration.

Provides easy and less painful entry into muscle Grasping and pinching the area aids needle penetration in patients with thick muscle.

Aspiration helps in checking if needle is in a blood vessel.

Injecting medication slowly helps the dispersal of medication into muscle tissue thus decreasing patients discomfort. Holding syringe steadily minimizes discomfort.

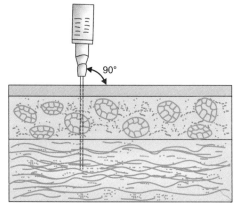

**Figure 8.6 (b):** Angle of needle insertion for intramuscular injection

*Contd...*

*Contd...*

| | | |
|---|---|---|
| 12 | Z-track technique: (Figure 8.6(c))<br>• Pull skin to one side, downward or laterally about an inch using non-dominant hand.<br>• Inject medication with airlock at 90 degree angle<br>• Hold needle in place for 10 sec<br>• Withdraw the needle and release the skin. | Allows medication to disperse evenly.<br>This leaves a zig-zag path that seals the needle track wherever tissue planes slide across each other.<br>Drug cannot escape from the muscle tissue. |

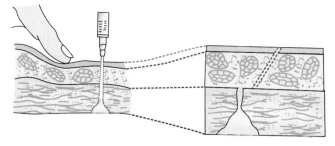

**Figure 8.6(c):** Z-track injection technique

| | | |
|---|---|---|
| 13 | Withdraw the needle slowly and steadily while supporting at the hub of syringe and needle. With non-dominant hand, support the skin surface using the cotton swab for applying counter traction at the site. | Supporting the skin surface with the cotton swab helps to reduce discomfort.Applying counter traction prevents pulling of tissues when needle is withdrawn. |
| 14 | Apply gentle pressure at the site with a dry sponge and if bleeding is present continue applying pressure till bleeding stops. Do not massage. | Massaging may irritate tissues at the injection site. |
| 15 | Discard the uncapped needle and syringe into appropriate receptacle. | |
| 16 | Remove gloves wash hands. | |
| 17 | Record procedure including the name of medication, dose, site and response of the patient. | Reduces chances of medication errors. |
| 18 | Assess effectiveness of medication. | |

## SPECIAL CONSIDERATION

1. For newborns, infants and small children the recommended site for intramuscular injection is the vastus lateralis.

# 8.7: ADMINISTERING BOLUS MEDICATIONS THROUGH INTRAVENOUS ROUTE

## DEFINITION

Introducing a single dose of concentrated medication directly into the systemic circulation.

An IV bolus may be given as follows:
a. Directly into a vein
b. Into an existing IV line through an injection port
c. Through a saline or heparin lock
   A saline lock consists of an indwelling needle or catheter attached to a plastic tube with a sealed injection port on the end.

## PURPOSES

1. Used in emergencies with critically unstable patient.
2. To achieve immediate and maximum effect of a medication.

## DISADVANTAGES

1. There is no time to correct in case of medication errors.
2. Direct irritation to the lining blood vessels.

## ARTICLES

1. Disposable gloves

### IV PUSH (EXISTING LINE)

2. Medication in ampoule or vial
3. Syringe (3 – 5 ml)
4. Sterile needle (optional)
5. Antiseptic swab
6. Wrist watch
7. Medication administration record.

### IV PUSH (INTRAVENOUS LOCK)

2. Medication in vial or ampoule
3. Syringe (1 – 5 ml)
4. Vial of heparin flush solution (1ml=100 units or 1 ml =10 units) depending on agency policy
5. Vial of normal saline
6. Sterile needles
7. Antiseptic swab
8. Medication administration record.

## PROCEDURE

| Nursing action | Rationale |
| --- | --- |
| 1. Check physician's order for name of medication, dosage, and route of administration | Ensures safety and accuracy in medication administration. |

*Contd...*

*Contd...*

| | | |
|---|---|---|
| 2. | Collect information necessary to administer drug safely including action, purpose, side effects, normal dose, time of peak onset, nursing implications. | Allows nurse to give drug safely and to monitor patient's response to therapy. |
| 3. | If drug is to be given through existing IV line, determine type of additive in IV solution if any. | IV medication may not be compatible with additives. |
| 4. | Assess condition of needle insertion site for signs of infiltration or phlebitis | Drugs should not be administered if site is edematous or inflamed. |
| 5. | Check patient's history of drug allergies. | IV bolus delivers drugs rapidly. Allergic reaction could prove fatal. |
| 6. | Assemble supplies in medication room. | Ensures sterile preparation of medication. |
| 7. | Wash hands and don gloves. | Reduces transmission of infection. |
| 8. | Prepare medication from vial or ampoule. | |
| 9. | Check patient's identification by asking name and compare with medication card. | Ensures that drug is administered to the correct patient. |
| 10. | IV Push (existing line) | |
| | a. Explain procedure to patient and encourage patient to report symptoms of discomfort at IV site. | Informs patient of planned therapies. |
| | b. Select injection port of IV tubing closest to patient. Whenever possible injection port should be a three-way port or other needleless device. | |
| | c. Connect syringe to IV line: In needleless system remove cap of needleless injection port. Clean port with antiseptic solution. Insert standard tip of syringe containing prepared medication. In needle system select port indicating site for needle insertion. Clean port with antiseptic swab. Insert small gauge needle of syringe containing drug through center of port. | Cleaning of port before insertion prevents introduction of microorganisms. Inserting a small gauge needle of syringe containing drug through center of port prevents damage to port diaphragm. |
| | d. Occlude the intravenous line by pinching tubing just above the injection port. Pull back gently on the syringe's plunger to aspirate for a blood return. | Ensures that medication is being delivered in the blood stream. |
| | e. After noting blood return, inject medication slowly over several minutes. | Rapid injection of an IV drug can be fatal. |
| | f. Observe IV site during injection for sudden swelling. | Determines development of infiltration into tissues surrounding vein |
| | g. Release tubing after injecting medication, withdraw syringe and recheck the fluid infusion rate. | Injection of a bolus may alter the rate of fluid infusion. Rapid fluid infusion can cause circulatory fluid overload. |
| 11. | Flush the three-way port in cases where medication is administered through a three-way port in which fluids are not flowing: | |
| | a. Heparin flush method | Flush solution keeps saline lock patent after drug is administered. |
| | • Prepare a syringe with 1 ml heparin flush solution. | |
| | • Attach small gauge needle to syringe | |
| | b. Saline flush method | Normal saline has been found to be effective in keeping intravenous lock patent. |
| | • Prepare syringe with 2ml of normal saline | |
| | • Attach small gauge needle to syringe. | |
| 12. | Dispose of uncapped needles and syringe in proper container. | Prevents accidental needle sticks. |
| 13. | Remove gloves and wash hands. | Reduces transmission of microorganisms. |

*Contd...*

*Contd...*

| | |
|---|---|
| 14. Observe patient closely for adverse reactions during administration and for several minutes thereafter. | IV medications act rapidly. |
| 15. Record drug, dose, route and time on medication forms. | Timely documentation prevents medication errors. |
| 16. Report any adverse reactions to nurse in-charge or physician. | Adverse reactions to IV bolus may necessitate emergency measures. |

## SPECIAL CONSIDERATIONS

1. Some IV medications can only be pushed safely when the patient is being continuously monitored for dysrhythmias, blood pressure changes or other adverse effects. So check the instructions before administering medication.
2. At times a saline or heparin lock will not yield a blood return even though the lock is patent.
3. If IV medication is incompatible with IV fluids, stop the IV fluids, clamp the IV line, flush with 10 ml of normal saline or sterile water, give the IV bolus over the appropriate amount of time, flush with another 10 ml of normal saline or sterile water at the same rate as the medication was administered and then restart the IV fluids at the prescribed rate.

# 8.8: INSTILLING MEDICATION INTO EAR

## PURPOSES

1. To soften ear wax for removing it.
2. To reduce localized inflammation and destroy infective organisms in the external ear canal.
3. To relieve pain.
4. To facilitate removal of foreign body.

## CONTRAINDICATION

1. Rupure of tympanic membrane.

## ARTICLES

1. Disposable gloves (optional)
2. Cotton tipped applicators
3. Medication bottle with dropper
4. Cotton balls
5. Kidney basin or paper bag
6. Bowl with normal saline (optional).

## PROCEDURE

| | Nursing action | Rationale |
|---|---|---|
| 1 | Assess for:<br>• Allergy to medication<br>• Redness/abrasion in the pinna/ meatus<br>• Type and amount of discharge<br>• Complaints of discomfort<br>• Ability to cooperate during procedure<br>• Specific drug action and side effects<br>• Patient's knowledge about medication to be administered. | Identifies contraindication for ear instillation. |
| 2 | Check medication order for name, dose, time, amount and ear to be treated. | Reduces risk of medication errors. |
| 3 | Identify patient and explain procedure, the purpose of medication and position to assume during and after instillation. | Reduces anxiety and promotes cooperation of patient. |
| 4 | Obtain assistance in case of children or infants, to immobilize them. | Prevents accidental injury due to sudden movement during the procedure. |
| 5 | Assist patient to a side lying position with ear being treated uppermost. | |
| 6 | Clean meatus of ear canal. Using cotton tipped applicators. Use normal saline if necessary. | Removes any discharge before instillation. |
| 7 | Warm container in hand or by placing it for a short time in warm water. | Promotes patient comfort and prevents vertigo and nausea. |
| 8 | Fill ear dropper partially with medication | |
| 9 | Straighten auditory canal. For an infant or child under 3 years pull pinna down and back. For an adult or child older than 3 years, pull pinna upward and backward. Figure 8.8(a) (i) and (ii) | Straightening the canal can ensure solution to flow the entire length of the canal. |

*Contd...*

*Contd...*

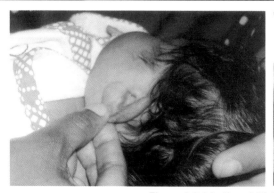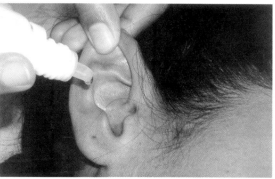

**Figure 8.8 (a):** (i) and (ii) Straightening the auditory canal

| | | |
|---|---|---|
| 10 | Instill correct number of drops along side of ear canal by holding the dropper one centimeter (½ inch) above ear canal. | Reduces risk of rupture of tympanic membrane. |
| 11 | Press gently and firmly a few times on the tragus of the ear. | Pressing on the tragus assists flow of medication into ear canal. |
| 12 | Instruct the patient to remain in side lying position for about 5 minutes. | Prevents drops from escaping and enables medication to reach all sides of canal. |
| 13 | Insert a small piece of cotton fluff loosely at the meatus of auditory canal for 15-20 minutes. | The cotton helps to retain medication when patient is upright. If pressed too tightly the cotton will interfere with the action of drug and movement of secretion. |
| 14 | Assess for patient's comfort, response and check for discharge/drainage from the ear. | |
| 15 | Replace medication and other articles. | |
| 16 | Wash hands. | Reduces spread of microorganisms. |
| 17 | Document medication administration, name of medication, no of drops administered and patient's response. | |

## SPECIAL CONSIDERATIONS

1.  Use sterile technique in administration of medication in case of perforation of the tympanic membrane
2.  Hydrocortisone ear drops are contraindicated in patients with fungal/viral infection in the ear.

## 8.9: INSTILLING MEDICATION INTO EYES

## PURPOSES

1. To treat infection
2. To instill medication before examination or surgery to eyes
3. To lubricate eyes
4. To stain cornea for identifing abrasions and scars.

## ARTICLES

1. Disposable gloves
2. Sterile cotton balls soaked in sterile normal saline
3. Medication
4. Dry cotton balls
5. Dry sterile dressing pad and paper tapes
6. Kidney tray.

## PROCEDURE

| | Nursing action | Rationale |
|---|---|---|
| 1 | Identify patient and assess for:<br>• Allergy to medication<br>• Appearance of eye and surrounding structures<br>• Lesions, exudate, erythema or swelling.<br>• Location and nature of any discharge.<br>• Level of consciousness and willingness to cooperate.<br>• Patient's knowledge about medication<br>• Use of contact lens. | Identifies contraindication for instillation of medication into eyes. |
| 2 | Check medication order<br>• Check physician's order for preparation, strength of medication, number of drops, frequency of instillation of medication and eye to be treated.<br>OD—Oculus Dexter (right eye)<br>OS—Oculus Sinister (left eye)<br>OU—Oculus Uterque (both eyes)<br>• Check expiry date and medication label. | Prevents medication error. |
| 3 | Prepare patient for treatment<br>• Check patient's identification and name<br>• Explain procedure<br>• Assist the patient to a comfortable position—sitting or lying with head slightly hyperextended<br>• Obtain assistance for immobilizing in case of young children | Reduces anxiety and ensures cooperation<br>Reduces errors.<br><br>Prevents accidental injury during medication administration. |
| 4 | Wash hands | Reduces spread of microorganisms. |
| 5 | Clean eyelid and eyelashes<br>• Don sterile gloves<br>• Use sterile cotton swab immersed in sterile normal saline and wipe from inner canthus to outer canthus | Cleaning the eye prevents secretions on eyelid and lashes being washed into the eye. Cleaning towards outer canthus prevents contaminants entering into the other eye and lacrimal duct. |

*Contd...*

*Contd...*

| | | |
|---|---|---|
| 6 | Administer eye medication | |
| | • Check ophthalmic preparation for name, strength, expiry date and number of drops in case of liquids. | Checking medication prevents medication error. |
| | • Instruct the patient to look upto the ceiling. Give the patient a dry sterile absorbent cotton ball. | Person is not likely to blink if looking up and in this position the cornea is protected by upper lid. A cotton ball can be used to wipe of excess ointment/ drug from eyelashes after instillation. |
| | • Expose the lower conjunctival sac by placing thumb or fingers of your non-dominant hand just below the eye on the zygomatic arch and gently draw down the skin on the cheek. If the tissues are edematous, handle the tissues carefully to avoid damaging them (Figure 8.9(a)). | Placing finger on the bony prominence avoids pressure to the eyeball and prevents person from blinking or squinting. |

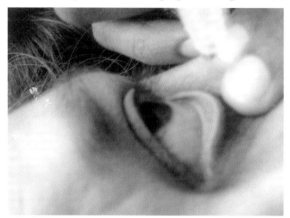

**Figure 8.9(a):** Exposing lower conjunctional sac

| | | |
|---|---|---|
| | Liquid medication: | |
| | • Discard the first drop of medication. | The first drop is considered to be contaminated |
| | • Approach the eye from the side and instill the correct number of drops onto the outer third of lower conjunctiva, holding the dropper 1-2 cm above the eye. | Patient is less likely to blink if a side approach is used. If drops fall directly on the cornea, it may cause injury. |
| | Eye ointment: | |
| | • Discard the first bead of ointment. | |
| | • Hold the tube above conjunctival sac, squeeze 2 cm of ointment from tube into lower conjunctival sac from inner canthus outward. | |
| 7 | Instruct patient to close eyelid and not to sqeeze them shut. | Squeezing can injure eye and push out medication. |
| 8 | Instruct patient to press on nasolacrimal duct for at least 30 seconds after instilling liquid medication. | Pressure prevents medication running down the duct. |
| 9 | Clean the eyelid as needed by wiping from inner canthus to outer canthus | Prevents spread of organisms into lacrimal duct. |
| 10 | Apply an eye pad if required and secure it with tape and instruct patient not to rub the eye. | Reduces risk of injury. |
| 11 | Assess patient response | |
| 12 | Replace medication | |
| 13 | Wash hands | |
| 14 | Document administration: Medication administered, no of drops, patient's response etc. | |

## SPECIAL CONSIDERATIONS

1. If more than one eyedrops (medications) are ordered, wait 5 minutes between each medication.
2. Instruct patient, on safety precautions if drops are meant for dilation of pupils.
3. If medication needs to be instilled into both eyes. Place in the unaffected eye first.

# 8.10: ADMINISTERING NASAL DROPS

## DEFINITION

Nasal instillation is the process by which a liquid is introduced into the nasal cavity drop by drop.

## PURPOSES

1. To treat allergies
2. To treat sinus infections
3. To treat nasal congestions
4. To give local anesthesia

## GENERAL INSTRUCTIONS

1. Medications are instilled only on written order from the doctor.
2. Avoid oil base solutions as nasal drops since it interferes with the normal ciliary action and may cause aspiration pneumonia.
3. Avoid the use of decongestant drops for a long period, because they become ineffective.
4. Administer drugs in correct concentration.
5. Identify the drug correctly and follow the rules for administration of medication.
6. Medical asepsis should be observed carefully throughout the procedure.

## ARTICLES

1. Prepared medication with clean dropper.
2. Pen light
3. Gloves
4. Facial tissues
5. Small pillow
6. Kidney tray
7. Wash cloth (optional)
8. Medication card.

## PROCEDURE

| | Nursing action | Rationale |
|---|---|---|
| 1 | Identify patient | Ensures that correct patient receives medication. |
| 2 | Review physician's order | Ensure safe and correct administration. |
| 3 | Determine which sinus is affected by referring to medical record. | Determines patient's position during drug instillation. |
| 4 | Assess patient's history of hypertension, heart disease, diabetes mellitus and hyperthyroidism. | These conditions can contraindicate use of decongestants that stimulate CNS side effects of transient hypertension, tachycardia, palpitations and headache. |
| 5 | Determine whether patient has any known allergies to nasal insillations. | Prevents complications. |
| 6 | Perform hand hygiene | Prevents infections. |
| 7 | Inspect conditions of nose and sinuses using penlight. Palpate sinuses for tenderness. | Provides baseline data to monitor effects of medication. Presence of discharge interferes with medication absorption. |

*Contd...*

*Contd...*

| 8 | Explain to patient the procedure including positioning and sensations to expect such as burning or stinging of mucosa or choking sensation as medication trickles into throat. | Helps patient anticipate experience of procedure to reduce anxiety. |
|---|---|---|
| 9 | Arrange supplies and medications at bedside. | Ensures smooth orderly procedure. |
| 10 | Apply gloves if patient has nasal drainage. | Reduces transmission of microorganisms. |
| 11 | Instruct patient to clear or blow nose gently unless contraindicated (increased intracranial pressure or nose bleeds). | Removes mucus and secretions that can block distribution of medication. |
| 12 | Administer nasal drops.<br>a. Assist patient to supine position<br>b. Position head properly<br>i. For access to posterior pharynx tilt patient's head backward.<br>ii. For access to ethmoid or sphenoid sinuses, tilt head back over edge of bed or place small pillow under patient's shoulder and tilt head back.<br>iii. Support patient's head with non-dominant hand.<br>iv. Instruct patient to breath through mouth. | Position provides access to nasal passages.<br><br>Position allows medication to drain into affected sinus.<br><br><br><br>Prevents straining of neck muscles.<br>Mouth breathing reduces chance of aspirating nasal drops. |

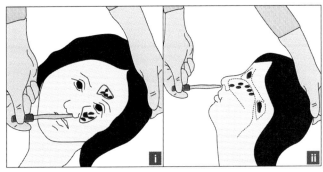

**Figure 8.10 (a):** Position for instilling nasal drops

| | c. Hold dropper 1cm (1/2 inch) above nares and instill prescribed number of drops towards midline of ethmoid bone (Figure 8.10 (a)).<br>d. Have patient remain in supine position for 5 minutes.<br>e. Offer facial tissue to blot running nose, but caution patient against blowing nose for several minutes. | Avoids contamination of dropper. Instilling toward ethmoid bone facilitates distribution of medication over nasal mucosa.<br>Prevents premature loss of medication through nares.<br>Allows maximal amount of medication to be absorbed. |
|---|---|---|
| 13 | Assist patient to a comfortable position after medication is absorbed. | Restores comfort. |
| 14 | Dispose of soiled supplies in proper container and perform hand hygiene. | Maintains neat orderly environment and reduces spread of microorganisms. |
| 15 | Observe patient for onset of side effects 15 to 30 minutes after administration. | Drugs absorbed through mucosa can cause systemic reactions. |
| 16 | Ask if patient is able to breath through nose after decongestant administration. It may be necessary to have patient occlude one nostril at a time and breath deeply. | Determines effectiveness of decongestant medication. |

*Contd...*

*Contd...*

| | | |
|---|---|---|
| 17 | Record medication name, concentration, number of drops, nostril into which medication was instilled, time of administration and patients response in nurses note. | Serves as a communication between the staff members. |
| 18 | Report any unusal systemic effects to the nurse-in-charge or physician. | |

## UNEXPECTED OUTCOMES

1. Patient begins wheezing or displays other signs of allergic reactions to drug.
2. Mucosa appears swollen and congestion is unrelieved.
3. Nasal mucosa remains inflamed and tender with discharge from nares.
4. Sinus headache.

# 8.11: ADMINISTERING METERED DOSE INHALATION

## DEFINITION

Metered dose inhalation is the process by which the patient inhales a specific or premeasured dose of aerosol medication by means of an inhaler.

## PURPOSES

1. To relieve inflammation and congestion of the mucous membranes.
2. To improve clearance of pulmonary secretions.
3. To act as a bronchodilator and mucolytic agent.

## ARTICLES

1. MDI (Metered dose inhaler with medication canister).
2. Facial tissues.

## PROCEDURE

| | Nursing action | Rationale |
|---|---|---|
| 1 | Review the physician's medication order, including patient's name, drug name, dosage, number of inhalation and time of administration. | Ensures safe and correct administration of medication. |
| 2 | Assess the patient's ability to hold and manipulate inhaler. | Impairment of grip strength, muscle strength or tremors of the hands interfere with ability to depress inhaler canister. |
| 3 | Assess drug schedule and number of inhalations prescribed for each dose. | Reduces risk of errors. |
| 4 | Instruct the patient to be in a comfortable environment by sitting in chair, in hospital room or at kitchen table at home. | |
| 5 | Allow the patient to manipulate inhaler and canister. Explain and demonstrate how canister fits into inhaler. | Patient must be familiar with how to use articles. |
| 6 | Explain metered dose and warn patient about overuse of inhaler, including drug side effects. | Patient must not arbitrarily decide to administer excessive inhalations because of risk of serious side effects.<br>If given in recommended doses, side effects are uncommon. |
| 7 | Explain steps used to administer inhaled dose of medication (Demonstrate steps when possible)<br>a. Remove cap and hold inhaler upright, grasping it with thumb and first two fingers.<br>b. Shake inhaler<br><br>c. Tilt head back slightly and breath out.<br>d. Position inhaler in one of the following ways:<br>i. Hold the inhaler 0.5-1inch (1-2 cm) away from mouth (Figure 8.11(a)) | Use of simple, step by step explanations allows patient to ask questions at any point during procedure.<br><br><br>Mixes medications evenly within solution so that aerosol drug concentration is uniform.<br>Maximizes airway exposure to medication from inhaler<br><br>Avoids rapid influx of inhaled medication and subsequent airway irritation. |

*Contd...*

*Contd...*

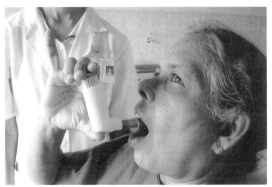

**Figure 8.11(a):** Positioning inhaler away from mouth

| | |
|---|---|
| ii. Optional: Attach spacer to mouthpiece of inhaler. | Eliminates rapid influx of particles from inhaled drugs, which reduces irritant properties and tendency to cough. Spacer is recommended for young children and older adults. |
| iii. Place the mouthpiece of inhaler or spacer in mouth. (Figure 8.11(b)) | Medication is distributed to airways during inhalation. |

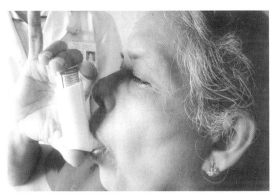

**Figure 8.11(b):** Placing mouthpiece of inhaler in mouth

| | |
|---|---|
| e. Press down on inhaler to release medications (One puff) while inhaling slowly. | Inhalation through mouth rather than nose draws medication more effectively into airways. As patient inhales particles of medication are delivered into airway. |
| f. Breath in slowly for 2-3 sec. | Allows tiny drops of aerosol spray to reach deeper branches of airways. |
| g. Hold breath for approximately 10 sec. | |
| h. Repeat puffs as ordered, waiting 1 min between puffs. | Allows maximal airway effect from first puff of medication. Therefore, airways are more open for second delivery. Thus, more particles are delivered directly into airways. |
| 8 If two inhaled medications are prescribed wait 5-10 min between inhalations as ordered by physician. | Drugs must be inhaled sequentially, usually bronchodilators are given first to maximize airway opening. Followed by other inhaled medications such as steroids. |
| 9 Explain that patient may feel gagging sensation in throat caused by droplets of medication on pharynx or tongue. | Results when inhalant is sprayed and inhaled incorrectly. |

*Contd...*

*Contd...*

| | |
|---|---|
| 10 Instruct the patient in removing medication canister and cleaning inhaler in warm water. | Accumulation of spray around mouthpiece can interfere with proper distribution during use. Accumulation at the mouthpiece increases risk of microorganism accumulation and oral infections. |
| 11 Ask if patient has any question. | Allows clarification of misconceptions or mis-understanding. |

## AFTER CARE OF THE PATIENT

1. Teach about cleanliness of inhaler.
2. Instruct the patient against repeating inhalations before next schedule.
3. Describe in nurses notes, the content of skill taught and patient's ability to perform skill.

## SPECIAL CONSIDERATION

1. Gargle with plain water after steroid inhalers to reduce chances of infection.
2. To check when the canister is to be replaced .
   a. Note the total number of puffs listed on the canister.
   b. Note the numbers of puffs ordered for the patient per day.
   c. Divide the total no of puffs available in the canister by number of puffs to be taken per day.
      This will give the total number of days for which the canister may last. Teach patient to replace the canister before this calculated date.
3. Newer delivery systems like dry powder inhalants are available which are simple to use. They contain dry powdered medication and are breath activated. An aerosol is created when patient inhales through reservoir containing dose.
4. Do not put inhaler in water.

## 8.12: ADMINISTERING RECTAL SUPPOSITORIES

### DEFINITION

Introduction of medication into the rectum in the form of suppository .

### PURPOSES

1. To stimulate peristalsis.
2. To promote defecation.
3. To act as analgesic and/or antipyretic.

### CONTRAINDICATIONS

1. Rectal surgery
2. Active rectal bleeding.

### ARTICLES

1. Rectal suppository
2. Lubricating jelly
3. Disposable gloves
4. Tissue paper
5. Kidney tray.

### PROCEDURE

| | Nursing action | Rationale |
|---|---|---|
| 1. | Review physician's order for patient's name and drug and explain the procedure to the patient | Ensures safe and correct administration of medication |
| 2. | Review patient information related to medication including action, purpose, side effects. | Allows nurse to administer drug correctly and to monitor patient's response. |
| 3. | Review medical record for history of rectal surgery or bleeding. | Identifies contraindication. |
| 4. | Review patient's knowledge of purpose of drug therapy and interest in self-administering suppository. | May indicate need for health teaching. Level of motivation influences teaching approach. |
| 5. | Provide privacy by pulling curtains. | Minimizes embarrassment in patient. |
| 6. | If patient is interested and capable of self-administration, provide instructions for it and send him to toilet with articles. | |
| 7. | Wash hands, arrange supplies at bedside and don gloves. | Reduces transfer of microorganisms, helps nurse to perform procedure in an organized manner. |
| 8. | Assist patient in assuming left lateral position with upper leg flexed. | Position exposes anus and helps patient to relax external anal sphincter. Left side lessens the likelihood of the suppository or faeces being expelled. |
| 9. | Keep patient draped with only anal area exposed. | Maintains privacy and facilitates relaxation. |
| 10. | Examine the condition of anus externally and palpate rectal walls as needed. | Determines presence of active bleeding. Palpation determines whether rectum is filled with faeces. |
| 11. | Remove suppository from foil wrap and lubricate rounded end with jelly. Lubricate gloved index finger of dominant hand. | Lubrication reduces friction as suppository enters rectal canal. |

*Contd...*

*Contd...*

| | |
|---|---|
| 12. Ask patient to take slow deep breaths through mouth and to relax anal sphincter. | Forcing suppository through constricted sphincter causes pain. |
| 13. Retract patient's buttocks with non-dominant hand. With gloved index finger of dominant hand, insert suppository gently through anus, past internal sphincter and against rectal wall 10 cm in adults, 5 cm in children and infants. | Suppository must be placed against rectal mucosa for eventual absorption and therapeutic action. |
| 14. Withdraw finger and wipe patient's anal area with tissue. | Provides comfort. |
| 15. Discard gloves turning them inside out and dispose in appropriate receptacle. | Reduces transfer of microorganisms. |
| 16. Ask patient to remain flat or on side for 5 minutes | Prevents expulsion of suppository. |
| 17. Check within 5 minutes to determine if suppository is in place. Instruct patient to retain suppository for 30 to 45 minutes (or as per manufacturer's instruction). | Reinsertion may be necessary if expelled. |
| 18. Ask if patient experienced localized anal or rectal discomfort during insertion | Determines whether insertion of suppository was irritating. |
| 19. Discard gloves and wash hands. | |
| 20. Record and report patient's response to medication including any unusual reactions. | Documents effect of medication. |

## SPECIAL CONSIDERATION

Instruct patient to walk if ambulatory to help promote peristalsis. Do not palpate rectum, if patient has had rectal surgery.

# 8.13: INSERTING MEDICATION INTO VAGINA

## DEFINITION

Introduction of medications into the vagina in the form of creams, jellies, foams, or suppositories.

## PURPOSES

1. To treat/prevent infections
2. To reduce inflammation
3. To relieve vaginal discomfort.

## ARTICLES

1. Triangular drape
2. Prescribed medication
3. Applicator with plunger in case of vaginal cream
4. Disposable gloves
5. Lubricant (in case of suppository)
6. Towel for wiping perineum
7. Mackintosh and towel for placing under buttocks.

## PROCEDURE

| | Nursing action | Rationale |
|---|---|---|
| 1. | Check medication order and identify the patient. Check the physician's order for specific medication ordered, its dosage and time of administration. | Reduces medication errors. Ensures that the right procedure is done on right patient. |
| 2. | Assess the patient for<br>• Allergy to medication<br>• Inflammation of external meatus/vagina<br>• Color, character and odour of vaginal discharge<br>• Complaints of vaginal discomfort. | |
| 3. | Explain procedure to the patient. Explain that insertion of medication is painless and will bring relief from pain, itching and discomfort. | Reduces anxiety and ensures cooperation |
| 4. | Encourage patient to perform procedure herself if she prefers. | |
| 5. | Instruct patient to empty bowel and bladder | Provides for comfort of patient and reduces injury to vaginal lining |
| 6. | Provide privacy | Reduces embarrassment. |
| 7. | Position the patient in dorsal recumbent /Sim's position and drape using triangular drape, so that only perineal area is exposed. | |
| 8. | Prepare articles, unwrap suppository and keep it ready on the opened wrapper. Fill applicator with prescribed cream, jelly or foam, as per manufacturer's instruction. | |
| 9. | Put on clean gloves | Protects nurse's hands from vaginal and perineal microorganisms. |
| 10. | Inspect perineum/vagina for any odour, discharge etc. | |

*Contd...*

*Contd...*

| | |
|---|---|
| 11. Provide perineal care to remove microorganisms. Encourage patient to perform her own perineal care in toilet if able. | Reduces chance of microorganisms moving into vagina |
| 12. Administer vaginal suppository, using one of the following methods:<br>a. Apply cream/foam and lubricate the rounded smooth end of suppository<br>• Lubricate your gloved index finger<br>• Expose the vaginal orifice by separating the labia with your non-dominant hand<br>• Insert suppository about 8 to 10 cm along posterior wall of vagina, or as far as it will go.<br>• Ask patient to remain lying in supine position for 5 to 10 minutes following insertion. The hip may also be elevated on a pillow<br>b. If using an applicator,<br>• Gently insert the applicator about 5 cm and slowly push the plunger until applicator is empty.<br>• Remove the applicator and place it on the towel<br>• Discard applicator if disposable, or clean it according to manufacturer's instruction.<br>• Ask patient to be in a supine position for 5 to 10 minutes following insertion.<br>• Ensure patient comfort. | |
| 13. Dry perineum using towel. | Ensures patient comfort. |
| 14. Apply a clean perineal pad if there is excessive drainage. | |
| 15. Remove gloves and wash hands. | Reduces risk of transmission of microorganisms. |
| 16. Dispose off all used articles and replace all reusable articles. | |
| 17. Document all relevant information. | Promotes communication between staff members. |

## 8.14: ADMINISTRATION OF MEDICATION THROUGH NASOGASTRIC TUBE

### DEFINITION

Administration of medications in liquid or powdered form through nasogastric tube.

### PURPOSE

To provide medications to patients who are unable to take it through oral route.

### ARTICLES REQUIRED

1. All articles required for tube feeding.
2. Medications to be administered
3. Mortar and pestle (if tablets are used)
4. Medicine containers.

### PROCEDURE

| | Nursing action | Rationale |
|---|---|---|
| 1 | Identify the patient and check physician's order. | Avoids medication error. |
| 2 | Allow liquid medications (if cold) to warm to room temperature. | Cold liquids cause discomfort to patient. |
| 3 | If tablets are to be administered crush it into fine powder and mix it in sufficient amount of water (follow oral medication administration principles in preparing and administering medications). | Prevents clogging of tube. |
| 4 | Wash hands and don gloves | Reduces transmission of microorganism and contamination of medicines. |
| 5 | Place mackintosh and towel over the chest. | Protects patient from spillage. |
| 6 | Elevate the head of bed 35 to 45 degree. | Protects the patient from aspiration. |
| 7 | Assess the placement of the tube (refer the procedure—nasogastric tube insertion). | |
| 8 | If placement of tube is correct, flush the tube with 15-30 ml water (adults) and 5-10 ml (children) before giving the medication. | Determines whether tube is clogged and helps in maintaining patency. |
| 9 | Administer the prepared medication in the same manner as feeding is administered. Administer each medication separately and flush with 5ml of water after each. Do not mix medications. | |
| 10 | After administering the prescribed medication, Flush the tubing with at least 30 cc of water. | Prevents clogging of feeding tube. |
| 11 | Observe patient for any adverse reactions. | |
| 12 | Record the procedure—total intake, medication administered, dose, time, etc. in the intake and output record as well as in the nurses notes. | |

### SPECIAL CONSIDERATIONS

1. If more than one medication needs to be administered it should be given separately and water should be used to flush between each drug.

2.  If the tube is connected to suction machine, keep it disconnected and clamped for 20-30 min  after administering medications.
3.  Disconnect a continuous tube feeding before giving medications and leave the tube clamped for  short period of time after the medication has been given according to agency protocol.
4.  Check the patient's record for fluid restrictions and total amount of fluids used for administering medication should be within the level of restriction.
5.  Medications should not be given with food.

# 8.15: APPLYING TOPICAL MEDICATIONS

## DEFINITION

It is the application of medication locally to the skin or mucous membranes in the form of lotion, ointments or liniments.

## PURPOSES

1. To protect, soothen or soften surface areas.
2. To warm an affected area and also for muscle relaxation.
3. To relieve itching
4. To check the growth of microorganisms.

## ARTICLES REQUIRED

A tray containing
1. Gloves
2. Cotton balls or gauze pieces
3. Medicine (ointment, lotion or liniment) in appropriate container.
4. Adhesive tape and dressing pad
5. Kidney tray.

## PROCEDURE

### APPLYING LOTIONS OR LINIMENTS

| | Nursing action | Rationale |
|---|---|---|
| 1 | Identify the patient and explain the procedure. | |
| 2 | Wash hands and don gloves on dominant hand. | Prevents spread of microorganisms. |
| 3 | Expose only the area where lotion/liniment is to be applied. | Keeps patient warm and prevents undue exposure. |
| 4 | Clean the area with soap and water and pat dry it if required. | Skin encrustation can hurbour microorganisms and previously applied medication remaining on the skin may reduce contact of medication with skin. |
| 5 | Apply skin preparation:<br>a. Powders—Make sure that the skin surface is dry and sprinkle evenly over the area till a fine thin layer covers the skin. Cover the area with dressing if required. | Moisture can cause the powder to stick and cause uneven distribution. |
| | b. Lotions—Shake the container and put a small amount of lotion on a gauze dressing pad and apply it evenly in the direction of hair growth. | Shaking the container ensures uniform distribution of the medication. |
| | c. Creams, ointments and pastes—Take a small quantity of medication in gloved hand. Smear it evenly over skin using long strokes in the direction of hair growth. Apply dressing if required. | Smearing medication evenly on the skin ensures uniform distribution. |
| | d. Aerosol spray—Shake the container well to mix contents. Hold the container at 15-30 cm away from the area and spray. Ensure that spray does not enter into eyes or nose. | Aerosol spray if enters into eyes or nose can cause adverse effects. |

*Contd...*

*Contd...*

| | |
|---|---|
| e. Transdermal patches—Select clean dry area which is free of air. Take the patch holding it without touching the adhesive edges and apply it firmly using palm of hand and press it for 10 seconds. Remove the patch at the appropriate time folding it with the medicated side in side. | Hair growth in the area of a application can affect the absorption of medication. Applying the patch for longer time than required can cause increased rate of absorption than required. |
| 6 Observe the area carefully for changes in color, swelling, appearance of a rash or other observable signs. | |

# Chapter 9

# Immobilization and Support

# 9.1: ASSISTING WITH APPLICATION OF SPLINTS

## DEFINITION

Application of an immobilizing device for supporting or securing specific part of body.

## PURPOSES

1. To support body part
2. To correct or prevent deformity
3. To provide stabilization
4. To enable application of traction
5. To provide first aid for fractured limb
7. To provide an erect posture for weight bearing
8. To manage sprains and strains.

## ARTICLES

1. Splint (Figure 9.1(a))
2. Cotton
3. Bandage
4. Adhesive

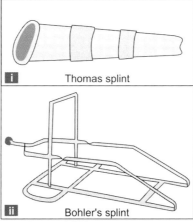

i    Thomas splint

ii    Bohler's splint

**Figure 9.1(a):** Types of splints

## PROCEDURE

|   | Nursing action | Rationale |
|---|---|---|
| 1. | Explain procedure to the patient | Helps in obtaining co-operation of the patient |
| 2. | Collect articles at bedside | Saves time and energy |
| 3. | Provide privacy and position body part in its functional position | Promotes comfort and good body mechanics. |
| 4. | Check distal pulse and record. | |
| 5. | Separate skin surfaces and pad adequately | Prevents maceration of skin surface |
| 6. | Pad bony prominences or hollow areas if present | Avoids friction and prevents necrosis |
| 7. | Immobilize joint above and below involved area | |
| 8. | Secure splint with bandage and strap away from injured area | |

*Contd...*

*Contd...*

| | | |
|---|---|---|
| 9. | Check neurovascular status | Identifies the neurological and circulatory complications at an early stage |
| 10. | Instruct patient and relative to inform about any discomfort or change in color of skin | |
| 11 | Remove and reapply splint if pain persists and swelling appears | Pressure can compress the nerves and blood vessels of the area. |
| 12 | Teach patients how to manage splint in home setting | |
| 13 | Document date and time of splinting, type of splint applied and purpose of applying such a splint, change in character of skin after applying, any discomfort felt by patient and action taken to relieve discomfort. | Documentation of procedure helps in identifying the problems patient has developed. |

## 9: 2: ASSISTING WITH APPLICATION OF SLINGS

### DEFINITION

Slings are used to provide support and protection for injured arms, wrists and hands or for immobilising an upperlimb.

### TYPES OF SLINGS

1. Arm slings
2. Elevation slings.

### ARM SLINGS

Arm slings are commonly used to support injuries to the upperlimb or to immobilize an upperlimb in case of chest injury.

### ELEVATION SLINGS

These are used to support a hand in well-raised position to control bleeding or to immobilise the upperlimb if there is a broken collar bone or there are rib injuries.

### PURPOSES

1. To support or immobilize parts of upper extremity.
2. To limit movement of upper extremity in presence of fracture, muscle strain or sprain and joint dislocation.
3. To prevent dependent edema
4. To control pain
5. To promote rest
6. To aid healing.

### ARTICLES

1. Pre-packaged sling or triangular bandage.
2. Safety pins.
3. Padding or flutted gauze squares.

### PROCEDURE

| | Nursing action | Rationale |
|---|---|---|
| 1 | Assess patient's presenting condition (stroke, fracture, dislocation). | Determines the motor and sensory status of affected extremity. |
| 2 | Observe condition of patient's upper extremity (mobility, presence of suture line, presence of cast, level of comfort, skin integrity). | Provides baseline data to determine changes in patient's condition. |
| 3 | Review patient's medical record for physician's prescription in relation to desired angle of forearm and other determinants. | Venous return, prevention of edema, and maintenance of functional alignment result from properly applied slings. Slings may be ordered round the clock or whenever patient is sitting or out of bed. |
| 4 | Identify patient's learning needs regarding condition and correct application of sling. | Indentifies areas for patient teaching for increasing patient's self-care ability. |
| 5 | Explain procedure | Reduces anxiety |

*Contd...*

*Contd...*

| | | |
|---|---|---|
| 6 | Teach skill to patient or significant others | Promotes coping ability and reduces stress. |
| 7 | Wash hands and provide privacy | Prevents cross-infections, reduces anxiety and maintains personal dignity. |
| 8 | Assess pulse on affected extremity | |
| 9 | Prepare patient:<br>(a) Position patient sitting or supine with forearm at angle with fingers higher than hand, hand higher than wrist, and wrist higher than forearm, all in anatomically correct alignment. | Ensures patient's co-operation facilitating rapid application of sling. |
| 10 | Open sling and place over patient's torso with binder centered under arm. Place longest side at wrist and apex of triangle extending beyond arm at elbow (Figure 9.2(a)). | Facilitates placement of closure beyond center of neck. Ensures support of forearm. |

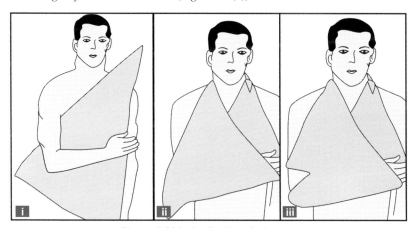

**Figure 9.2(a):** Application of sling

| | | |
|---|---|---|
| 11 | Bring the binder to level pointing upward over neck on affected side of body, continuing around patient's neck to affected side. At this point the longest side of triangle will extend straight down in vertical line on unaffected side of body. | Provides support to the patient's affected side as the sling is applied.<br>Prevents pressure on cervical spinal nerves. |
| 12 | Bring lower binder point over forearm and hand up- to neck on affected side. | Prepares sling to maintain optimum support to affected arm. |
| 13 | Reassess angle of forearm and adjust position if needed. | Proper positioning facilitates venous return and reduction of edema of digits. |
| 14 | Secure closure of sling at shoulder level on unaffected side using square knot, and fold remaining loose areas of binder around elbow and maintain fold and secure with safetypin. | Prevents pressure from knot on affected shoulder, Provides support to elbow and maintains appropriate alignment. |
| 15 | Apply padding as needed. | Reduces localized skin pressure: prevents cervical flexion related to pressure. Avoids excoriation of skin. |
| 16 | Inspect applied sling for adequacy of support, position of lower arm above level of elbow and avoidance of pressure on cervical vertebra. | Maintains proper alignment of affected arm. |
| 17 | Wash hands | Reduces transmission of microorganisms. |
| 18 | Evaluate distal pulses, sensation to fingers and condition of skin. | Determines adequacy of neurovascular status to distal area. |

*Contd...*

*Contd...*

| 19 | Inspect alignment of shoulder and extremity. | Determines adequacy of support and alignment provided by sling. |
|---|---|---|
| 20 | Question patient regarding level of comfort. | Identifies presence of any pain or discomfort. |
| 21 | Report patient's responses to application of sling | Maintains continuity of care and denotes patient's response to sling application. |
| 22 | Record alignment, circulation, sensation and skin integrity of affected extremity. | Denotes the presence or absence of complications related to application of sling. |

# 9.3: ASSISTING WITH APPLICATION OF SKIN TRACTION

## DEFINITION

A non-surgical procedure that makes use of adhesive straps slings and halters applied to skin for attachment of weight, to exert indirect pull or traction on underlying structures.

## PURPOSES

1. To immobilize a part requiring partial or temporary immobilization.
2. To reduce fractures and dislocations in children.
3. To reduce fractures in adults temporarily before definitive treatment is given.
4. To correct flexion deformities of knee or hip.

## ARTICLES

A tray containing:
1. Adhesive plaster
2. Scissors
3. Measuring tape
4. Spreader
5. Roller bandages
6. Tincture benzoin
7. Cotton swabs
8. Bath sheet
9. Kidney tray.

## OTHER ARTICLES

1. Traction ropes
2. Cross bars and clamps to fix pulleys
3. Bed blocks and weights
4. Balkan frame with trapeze bar.
5. Bed cradle
6. Thomas splint.

## TYPES OF TRACTION

1. Bryant's traction: Vertically held type of bilateral traction to the legs (Figure 9.3(a)).
2. Buck's extension: Horizontally applied unilateral traction (Figure 9.3(b)).
3. Contrel's traction: Skin traction consisting of two separate forms: Head halter and pelvic belt. Occasionally used as a preoperative treatment to help to straighten spinal curvatures before insertion of skeletal rods for correction of scoliosis.
4. Dunlop's traction: Simultaneous horizontal form of Buck's extension to the humerus with an accompanying vertical Buck's extension to the forearm.
5. Head halter: Traction involves a specially shaped halter with cut out areas for the ears, face and top of the head (Figure 9.3(c))
6. Pelvic traction: Traction consisting of a girdle-like belt that fits around the lumbosacral and abdominal areas, fastening in the middle of the abdomen with pressure sensitive straps or buckles (Figure 9.3(d)).
   This traction basically serves to keep the patient in bed, thus relieving inflammation and irritation of injuries, nerves or muscles.

7. Pelvic sling: Traction consisting of a hammock-like belt where-in the sling cradles the pelvis in its boundaries for treatment of one or more fractures of the pelvic bones.

8. Russell's traction: This is a balanced traction arrangement of pulleys, slings and weights used to treat knee or hip injuries in adult and to reduce femur fracture in children (Figure 9.3(e)).

   The weights used in application of skin traction are;

   In children:        : 1 –2lbs in Bryant's traction
   
                           : 7 – 10lbs for head halter traction
   
                           : 5 – 7lbs for Buck's extension
   
   Adult                     : 7 – 10lbs for Dunlop's traction
   
                           : 10 – 15lbs for pelvic belt traction
   
                           : 10 – 20lbs for pelvic sling

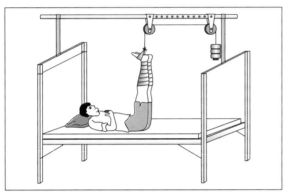

Figure 9.3(a): Bryant's traction

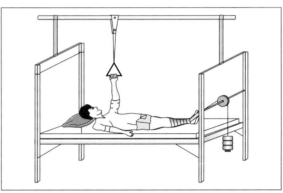

Figure 9.3(b): Buck's extension

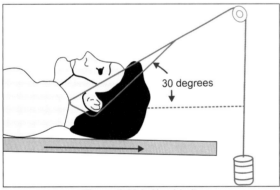

Figure 9.3(c): Head halter

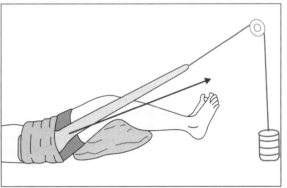

Figure 9.3(d): Pelvic traction

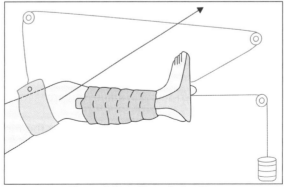

Figure 9.3(e): Russel's traction

# Immobilization and Support

## GUIDELINES FOR USE OF TRACTION

1. Maintain the established line of pull
2. Prevent friction
3. Maintain counter traction
4. Maintain continuous traction unless otherwise ordered.
5. Maintain correct body alignment.

## PROCEDURE

| | Nursing action | Rationale |
|---|---|---|
| 1. | Assess patient's overall health including degree of mobility | Determines patient's health status and ability to tolerate traction |
| 2. | Assess condition of specific tissues to be placed in traction. Note skin condition, excessive hair, bruises and other lesions.<br>a. **Head halter**: asseses head, ears, chin and neck.<br>b. **Bryant's traction**: assess both legs.<br>c. **Buck's extension**: assess one or both legs.<br>d. **Dunlop's traction**: assess arm and forearm.<br>e. **Pelvic belt**: assess lower back and abdomen.<br>f. **Pelvic sling**: assess back and abdomen<br>g. **Russell's traction**: assess lower limbs. | Determines ability of local tissues to tolerate traction |
| 3. | Assess patient's understanding of reason for traction | Determines concerns, acceptance and need for instruction |
| 4. | Assess patient's level of pain | Serves as baseline for later comparison |
| 5. | Explain procedure to patient, including traction set up and mobility restrictions | Promotes co-operation and reduces anxiety |
| 6. | Prepare patient and area of body to be in traction<br>a. **Head halter**: Cleanse face and neck. For male patient shave face unless he prefers to keep beard<br>b. **Bryant's traction**: Cleanse both legs | Lessens irritation under head halter |
| 7. | Position patient as requested by physician:<br>a. **Head halter**: patient flat on back<br>b. **Bryant's extension**: Child flat on back<br>c. **Buck's traction**: patient on back, head of bed flat or elevated 30 degree<br>d. **Dunlop traction**: patient flat on back<br>e. **Pelvic belt**: patient flat on back<br>f. **Pelvic sling**: patient flat on side or back<br>g. **Russell's traction**: patient on back; head of bed slightly elevated | Position varies with part of body to be placed on traction, plus effects of weight and gravity |
| 8. | Assist with application of specific head halter, adhesive strips and elastic bandages and pelvic belt or sling as needed. Nurse may be asked to hold patient in desired position or apply halter, strips or elastic bandages while physician and other assistants hold patient's tissues in desired position. | For lower extremity adhesive strips are applied beginning below head of fibula on lateral surface of leg to avoid pressure over peroneal nerve. Ensure proper alignment of body parts under traction. Elastic bandages are applied from distal to proximal to promote venous return. |
| 9. | Assist with attachment of spreader bars, ropes and pulleys. Ropes are tied securely in knot and passed in grooves of pulleys to weights | Provides proper weighted traction for extremity alignment |

*Contd...*

*Contd...*

| | |
|---|---|
| 10. When all traction materials and spread bars are in place, weights are placed on weight holder and hooked to loop in rope till it is taut. Physician determines exact amount of weight to be applied and position to be maintained by patient. | Traction is slowly established to avoid involuntary muscle spasm or pain for patient. Weight should be sufficient to create enough pull to overcome muscle spasm, but not to cause distraction or marked increase in pain |
| 11. Before physician leaves, check patient's position and ask about additional permissible positions for patient in bed. | Ensures safety of care and position for effective traction |
|     a. **Head halter:** Patient stay flat on back, or head of bed may be elevated 15-20 degree if ordered | Angle of pull may allow head to be up to use body weight as counter traction |
|     b. **Bryant's traction:** Baby or child must stay on back at all times. Buttocks are held slightly off bed if traction weight is correct amount | Child cannot turn to side or abdomen because traction would be ineffective and reinjury could occur |
|     c. **Buck's extension**: Patient may be allowed to turn to unaffected side for brief period. Pillow placed under leg in traction may be used only when patient is on side. | Positioning on side permits back care and rest to tissues. Pillows under legs in traction create friction and should not be used because they lessen traction effectiveness. |
|     d. **Dunlop's traction**: Patient must lie on back. Bed may be tilted on low shock blocks towards side opposite traction. Head of bed is kept flat. | Tilting uses body for some counter traction<br>Flexion of hips and knees relaxes lumbosacral muscles to lessen spasms |
|     e. **Pelvic sling:** Patient lies on back when in sling and should have enough weight attached to raise buttocks slightly off bed. If sling is off, it can be used carefully as turning sheet if patient's fractures permit side lying | Hammock effect of sling is most effective when patient is on back. Sling must be removed for placement of bedpan |
|     f. **Russell's traction**: Patient lies on back, head of bed may be elevated to 25 to 30 degree depending on injury | Low fowler's position creates most effective traction pull |
| 12. Ask patient how traction is affecting injured tissues if patient is able to respond. Babies or young children may cry when weights are initially applied but may soon ease crying and appear more comfortable | Initial reaction may be slight increase in soreness or pain until patient is able to relax and allow traction to perform as designed |
| 13. Place siderails elevated as appropriate. Patient in Bryant's traction should always have some one in attendance | Promotes patient's safety |
| 14. Gather unused materials and return to storage areas | |
| 15. Wash hands | Reduces transmission of microorganisms |
| 16. Observe entire skin traction set up and its functioning, check all knots, ropes in pulleys, weight on weight holder, whether apparatus is hanging freely, position of halter sling, belt or other material for specific traction | Reassessment is necessary to determine if traction is functioning as designed or described or to make needed adjustments. |
| 17. Assess condition of skin around straps or bandages | Ensures early identification of irritation or breakdown |
| 18. Ask if patient is experiencing pain or muscle burning | Indicates misalignment of bones or presence of muscles spasms |
| 19. Conduct neuromuscular checks every 1-2 hours initially, then every 4 hours if patient is stabilizing | Provides objective data concerning peripheral perfusion to tissues |
| 20 Observe patient's participation in self care | Patient may refrain from activity unnecessarily |
| 21. Record type of traction, site to which applied, amount of weight, person applying traction, time, patient's response and other pertinent data in nurse's notes. | Ensures continuity of care and provides documentation for legal consideration |

*Contd...*

*Contd...*

| | |
|---|---|
| 22. Record traction functioning every shift. Observe all ropes, pulleys weights and strings at the beginning of shift and after turning or position changes or if traction is removed for providing nursing care. | Safety, continuity of care and legal factors require recording of all details. |

## SPECIAL CONSIDERATIONS

1. If institution policies or physician's order specify, remove traction for skin care for short periods. If removed for skin care, patient is out of traction only for 10 to 15 minutes before it is reapplied.
2. Muscles and joints may be weakened from bedrest or traction and need time to regain strength.

## 9.4: APPLYING BANDAGES

## DEFINITION

Bandaging is the process of covering a wound or injured part using various materials such as gauze, elasticized knit, flannel or muslin.

## PURPOSES

1. To support the wound
2. To immobilize a fracture or dislocation
3. To immobilize an injured part so as to relieve pain
4. To prevent contamination of a wound
5. To control hemorrhage and to improve venous blood flow from lower extremites by applying pressure
6. To secure a dressing
7. To maintain splints in position
8. To retain warmth (e.g. a flannel bandage on a rheumatoid joint)
9. To prevent or reduce swelling.

## TYPES OF BANDAGES

1. Triangular bandage
2. Roller bandage
3. Special bandages
   a. Many tailed
   b. "T" Bandage

## ARTICLES

1. Roller bandages (according to the body part) refer table below

| Part to be bandaged | Width |
|---|---|
| 1. Fingers | 1 inch |
| 2. Arm | 2 to 2.5 inches |
| 3. Leg | 3 to 3.5 inches |
| 4. Trunk | 4 to 6 inches |
| 5. Head | 2 inches |

2. Scissors
3. Safetypin/adhesive strip

## PRINCIPLES OF BANDAGING

1. Use a tightly rolled bandage of the correct width
2. Support the part to be bandaged throughout the procedure.
3. Always stand in front of the patient, except when applying a capeline bandage.
4. Bandage a limb in the position in which it is to remain, e.g. forearm and hand should be prone.
5. Hold the bandage with the head of roll uppermost and apply the outer surface of the bandage to the part, never unroll more than a few inches of bandage at a time
6. Apply bandage from within outwards and from below upwards maintaining even pressure throughout.
7. Begin the bandage with a firm oblique turn to fix it and allow each successive turn to cover two thirds of the previous one with the free edges lying parallel.

8. Make any reverses or crossing line on the outer side of the limb except, when this brings the bandage over a wound or bony prominence, in which case, it must be on the front of the limb.
9. Pad the axilla or groin when bandaging these parts, so that two surfaces of skin do not touch each other beneath the bandage.
10. Finish off with a straight turn above the part, hold the end and fasten with the safetypin.

## CIRCULAR TURN

Used chiefly to anchor bandages or to bandage certain areas, such as the proximal aspect of a finger or a wrist.

| | Steps in procedure | Rationale |
|---|---|---|
| 1 | Apply the end of bandage to the part of the body to be bandaged | |
| 2 | Encircle the body part a few times or as close as needed, each turn directly covering the previous turn. | Provides even support to the area. |
| 3 | Secure the end of bandage with tape, metal clips or a safetypin over an uninjured area. | Clips and pins can be uncomfortable when situated over an injured area. |

## SPIRAL TURN/SIMPLE SPIRAL (FIGURE 9.4A (i))

Spiral turns are used to bandage parts of the body that are fairly uniform in circumference such as the upper arm or upper leg.

| | | |
|---|---|---|
| 1 | Make two circular turns to anchor the bandage | |
| 2 | Continue spiral turns at about a 30 degree angle, each turn, overlapping the preceding one by two thirds the width of the bandage | |
| 3 | End the bandage with two circular turns | |

## SPIRAL REVERSE TURN (FIGURE 9.4A (ii))

Spiral reverse turns are used to bandage cylindrical parts of the body that are not uniform in circumference such as the lower leg or forearm.

| | | |
|---|---|---|
| 1 | Make two circular turns to anchor the bandage and bring the bandage upward at about a 30 degree angle | |
| 2 | Place the thumb of the free hand on the upper edge of the bandage | The thumb will hold the bandage while it is folded on itself. |
| 3 | Unroll the bandage around about 15 cm (6 inches) then turn the hand so that the bandage falls over itself. | |
| 4 | Continue the bandage around the limb, overlapping each previous turn by two thirds the width of the bandage, make each bandage turn at the same position on the limb so that the turns of the bandage will be aligned. | |
| 5 | End the bandage with two circular turns and secure | |

## SPICA

The spica is a form of figure of eight in which one turn is very much larger than the other. It is used for joints at right angles to the body, e.g. shoulder, groin and thumb.

## ELBOW BANDAGE (FIGURE OF EIGHT) (FIGURE 9.4A (iii))

| | | |
|---|---|---|
| 1 | Bend the elbow at right angles | |
| 2 | Lay the outerside of the bandage on the innerside of the joint and take two straight turns carrying the bandage over the elbow tip and around the elbow. | Two turns are taken to fix the bandage to the body part. |
| 3 | Make a second turn to encircle forearm and the upper arm. | |
| 4 | Ensure the first turn is covered 1/3rd of the width of the bandage below and above. | By covering 1/3rd below and above, remaining 1/3rd is exposed. |
| 5 | Continue bandaging, covering 2/3rd of the previous turn until the entire dressing is secured. | |
| 6 | Complete bandaging by taking two circular turns above and secure it with safetypin or tape. | |

## KNEE BANDAGE (FIGURE OF EIGHT) (FIGURE 9.4A (iv))

| | | |
|---|---|---|
| 1 | Flex the knee and lay the outer side of the bandage against the inner side of the knee (medial) | |
| 2 | Take two straight/circular turns over the knee cap | This makes the bandage to go around the knee and secures it firmly. |
| 3 | Take a turn below and above covering 1/3rds of the previous turn. | Ensures that the margins of the bandage covering the knee cap are covered. |
| 4 | Continue the turns below and above the joint until the whole knee is covered. | |
| 5 | Secure the bandage by completing with two circular turns around the thigh. | |
| 6 | Fix the end with adhesive tape or safetypin. | |

## CAPELINE (HEAD) BANDAGE (FIGURE 9.4A (v))

This bandage is sometimes used when the whole scalp is to be covered. A double headed roller bandage is used.

| | | |
|---|---|---|
| 1 | Position the patient to sit on a stool or chair & stand behind the patient. | This position will be convenient to apply the head bandage. |
| 2 | Place the center of the outer surface of the bandage in the center of the forehead, the lower border of the bandage lying just above the eyebrows. | |
| 3 | Bring the head of the bandage around over the temples and above the ears to the nape of the neck when the ends are crossed. | Ensures that the ear is not covered. |
| 4 | Bring the upper bandage around the head and the other head of bandage over the center of the top of the scalp and then to the root of the nose. | |
| 5 | Bring the bandage which circles the victim's head over the forehead, covering and fixing the bandage which crosses the scalp. This bandage is then brought back over the scalp. | |
| 6 | Ensure that each turn of the bandage covers 2/3rd of the previous turn. | Adheres snugly to the body part (head) and also stays firm. |

*Contd...*

*Contd...*

| 7 | Cross it again at the back and fix using the encircling bandage and turn back over the scalp to the opposite side at the central line, now covering the other margin of its original turn. | |
|---|---|---|
| 8 | Repeat the backward and forward turns to alternate side of the center, each one being in turn fixed by the encircling bandage until the whole scalp is covered. | |
| 9 | End the bandging by taking two circular turns round the head | This will secure the turns of the bandage. |
| 10 | Secure it with adhesive tape or safety pin over the forehead. | |

## EAR BANDAGE (FIGURE 9.4A (vi))

This bandage is used to secure the dressing of the ear.

| 1 | Lay the outer surface of the bandage against the forehead and carry the bandage round the head in two circular turns, bandaging away from the injured ear. |
|---|---|
| 2 | Carry the bandage round the back of the head on the unaffected side and then down the nape of the neck. |
| 3 | Repeat the turns with each turn being slightly higher than the previous one. |
| 4 | Bring the bandage slightly lower as it covers the hair. |
| 5 | Continue the turns until the whole ear on the affected side is covered and complete the bandage by two straight/circular turns around the forehead. |
| 6 | Secure it with adhesive tape or safety-pin, where all the turns cross one another. |

## SPECIAL CONSIDERATION

The bandage can also be taken around the forehead between each turn covering the dressing, but this makes a heavy bulk around the head which is not really necessary.

## EYE BANDAGE (FIGURE 9.4A (vii))

| 1 | Lay the outer surface of the bandage against the forehead and take two circular turns around the head bandaging away from the injured eye. |
|---|---|
| 2 | Carry the bandage, round the head until it reaches the eye on the affected side. |
| 3 | Take it obliquely to the back of the head, under the prominence on the back of the skull and from there bring it upwards beneath the eye of the affected side. |
| 4 | Take it further over the pad of the eye to a circular turn and continue over the head to the starting point. |
| 5 | Repeat this turn 2 or 3 times until the dressing is covered. |
| 6 | Finish with the safetypin just above the unaffected eye. |

## JAW BANDAGE

A narrow strip of material about 4 feet long or a narrow fold of triangular bandage can be used for a jaw bandage.

| | |
|---|---|
| 1 | Place the center of the bandage under the chin. |
| 2 | Carry one end upwards over the top of the head and cross with the other end above the ear. |
| 3 | Carry the shorter end across the front of the forehead and the larger end in the opposite direction round the back of the head. |
| 4 | Tie the ends above the other ear over forehead. |

## SHOULDER (SPICA) (FIGURE 9.4A (viii))

| | |
|---|---|
| 1 | Place a small pad of cottonwool in the affected axilla. |
| 2 | Take 3-4 inch bandage and fix it with spiral turns round the upper part of the arm. |
| 3 | Take 2 or 3 reverse spiral turns round the upper arm until the bandage reaches the point of the shoulder. |
| 4 | Carry the bandage over the shoulder across the back and under the opposite armpit. |
| 5 | Bring it across the chest and arm round under the armpit and over the shoulder again, covering 2/3rds of the previous turn. |
| 6 | Repeat the turns until the whole shoulder is covered. |
| 7 | Secure the bandage using a pin over the injured shoulder. |

## THUMB (SPICA) (FIGURE 9.4A (ix))

| | |
|---|---|
| 1 | Place the hand so that the back of the thumb is uppermost (dorsal side of the thumb above). |
| 2 | Take two circular turns round the wrist and carry the bandage over the back of the thumb. |
| 3 | Encircle the thumb with one or two straight turns so that the lower border of the bandage is level with the root of the nail. |
| 4 | Carry the bandage back over the back of the hand, round the wrist and repeat the figure of eight turns round the thumb. |
| 5 | Ensure the body of the thumb is completely covered. |
| 6 | Complete the bandage with two straight turns, round the wrist and secure it with the pin or adhesive tape. |

## FINGER BANDAGE (WITHOUT COVERING THE FINGERTIP) (FIGURE 9.4A (x))

| | |
|---|---|
| 1 | With the hand pronated fix the bandage by two circular turns round the wrist. |
| 2 | Carry the bandage obliquely over the back of the hand to the base of the finger to be bandaged. |
| 3 | Take the head of roll to the fingers in order and start from the side of little finger. |

*Contd...*

*Contd...*

| 4 | Take one spiral turn to the base of the finger and then cover the finger by simple spiral turns. |
|---|---|
| 5 | Then carry the bandage across the back of the hand to the wrist and complete it with two straight turns round the wrist. |
| 6 | Secure the bandage by safetypin or adhesive tape. |
| 7 | If more than one finger is to be bandaged take a turn round the wrist between each two fingers and continue as above until the bandage is complete. |

## FINGER BANDAGE (TO COVER THE FINGERTIP) (FIGURE 9.4A (xi))

| 1 | Repeat steps 1-3 as mentioned in the above procedure. |
|---|---|
| 2 | Take the bandage straight upto the back of the finger and over the middle of the tip and down the front to the level of the second joint. |
| 3 | Hold the turns at the back and in front and with the fingers of the other hand, make two more turns over the tip of the finger one on either side of the first turn. |
| 4 | Fix the loop with the straight circular turn as near to the tip as possible and then cover the finger by simple spiral turn |
| 5 | Take simple spiral turns from medial to lateral aspect of the finger |
| 6 | Take two straight turns round the wrist and complete as before or continue to next finger. |

## SPICA OF HIP (FIGURE 9.4A (xii))

| 1 | Place the outside of the bandage on the inner side of the thigh about 6 inches below the groin. |
|---|---|
| 2 | Carry the bandage horizontally round the limb and make 3 or 4 ascending reverse spiral turns round the thigh. |
| 3 | Carry the bandage from medial to lateral over the front of the groin and up round the hip and back, passing over the prominence and the hip bone over the opposite side. |
| 4 | Bring the bandage down, over the abdomen to the outer side of the thigh and repeat the figure of eight round the body and the thigh until the hip is covered. |

## SPICA OF GROIN BANDAGE (FIGURE 9.4A (xiii))

| 1 | Place the outside of the bandage on the inner side of the thigh. |
|---|---|
| 2 | Carry the bandage horizontally round the limb in two circular turns. |
| 3 | Carry the bandage from medial to lateral aspect up towards the hip and to the back passing over the prominence of the hip bone on the opposite side. |
| 4 | Bring the bandage down, over the abdomen to the outer side of the thigh and repeat the figure of eight round the body and the thigh covering the 2/3rds of the previous turn, until the groin is covered. |
| 5 | The crossings are made over the front of the groin. |

*Contd...*

*Contd...*

| 6 | Secure the bandage on the unaffected side over the abdomen, with a safetypin or an adhesive tape. |
|---|---|

## DOUBLE SPICA OF GROIN BANDAGE

| 1 | Lay the outer surface of the bandage over the right groin and pass the bandage round the thigh, carrying it up over the front of the right groin to the left hip. |
|---|---|
| 2 | Carry the bandage round the back and right hip and over the lower part of the abdomen to the outer side of the thigh. |
| 3 | Pass the bandage under the thigh upto left groin and round the back and right hip and down again to the innerside of the right thigh. |
| 4 | Repeat these turns on either sides until both groins are covered. Each turn being slightly higher and covering 2/3rds of the previous one. |
| 5 | Secure the bandage over the abdomen by safetypin or adhesive tape. |

## STUMP BANDAGE (FIGURE 9.4A (xiv))

| 1 | Use a 4 inch bandage<br>Make two circular turns round the limb above the stump. |
|---|---|
| 2 | Place the end in the center of the upper side of the limb and carry the bandage over the center of the stump to the same level behind. |
| 3 | Hold the turns at the back and in front with the thumb and fingers of the other hand. |
| 4 | Repeat the recurrent turns over the end of the stump first and on the stump, on the left and on the right side of the original turns until the whole dressing is covered. |
| 5 | Fix the loops with straight turns round the stump and cover the dressing completely. |
| 6 | Secure it with a safetypin or adhesive tape. |

## FOOT AND ANKLE BANDAGE (FIGURE OF EIGHT) (FIGURE 9.4A (xv))

| 1 | Make two circular turns round the ankle to fix the bandage. |
|---|---|
| 2 | Take an oblique turn across the foot to the root of little toe. |
| 3 | Make one horizontal turn round the foot at this level and then carry the bandage back over the foot and take a turn round the ankle just above the heel. |
| 4 | Repeat this figure of eight turns round the foot and ankle each turn overlapping the previous one by 2/3rds of its width |
| 5 | Secure the bandage with two circular turns around the ankle with pin or tape. |

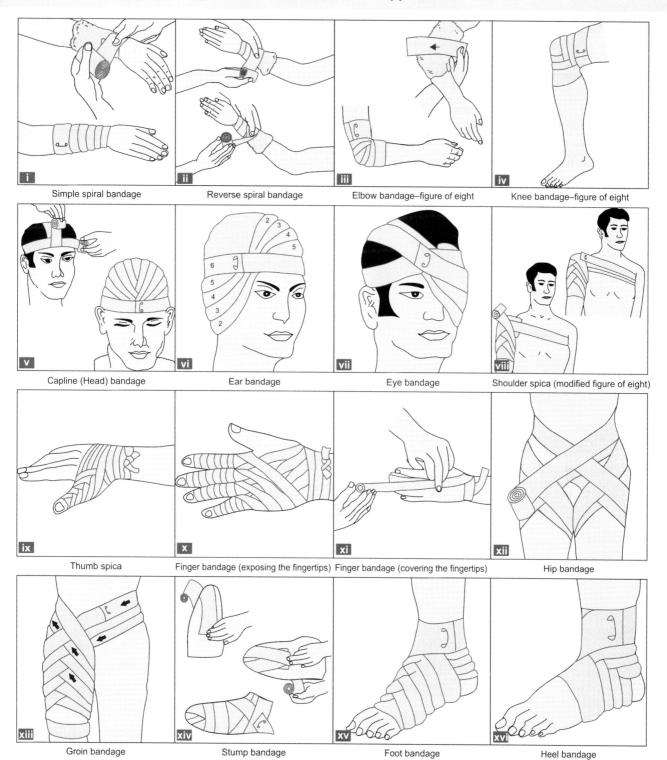

**Figure 9.4(a) (i to xvi):** Applying bandage illustrated

## HEEL BANDAGE (FIGURE 9.4A(xvi))

| | | |
|---|---|---|
| 1 | Keep the foot at right angles | |
| 2 | Start two circular turns on centre of the heel, carry it round the foot below the tip of the heel. | Tip of the heel is well covered |
| 3 | Bring the bandage over the ankle around the leg, below and then above the previous turn covering 1/3rd on either side. | |
| 4 | Repeat the turns by covering 2/3rds of the previous turn. | |
| 5 | Complete it by two circular turns above the ankle and secure it with pin or adhesive tape. | |

# 9.5: APPLYING BINDERS

## DEFINITION

Binders are special wide bandages used for supporting specific parts of body and large dressings.

## TYPES OF BINDERS

a. Abdominal binders
   1. Large rectangular piece of heavy cotton, muslin or flannel, which can be pinned at the center to fit the patient. (Figure 9.5(a))
   2. Synthetic binder with adhering straps, hooks and eyes.
   3. Scultetus binders – consists of a rectangular piece of strong cloth with many tails attached to the two longer sides. Used for support of abdominal (Figure 9.5(b)) musculature and to prevent wound dehiscence and evisceration following abdominal surgery.
b. T. binder
   1. Single tailed binder (Figure 9.5(c)).
   2. Double tailed binder.
c. Breast binder

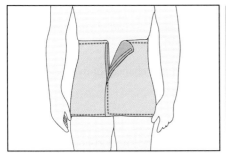

Figure 9.5(a): Abdominal binder—
Large rectangular

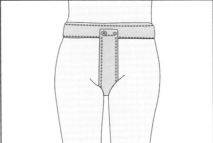

Figure 9.5(b): T-binder

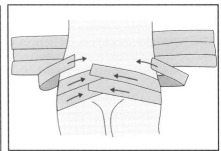

Figure 9.5(c): Scultetus (many-
tailed) binder

### A. ABDOMINAL BINDER/LARGE, RECTANGULAR

Abdominal binders are used primarily to provide support following abdominal surgery and to secure dressings.

## ARTICLES

1. Binder
2. Safetypins or clips.

## PROCEDURE

| | Nursing action | Rationale |
|---|---|---|
| 1. | Identify patient with need for support of abdomen. Assess ability to breathe deeply and cough effectively. | Baseline assessment determines patient's ability to breath and cough. |
| 2. | Inspect skin for actual or potential alterations in integrity. Observe for irritation, abrasions or skin surfaces that rub against each other. | Actual impairments in skin integrity can be worsened with application of binder. Binder can cause pressure and excoriation. |
| 3. | Review medical record if medical prescription for particular binder is required and reasons for application. | Application of supportive binder may be based on nursing judgement. In some situations physician's input is required. |

*Contd...*

*Contd...*

| | | |
|---|---|---|
| 4. | Explain to the patient about procedure and the need for application of binder. | |
| 5. | Gather necessary data regarding size of patient and appropriate binder. | Ensures proper fitting of binder. |
| 6. | Prepare necessary supplies<br>a. Abdominal binder of correct size (cloth or elastic)<br>b. Safetypins | Binder must be large enough to surround abdomen and overlap to secure closure. |
| 7. | Close curtains or room door | Promotes understanding and provides privacy. |
| 8. | Wash hands | Maintains medical asepsis and prevents infection. |
| 9. | Apply abdominal binder:<br>a. Position patient with head slightly elevated and knees slightly flexed.<br>b. Fan-fold far side of binder towards midline of binder<br>c. Instruct and assist patient to roll away from you toward raised side rail while firmly supporting abdominal incision and dressing with hands.<br>d. Place fan-folded ends of binder under patient.<br><br>e. Instruct patient to roll over folded ends.<br>f. Unfold and stretch ends out smoothly on far side of bed (binder should extend from just above symphysis pubis to just below costal margin).<br>g. Instruct patient to roll back into supine position.<br><br>h. Adjust binder so that supine patient is centered over binder using symphysis pubis and costal margins as lower and upper landmarks.<br>i. Pull distal end of binder over center of patient's abdomen. While maintaining tension on that end of binder, pull opposite ends of binder over center and secure with Velcro closure tabs or safetypins.<br>j. Assess patient's ability to breath deeply and cough effectively.<br>k. Ask patient about comfort level.<br>l. Adjust binder as necessary.<br>m. Record the procedure. | Minimizes muscular tension on abdominal wall.<br><br><br>Reduces pain and discomfort.<br><br><br><br>Permits placement and centering of binder with minimal discomfort.<br><br>Facilitates chest expansion and adequate wound support when binder is closed.<br><br>Proper placement reduces chances of decreased lung expansion.<br><br><br><br>Provides continuous wound support and comfort.<br><br><br><br>Determines effective ventilation |

## B. T. BINDER

T. binder is used primarily to secure rectal or perineal dressings. Double T. binder is used for males and single T. binder is used for females

## ARTICLES

1. T. binder
2. Safetypins.

## PROCEDURE

| | Nursing action | Rationale |
|---|---|---|
| 1 | Review medical record if medical prescription for particular binder is required and reasons for application. | Application of supportive binder may be based on nursing judgement. In some situations physician's input is required. |

*Contd...*

*Contd...*

| | | |
|---|---|---|
| 2 | Explain to the patient about procedure and the need for application of binder. | |
| 3. | Assist patient to dorsal recumbent position. | |
| 4. | Have patient raise hips and place horizontal band around waist with vertical tails extending past buttocks. Overlap waistband in front and secure with safetypins. | Minimizes muscular tension on perineal organs and secures binder around patient. |
| 5. | *Single tailed binder:* Bring remaining vertical strip over perineal dressing and continue up and under to center of horizontal band. Bring ends over waist band and secure vertical and horizontal band together with safetypin. *Double tailed binder:* Bring remaining vertical strips over perineal or suprapubic dressing with each tail supporting one side of scrotum and proceeding upward on either side of penis. Continue drawing ends behind and then downward in front of horizontal band. Secure all thickness with a safetypin | |
| 6. | Assess comfort level with patient in lying, sitting and standing positions. Readjust front pins as necessary. Increase padding if any area rubs against surrounding tissues. | Determines efficacy of binder to maintain dressings and support perineal structures. |
| 7. | Instruct patient regarding removal of binder before defecating or urinating and need to replace binder afterwards. | Cleanliness of binder reduces of chances infection. |
| 8. | Record the procedure in Nurses' notes | Gives information about patient's response. |

## C. BREAST BINDER

A breast binder looks like a tight fitting sleeveless vest and is used to apply pressure to the breasts.

## PURPOSES

1. To provide support after surgery.
2. To support breasts for comfort in case of engorgement.
3. To secure dressing.
4. To compress breasts to help in suppression of lactation following fetal loss or neonatal death.

## ARTICLES

1. Breast binder
2. Dressing pads or breast pads if padding is required.

## PROCEDURE

| | Nursing action | Rationale |
|---|---|---|
| 1. | Review medical record if medical prescription for particular binder is required and reasons for application. | Application of supportive binder may be based on nursing judgement. In some situations physician's input is required. |
| 2. | Explain to the patient about procedure and the need for application of binder. | |
| 3. | Assist patient to supine position in bed. | Maintains normal anatomical alignment of breasts and facilitates healing and comfort. |

*Contd...*

*Contd...*

| 4. | Pad area under breasts if necessary. | Prevents skin contact with under surface. |
|---|---|---|
| 5. | Place binder under torso with the center of binder at midline. | |
| 6. | Bring the farther end over patient's breasts, take the near end and place over the first one. | |
| 7. | Using Velcro closure tabs, secure binder at nipple level first, continue closure process above and then below nipple line until entire binder is closed. | Reduces risk of uneven pressure or localized irritation. |
| 8. | Bring the shoulder straps over on either side to the front and fix to the upper border of binder. | |
| 9. | Make appropriate adjustments including individualizing the fit of shoulder straps. | Maintains support to patient's breasts. |
| 10. | Instruct and observe skill development in self- care related to reapplying breast binder. | Self-care is an integral aspect of discharge planning. |
| 11. | Wash hands | Prevents cross infection. |
| 12. | Observe underlying skin for integrity circulation and characteristics of the wound (if present) and comfort level of patient. | • Determines that binder has not resulted in irritation of skin or underlying organs.<br>• Binders should not impede breathing or increase discomfort. |
| 13. | Record application of binder, condition of skin and circulation, integrity of dressings and comfort level. | Documents procedure. Baseline data ensures continuity of care. |

## Key points in the use of binders are:

1. Binders are applied so that firm, even pressure is exerted.
2. Binders should not impair neuromuscular or pulmonary functions.
3. Since binders are not attached to the skin they slip out of place easily and may require periodic reapplication.
4. Wrinkled binders are uncomfortable and may cause tissue damage.
5. Binders are secured so that there is no movement and friction against underlying skin surfaces.
6. Pins or knots are placed away from wound edges or tender areas.
7. Binders are applied with the body part in anatomical alignment and with joints in position of function.
8. Soiled or moist binders may promote infection if applied over skin surfaces that are not intact.
9. The skin surfaces underneath a binder should be inspected at frequent intervals.
10. Neurovascular integrity of areas distal to the binder should be assessed at frequent intervals.
11. Binders that cause discomfort should be removed and reapplied.
12. Talcum powder may be applied to skin surface.

# 9.6: ASSISTING WITH APPLICATION OF PLASTER OF PARIS (POP)

## DEFINITION

A plaster cast is a rigid immobilizing device that is moulded to contours of body to encase an injured part.

## PURPOSES

1. To immobilize a body part in specific position.
2. To apply uniform pressure or encase soft tissue.
3. To correct or prevent deformity.
4. To provide support/stability for weakened joints.
5. To immobilize a reduced fracture.

## TYPES

1. Short arm cast (wrist plaster).
2. Long arm cast (above-elbow plaster).
3. Arm cylinder cast.
4. Short leg cast (below knee plaster).
5. Long leg cast (above-knee plaster).
6. Leg cylinder cast.
7. Shoulder spica cast.
8. Minerva cast.
9. Bivalved cased.

## ARTICLES

Tray containing
1. Plaster bandages
2. Stockinette
3. Short trimming knife
4. Scissors
5. Dressing supplies
6. Measuring tape
7. Protective sheet
8. Plastic apron/gown
9. Gloves
10. Newspaper
11. Bowl of warm water and washcloth
12. Fracture table.

## PROCEDURE

| | Nursing action | Rationale |
|---|---|---|
| 1. | Assess patient's health status, including conditions affecting wound healing(e. g. diabetes, malnutrition) | Patient's health status is pertinent to potential healing of tissues enclosed by cast. |
| 2. | Explain to patient the purpose and procedure of cast application, according to his level of understanding. | Relieves patient's anxiety and helps nurse determine whether additional information is needed. |

*Contd...*

*Contd...*

| | | |
|---|---|---|
| 3. | Assess condition of tissues to be in the cast including circulation to extremities. Note presence of skin breakdown, bruising, rash and irritation. Skin of babies, children and older persons may contain less subcutaneous fat. | Determines need for additional skin care before cast application. |
| 4. | Determine patient's pain status. | Fractures are painful. Patient's responses vary as does need for analgesic. |
| 5. | Protect patient's cloth with protective sheet. | Prevents soiling. |
| 6. | Administer analgesics 20-30 minutes before cast application. | Reduces pain during cast application. |
| 7. | Wash hands and don gloves. | Reduces transmission of microorganisms. Synthetic cast can leave glue-like stain on hands. |
| 8. | Position patient as desired. Patient may be lying; sitting or standing depending on type and body part to be casted. | Parts to be put in cast must be supported and placed in optimal position for cast application. |
| 9. | Prepare skin for cast if necessary; may involve cleansing with soap and water, changing dressing and trimming or shaving long hair. Use gentle strokes to maintain skin integrity. | Reduces complications to underlying tissues after casting. Gentle manipulation prevents pain or additional injury. |
| 10. | Place stockinette over the skin where casting material will be applied (Figure 9.6(a)). | Reduces skin irritation. |

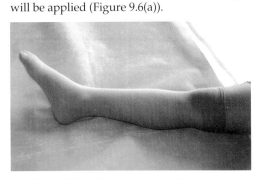

Figure 9.6(a): Placing stockenette over skin

| | | |
|---|---|---|
| 11. | Wrap the site with cast padding (Figure 9.6(b)). | |

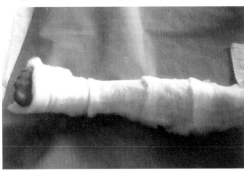

Figure 9.6(b): Padding the cast site

| | | |
|---|---|---|
| 12. | Depending on type of cast material being applied do one of the following:<br>a  Hold plaster roll under water in a casting bucket or plastic basin until bubbles stop, then squeeze slightly and hand over to person applying cast (Figure 9.6(c)). | Dampened plaster rolls are unrolled and molded to fit part being casted. Some have resin for easy moldability |

*Contd...*

*Contd...*

| | |
|---|---|
| b Submerge synthetic cast roll in lukewarm water for 10-15 seconds, sqeeze to remove excess water. | Initiates chemical reaction that produces heat and hardens the cast roll. |
| c Hold body part or parts to be put in cast in position requested for applying cast. | Support of body part may involve applying slight manual traction if desired to maintain optimal position. |

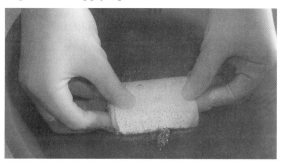

**Figure 9.6(c):** Holding plaster roll under water

| | |
|---|---|
| 13 Continue to apply dampened rolls of plaster to hold parts as necessary until cast is finished (Figure 9.6(d)). | Plaster must be of sufficient thickness to give strength to cast. |

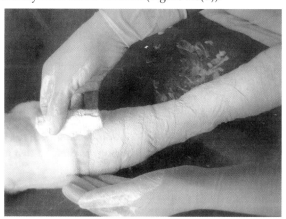

**Figure 9.6(d):** Applying plaster rolls

| | |
|---|---|
| 14. Assist with "finishing" the cast by folding stockinette or other padding down the outer edge of cast to provide smooth edge to cast. Damp plaster is then rolled over padding to hold it securely outside cast (Figure 9.6(e)). | Smooth edges lessen possible skin irritation. Finishing cast with stockinette provides smooth edges. "Petaling" is not required when cast is dry. |

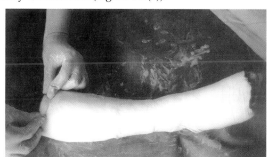

**Figure 9.6(e):** Finishing of the cast application

*Contd...*

*Contd...*

| | | |
|---|---|---|
| 15 | Supply scissors to trim plaster roll around thumb, finger or toes as necessary. | Casts should be snug but should not constrict joint movement or circulation. |
| 16 | Depending on tissues casted, do one of the following<br>  a. Place damp cast on cloth covered pillows to prevent deformation or pressure points as it sets.<br>  b. Handle the damp plaster cast with only the palm of the hand and not the fingers. | Pillows or soft areas prevent cast from hardening in undesirable position.<br>Handling plaster cast with fingers can cause indentation. |
| 17 | Remove and dispose of gloves. Assist with transfer of patient to stretcher or wheelchair for return to nursing unit. | Safety in transfer requires use of pillows to support cast, siderails, restraints and sufficient personnel to support patient and cast. |
| 18 | Clean equipment used, return to usual place; discard used materials and wash hands. | Facilitates use of article and area for next patient.<br>Reduces transmission of infection |
| 19 | Explain purposes of exposure for faster drying. Use elevation if pertinent, apply icebags if ordered, or use fans or hairdryer set to cool settings to facilitate drying. | Cast must dry from inside out for thorough drying.<br>Elevation and use of ice decreases edema formation. |
| 20 | Have patient turn every 2-3 hours. | Prevents any one area of cast from receiving continuous pressure.<br>Avoids indentation of the cast. |
| 21 | Observe patients for signs of pain or anxiety; hyperventilation, swallowing air, tachycardia or BP increase. | These are signs of development of "cast syndrome" which may occur when body cast is applied. |
| 22 | Assess neurovascular status by performing neurovascular checks:<br><br>  a. Observe colour of tissues distal to cast<br><br><br><br>  b. Observe for odema distal to cast<br>  c. Feel temperature of tissues above and below the cast<br><br>  d. Palpate the distal pulses of the casted extremity. Note presence and strength of pulse<br>  e. Ask patient to move parts distal to cast in ROM if possible if patient cannot do active ROM, perform passive ROM on these joints noting responses or complaints of increased pain<br>  f. Ask patient to describe sensations or feelings of tissue in cast; listen for descriptions such as pins and needles, asleep, numb, burning or throbbing. | Neurovascular status determines circulation and oxygenation of tissues<br>Pink color indicates that arterial pressure is normal, pallor signifies decreased blood supply, bluish color signifies reduced venous circulation.<br>Edema results from trauma or venous stasis<br>Warmth of tissues distal or proximal to cast usually indicates adequate perfusion<br>Weak or absent pulses may indicate decreased circulation to casted area<br>Range of motion should be possible within limitations imposed by casts<br>Passive movements decrease oedema<br>May signify pressure or anoxia affecting normal transmission of nerve impulses. |
| 23 | Record application of cast and condition of skin and circulation status. | |
| 24 | Record patients ability or inability to perform ADL and specific requirements for care. | Independence is valued for continuity of care and self care. |

**Table 9.6.1:** Complications of plaster cast

| | Complications | Signs and symptoms |
|---|---|---|
| 1 | Impaired blood flow | • Absence of pulse in the extremity below the plaster cast.<br>• Blanching or cyanosis of the skin<br>• Pain<br>• Coldness of the skin<br>• Swelling<br>• Numbness |
| 2 | Nerve damage | • Persistent and increasing pain<br>• Numbness<br>• Motor paralysis |
| 3 | Tissue necrosis and infection | • Unpleasant odour<br>• Feeling of " hot " sensation<br>• Drainage through the cast<br>• Sudden unexplained elevation of body temperature. |
| 4 | Volkman's Ischemic contracture | All the signs and symptoms of impaired blood flow<br>• Absence of radial/pedal pulse<br>• Infarction and necrosis of the muscle<br>• Absence of finger/toe movement'<br>• Absence of pain which was intense in the beginning. |
| 5 | Cast syndrome | • Prolonged nausea and vomiting<br>• Abdominal distention<br>• Vague abdominal pain |
| 6 | Complication due to immobility | • Hypostatic pneumonia<br>• Footdrop<br>• Renal calculi<br>• Decubitus ulcers on pressure points<br>• Stiffness of joints<br>• Constipation and retention of urine<br>• Lethargy, loneliness and depression, insomnia |
| 7 | Surgical complications | Phlebothrombosis and pulmonary embolism wound infection. |

## SPECIAL CONSIDERATIONS

1. It is important to inform the patient that sensation of heat may occur at the time of drying of the plaster cast.
2. Plaster cast is never applied over areas with open wounds.

\* **Petaling:** Application of adhesive tape three or four inches in length by tucking the straight end inside the cast and by bringing the rounded end over the cast edge to the outside.

## 9.7: PINSITE CARE IN SKELETAL TRACTION

Skin care to be carried out at the site of pin insertion for patients on skeletal traction at regular intervals to detect and prevent infection.

## ARTICLES

1. Sterile dressing tray
2. Normal saline solution
3. Hydrogen peroxide
4. Sterile gloves
5. Disposable gloves
6. Povidone-iodine solution
7. Sterile cotton balls and gauze pieces
8. K-basin.

## PROCEDURE

|  | Nursing action | Rationale |
|---|---|---|
| 1 | Wash hands and don disposable- gloves. | Reduces transmission of infection. |
| 2 | Open dressing tray. | |
| 3 | Pour normal saline and hydrogen peroxide in 1:1 dilution in a cup. Pour povidone iodine in another cup. | |
| 4 | Remove old gauze dressing around pinsite and discard. | |
| 5 | Remove disposable gloves and don sterile gloves. | Aseptic technique reduces transmission of infection. |
| 6 | Begin by cleaning pins on one side of extremity, then do the same on the other side. | Prevents cross contamination. |
| 7 | Clean first with hydrogen peroxide and saline. | Removes crust from pinsite. |
| 8 | Soak sterile gauze in povidone iodine solution, squeeze and wrap around each pinsite. | Reduces bacterial growth. |
| 9 | Ensure that all the pinsites are covered. | |
| 10 | Remove gloves and replace articles. | |
| 11 | Record the condition of pinsite, any discharge or bleeding if present. Look for any induration. Record type of solution used and patient's compliance. | Provides data for evaluating wound healing. |

# 9.8: ASSISTING WITH WALKING USING WALKER AND CANE

## WALKER

A walker is a light weight metal frame (Usually aluminium) with four legs. It provides a sense of security and support. Walker is used by patients who are able to bear partial weight.

Walkers are of several types specified according to the arm strength and balance of the patient.

*Patient's requirements to use walker:*
1. Partial strength in both hands and wrists.
2. Strong elbow extensors such as triceps brachi
3. Strong shoulder depressors such as the pectoralis minor.
4. Ability to bear at least partial weight on both legs.

## PROCEDURE

| | Nursing action | Rationale |
|---|---|---|
| 1 | Explain the method of using walker. | Prevents anxiety and helps in obtaining co-operation of the patient. |
| 2 | Instruct patient to wear nonskid shoe or slipper. | Prevents falling. |
| 3 | Instruct patient not to use walker on stairs. | |
| 4 | Have patient stand in center of walker and grasp handgrips on upperbars (Figure 9.8(a)). | Patient balances self before attempting to walk. |

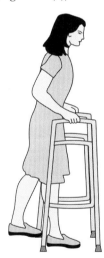

Figure 9.8(a): Positioning with walker

| | | |
|---|---|---|
| 5 | Lift walker, and move it 6-8 inches forward, making sure all four feet of the walker stays on the floor. Take a step forward with one foot. Then follow through with the other leg. | Provides broad base of support between walker and patient. Patient then moves center of gravity towards the walker. Keeping all four feet of the walker on the floor is necessary to prevent tipping of the walker. |
| 6 | If there is unilateral weakness, after the walker is advanced, instruct the patient to step forward with the weaker leg, support self with the arms, and follow through with the uninvolved leg. If patient is unable to bear weight on one leg, after advancing walker, have the patient swing onto it, supporting weight on hands. | |

## CANE WALKING

Canes are light weight, easily movable devices that are made of wood or metal. They provide less support than a walker and are less stable.

A person's cane length is equal to the distance between the greater trochanter and the floor (56 – 97 cm).

### TYPES OF CANES

1. Single-ended canes with half-circle handles:
   Recommended for patients requiring minimal support and those who will be using stairs frequently **(**Figure 9.8 (b)i).
2. Single-ended canes with straight handles:
   Recommended for patient with hand weakness because the handgrip is easier to hold but not recommended for patients with poor balance (Figure 9.8 (b)ii).
3. Canes with three or four prongs: (Qwad cane)
   Provides a wide base of support and it is recommended for patients with poor balance (Figure 9.8 (b)iii).

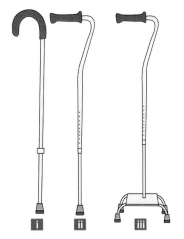

i. Single ended cane with half circle handles
ii. Single ended cane with straight handle
iii. Qwad cane

**Figure 9.8(b):** Types of canes

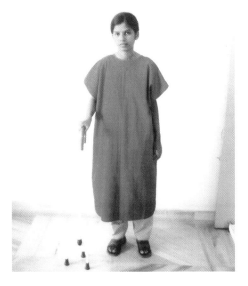

**Figure 9.8(c):** Positioning with cane

## PROCEDURE

| | Nursing action | Rationale |
|---|---|---|
| 1 | Instruct patient to stand with weight, evenly distributed between the feet and the cane. | |
| 2 | The cane is held on the patient's stronger side. Instruct patient to position cane 6″ laterally and 6″ anterior of the near foot. Ensure that flexion of elbow joint is maintained at 30 degree (Figure 9.8(c)). | Helps in improving stability. |
| 3 | Instruct the patient to advance the cane 4-12 inches while supporting the weight on the stronger leg. | |
| 4 | Supporting weight on the stronger leg and the cane, the patient advances the weaker foot forward, parallel with the cane | Helps in improving stability. |

*Contd...*

*Contd...*

| | | |
|---|---|---|
| 5 | Supporting weight on the weaker leg and the cane, the patient next advances the stronger leg forward ahead of the cane. | Helps in improving stability. |
| 6 | The weaker leg is moved forward until even with the stronger leg, and the cane is once again advanced. | |
| 7 | Instruct patient to position their canes with-in easy reach, when they sit down, so that they can rise easily. | |
| 8 | Teach patients to stand erect when walking with a cane and not lean over the cane. | |

## SPECIAL CONSIDERATIONS

1  The patient should be taught to examine the frame daily when inspecting a walker .The patient should observe for signs of bending or deformation of the frame, protruding screws that can scratch and loose or missing screws that can weaken the joints of the frame. Handgrips should be assessed for any cracks or signs of being loose.

2. Use caution when attempting to ambulate a patient who has already been given an antihypertensive or analgesic medication because the medication may cause dizziness or instability.

3. Caution should be used if the patient uses a walker on uneven terrain or on inclines.

4. Care must be taken if the patient has IV line, urinary catheter, etc.

When patient is ambulating with or without assistive device emphasize need to always look ahead to prevent injuries and maintain a good posture.

# 9.9: ASSISTING WITH CRUTCH WALKING

## DEFINITION

Assisting patient to walk using crutches while providing support and balance and as a convenient method of getting from one place to another.

## PREPARATORY EXERCISES

### QUADRICEPS SETTING

Instruct patient to contract quadriceps muscles while attempting to push popliteal area against mattress and simultaneously raising heel. Contract for a count of 5 and relax for next count of 5.

### GLUTEAL SETTING

Instruct patient to contract buttocks for a count of 5 and relax for a count of 5.

### SIT-UPS

While in sitting position, instruct patient to raise body from chair by pushing hands against chairseat or bed.

### PUSH-UPS

Instruct patient to push self up from prone position.

### PULL-UPS

Instruct patient to lift self up with help of trapeze.

### TYPES OF CRUTCHES

1. The axillary crutch: The axillary cructh is frequently used by patients of all ages on a short-term basis.
2. The Lofstrand crutch: It has a handgrip and a metal band that fits around the patient's forearm. Both the metal band and the hand grip are adjusted to fit the patient's height. This crutch is useful for patients with permanent disability.

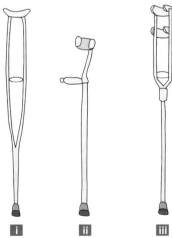

i.   Axillary crutch
ii.  Lofstrand crutch
iii. Platform/elbow extensor crutch

**Figure 9.9(a):** Types of crutches

3. The platform crutch: It is used by patients who are unable to bear weight on their wrists. It has a horizontal trough on which the patient can rest their forearms and wrists and a vertical handle for the patient to grip.

## PROCEDURE

| | Nursing action | Rationale |
|---|---|---|
| 1 | Review patient's chart:<br>a. Patient's medical history.<br><br>b. Patient's previous activity level.<br><br>c. Current activity order | Identifies factors that influence the patient's ambulation activity.<br>Identifies patient's previous activity level. Patient may tire easily or may be prone to orthostatic hypotension<br>Verifies if an ambulation aid is needed along with specifying the amount of activity permitted. |
| 2 | Assess patient's physical readiness:<br>a. Vital signs and orientation to time, place and person. | Ambulation following immobility can be fatiguing and stressful. An oriented patient is able to understand instructions. |
| 3 | Assess patient for any visual, perceptual or sensory deficits. | Determines if patient can use assistive device safely. Ambulation after immobility can be fatiguing and stressful. |
| 4 | Explain reasons for exercise and demostrate specific gait technique to patient or caregiver. | Teaching and demonstration enhances learning, reduces anxiety and encourages co-operation. |
| 5 | Schedule ambulation around patient's other activities. | Schedule time between activities so that patient does not become too fatigued. |
| 6 | Place bed in low position and slowly assist patient to upright position. Let patient sit or stand for a few minutes until balance is gained. | Prevents orthostatic hypotension and potential injuries. |
| 7 | If ambulation device is used, make sure it is of appropriate height.<br>a. Crutch measurement includes three areas: Patient's height, distance between crutchpad and axilla and angle of elbow flexion. Use one of two methods: | Promotes optimal support and stability.<br>Radial nerve passes under axillary area superficially. If crutch is too long, it can cause pressure on axilla. Injury to nerve causes paralysis of elbow and wrist extensors commonly called as crutch palsy. Also if |

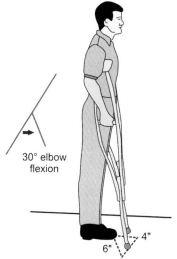

30° elbow flexion

4"

6"

**Figure 9.9(b):** Standing position with crutches

*Contd...*

*Contd...*

Standing: position crutches with crutch tips at a point 4-6 inches (14-15 cm) to side and 4-6 inches in front of patient's feet and crutchpads 1 ½-2 inches (4-5 cm) below axilla. Crutch pads should be 3-4 fingers width under axilla. with crutch tips positioned 6 inches (15 cm) lateral to patient's heel (Figure 9.9(b)).

b. With either method, elbows should be flexed 15-30 degrees. Elbow flexion is verified with goniometer.

crutch is too long, shoulders are forced upward and patient cannot push body, off the ground. If ambulation device is too short, patient will bent over and will be uncomfortable.

-Instruct patient to report any tingling or numbness in the upper torso. This may mean that crutches are being used incorrectly or they are of wrong size.

-For following correct crutch adjustment, two or three fingers should fit between top of crutch and axilla. If handgrip is too low, radial nerve can be damaged. If handpiece is too high, patient's elbow is sharply flexed and strength and stability of arms are decreased.

---

8  Assist patient in crutch walking by choosing appropriate gait.

To use crutches, patient supports self with hands and arms. Therefore strength in arm and shoulder muscles and ability to balance body in upright position and stamina are necessary. Type of gait patient uses in crutch walking depends on amount of weight patient is able to support with one or both legs.

a. **Four point gait:** This is the most stable of crutch gaits because it provides at least three points of support at all times. Requires weight bearing on both legs.

Improves patient's balance by providing wider base of support. Posture should be erect, head and neck should be straight, vertebrae straight and hips and knees extended.

• Begin in tripod position. Crutches are placed 6 inches in front and 6 inches to side of each foot (Figure 9.9(c))

Crutch and foot position are similar to arm and foot position during normal walking.

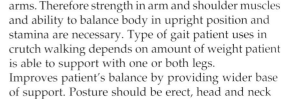

**Figure 9.9(c):** Tripod position

• Move right crutch forward 4-6 inches.
• Move left foot forward level to left crutch
• Move left crutch forward 4-6 inches.
• Move right foot forward to level of right crutch (Figure 9.9 (d))
• Repeat above sequence.

*Contd...*

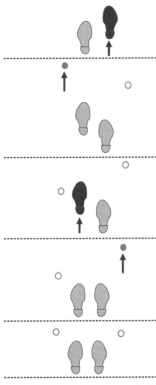

**Figure 9.9(d):** Four point gait—alternating gait. Shaded feet and crutch tips show foot and crutch tip moved in each of the four phases

b. **Three-point gait:** Requires patient to bear all weight on one foot. Weight is borne on uninvolved leg, then on both crutches.
   Affected leg does not touch ground during early phase of three point gait. May be useful for patient with broken leg or sprained ankles
   • Begin in tripod position
   • Advance both crutches and affected leg (Figure 9.9(e)).

Improves patients balance by providing wide base of support.

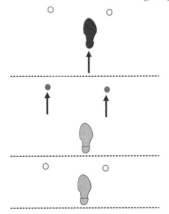

**Figure 9.9(e):** Three point gait: Weight borne on unaffected leg. Shaded foot and crutch tips show weight bearing in each phase

- Move stronger leg forward.
- Repeat sequence.

c. **Two-point gait:** (Figure 9.9(f))

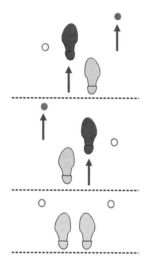

**Figure 9.9(f):** Two point gait: Weight borne partially on each foot and each crutch, advancing with opposing leg. Shaded areas show leg and crutch tip bearing weight.

Requires at least partial weight bearing on each foot.
Is faster than the four point gait. Requires more balance because only twopoints support body at one time.

- Begin in tripod position
- Move left crutch and right foot forward.
- Move right crutch and left foot forward.
- Repeat sequences.

d. **Swing to gait:** Frequently used by patients whose lower extremities are paralysed or who wear weight supporting braces on their legs

1. Move both crutches forward.
- Lift and swing leg to crutches, letting crutches support body weight.
- Repeat two previous steps.

e. **Swing-through gait:** Requires that patient have the ability to sustain partial weight bearing on both feet.
- Move both crutches forward
- Lift and swing legs through and beyond crutches.

Improves patients balance by providing wider base of support.
Crutch movements are similar to arm movement during normal walking.

Initial placement of crutches is to increase the patient's base of support so that when the body swings forward.The patient is moving the center of gravity toward the additional support provided by the crutches.

---

9   Assist patient in climbing stairs with crutches: (Figure 9.9(g))

a. Begin a tripod position

b. Patient transfers bodyweight to crutches.

c. Patient advances unaffected leg to stair.

d. Then advance affected leg and crutches
e. Repeat sequence until patient reaches top of stairs.

Improves patient balance by providing wider base of support.
Prepares patient to transfer weight to unaffected leg when ascending first stair.
Crutches adds support to affected leg. Patient then shifts weight from crutches to unaffected leg.
Maintains balance and provides wide base of support.

*Contd...*

*Contd...*

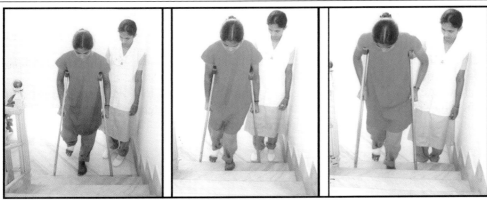

**Figure 9.9(g):** Ascending stairs with crutches

10  Assist patient in descending stairs with crutches: (Figure 9.9(h))

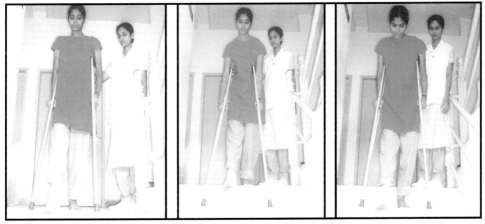

**Figure 9.9(h):** Descending stairs with crutches

| | |
|---|---|
| a. Begin in tripod position | Prepares patient to release support of body weight maintained by crutches. |
| b. Patient transfers body weight to unaffected leg. | Maintains patient's balance and base of support. |
| c. Move crutches to stairs and instruct patient to begin to transfer body weight to crutches and move affected leg forward. | |
| d. Patient moves unaffected leg to stair and align with crutches. | Maintains patient's balance and provides base of support. |
| e. Repeat sequence until stairs are descended. | |
| 11  Record in nurse's progress notes- type of gait patient used, amount of assistance required, distance walked and patient's tolerance of activity. | Documents technique used and patient's progress while using technique. |

## FOLLOW-UP ACTIVITIES

1. Inspect rubber tips on bottom of ambulation device frequently.
2. If wooden crutch is used, examine it for cracks.
3. Remove obstacles from pathways, including throw rigs, and wipe up any spills immediately.
4. Avoid large crowds.
5. Instruct patient to continue muscle strengthening exercise at home.

## TEACHING STRATEGIES

- Teach patient with axillary crutches about the dangers of pressure on the axillae, which occurs when leaning on the crutches to support body weight.
- Instruct patient to routinely inspect crutch tips.
  Rubber tips should be securely attached to the crutches. When tips are worn, they should be replaced. Rubber crutch tips increase surface friction and help prevent slipping.
- Explain that cructh tips should remain dry. Water decreases surface friction and increases the risk of slipping.
- Show patient how to inspect the structure of the crutches. Cracks in a wooden crutch decrease its ability to support weight. Bends in aluminium crutches can alter body alignment.

# Chapter 10

# Skin Integrity and Wound Care

# 10.1: PERFORMING A WOUND DRESSING

## DEFINITION

Cleansing a wound or incision and applying sterile protective covering using aseptic technique.

## PURPOSES

1. To protect the wound from contamination with microorganisms.
2. To promote wound granulation and healing.
3. To support or splint the wound site.
4. To promote thermal insulation to the wound surface.
5. To provide for maintenance of high humidity between the wound and dressing.
6. To promote physical, psychological and aesthetic comfort.

## ARTICLES

### STERILE DRESSING TRAY CONTAINING

- i. Artery forceps-1 (2, for extensive or infected wounds.).
- ii. Thumb forceps - 1
- iii. Cotton swabs.
- iv. Gauze pieces.
- v. Gallipot for cleansing solution.
- vi. Surgical pads.
- vii. Kidney tray.
- viii. Sterile scissors.

### A CLEAN TRAY CONTAINING

- i. Clean gloves.
- ii. Sterile gloves.
- iii. Cleaning solution (Normal Saline).
- iv. Ordered medications.
- v. Adhesive plaster.
- vi. Bandage scissors.
- vii. Plastic bag.
- viii. Waterproof pad or mackintosh.
- ix. Culture tubes (optional).

* For Major wound dressing a larger dressing pack with additional articles may be required.

## PROCEDURE

| | Nursing action | Rationale |
|---|---|---|
| 1. | Identify the patient | |
| 2. | Inform patient of dressing change, explain procedure and have patient lie in bed. | Encourages patient co-operation. |
| 3. | Gather equipment and arrange at the bedside. | An organized approach will save time and energy. |
| 4. | Wash hands | Reduces spread of microorganisms. |

*Contd...*

# Skin Integrity and Wound Care

*Contd...*

| | | |
|---|---|---|
| 5. | Check physician's order for dressing change and any specific instruction. | Clarifies type of dressing. |
| 6. | Close door or curtains and place waterproof pad on bed beneath area of dressing. | Provides privacy and prevents soiling of linen. |
| 7. | Assist patient to comfortable position that provides easy access to wound area. | Provides for comfort. |
| 8. | Place opened, cuffed plastic bag near working area. | Reduces risk of contamination from soiled dressing and used cotton balls. |
| 9. | Loosen tapes on dressing (if tape is soiled, don clean gloves before loosening the tape) | Removal of tape is easier before wearing gloves. |
| 10. | Don clean disposable gloves and remove soiled dressings carefully from more clean to less clean area. (if dressing is adherent to the skin, moisten it by pouring small amount of normal saline.) Keep soiled side of dressing away from patient's view. | Protects nurse from contamination . Cautious removal of dressing is less painful for the patient. Moistened dressing is easier to remove. Reduces anxiety of patient. |
| 11. | Assess the amount, color and odor of drainage. | Helps for identifying the wound healing process. |
| 12 | Discard dressing in disposal bag. Pull off gloves inside out and discard in appropriate receptacle. | Prevents spread of microorganisms. |
| 13. | Using sterile technique, open sterile dressing tray and arrange supplies on work area. | Keeps supplies within easy reach and maintains sterility |
| 14. | Open cleaning solution and pour into the sterile gallipot/cup over the cotton balls. | |
| 15. | Don sterile gloves. | Maintains asepsis. |
| 16. | Pick up soaked cotton using artery forceps. | |
| 17. i. | For a surgical wound, clean from top to bottom or from center outward (Figure 10.1(a)). In contaminated wound clean from periphery to center (circular motion for cleaning circular wound) | Moving from least to most contaminated area prevents spread of microorganisms to less infected area. |

Figure10.1 (a): Methods of cleansing a wound site

ii. Use one cotton swab/gauze sponge for each wipe, discarding each by dropping into the plastic bag after wiping. Do not touch the plastic bag with forceps.
iii. If a drain is present, clean around it, moving from center outward in a circular motion.

*Contd...*

*Contd...*

| | |
|---|---|
| iv. Dry the wound using sponge in same motion | Moisture provides medium for growth of microorganisms and drying the wound may retard the growth of organisms and improve healing process. |
| 18. Apply medication ordered (ointment) to the wound on a dry sterile gauze. Apply a layer of sterile dressing over wound. | Additional dressing serves as a wick for drainage. |
| 19. Place a sterile gauze slit on side under and around the drain (use precut gauze or cut one using sterile scissors). | Drainage is absorbed and surrounding skin area is protected. |
| 20. Apply a second layer of gauze to wound site and a surgical pad as the outer most layer. | Provides for absorption of wound drainage and protection from microorganisms. |
| 21. Remove gloves from inside out and discard in plastic waste bag. Apply adhesive tape to secure the dressing (Figure10.1(b and c)). | Tape is easier to apply after gloves have been removed. |

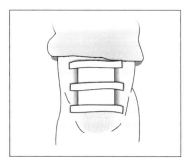

**Figure 10.1(b):** Strips of tape placed at the ends of dressing

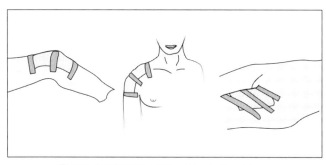

**Figure 10.1(c):** Dressing over moving parts

| | |
|---|---|
| 22. Wash reusable articles to be sent for sterilization. | |
| 23. Wash hands, remove all articles and make patient comfortable. | Prevents spread of infection. |
| 24. Record dressing change, appearance of wound and describe any drainage in the chart. | Provides accurate documentation of procedure. |

# 10: 2: DRESSING A BURNS WOUND

## DEFINITION

Cleaning a burns wound with normal saline using aseptic technique for removal of exudates and applying anti-bacterial agent.

## PURPOSES

1. To enhance wound healing
2. To reduce pain
3. To prevent complications
4. To perform wound debridement.

## ARTICLES

Dressing trolley with
1. Dressing pack
2. Sterile bandages in a bin
3. Sterile dressing pads in a bin
4. Sterile vaseline gauze
5. Silver sulpha diazene 1%
6. Sterile normal saline
7. Cheatle forceps
8. Adhesive tape and scissors
9. Sterile scissors
10. Sterile sheets
11. Receptacle for waste.

## TYPES OF WOUND DRESSING

1. Open dressing
2. Closed dressing.

### OPEN METHOD

The antimicrobial cream is applied with a gloved hand and the wound is left open to the air without gauze dressing. The cream is reapplied as needed.

*Advantages*

a. Increased visibility of the wound
b. Freedom for joint mobility.

*Disadvantages*

Increased chance of hypothermia.

### CLOSED METHOD

In closed method, gauze dressing is impregnated with antimicrobial cream and applied to the wound.

*Advantages*

a. Decrease in evaporative fluid and heat loss from wound surface.
b. Gauze dressing aids in debridement.

*Disadvantages*

a. Mobility limitations
b. Wound assessment is limited.

## PROCEDURE

| | Nursing action | Rationale |
|---|---|---|
| 1 | Explain procedure to patient | Helps in obtaining co-operation of patient. |
| 2 | Instruct patient to have a shower bath | Dressings that adhere to burns wound can be removed comfortably when it is moistened. |
| 3 | Administer analgesics about 20 minutes before procedure as per physician's instructions. | Minimizes pain during dressing. |
| 4 | Provide privacy and give psychological support to patient. | Prevents embarassment to the patient. |
| 5 | Regulate temperature of the room at 24 degree centigrade (80 degree fahrenheit) and humidity at 40–50% if possible. | Portable humidifiers can be used to obtain optimal humidity. |
| 6 | Put on mask and cap | |
| 7 | Scrub hands and don sterile gown, gloves and goggles if available | Prevents transmission of microorganisms. |
| 8 | Clean and debride the wound using sterile scissors and forceps. Trim loose eschar and separate devitalized skin. | Removes debris, any remaining topical agent, exudates and dead skin. Increases viability and vascularity of wound. |
| 9 | Inspect wound and surrounding area. | |
| 10 | Apply topical medications over the wound. | |
| 11 | If closed method is used for dressing, cover the wound with vaseline gauze and place sterile dressing pad. | |
| 12 | Apply bandage over the dressing pad | |
| 13 | Wash reusable articles to be sent for autoclaving. | Autoclaving destroys microorganisms and spores. |
| 14 | Discard gloves and gown and wash hands. | |
| 15 | Record procedure and note the odour, color, size, amount of exudate, signs of epithelialization and any change from previous dressing | Gives information about the patient's response and wound healing. |

## TOPICAL ANTIMICROBIAL AGENTS FOR BURNS

1. Silver sulfadizane 1%.
2. Mefenide acetate 10% cream or 5% solution.
3. Silvernitrate 0.5% solution.
4. Povidone Iodine 1%.

# Skin Integrity and Wound Care

Table 10.2.1: Antimicrobial agents used in burns

| Topical agent | Description and indications | Disadvantages | Nursing Implications |
|---|---|---|---|
| 1. Silver sulphadiazine 1% | A white crystalline, highly insoluble opaque, odorless water-soluble cream. Exerts antimicrobial effect at level of cell membrane and cell wall against gram-negative and gram-positive bacteria and yeast | May increase possibility of kernicterus. Not to be used in pregnant women in last trimster<br>- Exposure to sunlight produces gray discoloration<br>- Transient leukopenia disappears after 2-3 days | - use with either open treatment, light or occlusive dressings<br>- apply with sterile gloved hand directly to wound or applied to gauze dressing 0.16 cm thickness of once or twice daily after thorough wound cleansing<br>- Silver sulphadiazine will be discontinued if WBCs are less than 1500 in an adult or less than 2000 in a child. WBC count usually recovers in 2-4 days and application may be resumed. |
| 2. Mafenide acetate 10% cream | Usually supplied in water miscible hydroscopic cream base | Painful during and for a while after application | Cream is applied with or without dressing. If possible, must be reapplied every 12 hours for therapeutic effectiveness |
| | Active against most gram-positive organisms | A potent carbonic anhydrase inhibitase resulting in metabolic acidodsis therefore not used in 20% total burns surface area or more. | |
| | Active against common gram-negative organisms which infect burn wound but has less fungal activity | Brisk alkaline diuresis and polyuria may result when used in patient with large burn surface area | Therapeutic solution concentration is maintained with bulky wet dressing. Rewet every 2-4 hours. Hypersensitivity is evidenced by maculopapular rash and treated with histamine or by discontinuing use. |
| | Haemolytic anemia is a rare complication | | Require careful monitoring of pulmonary status and acid–base fluid balance. |
| 3. Silver nirate 0.5% solution | Clear solution with low toxicity and significant antimicrobial effect against common burn wound pathogens.<br>Non-allergic and not usually painful on application.<br><br>Best use us prophylaxis against infection. | Can cause elctrolyte abnormalities depleting serum sodium, chloride, potassium and magnesium<br><br>Stains normal skin brown or black | Monitor electolyte balance carefully, supplementation with potassium and sodium salt is routinely needed for patients with extensive burns. Use bulky dressings, rewet every 2-4 hours to maintaion therapeutic concentration. Maintains patient warm and minimizes transient evaporative water loss with dry top layer such as stockinette or bath blanket. |

## 10.3: REMOVAL OF SUTURES AND STAPLES

**Sutures** are threads used to sew body tissues together.

Sutures used to attach tissues beneath the skin are often made of an absorbable material that disappears in several days.

Skin sutures are made of a variety of nonabsorbable materials such as silk, cotton, linen, wire, nylon and dacron. Staples are also available.

**Staples**——are a type of outer skin closure that causes less trauma to tissues than sutures and provide extra strength.

## TYPES OF SUTURING TECHNIQUES/METHODS

1. Plain interrupted
2. Mattress interrupted
3. Plain continuous
4. Mattress continuous
5. Retention sutures.

## ARTICLES

A Tray containing:
1. Suture removal kit (sterile)
   a. Sterile scissors/staple remover as indicated.
   b. Sterile forceps
   c. Antiseptic swab packets.
2. Gauze pieces
3. Clean gloves (1 pair)
4. Sterile gloves (1 pair)
5. Disinfectant- Surgical spirit and povidone iodine.
6. Kidney tray.

## PROCEDURE

| | Nursing action | Rationale |
|---|---|---|
| 1 | Explain procedure to patient and describe the sensations that will be experienced such as a pulling or slightly uncomfortable experience. | Helps in obtaining cooperation of patient. |
| 2 | Use sterile techniques. | Prevents spread of infection |
| 3 | Check for physician's order. | Acts as a guideline for suture removal. |
| 4 | Arrange all needed equipments at bedside. | Saves time, energy and effort |
| 5 | Provide privacy. | Prevents embarrassment |
| 6 | Wash hands. | Prevents risk of transmission of micro organisms. |
| 7 | Position the patient so that the dressing or incision is exposed. | |
| 8 | Open sterile suture removal kit. Prepare a sterile field and place supplies on it. | Ensures aspectic technqiue |
| 9 | Don clean gloves. | |
| 10 | Remove and discard any dressing covering the wound. | Removes potentially contaminated materials. |
| 11 | Inspect the wound for signs of dehiscence and infection. | |

*Contd...*

*Contd...*

| | | |
|---|---|---|
| 12 | Wash hands, don sterile gloves. | Prevents infection. |
| 13 | Clean sutures with spirit swabs moving from proximal to distal end. Discard swabs after wiping each surface once. | Cleaning and antiseptic action of alcohol removes surface microorganisms from the wound site. |
| 14 | Removal of plain interrupted sutures:<br>a. Place dry sterile gauze near the wound.<br>b. Grasp the suture at the knot with a pair of forceps.<br>c. Place the curved tip of the suture scissors under the suture. as close to the skin as possible, either on the side opposite the knot or directly under the knot and cut the suture. Sutures are cut as close to the skin as possible on one side of the visible part (Figure 10.3(a)). | Suture material that is visible to the eye is in contact with resident bacteria of skin and must not be pulled beneath the skin during removal. Suture material that is beneath the skin is considered free from bacteria. |

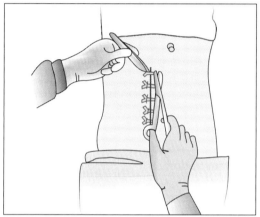

**Figure 10.3 (a):** Removing sutures

| | | |
|---|---|---|
| | d. With the forceps, pull the suture out in one piece. Inspect the suture carefully to make sure that all suture materials are removed. | Suture material left beneath the skin acts as a foreign body and causes inflammation. |
| 15 | Apply steri strips on the wound or clean with betadine after removing sutures as orderded by physician. | Steri strips hold the incision edges together and promote supports in healing of the wound. |
| 16 | Instruct the client about follow-up if wound discharge appears. | |
| 17 | Place dressing over the incision if ordered. | Provides a protective covering. |
| 18 | Reposition the client, wash and replace articles. | Gives neat appearance of the work area. |
| 19 | Wash hands | Prevents spread of infection |
| 20 | Document the number of sutures removed, the condition of the incision, evidence of dehiscence or infection and time of the procedure. | Acts as a communication between staff members. |

## SPECIFIC INSTRUCTIONS FOR STAPLE REMOVAL

1. As directed on the package, gently position the sterile staple remover under the staple to be removed (Figure 10.3 (b)).

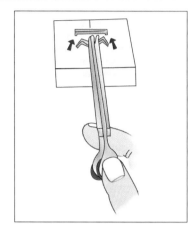

**Figure 10.3(b):** Removing staples

2. Firmly close the staple remover to straighten the staple ends (do not lift upward while disengaging staple ends).
3. Carefully lift the clips upward with the closed staple remover to remove them from the incision line. It may be necessary to remove one end of the staple and then the other if it does not easily lift out.

## SPECIAL CONSIDERATIONS

1. Abdominal belts or many tailed bandages may be applied on the abdomen after removal of abdominal sutures in obese patients to prevent wound dehiscence and evisceration.
2. Patient should be instructed not to strain the part, e.g. not to cough or lift heavy weights in case of abdominal sutures.

# 10.4: PERFORMING A WOUND IRRIGATION

## DEFINITION

Flushing the wound with large amount of sterile fluid.

## PURPOSES

1. To clean the area from pathogens and debris
2. To apply local heat
3. To irrigate with antiseptic solution.

## ARTICLES

1. Irrigant/cleansing solution as ordered, usually 200-500 ml depending on the size of wound
2. Asepto syringe for large wound or 40 ml syringe with 19G needle or sterile soft angio-catheter
3. Clean gloves
4. Sterile gloves
5. Waterproof underpad
6. Dressing supplies
7. Disposable waterproof bag
8. Gown
9. Goggles
10. Sterile soft catheter
11. Sterile dressing set
12. Sterile basin.

## PROCEDURE

| | Nursing action | Rationale |
|---|---|---|
| 1 | Check physician's order for wound irrigation and type of solution to be used. | Physician's order clarifies procedure and type of supplies required. Open wound irrigation requires medical order including type of solutions to be used. |
| 2 | Explain procedure to patient | Explanation facilitates patient's cooperation. |
| 3 | Assess patient's level of pain. Administer prescribed analgesic 30-45 min before starting wound irrigation procedure. | Reduces pain and permits patient to tolerate the procedure better. |
| 4 | Assess recent recording of signs and symptoms related to patient's open wound<br>a. Condition of skin and wound<br>b. Elevation of body temperature<br>c. Drainage from wound<br>d. Odour<br>e. Consistency of drainage<br>f. Size of wound including depth, length and width | Data are used as base line to identify change in condition of wound<br><br>May indicate response to infection<br>Amount will decrease as healing takes place<br>Strong odour indicates infection process<br>Leucocytes produce thick drainage.<br>Determines stage of healing |
| 5 | Perform handwashing | Reduces transmission of microorganisms |
| 6 | Position patient comfortably to permit gravitational flow of irrigating solution through wound and into collection receptacle. | Gravity directs flow of fluid from least contaminated to more contaminated area. Waterproof pad protects patient and bed linen |
| 7 | Warm irrigation solution to approximate body temperature. | Warm solution increases comfort and reduces vaso constriction response in tissues. |

*Contd...*

*Contd...*

| | | |
|---|---|---|
| 8 | Form a cuff of waterproof bag and place it near bed. | Cuffing helps to maintain large opening, thereby permitting placement of contaminated dressing without touching refuse bag itself. |
| 9 | Close room door and pull curtains. | Maintains privacy. |
| 10 | Apply gown and goggles if needed. | Protects nurse from, splashes or sprays of blood and body fluids. |
| 11 | Put on clean gloves and remove soiled dressings and discard in waterproof bag. Discard gloves. | Reduces transmission of microorganisms. |
| 12 | Open sterile dressings and supplies on work area using aseptic technique. | Supplies are within easy reach and sterility is maintained. |
| 13 | Put on sterile gloves. | Maintains surgical asepsis |
| 14 | Position the sterile basin below the wound to collect irrigation fluid with dominant hand. | Irrigation is facilitated and patient and bed linen are protected from contaminated fluid. |
| 15 | Irrigate wound<br>a. Wound with wide opening:<br>• Fill 35 ml syringe with irrigation solution | irrigating wound helps remove debris and facilitates healing by secondary intention. |
| | • Attach 19 gauge needle or angio-catheter | Provides ideal pressure for cleansing and removal of debris. |
| | • Hold syringe tip 2.5 cm above upper end of wound and over area being cleansed (Figure 10.4 (a)). | Prevents syringe contamination. Careful placement of the syringe prevents unsafe pressure of the flowing solution. |
| | • Using continuous pressure, flush wound; repeat steps until solution draining into basin is clear. | Clear solution indicates that all debris has been removed. |

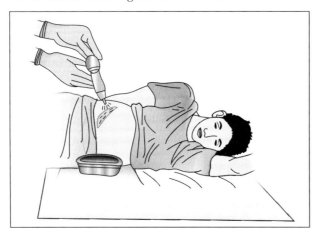

**Figure 10.4 (a):** Wound irrigation using asepto syringe

| | | |
|---|---|---|
| | b. Deep wound with very small opening<br>• Attach soft angio-catheter to filled irrigating syringe | Catheter permits direct flow of irrigant into wound. Expect wound to take longer time to empty when opening is small. |
| | • Lubricate tip of catheter with irrigating solution then gently insert tip of catheter and pull out about 1cm (1/2 inch). | Helps in easy entry of catheter.<br>Removes tip from fragile inner wall of wound |
| | • Use slow continuous pressure to flush wound. | |

*Contd...*

*Contd...*

| | | |
|---|---|---|
| | • Pinch off catheter just below Syringe while keeping catheter in place. <br> • Remove and refill syringe. Reconnect to catheter and repeat until solution draining into basin is clear. | Avoids contamination of sterile solution. |
| 16 | Dry wound edges with gauze. | Prevents maceration of surrounding tissues caused by excess moisture. |
| 17 | Apply appropriate dressing. | Maintains protective barrier and healing environment for wound. |
| 18 | Remove gloves, mask, goggles and gown. | Prevents transfer of microorganisms. |
| 19 | Dispose of soiled equipment and soiled supplies. Perform handwashing. | Reduces transmission of microorganisms. |
| 20 | Assist patient to comfortable position. | |
| 21 | Assess type of tissue in the wound bed. | Identifies wound healing progress and determines type of wound cleansing needed. |
| 22 | Inspect dressing periodically | Determines patient's response to wound irrigation and need to modify plan of care. |
| 23 | Evaluate skin integrity | Determines if extension of wound has occurred |
| 24 | Observe for presence of retained irrigant | Retained irrigant is a medium for bacterial growth and subsequent infection. |
| 25 | Record wound irrigation and patient responses in progress notes. | |
| 26 | Report any evidence of fresh bleeding, sharp increase in pain, retension of irrigant or signs of shock to physician. | |

## SPECIAL CONSIDERATIONS

1. Consider culturing a wound if it has foul odour, inflammation surrounding the wound, purulent drainage from wound or fever.
2. If insertion of packing is ordered
   a. Use sterile forceps to insert sterile packing into wound gently.
   b. Be careful not to pack wound excessively because this may impede blood flow and delay healing.
   c. Cut packing material with sterile scissors.
   d. Allow a small strip of packing to protrude from small and deep wounds to facilitate removal.
3. The wound may be anesthetized first if the patient cannot tolerate the wound irrigation and cleansing
4. A catheter tip syringe may be used to create a hydraulic action.
5. Devitalized tissue and foreign matter are removed. Devitalized tissue inhibits wound healing and enhances chances of bacterial infection.
6. Obtain culture if needed after cleansing with non-bacteriostatic saline.

# Chapter 11

# Advanced Clinical Procedures

# 11.1: RECORDING AN ELECTROCARDIOGRAM

## DEFINITION

Electrocardiogram is a graphical recording of electrical activity of the heart detected by means of surface electrodes and measured by using a galvanometer.

## PURPOSES

1. To assess the cardiac function (rate, rhythm and conduction).
2. To diagnose cardiac rhythm disorders (e.g. heart block, dysrhythmias).
3. To diagnose cardiac diseases (e.g. myocardial infarction)
4. To detect electrolyte imbalance (e.g. hyperkalemia, hypokalemia, etc).
5. To evaluate effects of treatment (e.g. administration of cardiac drugs).

## ARTICLES

1. ECG machine.
2. Electrodes for 12 lead ECG.
3. Electroconductive gel.
4. Front open gown or shirt for patient.
5. Tissue paper.

## PROCEDURE

|  | Nursing action | Rationale |
|---|---|---|
| 1 | Explain the purpose of ECG and procedure to the patient. Reassure patient that procedure is painless and safe. | Helps to gain patient's co-operation and reduces anxiety regarding procedure. |
| 2 | Ask female patients to remove all tight fitting clothing around the chest. Assist patient to put on a front open loose gown or shirt. | Procedure requires placement of electrodes over chest area. |
| 3 | Ensure that the ECG machine is in functioning order. | |
| 4 | Ensure proper standardization of machine<br>a. Set paper speed at 25 mm/min.<br>b. Provide standard 1 mv signal to ECG machine so that the spike made will be 10 mm or 2 large squares in height.<br>c. Ensure that the machine is properly earthed. | Proper standardization of machine ensures a precise recording of ECG. |
| 5 | Ask the patient to lie in supine position and be as relaxed as possible.<br>If the patient needs to be transported to the ECG department, transport him on a trolley. Never allow him to walk till diagnosis is confirmed. | Rigid posture and contraction of muscles may result in artifacts on ECG record. |
| 6 | Provide privacy by pulling the curtains around the patient. | Procedure requires exposing chest area, which is embarrassing for the patient. |
| 7 | Expose chest completely. Apply electroconductive gel on lead placement sites and position all electrodes appropriately.<br>a. Check for color codes of limb leads and connect limb electrodes to all four extremities as per the manufacturer's code. | |

*Contd...*

*Contd...*

b.  Place suction electrodes at appropriate sites (Figure 11.1(a)).
    V1——4th intercostal space on the right side, parasternal)
    V2——4th intercostal space on the left side, parasternal
    V3——midway between V2 and V4
    V4——5th intercostal space on left side in the mid clavicular line.
    V5——5th intercostal space on left side in the anterior axillary line.
    V6——5th intercostal space on left side in the mid axillary line.

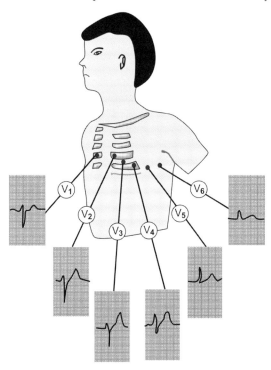

**Figure 11.1(a):** Sites for chest lead placement

c.  Ensure proper contact between the lead and skin. Shaving of the chest may be required in case of male patient's | Proper contact between skin and electrodoes and proper placement of electrodes are very essential for obtaining a good recording.

---

8  Instruct the patient that you are going to start the recording and he/she should lie still in the bed without moving till the recording is complete, which may take 5-10 minutes. | Patient movement during recording causes artifacts on ECG record.

---

9  Record the ECG:
a.  Manual recording:
    i.   Record limb leads (I, II, III, AVR, AVL, AVF) by advancing the machine settings to the respective leads.
    ii.  To record chest leads (V1-V6) advance the suction in electrode to next position after recording each lead. (ensure that machine is set for chest lead recording).
    iii. Record long lead II.

*Contd...*

*Contd...*

| | | |
|---|---|---|
| | b. Automatic recording:<br> i. Place limb as well as all chest electrodes in position and ask for autorecording. | |
| 10 | Check the ECG record for appropriateness and presence of artifacts if any. | In case of inappropriate recording or presence of artifacts, recording needs to be repeated. |
| 11 | Inform patient that ECG recording is completed. | |
| 12 | Remove electrodes from all four limbs and chest. Wipe off the electroconductive gel using tissue papers. Assist patient in dressing. | |
| 13 | Wipe off the electroconductive gel from electrodes. | After drying, the gel forms a crust over the electrodes which may interfere with future recording. |
| 14 | Label the ECG:<br> i. Write patient's full name, inpatient/out patient number, date and time of recording.<br> ii. Record lead identification in case of manual records.<br> iii. A standard lead should be labelled and pasted on ECG card when manual records are obtained. | Provides accurate identification data. |
| 15 | Read and report ECG as follows:<br> i. Rhythm<br> ii. Conduction intervals<br> iii. Cardiac axis<br> iv. A discription of the QRS complexes.<br> v. A description of the ST segments and T waves. | Helps to identify obvious gross abnormalities. |
| 16 | Show ECG record to physician as soon as possible so that further treatment orders can be obtained if any. | |

## SPECIAL CONSIDERATIONS

Note that the following can cause poor ECG signal and or artifacts on an ECG record.
1. Oily, dirty and scaly skin.
2. Dirty or encrusted electrodes .
4. Improper application of electrodes.
5. Loose or dislodged electrodes.
6. Patient's movement
7. Muscle tremor
8. Broken cable wire.
9. Faulty grounding
10. Faulty articles.

# 11.2: ASSISTING WITH AN ARTERIAL PUNCTURE

## DEFINITION

Assisting for collection of blood sample from an artery by performing an arterial puncture.

## PURPOSES

1. For accurate assessment of acid-base status.
2. For assessing degree of oxygenation of blood and adequacy of alveolar ventilation
3. For starting continuous arterial blood pressure monitoring in an emergency.

## ARTICLES

1. 1 ml or 2 ml disposable syringe
2. Disposable needles size 20 gauge
3. Leur-Lock for syringe
4. Heparin 1:1000
5. Alcohol swab
6. Crushed ice in specimen bag
7. Disposable gloves and disposable probes
8. Arterial catheter for continuous pressure monitoring.
9. Waterproof pad.

## PROCEDURE

| | Nursing action | Rationale |
|---|---|---|
| 1. | Identify patient by asking name and explain procedure to patient. | Helps in obtaining cooperation. |
| 2. | Record patient's inspired oxygen concentration. | Degree of hypoxemia cannot be assessed without knowing the inspired oxygen concentration. |
| 3. | Check patient's temperature. | Hypothermia or hyperthermia influences oxygen release from hemoglobin. |
| 4. | Heparinize the 2 ml syringe <br> a. Withdraw heparin into syringe to wet the plunger and fill dead space in the needle <br> b. Hold syringe in an upright position and expel excess heparin and air bubbles | This action coats the interior of the syringe with heparin to prevent clotting. <br> Air remaining in the syringe may affect measurement of $PaO_2$. Heparin in the syringe may affect measurement of pH. |
| 5. | Wash hands, and don gloves. | Prevents infection |
| 6. | Palpate the radial, brachial or femoral artery. | The radial artery is the preferred site of puncture. Arterial puncture is performed in areas where good pulse is palpable. |
| 7. | If radial artery is selected for puncture, perform the Allen test <br><br> a. Obliterate the radial and ulnar pulses simultaneously by pressing on both blood vessels at the wrist. <br> b. Ask patient to clench and unclench fist until blanching of skin occurs. <br> c. Release pressure on ulnar artery (while still compressing radial artery) watch for return of skin color within 15 seconds. | The Allen test is a simple method for assessing collateral circulation in the hand. <br> Impedes arterial blood flow in the hand. <br><br> Forces blood from the hand. <br><br> Identifies that ulnar artery alone is capable of supplying blood to the hand while radial artery is occluded |

*Contd...*

*Contd...*

| | |
|---|---|
| Note: If the ulnar artery does not have sufficient blood supply to perfuse entire hand, the radial artery should not be used). | |
| d. Obliterate the radial and ulnar pulses simultaneously at the wrist | |
| e. Elevate patient's hand above heart and squeeze or compress hand until blanching occurs | |
| f. Lower patient's hand while still compressing the ulnar artery and watch for return of skin color. | Identifies that radial artery alone is capable of supplying blood to the hand while ulnar artery is occluded. |
| 8. For a radial puncture, place a small towel under the patient's wrist. | Makes the artery more accessible |
| 9. Place waterproof pad under forearms. | Protects the bed linen. |
| 10. Feel along the course of radial artery and palpate for maximum pulsation with the middle and index fingers. | The wrist should be stabilized to allow for better control of the needle. Prepare the skin with germicide. The skin and subcutaneous tissues may be infiltrated with a local anesthetic agent. Prevents entry of microorganisms. |
| 11. The needle is at a 45-60 degree angle to the skin surface and is advanced into the artery. Once the artery is punctured, arterial pressure will push up the piston of the syringe and a pulsating flow of blood will fill the syringe (Figure 11.2 (a)) | The arterial pressure will cause the syringe to be filled within few seconds. |

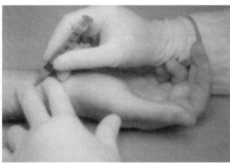

**Figure 11.2(a):** Puncturing radial artery

| | |
|---|---|
| 12 After blood is obtained withdraw needle and apply firm pressure over the puncture site with a dry sponge for 5 minutes (Figure 11.2(b)) | Significant bleeding can occur because of the pressure in the artery |

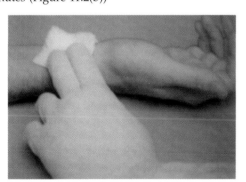

**Figure 11.2(b):** Applying pressure over puncture site

*Contd...*

*Contd...*

| | | |
|---|---|---|
| 13 | Remove air bubbles from syringe and needle. Insert needle into the rubber stopper placed on the flat surface. Do not hold the rubber stopper. | Immediate capping of needle prevents room air from mixing with blood specimen. Holding rubber stopper in one hand may lead to needle stick injury. |
| 14 | Place the capped syringe in the container of ice. | Icing the syringe will prevent false results. |
| 15 | Maintain firm pressure on the puncture site for 5 minutes. If the patient is on anticoagulant therapy apply direct pressure over puncture site for 10-15 minutes and then apply a firm pressure dressing. | Firm pressure on the puncture site prevents further bleeding and hematoma formation. |
| 16 | For patients requiring serial monitoring of arterial blood, an arterial catheter is attached to the radial or femoral artery. | All connections must be tight to avoid disconnection and rapid blood loss. The arterial line also allows for direct blood pressure monitoring in critically ill patients. |
| 17 | Send labelled, iced specimen to the laboratory immediately with duly filled request. | Blood gas analysis should be done as soon as possible because $PaO_2$ and pH can change rapidly. |
| 18 | Palpate the pulse (distal to the puncture site), inspect the puncture site and assess for reduced temperature, cold, numbness, tingling or discoloration. | Hematoma and arterial thrombosis are complications |
| 19 | Change ventilator settings, inspired oxygen concentration or type and setting of respiratory therapy equipment as indicated by the results. | The $PaO_2$ results will determine whether to maintain, increase or decrease the FiO2. The $PaO_2$ and pH results will dictate if any changes are needed in tidal volume or rate of patient's ventilator. |

## NORMAL VALUES

### pH

Normal: 7.35-7.45
Acidemia <7.35
Alkalemia >7.45

### $PaCO_2$

Normal:35-45 mmHg
Respiratory acidosis >45mmHg
Respiratory Alkalosis <35mmHg

### $HCO_3$

Normal: 22-26 mEq/L
Metabolic acidosis < 22 mEq/L
Metabolic alkalosis > 26 mEq/L

### $PaO_2$

Normal: 80-100 mmHg.
Oxygen saturation: 96-100%
Base excess: $\pm$ 2.0 mEq/L

# 11.3: PREPARATION OF AND ASSISTING FOR CARDIAC CATHETERIZATION

## DEFINITION

An invasive diagnostic procedures in which one or more catheters are introduced into heart and selected blood vessels, to measure pressures and to determine oxygen saturation in the various heart chambers.

## PURPOSES

1. To assess patency of coronary arteries
2. To decide on appropriate treatment, e.g. PTCA/CABG if atherosclerosis is present.
3. To measure pressures in various chambers of the heart
4. To obtain blood samples for measurement of hematocrit and oxygen saturation
5. To confirm diagnosis of heart disease and to determine the extent to which the disease has affected structure and function of heart.
6. To obtain clear picture of cardiac anatomy prior to heart surgery.
7. To determine cardiac output.
8. To obtain endocardial biopsies.
9. To allow infusion of fibrinolytic agents directly into the occluded coronary artery to restore coronary blood flow.
10. To detect shunts.

## RIGHT HEART CATHETERIZATION

Passing a radiopaque catheter from antecubital or femoral vein into the right atrium, right ventricle and pulmonary vasculature.

## LEFT HEART CATHETERIZATION

Insertion of a catheter into right brachial artery or femoral artery, ascending aorta and into left ventricle. It can also be performed trans-septally from right atrium into left atrium and then left ventricle.

## ARTICLES

1. Cardiac monitor
2. Pressure monitoring device
3. Fluoroscope
4. Sterile radiopaque cardiac catheters
5. Radiopaque dye
6. Sterile linen for draping
7. Cleaning solutions
8. Sterile gloves
9. Cardiac catheterization pack
10. Cut down set
11. Scalpel blade
12. Emergency articles
13. Sterile gown
14. Local anesthetic agent
15. Sterile syringes and needles.

## CONTRAINDICATIONS

1. Pregnancy because of radioactive iodine crossing the blood placental barrier
2. Cardiomyopathy

3. Severe dysrhythmias
4. Uncontrolled congestive heart failure
5. Patient allergic to local anesthesia, iodine or radiopaque contrast material
6. Bleeding disorders.

## PROCEDURE

| | Nursing action | Rationale |
|---|---|---|
| 1. | Assess patient's knowledge of procedure and explain procedure to patient. | Allays anxiety and ensures co-operation of patient. |
| 2. | Assess vital signs including peripheral pulses, heart and lung sounds and body weight. | Provides baseline data for comparison of findings during and after the procedure. |
| 3. | Determine whether right or left heart is being studied. | Enables nurse to anticipate patient teaching needs and post procedure interventions. |
| 4. | Assess whether patient has signed consent forms. | Both types of procedures usually require informed consent to reduce legal risk. |
| 5. | Assess time of last ingested fluid or food. Patient should be NPO for 6-8 hours before the procedure. | Prevents possible aspiration since patient is sedated for the procedure. Excessive hydration causes dilution of the contrast medium which makes structures more difficult to visualize. |
| 6. | Assess if patient is allergic to iodine dye. If so notify the cardiologist or radiologist | An iodine-based radiopaque contrast medium may be used during the procedure, however a hypo allergic contrast medium is more frequently used. |
| 7. | Assess blood count, platelets and prothrombin time, electrolytes, BUN, creatinine levels etc prior to the procedure. | Abnormal findings might contraindicate the procedure since hemorrhage or renal failure may occur. |
| 8. | Review physicians order for pre-procedural medication:<br>**a.** Atropine (contraindicated in glaucoma).<br><br>**b.** Benadryl<br>**c.** Sedative | <br>Decreases or prevents bradycardia, caused by vagal stimulation and decreases oral secretions<br>Prophylaxis against allergic reaction to dye.<br>Decreases anxiety and promotes relaxation |
| 9. | Mark distal pulses. | Enables easy reference after procedure |
| 10. | Instruct the patient to empty his/her bladder. | Ensures that patient will be comfortable during procedure. |
| 11. | Wash hands and prepare area as for surgical procedure. | Reduces transmission of microorganisms. |
| 12. | Don mask, goggles, sterile gown, cap and gloves. Drape patient with sterile drapes. | Protects nurse from risk of infection. Maintains surgical asepsis. |
| 13. | Assist in anesthetizing the skin overlying the arterial puncture site | Provides local anesthesia to areas of incision or puncture site. |
| 14 | Assist in performing needle puncture of artery, inserting guide wire through needle and threading angiographic catheter. Cardiologist advances catheter to desired artery or cardiac chamber and inject contrast medium. | Permits access to artery and prevents coiling of catheter in artery. Permits radiographic visualization of structure, aneurysms, occlusions or anomalies. |
| 15 | Explain to patient that he will experience a feeling of heat, flushing of face and a desire to cough during dye injection and X-ray films will be taken rapidly at this time. | Permits radiographic records of visualization of dye through artery as well as any abnormalities present. Reduces anxiety of patient. |

*Contd...*

*Contd...*

| 16 | Withdraw catheter after the entire procedure is over and apply pressure to puncture site for at least 10-20 minutes. Assess puncture site for hematoma formation at site and increase in pain/tenderness. | Provides data related to cardiac output, CVP, ventricular pressure and pulmonary artery pressure. Pressure on puncture site promotes clotting and prevents bleeding. |
|----|----|----|
| 17 | Apply pressure dressing over puncture site. | Prevents bleeding. |
| 18 | Monitor vital signs, apical and peripheral pulses, auscultate heart and lungs after cardiac catheterization every 15 minutes until stable and compare with baseline values | Verifies patient's physiologic status and evaluates effect of procedure on physiologic functions. |
| 19 | Assess patient for possible delayed reaction to iodine dye, like dyspnea, hives, tachycardia or rash. | Reaction may occur up to few hours after injection of dye. |
| 20 | Assess post procedure laboratory values such as blood count, prothrombin time, electrolytes, blood count and creatinine | Changes in laboratory values may indicate the onset of complications. |
| 21 | Instruct patient about strict bedrest for 12-24 hours and to keep affected extremity straight for 12 hours. | Prevents bleeding. |
| 22 | Encourage fluid intake | Promotes excretion of dye. |
| 23 | Record type of cardiac catheterization done and patient's tolerance of the procedure | Documents patients response to invasive procedure. |
| 24 | Record type of dressing, amount and type of drainage and presence of pain or discomfort | Provides baseline data for determining patients' progress. |

## SPECIAL CONSIDERATIONS

1. Check for symptoms like nausea, hypotension, bradycardia, etc. which indicate vagal stimulation.
2. Evaluate for signs and symptoms of myocardial infarction, also check for back pain or groin pain which may indicate retroperitoneal bleeding.

# 11: 4: PREPARATION OF AND ASSISTING FOR PACEMAKER IMPLANTATION

## DEFINITION

A pacemaker is an electronic device that provides repetitive electrical stimuli to heart muscles when the patient's intrinsic pacemaker fails to provide a perfusing rhythm.

## CLASSIFICATION OF PACEMAKERS

1. Temporary pacemaker (external pacemaker)
2. Permanent pacemaker (Internal pacemaker).

### TEMPORARY PACEMAKER

Pulse generators are outside the body and this is used for short-term therapy (Figure 11.4(a)).

Temporary pacemakers are used frequently during emergency situtations requiring immediate cardiac pacing.

Temporary pacing systems use batteries, which need replacement based on use of device. The transcutaneous system has rechargeable battery circuit.

### Classification of Temporary Pacemakers

a. Non-invasive pacing (Transcutaneous)
b. Transvenous invasive pacing (Endocardial) (Figure 11.4(b))
c. Transthoracic invasive pacing (Epicardial)

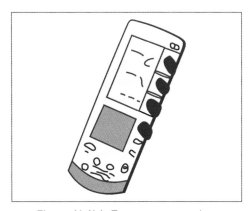

Figure 11.4(a): Temporary pacemaker

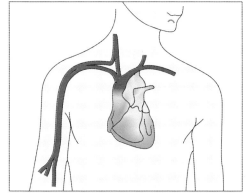

Figure 11.4(b):Temporary pacemaker lead placement

## INDICATIONS

1. Symptomatic bradydysrhythmias.
2. During diagnostic testing:
   Cardiac catheterization
   Electrophysiological studies
   Percutaneous transluminal coronary angioplasty.
3. Before permanent pacing
4. Postoperatively following major cardiac surgeries
5. Post myocardial infarction
6. Prophylaxis after open heart surgery
7. Suppression of ectopic activity.

# PROCEDURE

Temporary pacing is usually performed in cardiac catheterization laboratory.

| | Nursing action | Rationale |
|---|---|---|
| 1 | Explain procedure to patient and family Explain that there will be a sensation of discomfort with external pacing. | Allays anxiety and helps in cooperation of patient. Discomfort is felt with each firing, but can be relieved by analgesics. |
| 2 | Get informed consent for procedure. | Informed consent protects the health care personnel from legalities relating to procedure. |
| 3 | Remove jewellery, dentures and contact lens. | Jewellery will act as a source of infection and may be lost during procedure. Removing dentures prevents trauma to patient if any emergency occurs. |
| 4 | Shave area depending upon the site selected. | Reduces risk of infection caused by microorganisms settling in hair follicles. |
| 5 | Provide clean gown. | Prevents unnecessary exposure. |
| 6 | Start good IV access with heparin lock. | Ensures a patent IV line to administer fluids and medications. |
| 7 | Record ECG before procedure and obtain a rhythm strip | Helps in comparison after procedure. |
| 8 | Administer premedication and send patient to cardiac catheterization lab with patient's chart, X-ray films, lab forms, ECG strip and other items depending upon agency policy. | Gives information about patient's baseline data. |
| 9 | Reassure the patient during procedure | Provides psychological support. |
| 10 | When the pacing catheter is in vein, alligator clips can be used to connect the exposed tip of the catheter to an ECG machine. Larger P waves are seen as the catheter passes through the atrium and larger QRS complexes when catheter is in ventricles. The stimulus and sensitivity settings are set and maintained according to cardiologist's orders. The electrode is taped or sutured at the insertion site. | Monitors the progression of catheter through the heart. |

*Postprocedure Care*

1. Check vital signs frequently.
2. Check for heart rhythm and emotional reactions to procedure and pacing.
3. Check whether connections are secured or not
4. Monitor battery and control setting.
5. Clean and dress incision site according to hospital policy.
6. Keep the pulse generator clean and dry and prevent mishandling.
7. Use rubber gloves when exposed wires are handled.
8. Enclose the pulse generator in a rubber glove to keep it dry.
9. Check electrical equipments for adequate grounding.
10. Keep patient in supine position and ask to maintain adduction of affected extremity for 12 hours.
11. Stabilize arm, catheter and pacemaker to an armboard and avoid movement of the arm above shoulder level to prevent dislodgment.
12. If the leg is the insertion site limit movement especially hip flexion and outward rotation.
13. Explain that bedrest for 24 hours and reduced activity for another 48 hours is required.
14. Connect patient to cardiac monitor and monitor rhythm.

**Table 11.4.1:** Pacemaker malfunctions and nursing interventions

| Problem | Possible Cause | Nursing Interventions |
|---|---|---|
| **I Failure to pace properly:**<br>1. Intermittent or complete absence of pacing artifact.<br><br>2. Rapid, inappropriate firing of pacemaker (pacemaker mediated tachycardia). | -Battery failure<br>-A break or loose connection anywhere along the system.<br>-Pulse generator failure.<br>-Circulatory failure.<br>-"oversensing" or "undersensing" by pacemaker. | • Replace pulse generator.<br>• Replace battery unit.<br>• Check and connect all connections between pulse generator and leads.<br>• Reduce or increase sensitivity threshold of pacemaker unit.<br>• Assess patient's tolerance of pacemaker failure.<br>• Have emergency medications at hand.<br>• Perform CPR if indicated. |
| **II Failure to capture:**<br>Pacing artifact present but is not followed by a QRS complex or P Wave. | • Decreased conductivity by the myocordial tissue due to electrolyte imbalance, infarction, drug toxicity, perforation or excessive fibrosis of tissue at electrode site.<br>• Lead displacement due to migration or idle manipulation of pulse generator ("Twiddlers syndrome"). | • Increase voltage by 1-2 mA<br>• Increase amplitude of pacemaker output<br>• Reposition patient to either side in an attempt to improve contact of electrode with endocardium. In temporary lead try moving arm if leadwire is inserted in antecubital area.<br>• Obtain chest film to determine lead position.<br>• Have emergency drugs at hand. Initiate CPR if necessary. |
| **III Failure to sense:**<br>Pacing artifact present despite the presence of QRS complexes and P waves.<br>A Competitive rhythm may develop | • Sensitivity threshold set too low.<br>-Intrinsic beats of too-low voltage may go undetected by pacemaker's sensing mechansim.<br>-Dislodged or fractured lead.<br>-Circulatory failure.<br>-Electromagnetic interference. | • Increase sensitivity threshold on pulse generator.<br>-Reposition patient.<br>-If patient's intrinsic rhythm/rate is adequate turn off pacemaker.<br>-Increase pacing rate to overdrive patient's intrinsic heart rate.<br>-Give antidysrhythmics to decrease ectopy.<br>-Notify physician.<br>-Obtain chestfilm to determine electrode placement. |
| **IV Over sensing:**<br>Pace maker senses electrical activity within the myocardium or myopotential. | • Sensitivity threshold set too high.<br>• T wave sending myopotentials.<br>• Electromagnetic interference<br>• Two leads touching. | • Decrease sensitivity threshold<br>• Correct conditions that produce large T waves |

## PERMANENT PACEMAKER

The pulse generator is implanted underneath the skin in subcutaneous tissue in the pectoral region below the clavicle and sometimes an abdominal site is selected, and electrical stimulation is passed to the heart through pacing catheters (Figure 11.4(c and d)).

Permanent pacing systems use reliable power sources such as lithium or nuclear batteries. Lithium batteries have a lifespan of 8-12 years and nuclear power sources have life span of 20 years.

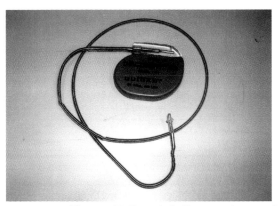 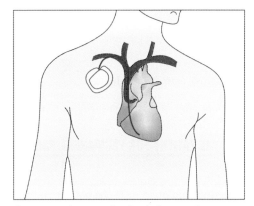

**Figures 11.4(c and d):** Permanent pacemaker and permanent pacemaker lead placement

### Indications

1. Irreversible complete heart block.
2. Left ventricular heart failure
3. Ectopic rhythms
4. Chronic atrial fibrillation,
5. Atrial flutter
6. Supraventricular tachycardia.
7. Hypersensitive carotid sinus syndrome
8. Sick sinus syndrome
9. Prophylactic implantation in patients after myocardial infarction complicated by advanced AV block, during the acute stages of infarction.

## TYPES OF PERMANENT PACEMAKERS

Pacemakers are classified by uniform codes according to a classification system.
The classification originally uses a three letter code.
a. The first letter denotes the cardiac chamber to be paced.
b. The second letter reflects the chamber to be sensed.
c. Third letter indicates the type of response to occur, that is sensed myocardial electrical activity will cause the pacemaker's impulse to be "triggered"
(T or "Inhibited"(I) or both
In clinical practice usually the three letter classification is used commonly.
For example, VVI pacemaker
V—Ventricle is paced.
V—Ventricle is sensed
I—The pacemaker will inhibit pacing when the patient's own impulse is sensed. Later two more categories were added ie programmability and rate modulation, and antitachydysrhythmia functions.

*Symbols used:*
A—Atrium
V—Ventricle
O—None
D—Dual(Both chambers)
T—Triggered
I—Inhibited

Table 11.4.2: Summary of pacemaker modalities

| Pacemaker type | NBG code | Atrium | Ventricle |
|---|---|---|---|
| Atrial asynchronous | AOO | Pace | …. |
| Ventricular asynchronous | VOO | …… | Pace |
| Atrial demand | AAI/AAT/AAIR | Pace & Sense | |
| Ventricular demand | VVI/VVT/VVIR | | Pace & Sense |
| Atrial synchronous | VAT | Sense | Pace |
| Atrial synchoronous, Ventricular inhibited | VDD | Sense | Pace & Sense |
| AV sequential | DVI/DVIR | Pace | Pace & Sense |
| Fully automatic | DDD/DDDR | Pace & Sense | Pace & Sense |

## PREPARATION OF THE PATIENT FOR PERMANENT PACEMAKER INSERTION

| | Nursing action | Rationale |
|---|---|---|
| 1 | Explain procedure and purpose to the patient and family and explain to him how he has to cooperate. | Allays anxiety and helps in obtaining cooperation of patient. |
| 2 | Get informed consent for procedure | Prevents litigation for health workers. |
| 3 | Explain about the need to avoid food and fluids for 8-10 hours prior to procedure. | An empty stomach prevents risk of aspiration during procedure. |
| 4 | Shave following areas:<br>a. Anterior chest from neck to umbilicus.<br>b. Nape of neck to loins of back<br>c. Both arms and axilla | Reduces risk of infection. |
| 5 | Advise to take bath with antiseptic scrub and water for 2 days before procedure and on the day of procedure. | Reduces risk of infection. |
| 6 | Provide clean gown | Prevents unnecessary exposure. |
| 7 | Remove jewellery, dentures and contact lens. | Jewellery acts as a source of infection. |
| 8 | Start good IV access with heparin lock | Ensures patent IV line to administer fluid and medications |
| 9 | Obtain a preoperative ECG | Helps in comparison study after procedure. |
| 10 | Administer prophylactic antibiotic as per physician's order | |
| 11 | Send the patient to O.T. with patient's chart, X-ray film, lab forms, ECG and others depending upon hospital policy. | Gives details about patient's baseline data. |

## PROCEDURE

Permanent pacing –This is indicated in long-term management of symptomatic or life-threatening dysrhythmias.

The surgeon inserts the pacing electrode either via the transvenous route or by direct application to the epicardial surface during thoracotomy. The surgeon places the permanent pulse generator into a small tunnel borrowed within the subcutaneous tissue below the right clavicle or less often the left clavicle.

The pulse generator is a small thermatically sealed (To prevent ingress of body fluids) lithium battery.

## POSTPROCEDURE CARE

1. Monitor vital signs and pacemaker function.
2. Explain about bedrest for 24 hours and reduced activity for another 48 hours.
3. Connect patient to cardiac monitor and check rhythm.
4. Check operative site for excessive swelling redness, bleeding, etc.
5. Check vital signs and wound hourly.

6. Discourage patient from vomiting, coughing or rolling on to affected side.
7. Continue ECG monitoring for 24 hours.

## RECORDING

Record the location and type of pacing lead, pacing mode, stimulus threshold, sensitivity setting, pacing rate and intervals, and intrinsic rhythm.

## PATIENT EDUCATION

1. Assess wound daily.
2. Report any signs of inflammation to the physician.
3. Avoid constrictive clothing which puts excessive pressure on the wound and pulse generator.
4. Avoid "toying" with pulse generator because this may cause pacemaker malfunction and local skin inflammation.
5. Explain to patient how to check pulse in wrist and instruct him to report sudden slowing or increase of pulse rate which indicates pacemaker malfunction.
6. Report any abnormal signs of dizziness, fatigue, swelling of ankles, legs, chestpain and shortness of breath.
7. "Avoid being near areas with high voltage, magnetic force field or radiation, standing near large running motors, high tension wires, power plants, radiotransmitters, large industrial magnets, welding machines, standing in open areas, during thunder storms, etc.
8. Safely operate most appliances and tools that are properly grounded and in good repair including microwave ovens, televisions and video recorders.
9. Show identification card and request scanning by hand scanner when passing through security gates.
10. Carry an identification card indicating manufacturer's name, pacemaker model and hospital where pacemaker was inserted.
11. Do not lift more than 5-10 pounds weight for the first 6 weeks after surgery.
12. Normal activity including sexual activity can be resumed in 6 weeks.
13. The importance of regular physician or clinic visits (for evaluation of pacemaker function and possible reprogramming) must be stressed.
14. Mobile phones should not be kept on affected side.
15. Keep incision dry for one week after implantation.
16. Avoid lifting operative side arm above shoulder level for one week after implantation.

## COMPLICATIONS

1. Local infection at the entry site of the leads for temporary pacing.
2. Bleeding and hematoma at the lead entry sites.
3. Hemothorax and pneumothorax from puncture of the subclavian vein.
4. Failure to sense.
5. Failure to capture.
6. Atrial and ventricular septal perforation.
7. Atelectasis.
8. Pericardial fluid accumulation.
9. Diaphragmatic stimulation (Hiccupping or twitching at the pacemaker site).

## SPECIAL CONSIDERATION

If external defibrillation is required it is essential that defibrillation paddles not be placed directly over an implanted device. Anteroposterior paddle position may be used.

# 11.5: PERFORMING A CARDIOPULMONARY RESUSCITATION (CPR)

## INTRODUCTION

Basic life support (BLS) is that particular phase of emergency cardiac care that either (1) prevents circulatory or respiratory arrest or insufficiency through prompt recognition and intervention or (2) externally supports the circulation and ventilation of a victim of cardiac or respiratory arrest through cardiopulmonary resuscitation (CPR).

## OBJECTIVE OF CPR

To provide oxygen to the brain, heart and other vital organs until appropriate definitive medical treatment (advanced cardiac life support) can restore normal heart and ventilatory action.

## INDICATIONS

1. Respiratory arrest resulting from drowning, stroke, foreign body, airway obstruction, smoke inhalation, drug overdose, electrocution, suffocation, myocardial infarction, injury from lightening and coma of any cause leading to airway obstruction.
2. Cardiac arrest.

## THE SEQUENCE OF BLS

**ABCs** of CPR are **A**irway, **B**reathing and **C**irculation and begins with an assessment phase to determine the need for action which include 'determine unresponsiveness,' 'determine breathlessness' and 'determine pulselessness' respectively.

## ARTICLES

1. Arrest board/back board/flat surface
2. Oral airway
3. A piece of lint to place over victim's mouth or oral barrier device for mouth to mouth respiration or a mask and ambubag.

## PROCEDURE

| Nursing action | Rationale |
|---|---|
| A   Determine unresponsiveness (Figure 11.5(a)) | |

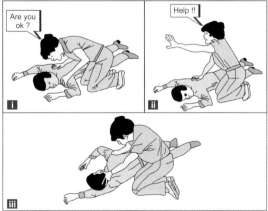

Figure 11.5(a): Determining unresponsiveness

*Contd...*

*Contd...*

| | | |
|---|---|---|
| 1 | Tap or gently shake patient while shouting "Are you Ok". | This will prevent injury from attempted resuscitation of a person who has not suffered a cardiac or respiratory arrest. |
| 2 | Check for breathing by keeping your cheek against the victim's nose and look at the chest for rise and fall and simultaneously listen and feel for exhaled breath against your cheek (Figure 11.5(b)). | CPR should not be administered to a patient with spontaneous respiration because of potential risk of injury. |

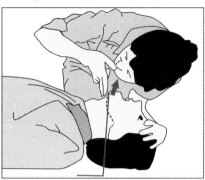

**Figure 11.5(b):** Determining breathlessness

| | | |
|---|---|---|
| 3 | Check for carotid pulse on one side for 5-10 seconds (Figure 11.5(c)). | Carotid pulse may persist when peripheral pulses are not palpable |

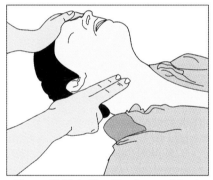

**Figure 11.5(c):** Checking for carotid pulse

| | | |
|---|---|---|
| 4 | Call for help in hospital set up. | Alerts other trained personnel. |
| 5 | Position the arrest board underneath the victim's chest (when arrest board is not available, place victim on firm, flat surface. | The arrest board provides a firm surface allowing for compression of the heart. |
| 6 | Kneel at victim's side | Allows performance of rescue breathing and chest compressions with efficiency. |
| 7 | Open victim's airway by using one of the following maneuvers.<br>a. Head tilt chin lift maneuver— Place one hand on victim's forehead and apply firm backward pressure with the palm to tilt the head back. Then place the fingers of the other hand under the bony part of the lower jaw near the chin and lift up to bring the jaw forward (Figure 11.5(d)).<br>b. Jaw thrust maneuver— Grasp the angles of the patient's lower jaw and lift with both hands, one on each side, displacing mandible forward (Figure 11.5(e)). | This supports the jaw and helps tilt the head back. This maneuver should not be performed for victims with suspected head and neck injuries.<br><br><br>Jaw thrust technique without head-tilt is the safest method for opening the airway in the presence of suspected neck injury. |

*Contd...*

*Contd...*

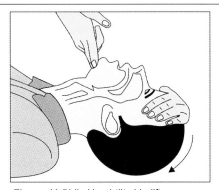

**Figure 11.5(d):** Head tilt-chin lift maneuver

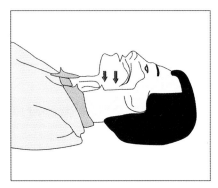

**Figure 11.5(e):** Jaw thrust maneuver

| | | |
|---|---|---|
| 8 | Place an airway if available | Keeps airway patent |
| 9 | i. Occlude nostrils with thumb and index finger of the hand on forehead that is tilting the head back. Form a seal over the patient's mouth using either your mouth or appropriate respiratory arrest device (ambubag and mask) and give two full breaths of approximately 0.5 to 2 seconds allowing time for both inspiration and expiration.<br><br>ii. Observe for rise and fall of the chest (Figure 11.5(f)). | Occluding the nostrils and forming a seal over the patient's mouth will prevent air leakage and provide full inflation of the lungs.<br>Excessive air volume and rapid respiratory flow rates can create pharyngeal pressure that is greater than oesophageal opening pressure. This will allow air into the stomach resulting in gastric distention and increased risk of vomiting. |

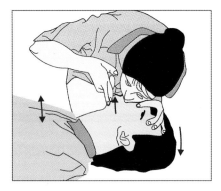

**Figure 11.5(f):** Providing mouth to mouth
respiration

*Contd...*

*Contd...*

| | | |
|---|---|---|
| 10 | Using the index finger of hand nearest to legs of patient locate the lower rib margin and move the fingers up to where the ribs connect to the sternum.<br>Place the middle finger of this hand on the notch and index finger next to it. Place the heel of the opposite hand next to the index finger on the sternum. Ensure that the long axis of the heel of hand is parallel to the long axis of the sternum (Figure 11.5(g)). Remove the first hand from the notch and place on top of the hand that is on the sternum. Extend or interlace fingers. Do not allow them to touch the chest. Keep arms straight with shoulders directly over the hands on sternum and lock elbows (Figure 11.5(h)). | Proper hand positioning ensures maximum compression of the heart and prevents injuries to liver and ribs. |

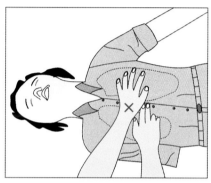

**Figure 11.5(g):** Positioning hands for chest compressions

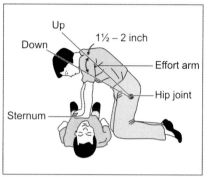

**Figure 11.5(h):** Position of rescuer during cardiac compressions

| | | |
|---|---|---|
| 11 | Compress the adult chest 1 ½ to 2 inches at the rate of approximately 100 per minute. | |
| 12 | Release the external chest compression completely and allow the chest to return to its normal position after each compression. The time allowed for release should be equal to the time required for compression. Do not lift hands off chest. | Release of external chest compression allows blood flow into the heart. Removing hands from the chest will result in more time required to locate the exact point for chest compressions. |
| 13 | Do 30 compressions and then perform two ventilations, re-evaluate the patient after four cycles (use the mnemonic 1 and 2 and 3 ——" to keep rhythm and timing). | Rescue breathing and chest compressions should be combined. |
| 14 | For CPR performed by one or two rescuers, the compression rate is 100 per minute.<br>The compression: Ventilation ratio is 30:2 | |
| 15 | While resuscitation proceeds, simultaneous efforts must be made to obtain and use special resuscitation equipment to manage breathing and circulation and provide definitive care. Definitive care includes defibrillation, pharmacotherapy for dysrhythmias and acid-base disturbances and ongoing monitoring and skilled care in an intensive care unit. | |

## WHEN TO STOP CPR

Guidelines for termination of resuscitation are:
1. Return of spontaneous circulation

2. Arrival of arrest team or medical help
3. If the rescuer becomes exhausted
4. When death is confirmed.

**Note:** The 2006 American heart association recommendation for chest compression – ventilation ratio is 30:2. The recommended rate until 2006 was 15:2. (Published on line on November 28, 2005). Reference www.american heart association.com

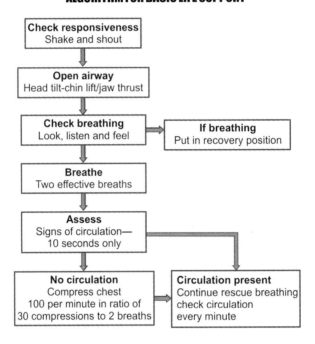

**ALGORITHM FOR BASIC LIFE SUPPORT**

# 11.6(A): PERFORMING DEFIBRILLATION AND ADVANCED CARDIAC LIFE SUPPORT (ACLS)

## DEFINITION

Defibrillation means delivering electrical current transthoracically through paddles to terminate lethal arrhythmias.

## PURPOSE

To treat lethal arrhythmias such as pulseless ventricular tachycardia and ventricular fibrillation.

## INDICATIONS

1. Ventricular fibrillation
2. Pulseless ventricular tachycardia.

## TYPES OF DEFIBRILLATORS (FIGURE 11.6(A))

1. Direct current defibrillator
2. Automated external defibrillator (AED)
3. Automatic implantable cardioverter—defibrillator (Figure 11.6 (b))

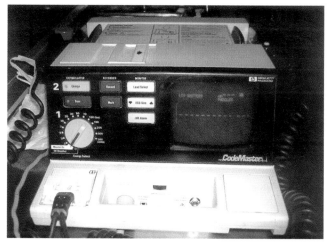

Figure 11.6(a): Direct current defibrillator

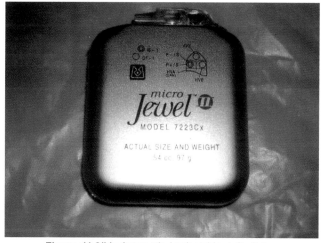

Figure 11.6(b): Automatic implantable defibrillator

### DIRECT CURRENT DEFIBRILLATOR

It delivers an electrical current of preset voltage to the heart through paddles placed on the chest wall.

### AUTOMATED EXTERNAL DEFIBRILLATOR (AED)

AED delivers shock to a patient after it identifies pulseless ventricular tachycardia and ventricular fibrillation. The device has two electrodes (pads) which has to be positioned over clean, dry skin. Position of electrodes is same as that of direct current defibrillator. These electrodes sense the electrical activity of heart and analyse the rhythm. If the rhythm is shockable one, the device gives visual and auditory signal and provides directions to the lay person to deliver shock.

### AUTOMATIC IMPLANTABLE CARDIOVERTER DEFIBRILLATOR (AICD)

The AICD is a device that delivers electric shock directly to the heart muscles in order to terminate lethal dysrthymias. It has a pulse generator and a sensor that continuously monitors rhythm and detects dysrhythmias. It automatically delivers a counter shock.

AICD is surgically implanted by lateral thoracotomy or median sternotomy, in subxiphoid or subintercostal regions.

## ARTICLES

1. DC defibrillator with paddles
2. Interface material (disposable conductive gel pads, electrode gels and paste)
3. Resuscitative article.

## PROCEDURE

| | Nursing action | Rationale |
|---|---|---|
| 1 | Explain procedure to the family | Allays anxiety and helps in cooperation |
| 2 | Position patient in supine without any pillow. | |
| 3 | Confirm ventricular tachycardia or ventricular fibrillation by checking monitor and patient's clinical condition. Defibrillation is to be started within 10 to 20 seconds of onset of arrhythmia. Remove oxygen from area. | Defibrillation should be done before myocardial cells are anoxic or acidotic. |
| 4 | Expose anterior chest. Start CPR immediately | |
| 5 | Apply interface material to the patient or to the paddles. The electrode paddles should be in firm contact with the patient's skin. | The interface material helps provide better conduction and prevents skin burns. Do not allow any paste on the skin between the electrodes. If the paste areas touch, the current may short circuit (severely burning the patient) and may not penetrate the heart. Saline pads are not recommended because the saline can easily drip making a path for the current. |
| 6 | Put on defibrillator and switch off synchronizer mode. | |
| 7 | The initial defibrillation should be 200-J of delivered energy. A second attempt at same level (200-300 J) should be given if first attempt is unsuccessful. A third attempt with an increase of energy level to 360-Joules should be attempted. Allow only approximately 5 seconds between the successive attempts to assess rhythm and pulse. | The shock is measured in joules or watt seconds. Less time between successive shock enhances effectiveness. High doses of shock causes myocardial damage. Transthoracic impedence is reduced with repeated delivery of shock. |
| 8 | Apply one electrode anteriorly at 2nd intercostal space to right of sternum and another paddle laterally at mid clavicular line on left side (apex). About 20 to 25 lb of pressure are applied to paddles to ensure good contact with the patient's skin (Figure 11.6(c). | The paddles are placed so the electrical discharge flows through as much myocardial mass as possible. If antero posterior paddles are used, the anterior paddle is held with pressure on the apex, while the patient lies on the posterior paddle under the left infrascapular region. In this method, the counter shock moves directly through heart (Figure 11.6(d)). |

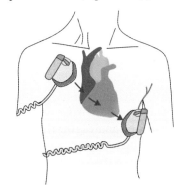

**Figure 11.6(c):** Paddle placement and current flow in defibrillation

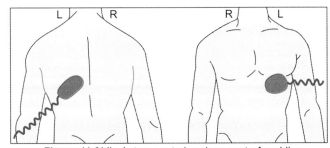

**Figure 11.6(d):** Antero-posterior placement of paddles

*Contd...*

*Contd...*

| 9 | Grasp the paddles by handles . | Handling the paddles safely will reduce the risk of electrical shock. |
|---|---|---|
| 10 | Charge the paddles. Once paddles are charged, give the command for personnel to stand clear off the patient and the bed. Call "clear" 3 times. With first call, see that you move away from bed and patient. With 2nd call, ensure that others are away and with 3rd call, look quickly to make sure all are clear from the patient and bed. | If a person touches the bed, he or she may act as a ground for the current and receive a shock especially if there are electrolyte solutions on the floor. |
| 11 | Push the discharge button in both paddles simultaneously. | |
| 12 | Reassess monitor for rhythm change, holding paddles on position over chest. | Determines rhythm of the heart. |
| 13 | If rhythm is not reverted back, deliver two more shocks in succession (200 – 300J, 360J). | |
| 14 | Resume CPR efforts until stable rhythm, spontaneous respiration, pulse and BP returns. | After the three attempts using difibrillator CPR efforts should be resumed. Total delay should be no more than 5 seconds to oxygenate the patient and restore circulation. |
| 15 | When ventricular tachycardia and ventricular fibrillation persists, administer emergency drugs injection adrenaline 1 mg and injection atropine and give CPR for one minute. Repeat defibrillation at 360 joules and continue procedure as per ACLS guidelines. | |
| 16 | Clean and replace paddles for next use. | |
| 17 | Record the procedure and effectiveness. | |
| 18 | Check for burns on the skin. | |

*Follow-up Activities*

1. After the patient is defibrillated and rhythm is restored lidocaine is usually given to prevent recurrent episodes.
2. Continue intensive monitoring .

## II. AUTOMATED EXTERNAL DEFIBRILLATOR

### PROCEDURE

| | Nursing action | Rationale |
|---|---|---|
| 1 | Ascertain unconsciousness and pulselessness. | |
| 2 | Position patient in supine position | |
| 3 | Start CPR while AED is being applied | |
| 4 | Place electrode on the patient's anterior chest, just below the right clavicle and below the left nipple. | Appropriate electrode position ensures passage of current through the majority of myocardium. |
| 5 | Turn AED on, follow audio or visual instruction from the AED | The AED will analyze the rhythm in 5 to 15 seconds and determine the need for defibrillation based on that analysis. It will then let the operator know how to proceed. |
| 6 | Suspend CPR or any movement of the patient during the analysis. | External movement will impair the AED accuracy in analyzing the rhythm. |

*Contd...*

*Contd...*

| | | |
|---|---|---|
| 7 | If after analyzing the rhythm a shock is advised, the AED will instruct the operator to prepare for a shock. It will charge the unit, give warning to "stand clear" and then deliver the stock. | |
| 8 | After the first shock, do not restart CPR. Allow the AED to reanalyze the rhythm. If a second shock is indicated the AED will proceed as above. Most AEDs will deliver 3 successive shocks. | Delivering the shock in rapid succession or "stacking" the shocks decreases thoracic impedance and enhances the effectiveness of defibrillation. |
| 9 | After the third shock is delivered, if there is no pulse, continue CPR for 1 minute then begin the analysis of procedure again. | The patient will have been pulseless by this time. Oxygenation and circulation must be restored or the patient's chances of survival decreases markedly. |
| 10 | If the patient regains a pulse, continue to support ventilation. Keep AED electrode attached and the unit on in case the patient loses consciousness again. | |

## COMPLICATIONS

1. Damage to myocardium due to repeated high energy electrical shocks.
2. Chest burns due to repeated high-energy discharges and poor contact between the paddles and the skin.
3. Electrocution of the bystanders.
4. Formation of short circuits between paddles due to excessive amount of conduction jelly applied on the paddles. This causes loss of electrical energy.

## NURSING CONSIDERATIONS

1. Defibrillation is an emergency procedure, the article should be kept ready at all times.
2. The conduction jelly should be kept along with defibrillator to prevent waste of time in search of jelly.
3. The defibrillator should be checked for its proper functioning every shift/every day.
4. When using paddles. Apply appropriate conductant between paddles. Do not substitute any other type of conductant like ultrasound gel.

# 11.6(B): ACLS ALGORITHM

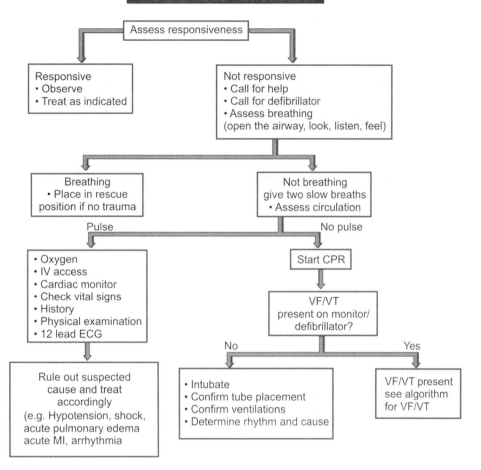

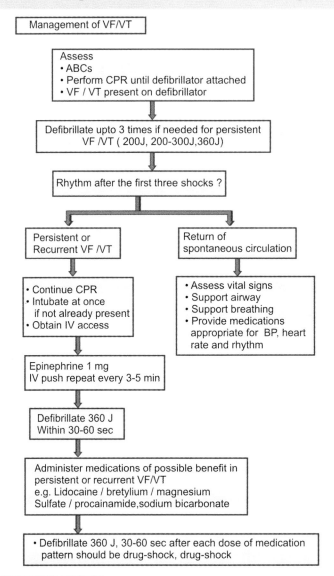

## MEDICATIONS ARE USED IN FOLLOWING DOSAGE

1. **Lidocaine**
   1.5 mg/kg IV push. Repeat in 3-5 min to total loading dose of 3 mg/kg: then use. Bretylium
2. **Bretylium**
   5 mg/kg IV push repeat in 5 min at 10 mg/kg
3. **Magnesium sulfate**
   1-2 g IV in torsades de pointes or suspected hypomagnesemic state or severe refractory VF
4. **Procainamide**
   30 mg/min in refactory VF (Maximum dose 17mg/kg)
5. **Sodium bicarbonate**
   1 mEq/ kg IV
   • If known preexisting bicarbonate responsive acidosis.
   • If overdose with tricyclic antidepressants
   • To alkalinize the urine in drug overdose.
   • Hypoxic lactic acidosis.

## 11. 7: ASSISTING WITH BRONCHOSCOPY

## DEFINITION

Assisting with direct inspection and examination of the larynx, trachea and bronchi through either a flexible fiber-optic bronchoscope or a rigid bronchoscope (Figure 11.7(a)).

The fiberoptic scope allows for more patient comfort and better visualization of smaller airways.

Rigid bronchoscopy is preferred for small children and endobronchial tumor resection.

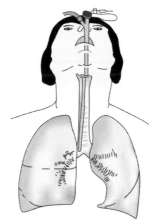

**Figure 11.7(a):** Bronchoscope inserted through trachea

## PURPOSES

I. **Diagnostic:**
   a. For examination of tissue.
   b. For further evaluation of a tumor for potential surgical resection.
   c. To collect tissue specimen for diagnosis.
   d. To evaluate bleeding sites.

II. **Therapeutic:**
   a. To remove foreign bodies
   b. To remove thick, viscous secretions
   c. To treat postoperative atelectasis
   d. To remove and destroy lesions.

## PROCEDURE

| | Nursing action | Rationale |
|---|---|---|
| 1 | Explain procedure to patient and family members. | Helps in obtaining cooperation and providing reassurance. |
| 2 | Obtain informed consent from patient. | Prevents legalities to the staff members. |
| 3 | Instruct patient to be on NPO for 6-12 hours before procedure. | Reduces risk of aspiration during procedure. |
| 4 | Remove dentures, contact lens and other prosthesis before procedure | Prevents interference with the procedure. |
| 5 | Administer pre-medications as per physician's instruction (usually atropine, sedative, and an opioid). | Inhibits vagal stimulation. |

*Contd...*

*Contd...*

| | | |
|---|---|---|
| 6 | Administer local anesthetic agent as per physician's order (general anesthesia may be needed for rigid bronchoscopy) | |
| 7 | Spray topical anesthetic- lignocaine on the pharynx or drop on the epiglottis and vocal cords and into the trachea. | Suppresses cough reflex and minimises discomfort. |
| 8 | Administer sedatives intravenously as prescribed. | |
| 9 | Instruct patient to lie supine with head hyperextended. | |
| 10 | Monitor vital signs, $O_2$ saturation, cardiac rhythm and reassure the client during the procedure. | |

## POSTPROCEDURE CARE

1. Monitor vital signs.
2. Observe the client for signs of respiratory distress including dyspnea, changes in respiratory rate, use of accessory muscles and absent lung sounds.
3. Inspect expectorated secretions for hemoptysis.
4. Keep patient on NPO until gag reflex returns.
5. Give ice chips and small sips of water when patient regains swallowing reflex.
6. Monitor lung sounds for 24 hours.
7. Assess for lethargy and confusion in elderly patients which may be due to large doses of lignocaine given during the procedure.
8. Instruct the patient and family (care givers) to report any shortness of breath or bleeding immediately.

## COMPLICATIONS

1. Pneumothorax
2. Dysrhythmias
3. Bronchospasm
4. Infection
5. Aspiration
6. Perforation.

## SPECIAL CONSIDERATION

Sedation to patients with respiratory insufficiency may precipitate respiratory arrest.

# 11: 8: ASSISTING WITH THORACENTESIS

## DEFINITION

Insertion of a needle into the pleural space to remove accumulated fluid and air using aseptic technique.

## PURPOSES

1. To remove air and fluid from pleural cavity
2. To decrease pressure on the lung tissue
3. To aspirate pleural fluid for diagnostic studies.
4. To instill medication into the pleural space.
5. To perform pleural biopsy.

## ARTICLES

I. **A pleural aspiration set containing:**
1. Sponge holding forceps(1)
2. Syringe(5 ml) and needle
3. Syringe(20 ml)with leur lock
4. Aspiration needles(no 16G)
5. Small bowls (2)
6. Dissecting forceps (1)
7. Artery forceps (1)
8. Specimen bottles and slides
9. Gown, mask and gloves
10. Sterile dressing towels
11. Cotton swabs, gauze pieces and pads
12. Scalpel blade.

II. **Clean tray containing**
1. Mackintosh and towel
2. Kidney tray and paper bag
3. Spirit, Iodine
4. Lignocaine 2%
5. Adhesive plaster and scissors
6. Tincture benzoin

III. **Other articles like**
1. Cardiac table
2. Pillows.

## PROCEDURE

| | Nursing action | Rationale |
|---|---|---|
| 1 | Identify patient and explain procedure to him and relatives. Explain that during procedure he may experience a sensation of deep pressure when fluid is aspirated | Allays anxiety and wins cooperation. |
| 2 | Review the chest X-ray | X-ray shows localization of fluid and air in pleural cavity for determining puncture site. |
| 3 | Obtain an informed consent from patient. | Avoids risk of legal complications. |

*Contd...*

*Contd...*

| | | |
|---|---|---|
| 4 | Instruct patient that he should not move during procedure | Any movement or coughing during procedure can cause injury to vital organs or blood vessels. |
| 5 | Position the patient comfortably<br>a. Sitting on the edge of bed with the feet supported, arms and head on pillows over the cardiac table.<br>b. Straddling a chair with arms and head resting on the back of the chair.<br>c. Lying on the unaffected side with the bed elevated 30-40 degree if patient is unable to assume sitting position. | An upright position facilitates localization of fluid at the base of the chest. |
| 6 | Expose the chest. The physician determines the site for aspiration by visualizing chest X-ray and performing chest percussion. If air is to be removed the site is usually in 2nd and 3rd intercostal space . If fluid is to be aspirated then site is usually in the 8th and 9th intercostal space. | Fluid usually localizes at the base of the chest. |
| 7 | Clean the site with antiseptic solution and assist the physician in administering local anesthesia | Reduces risk of infection. |
| 8 | The physician introduces the thoracentesis needle. Instruct the patient to hold his breath when needle is inserted. | Respiratory movement can cause risk of puncture to vital organs. |
| 9 | When needle is in pleural space, physician aspirates pleural fluid with syringe. Assist in collecting specimen in sterile containers.<br>• A 20 ml syringe with a three-way adapter is attached to needle. The tubing which leads to the receptacle is attached to the third port of the three-way adapter.<br>• If a considerable quantity of fluid is to be removed, the needle is held in place on the chest wall with a small hemostat. | The three-way adapter helps in preventing air from entering the pleural cavity when large volumes of fluid is removed.<br>Hemostat steadies the needle on the chest wall.Sudden chest pain or shoulder pain indicates that the needle point is irritating pleural cavity. |
| 10 | For therapeutic purpose usually 1000-1200 ml of fluid is removed and for diagnostic purpose 30-60 ml of fluid is removed. Encourage patient to remain still during the procedure and monitor vital signs. | |
| 11 | After needle is withdrawn, apply tincture benzoin seal and pressure dressing over the site. | Pressure dressing prevents risk of bleeding, leakage and infection at site. |
| 12 | Position patient in bed with affected side up. He should remain in bed for 4-6 hours after procedure. | This position minimises risk of possible fluid leakage |
| 13 | Monitor vital signs every half an hour for 4-6 hours or till steady. Observe patient for complications such as shock, fainting, low blood pressure, rapid pulse, rapid respiration, uncontrolled cough and blood tinged frothy sputum. Check breath sounds in all lung fields. | Complications may occur because of accidental puncture of vital organs or blood vessels. |
| 14 | Record the procedure with total amount of fluid withdrawn, colour, nature and signs of complications. | |
| 15 | Send labelled specimen to laboratory. | |
| 16 | Instruct patient to do deep breathing and coughing exercises. Demonstrate and teach these excercises to patient. | Deep breathing and coughing promotes lung expansion. |
| 17 | Have a chest X-ray if indicated. | |
| 18 | Wash articles used for thoracentesis in cold water and then in warm soapy water. Rinse, dry and send for autoclaving. Wear gloves while washing. | |

# 11.9: PERFORMING AN OROPHARYNGEAL SUCTIONING

## DEFINITION

Oropharyngeal suctioning is the process of removing secretions from the oral cavity and pharynx.

## PURPOSES

1. To remove secretions that obstruct the airway
2. To facilitate ventilation
3. To obtain secretions for diagnostic purposes
4. To prevent infection that may result from accumulated secretions

## ARTICLES

1. Appropriate size sterile suction catheter (smallest diameter that will remove secretions effectively) 12=18 Fr or Yankauer catheter (special catheter for oropharyngeal suctioning)
2. Portable or wall suction unit with connecting tubing and Y- connector
3. Sterile water/Normal saline in a sterile bowl
4. Clean disposable gloves
5. Face mask
6. Nasal or oral airway if indicated
7. Towel or waterproof pad.

## PROCEDURE

| | Nursing action | Rationale |
|---|---|---|
| 1 | Assess for signs and symptoms indicating presence of upper airway secretions: gurgling respirations, restlessness, drooling, etc. | Physical signs and symptoms result from decreased oxygen to tissues as well as pooling of secretions in upper airway |
| 2 | Explain to the client that suctioning will stimulate the cough, gag or sneeze reflex | Helps in obtaining cooperation of patient and relieves patients anxiety |
| 3 | Explain importance of and encourage coughing during procedure | Facilitates removal of secretion and frequency and duration of future suctioning |
| 4 | Assemble articles. | Provides for organized approach |
| 5 | Adjust bed to comfortable working position. Lower side rails closer to you, place the patient in a semi- Fowler's position if conscious.<br>An unconscious patient should be placed in lateral position facing you. | • Having the patient in a sitting position helps him/her to cough and makes breathing easier<br>• Gravity facilitates the insertion of the catheter<br>• Lateral position prevents the airway from becoming obstructed and promoted drainage of secretions |
| 6 | Place towel or waterproof pad across patient's chest | • Protects bed linen |
| 7 | Wear mask or face shield | • Suction may cause splashing of body fluids |
| 8 | Turn on suction and adjust to appropriate pressure<br><br>a. Wall unit<br>  Adult——100-120 mm of Hg<br>  Child—— 95-110 mm Hg<br>  Infant——50-95 mm Hg | Negative pressure must be at a safe level or pneumothorax may occur |

*Contd...*

*Contd...*

| | | |
|---|---|---|
| | b. Portable unit<br>Adult ——10-15 mm Hg<br>Child —— 5-10 mm Hg<br>Infant ——2-5 mm Hg | |
| 9 | Wash hands | Reduces transmission of microorganisms |
| 10 | Perform oropharyngeal suctioning (Figure 11.9(a))<br>a. Apply clean disposable gloves<br>b. Connect one end of connecting tubing to suction machine and other to suction catheter, fill sterile bowl with sterile water<br>c. Suction small amount of sterile water from bowl<br>d. Remove oxygen mask, if present<br>e. Insert catheter into mouth along gum line to pharynx. Move catheter in oral cavity until secretions are cleared. Encourage client to cough during suctioning.<br>f. Replace oxygen mask<br>g. Rinse catheter with water in bowl until connecting tubing is cleared of secretions. Turn off suction | <br><br>Prepares suction apparatus<br><br><br>Ensures equipment function and lubricates catheter<br><br>Provides continuous suction. Care must be taken not to allow suction tip to invaginate oral mucosal surfaces.<br><br><br>Rinses catheter and reduces probability of transmission of microorganisms. |

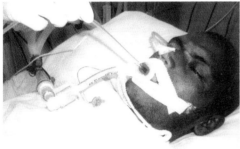

**Figure 11.9(a):** Oropharyngeal suctioning

| | | |
|---|---|---|
| 11 | Reassess client's respiratory status | Directs nurse to initiate or cease intervention. |
| 12 | Remove towel, place in laundry bag.<br>Remove gloves and dispose in appropriate receptacle | Reduces transmission of microorganisms |
| 13 | Reposition client: Sim's position encourages drainage and should be used if client has decreased level of consciousness | Facilitates drainage of oral secretions |
| 14 | Wash and rinse used articles with warm soapy water and dry with paper towels | |
| 15 | Place catheter in clean dry area | |
| 16 | Wash hands | Reduces transmission of organisms to other clients |
| 17 | Document the procedure in nurses record | Provides for communication between staff members. |

## SPECIAL CONSIDERATION

- For patients who have undergone oropharyngeal surgery, the procedure has to be performed using strict aseptic technique.
- A suction attempt should last only 10-15 seconds. During this time, the catheter is inserted, the suction applied and discontinued and the catheter removed.
- Allow 20 to 50 seconds intervals between each suction and limit suction to 5 minutes in total.

## 11.10: ASSISTING WITH ENDOTRACHEAL INTUBATION

### DEFINITION

Assisting in passing of a slender hollow tube into the trachea through nose or mouth using aseptic technique to facilitate artificial ventilation and resuscitation.

### PURPOSES

1. To treat acute respiratory failure, persistent hypoxemia, persistent rise in $pCO_2$
2. To maintain patent airway
3. To ensure adequate oxygenation
4. To provide ventilatory assistance when indicated.

### INDICATIONS

1. CNS depression
2. Neuromuscular disease
3. Chest wall injury
4. Upper airway obstruction
5. Anticipated upper airway obstruction (edema, soft tissue swelling due to head and neck trauma. Postoperative head and neck surgeries, decreased level of consciousness
6. Aspiration prophylaxis
7. Fracture of cervical, vertebral and spinal cord injury.

### COMPLICATIONS

1. Laryngeal/tracheal injury
2. Pulmonary infection and sepsis
3. Dependence on artificial airway.

### ARTICLES

1. Sandbag /towel roll
2. Suction apparatus with tubing
3. Suction catheter (Fr-14)
4. Ambubag and mask
5. Oxygen source and tubing
6. Laryngoscope with appropriate size blade
7. Magill's forceps
8. Endotracheal tubes of appropriate size (Figure 11.10a)
9. Stilette
10. Xylocaine jelly
11. Plastic syringe 10 ml
12. Oral airway
13. Cotton tape/Dynaplast
14. Gloves
15. Facemask

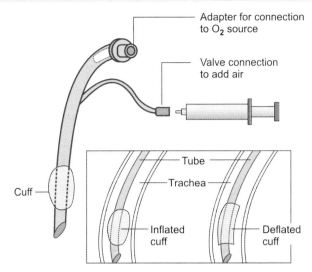

Adapter for connection
to O₂ source

Valve connection
to add air

Tube

Trachea

Cuff

Inflated
cuff

Deflated
cuff

**Figure 11.10(a):** Parts of an endotracheal tube

## PROCEDURE

| | Nursing action | Rationale |
|---|---|---|
| 1 | Explain procedure to the patient if conscious and get consent from patient and relatives. | Promotes acceptance of procedure and cooperation for procedure from patient. |
| 2 | Place patient in supine position with head extended by keeping sandbag or towel roll under neck. | Promotes access to trachea. |
| 3 | Check for loose teeth/dentures, if so remove with Magill's forceps. | Avoids danger of loose teeth causing airway obstruction. |
| 4 | Seal mouth and nose with mask and AMBU bag and initiate bagging with oxygen. | |
| 5 | Provide laryngoscope to doctor. | |
| 6 | Suction oral cavity. | Provides a clear field of work and prevents aspiration when performing oral tracheal insertion. |
| 7 | Provide lubricated endotracheal tube with stilette *in situ*. | Facilitates insertion without chances of injury. |
| 8 | Press crico-thyroid cartilage with thumb and index finger against esophagus. | Permits clear visualization of oropharynx for insertion |
| 9 | Assist while endotracheal tube is introduced into trachea and remove stilette. The tube when inserted should have the 22 cm marking at the incisor teeth and tube should be fixed at the midline to prevent pressure ulcer at the angle of the mouth (Figure 11.10(b)). | |

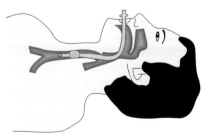

**Figure 11.10(b):** Endotracheal tube in place

*Contd...*

*Contd...*

| | | |
|---|---|---|
| 10 | Verify placement of tube by auscultation, listening/feeling for airflow through tube and observe for bilateral chest movements. | Confirms tube placement. |
| 11 | Connect Ambubag with oxygen attached to endotracheal tube and continue bagging. | |
| 12 | Inflate cuff of the endotracheal tube with 10 ml of air | Prevents chances of tube displacement and aspiration. |
| 13 | Insert an oral airway and apply endotracheal suctioning if necessary | |
| 14 | Fix endotracheal tube in position by using adhesive tape. (Figure 11.10(c)) | |

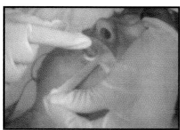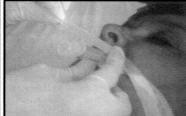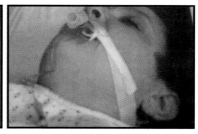

**Figure 11.10(c):** Fixing the endotracheal tube

| | |
|---|---|
| 15 | Connect to ventilator if needed |

Postprocedural care:
1. Place patient in lateral position
2. Arrange for chest X-ray to be taken in order to check placement of ET tube
3. Apply endotracheal suctioning if secretions are present.
4. Watch for chest movements, ET tube kinking, obstruction with secretion and blood, leakage of tube cuff, change in position of tube and over inflation of cuff.
5. Document type and size of tube used, chest movements, vital signs and patient's tolerance to procedure.
6. Check ABG periodically.

## SPECIAL CONSIDERATIONS

Check cuff pressure using manometer (if available) for detecting under inflation or over inflation of cuff. If under inflated, it can lead to aspiration and displacement of tube. Over inflation can lead to tracheal injury and ulceration leading to stenosis.

# 11.11A: ASSISTING WITH TRACHEOSTOMY

## DEFINITION

Assisting in creating a surgical opening into anterior wall of trachea and inserting a tube to maintain patent airway.

## PURPOSES

1. To bypass upper airway obstruction and trauma
2. To remove tracheobronchial secretions
3. To promote long-term use of mechanical ventilation
4. To prevent aspiration of oral or gastric secretion in unconscious or paralyzed patient
5. To replace endotracheal tube when long-term mechanical ventilation is required.

## ARTICLES

### TRACHEOSTOMY SET CONTAINING

1. Toothed dissecting forceps-1
2. Curved mosquito forceps-2
3. Straight mosquito forceps-2
4. Artery forceps-2
5. Allis forceps-2
6. Needle holder
7. Double hook retractors-2
8. Blunt hook
9. Cricoid hook
10. Sharp scissors
11. Tracheal dilator
12. Gall-pots-2
13. Cutting edge suture needle with cotton thread
14. Dressing forceps
15. Vaseline gauze

### A CLEAN TRAY CONTAINING

1. Suction catheter with connection
2. Hand towel
3. Kidney basin
4. Scalpel blade
5. Gloves
6. Mask
7. Apron
8. Antiseptic solution
9. Local anesthetic (Xylocaine 2%)
10. Syringes
11. Needles
12. Sandbag
13. Spot light
14. Tracheostomy tube (Figure 11.11(a))

Cuffless                                    Cuffed

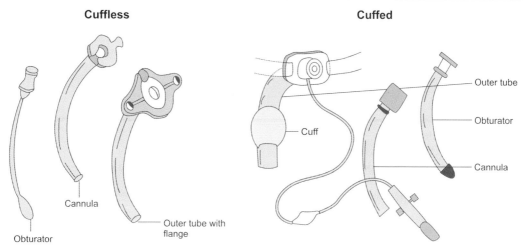

**Figure 11.11(a):** Types of tracheostomy tube

# PROCEDURE

| Nursing action | Rationale |
| --- | --- |
| 1. Explain procedure to the patient if conscious and get consent from patient and relatives. | Allays anxiety and facilitates patient co-operation. |
| 2 Place patient in supine position with full extension of neck and head. | Promotes visualization of site of insertion for the procedure. |
| 3 Remove gown and expose neck. | |
| 4 Keep suction and oxygen ready for use. | Facilitates timely use of articles. |
| 5 Assist in preparing skin and administering local anesthetic | Reduces risk of infection . Reduces sensation of pain. |
| 6 Assist in and support patient as incision is made and provide. suitable tracheostomy tube for insertion. | |
| 7 Assist in securing tracheostomy tube to neck while tying with tape. | Reduces chance of tube displacement. |
| 8 Assist while tube is being sutured in place. | Reduces chance of tube displacement. |
| 9 Place vaseline gauze around tube. | |
| 10 Assist patient to a comfortable position. | |
| 11 Replace equipment. | |
| 12 Document time, tube size, purpose of tracheostomy and patient's condition. | |

# POSTPROCEDURAL CARE

1. Connect to ventilator (if needed)
2. Place patient in semi-Fowler's position
3. Check vital signs
4. Administer analgesics and sedatives as per order
5. Watch for complications like bleeding, respiratory failure and blockage of tracheostomy tube with secretions
6. If metal tube is inserted, leave the stillete in a sterile tray at the bedside.
7. Keep suction apparatus and suction tube ready at bedside.

# 11.11B: PROVIDING TRACHEOSTOMY CARE

## DEFINITION

Tracheostomy care includes changing a tracheostomy inner tube, cleaning tracheostomy site and changing dressing around the site.

## PURPOSES

1. To maintain airway patency
2. To prevent infection at the tracheostomy site
3. To facilitate healing and prevent skin excoriation around the tracheostomy site
4. To promote comfort
5. To assess condition of ostomy.

## EQUIPMENT

I. Tracheostomy care kit containing
   1. Gallipots (3)
   2. Sterile towel
   3. Sterile nylon brush/Tube brush
   4. Sterile gauze squares
   5. Cotton twill ties or tracheostomy tie tapes
   6. Sterile bowl for solution
II. A clean tray containing:
   1. Sterile suction catheter
   2. Hydrogen peroxide
   3. Normal saline
   4. Sterile gloves-2 pairs
   5. Clean scissors
   6. Face mask and eye shield (optional)
   7. K Basin
   8. Waterproof pad
III. Suction apparatus

## PROCEDURE

| | Nursing action | Rationale |
|---|---|---|
| 1 | Assess condition of stoma: (Redness, swelling, character of secretions, presence of purulence or bleeding. | Presence of any of these indicates infection and culture examination may be warranted. |
| 2 | Examine neck for subcutaneous emphysema evidenced by crepitus around the ostomy site. | Indicates air leak into subcutaneous tissue. |
| 3 | Explain procedure to the patient and teach means of communication such as eye blinking or raising a finger to indicate pain or distress. | Obtains cooperation from patient. |
| 4 | Assist patient to a Fowler's position and place waterproof pad on chest. | Promotes lung expansion. Prevents soiling of linen. |
| 5 | Wash hands thoroughly. | Prevents cross-infection. |
| 6 | Assemble equipments, <br> a. Open the sterile tracheostomy kit, pour hydrogen peroxide and sterile normal saline in separate gallipots. | Hydrogen peroxide and saline removes mucus and crust which promote bacterial growth. |

*Contd...*

*Contd...*

| | | |
|---|---|---|
| | b. Open other sterile supplies as needed including sterile applicators, suction kit and tracheostomy care kit (dressing kit). | Enhances performance phase of procedure. |
| | c. Put on face mask and eye shield. | Protects the nurse. |
| 7 | Don sterile gloves. Place sterile towel on patient's chest. | Maintains aseptic technique. |
| 8 | Suction the full length of tracheostomy tube and pharynx thoroughly. | Removes secretions. |
| 9 | Rinse the suction catheter and discard it. | |
| 10 | Unlock the inner cannula (if present) and remove it by gently pulling it out towards you in line with its curvature. Place the inner cannula in the bowl with hydrogen peroxide solution (Applicable for tubes having inner and outer cannula). | Hydrogen peroxide moistens and loosens dried secretions. |
| 11 | Remove the soiled tracheostomy dressing, discard the dressing and gloves. | |
| 12 | Don a second pair of sterile gloves. | |
| 13 | Clean the flange of the tube using sterile applicators or gauze moistened with hydrogen peroxide and then with normal saline. Use each applicator once only. | Using the applicator or gauze once only, avoids contaminating a clean area with a soiled gauze. |
| 14 | Clean the stoma area with gauze (make only a single sweep with each gauze sponge before discarding)<br>• Half strength hydrogen peroxide (mixed with normal saline) may be used.<br>• Thoroughly rinse the cleaned area using gauze squares moistened with sterile normal saline. | Hydrogen peroxide helps to loosen dry crusted secretions.<br>Hydrogen peroxide is irritating to the skin and inhibits healing if not removed thoroughly. |
| 15 | Dry the stoma tube with dry sterile gauze<br>An infected wound may be cleaned with gauze saturated with an antiseptic solution, then dried.<br>A thin layer of antibiotic ointment may be applied to the stoma with a cotton swab. | May help to clear the wound infection. |
| 16 | Cleaning the inner cannula<br>• Remove the inner cannula from the soaking solution.<br>• Clean the lumen and entire cannula thoroughly using the brush.<br>• Rinse the cleaned cannula by rinsing it with sterile normal saline (agitating the cannula in the container with saline cleans it well).<br>• Gently tap the cannula against the inside of the sterile saline container after rinsing. | Thorough rinsing is important to remove hydrogen peroxide from inner cannula.<br><br>Removes solution adhering on the cannula. |
| 17 | Replace the inner cannula and secure it in place<br>• Insert the inner cannula by grasping the outer flange and pushing in the direction of its curvature.<br>• Lock the cannula in place by turning the lock (if present) into position. | This secures the flange of the inner cannula to the outer cannula. |
| 18 | Apply sterile dressing<br>• Open and refold a 4 x 4 gauze dressing into a 'V' shape and place under the flange of the tracheostomy tube. Do not cut gauze pieces (Figure 11.11(b)).<br>• Ensure that the tracheostomy tube is securely supported while applying dressing. | Avoid using cotton –filled 4 x 4 gauze. Cotton or gauze fiber can be aspirated by the patient potentially creating a tracheal abscess.<br>Excessive movement of the tracheostomy tube irritates the trachea. |

*Contd...*

*Contd...*

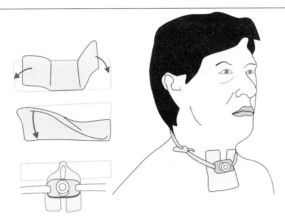

**Figure 11.11(b):** Method of folding gauze square for placement under faceplate

| | |
|---|---|
| 19 Change the tracheostomy ties | |
| a. Leave the soiled tape in place until the new one is applied | Leaving tape in place ensures that tube will not be expelled if patient coughs or moves. |
| b. Cut a piece of tape that is twice the neck circumference plus 10 cm. Cut the ends of tape diagonally. | This action provides a secure attachment with knot. Diagonal cut facilitates insertion of tape into openings of faceplate. |
| c. Apply the new tape | |
| • Grasp slit end of clean tape and pull it through opening on one side of the tracheostomy tube. | |
| • Pull the other end of the tape securely through the slit end of the tracheostomy tube on the other side (Figure 11.11(c)). | |
| • Tie the tapes at the side of the neck in a square knot. | |
| • Alternate knot from side to side each time tapes are changed | Prevents irritation and aids in rotation of pressure site |
| • Ties should be tight enough to keep tube securely in the stoma, and loose enough to permit two fingers to fit between the tape and neck. | Excessive tightness compresses jugular veins, decreases blood circulation to the skin and results in discomfort for patient. |

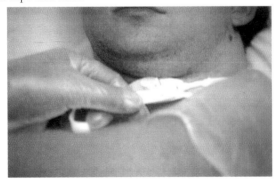

**Figure 11.11(c):** Changing tracheostomy ties/tapes

d. Remove old tapes carefully.

20. Document all relevant information in the chart
   • Suctioning done
   • Tracheostomy care carried out
   • Dressing change and
   • Observations

## SPECIAL CONSIDERATIONS

1. Tracheostomy dressing should be done every 8 hours or whenever dressings are soiled

2. Tracheostomy tubes may come with disposable inner cannula or without the inner cannula. If disposable inner cannula is present then replace the one that is inside with a new one.

3. If only single lumen is present, then suction the tracheostomy tube and clean the neck plate and tracheostomy site.

# 11.12: PERFORMING AN ENDOTRACHEAL/TRACHEAL SUCTIONING

## DEFINITION

Removal of secretions from tracheobronchial tree throught an endotracheal tube with the help of a mechanical suction device.

## PURPOSES

1. To maintain a patent airway by removing secretions
2. To prevent lower respiratory tract infection from retained secretions.

## ARTICLES

Assemble the following articles and obtain a pre-packaged suctioning kit:

A clean tray containing:

1. Sterile suction catheters with cover      No 12-16 Fr- adult
                                             No 8-10 Fr- child
2. Sterile water/ normal saline in a container
3. Sterile gloves
4. Mask
5. Face shield and gown if appropriate
6. Kidney tray
7. Alcohol swabs
8. Stethoscope

A sterile tray containing:

1. Sterile towel
2. Bowl
3. Gauze pieces

## ADDITIONAL ARTICLES

1. Resuscitation bag with a reservoir connected to 100% oxygen source.
2. Suction source - portable suction machine or wall suction unit.

## PROCEDURE

| | Nursing action | Rationale |
|---|---|---|
| 1 | Assess depth and rate of respiration, auscultate breath sounds. Monitor heart rate if patient is on continuous cardiac monitoring. If arterial blood gases are done routinely, check the baseline value. | Determines need for suctioning. |
| 2 | Explain the procedure and what the patient should be expecting during the procedure to the patient if conscious/relatives. | Thorough explanation lessens patient's anxiety and promotes cooperation. |
| 3 | Assist the patient to a semi-Fowlers or Fowlers position if conscious. An unconsiuous patient should be placed in the lateral position facing you. | Sitting position helps patient to cough and breath more easily. The position also uses gravity to aid in the insertion of catheter. Lateral position prevents the airway from becoming obstructed and promotes drainage of secretions. |
| 4 | Assemble equipment, check function of suction apparatus and manual resuscitation bag connected to 100% oxygen source | Make sure that all equipments are functional before sterile technique is instituted to prevent interruptions, use of 100% oxygen will help to prevent hypoxia |

*Contd...*

*Contd...*

| | | |
|---|---|---|
| 5 | Wear mask and wash hands thoroughly. | Prevents infection. |
| 6 | Open sterile tray. Take the towel and place in a bib like fashion on patient's chest. Open alcohol swab and place on corner of towel. Place small amount of sterile, water-soluble jelly on towel. | |
| 7 | Open sterile catheter pack and place catheter into sterile tray. Fill the bowl with sterile water. | |
| 8 | If the patient is on mechanical ventilator, make sure that disconnection of ventilator attachment may be made with one hand. | |
| 9 | Don sterile gloves. Designate one hand as clean hand for disconnecting, bagging and working the suction control. Usually the dominant hand is kept sterile and will be used to thread the suction catheter (Figure 11.12(a)). | The hand designated as sterile must remain uncontaminated so organisms are not introduced into the lungs. The other gloved hand protects the nurse from infection. |

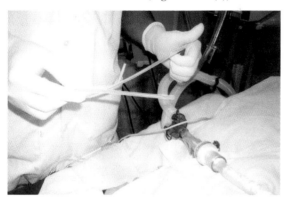

**Figure 11.12(a):** Dominant hand kept sterile to thread the catheter

| | | |
|---|---|---|
| 10 | Connect suction catheter to the suction source | |
| 11 | Using clean hand, disconnect the patient from ventilator, CPAP device or other oxygen source (Place the ventilator connector on the sterile towel and flip a corner of the towel over the connection to prevent fluid from spraying to the area | Prevents contamination of the connection |
| 12 | Ventilate and oxygenate the patient with the resuscitation bag, compressing firmly and as completely as possible approximately 4-5 times with clean hand. In spontaneously breathing patient, co-ordinate manual ventilations with the patient's own inspiratory effort. [when possible get a nurse or a respiratory therapist to do the bagging] | Ventilation before suctioning helps prevent hypoxia Attempting to ventilate against the patient's own respiratory efforts may result in high airway pressure, predisposing the patient to barotrauma |
| 13 | Lubricate the catheter by dipping it into the container of sterile saline/water (except silicon catheters). | Lubrication promotes easy insertion. Silicon catheters do not require lubrication. |
| 14 | Turn on suction source with clean hand. | |
| 15 | Pinch the catheter if there is no 'Y' port and insert it in tracheal/ endotracheal tube. Insert the catheter about 12.5 cm (5 inches) for adults, less for children or until the patient coughs or you feel resistance (Figure 11.12(b)). | Using suction while inserting catheter can cause trauma to mucosa and removes oxygen from the respiratory tract. Resistance usually means that the catheter tip has reached the carina. If resistance is felt, the catheter should be withdrawn 1-2 cm before applying suction |

*Contd...*

*Contd...*

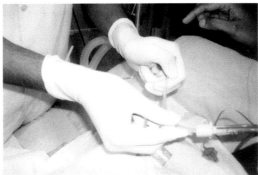

**Figure 11.12(b):** Pinching the catheter while inserting

| 16 | Apply suction by releasing thumb from Y port or by releasing the pinch on the catheter. Gently rotate catheter with thumb and index finger of sterile gloved hand as catheter is being withdrawn (Figure 11.12(c)) | Turning the catheter while withdrawing helps clean surface of respiratory tract and prevents injury to tracheal mucosa. |
|----|----|----|

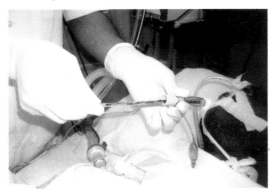

**Figure 11.12(c):** Endotracheal suctioning – Applying suction

| 17 | Apply suction for only a maximum of 10 seconds. Hyperventilate 3 to 5 times between suctioning or encourage patient to cough and deep breath between suctioning. | Suctioning for longer than 10 seconds may result in hypoxia. Hyperventilation reoxygenates the lungs |
|----|----|----|
| 18 | Rinse catheter between suction passes by inserting tip in cup of sterile water and apply suction. | Flushing cleans and clears catheter and lubricates it for next insertion. |
| 19 | Repeat suctioning as needed and according to patient's tolerance of procedure. Allow patient to take rest at least for one minute between suctioning and replace oxygen delivery set up if necessary. No more than four suction passes should be made per suctioning episode. | Allowing time interval and replacing oxygen delivery set up helps compensate for hypoxia induced by the previous suctioning. Irritation from multiple suctioning results in an increased amount of secretions. |
| 20 | When the airway becomes clear, return the patient to the ventilator or apply CPAP or other oxygen delivery devices. | |
| 21 | Suction oral secretions from the oropharynx. | Removes accumulated oral secretions. |
| 22 | When procedure is completed, turn off suction and disconnect catheter from suction tubing. Remove gloves inside out and dispose off gloves and catheter in proper receptacle. | Prevents transmission of microorganisms. |

*Contd...*

*Contd...*

| | | |
|---|---|---|
| 23 | Replace the articles, clean elbow fitting of resuscitation bag with alcohol; cover with a sterile glove or sterile 4 x 4 gauze and wash hands. | |
| 24 | Position patient comfortably. Auscultate over lung area. | Auscultation helps to determine whether respiratory passageways are cleared of secretions. |
| 25 | Record the time of suctioning and nature and amount of secretions. Also note the character of patient's respirations before and after suctioning. | Provides accurate documentation and provides for comprehensive care. |
| 26 | Perform oral hygiene procedure if required. | Respiratory secretions that accumulate are irritating to mucous membranes and unpleasant for the patient. |

## SPECIAL CONSIDERATIONS

1. The outer diameter of the suction catheter should be no greater than one half the inner diameter of the artificial airway
2. Suctioning should be discontinued and oxygen applied or manual ventilation reinstituted if during the suction procedure the heart rate decreases by 20 beats per minute or increases by 40 beats per minute or blood pressure drops, or cardiac dysrhythmia is noted. Suctioning may cause hypoxemia and vagal stimulation
3. Some clinicians believe that removal of secretions may be facilitated with saline instillation in endotracheal/tracheal tube which is followed by vigorous bagging.

**Table 11.12.1:** Amount of negative pressure necessary for suctioning

| | Portable suction machine | Wall suction unit |
|---|---|---|
| Adult | 8-15 mmHg | 100-120 mmHg |
| Children | 5-8 mmHg | 50-100 mmHg |
| Infants | 3-5 mmHg | 40-60 mmHg |

## 11.13: CONNECTING AND CHANGING INTERCOSTAL DRAINAGE (ICD) BOTTLES

### MEANING

It refers to the replacement of existing intercostal drainage bottle with a new one using aseptic technique.

### PURPOSE

1. To maintain and enable the system to continue functioning effectively.

### INDICATIONS

1. Disconnection of the tube
2. Broken container
3. To empty the bottle when it is full.

### ARTICLES

1. Clean trolley
2. Chest drainage bottle holder
3. Sterile chest drainage bottle with two way or three-way cork
4. Long and short tubes (plastic/glass)
5. Sterile water or sterile normal saline
6. Sterile pint measure (optional)
7. Clean clamps – 2 Nos (tips covered with rubber)
8. Sterile dressing set
9. Sterile gloves
10. Clean mask
11. Waterproof adhesive tape
12. Scissors
13. Receptacle for soiled disposable items.

### PROCEDURE

| | Nursing action | Rationale |
|---|---|---|
| 1. | Check physician's order and nursing care plan for specific instructions. | |
| 2. | Identify the patient and explain procedure to the patient and relatives. | Allays fear and gains patient's confidence and cooperation. |
| 3. | Monitor vital signs. | Provides baseline to compare with changes after procedure. |
| 4. | Assemble equipment. | Saves time and energy. |
| 5. | Provide privacy. | |
| 6. | Wash hands and don sterile gloves. | |
| 7. | Prepare chest drainage bottle<br>a. For one bottle system<br>• Open a sterile two-way bottle and add sterile water. Ensure that the distal end of the long tube is immersed in 2 to 3 cm of water. | The depth of tube submersion determines the amount of suction. |

*Contd...*

*Contd...*

- Mark the water level in the bottle
- Insert long and short tubes through the two-way cork into the bottle (Figure 11.13(a))

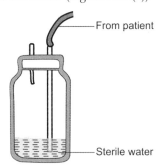

From patient

Sterile water

**Figure 11.13(a):** One bottle system

b. For two bottle system
In case of two-bottle system the first bottle is used to collect fluid and air from pleural space and the second bottle serves as water seal chamber (Figure 11.13(b)).
To change these bottles:
- Prepare the water seal chamber as mentioned above
- Prepare another empty, sterile, two-way bottle with two short tubes.
- Connect the two bottles as shown in Figure 11.13(b).

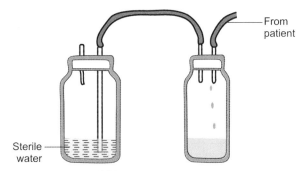

From patient

Sterile water

**Figure 11.13(b):** Two bottle system

c. Three bottle system
In case of three bottle system, the first bottle is used to collect fluid and air from pleural space, second bottle serves as water seal and the third bottle is to control the amount of suction applied (Figure 11.13 (c))
- Prepare the first and second bottles as in two bottle system
- Add 20 cm of sterile water in the third sterile bottle.
- Insert two short tubes and long tube through the three-way cork into the bottle
- Connect the bottles as shown in Figure 11.13(c).

*Contd...*

*Contd...*

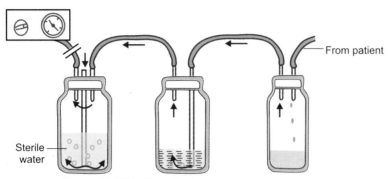

**Figure 11.13(c):** Three bottle system

| | | |
|---|---|---|
| 8. | Ensure that bottles are kept in the bottle holder. | Prevents risk of accidental breakage |
| 9. | Place the patient in a comfortable sitting position | Enables free access to the site. |
| 10. | Clamp the intercostal drainage tubing by using two clamps. One clamp is positioned 1 ½ to 2 ½ inches from insertion site and the second clamp is placed one inch down from the other one | Prevents air entering into pleural cavity. |
| 11. | Disconnect old bottle/bottles from the chest tube | |
| 12. | Reconnect new bottle/ bottles as shown in figure | |
| 13. | Maintain bottle /bottles at 0.5 – 1m below the patient's chest | Prevents water being sucked into the chest. |
| 14. | Release clamps from chest tube. | Prolonged clamping may lead to the development of tension pneumothorax. |
| 15. | Watch for repeated fluctuation in the water level in the distal end of chest tube (tidaling). | These fluctuations correspond to the patient's breathing and indicates that the system is patent. Absence of fluctuation indicates that the chest tube is blocked or the lung is re-expanded. This can be confirmed by percussion, auscultation and chest radiography. |
| 16. | Loosely fasten the chest drainage tube to patient's clothing. | Prevents dragging of the chest tube. |
| 17. | Position patient comfortably on the bed. | |
| 18. | Wash and dry hands. | Prevents transmission of infection. |
| 19. | Record procedure. | Acts as communication among staff members. |
| 20. | Continue monitoring the patient. | Helps to know the response to new system. |

## SPECIAL CONSIDERATIONS

1. Milking or stripping the chest tube is controversial as it may create excessive negative pressure, so it is not recommended nowadays.
2. Extra set of sterile containers and connection should always be available
3. Regular, frequent, staged coughing and deep breathing are important since they increase the intrapleural pressure and force air and fluid to drain out of the cavity and thus promoting lung expansion.
4. Drainage exceeding 100 ml/hour or a change in drainage to a bright red color, indicates fresh bleeding and requires immediate notification to the physician.
5. Always keep two clamps near bedside, to use in case of accidental disconnection or breakage of system.
6. In case of accidental breakage of bottles, the tubes should be immersed in a bottle with sterile saline or sterile water.
7. If there is accidental displacement of chest tubes, nurse should cover the site with a sterile Vaseline gauze pad.

## 11.14: ASSISTING WITH REMOVAL OF CHEST DRAINAGE TUBES

### DEFINITION

Removal of chest drainage tube in aseptic manner after full lung expansion has taken place .

### ARTICLES

1. Suture removal set
2. Dressing set
   * Petrolatum on a gauze piece
   * 4x4 gauze dressing
3. Clean tray with
   * Sterile disposable gloves
   * Chest tube clamp
   * Povidone iodine
   * Normal saline
   * Ether
   * Adhesive tape
   * Elastic bandage
   * Scissors
   * Kidney tray
4. Disposable waterproof absorbing pads.
5. Chest tube clamps.

### PROCEDURE

| | Nursing action | Rationale |
|---|---|---|
| 1. | Ensure that lung re-expansion is complete by noting the signs | |
| | a. Chest X-ray reveals total lung re-expansion | |
| | b. Water seal fluctuation has stopped for 24 hours | Pleura of the expanded lung seals the holes on the internal tip of the chest tube, halting fluctuation in the water seal. This can be expected 2-3 days after chest tube insertion. |
| | c. Drainage is decreased to less than 50 ml /day | Drainage has been reduced, allowing the lungs to re-expand |
| | d. Percussion reveals tympany | Normal percussion sound occurs with re-expansion |
| 2. | Clamp chest tube for 12 – 24 hours before removal or as ordered by the physician. Assess for changes in vital signs, chest pain and level of apprehension. | Physician orders tube clamping before removal to assess patient's tolerance. |
| 3. | Explain procedure to patient. | Reduces anxiety and promotes patient's co-operation. |
| 4. | Administer prescribed medication for pain relief about 30 minutes before procedure. | Reduces discomfort and relaxes patient. |
| 5. | Assist patient to sit on edge of bed or to lie on the unattached side. | Physician prescribes patient's position to facilitate tube removal. |
| 6. | Support patient physically and emotionally while physician removes dressing and clips or sutures. | Reduces anxiety and promotes co-operation. |
| 7. | Physician prepares an occlusive dressing of petroleum gauze on a pressure dressing and sets it aside on a sterile field. | Essential to prepare in advance for quick application to the wound upon tube withdrawal. |

*Contd...*

*Contd...*

| | | |
|---|---|---|
| 8. | Tell the patient to take a deep breath and hold it or exhale completely and hold it. | Prevents air from being sucked into chest as the tube is removed. |
| 9. | Physician quickly pulls out the chest tube while patient is holding his breath. | Prevents entry of air through the chest wound. |
| 10. | Quickly apply prepared dressing over the wound and firmly secure it in position with elastic bandage. | Keeps wound aseptic. Prevents entry of air into the chest. Wound closure occurs spontaneously. Clips or sutures aid in skin closure. |
| 11. | Assist patient to a comfortable position. | Assures that the patient is comfortable. |
| 12. | Remove used equipment from bedside with gloved hands. | Prevents spread of microorganisms. |
| 13. | Remove gloves and wash hands. | Reduces transmission of microorganism. |
| 14. | Observe patient for subcutaneous emphysema or respiratory distress during the first few hours after the removal | Provides for early notification of physician if adverse symptoms occur. Chest tube may need to be re-inserted. |
| 15. | Assess patient's vital signs and psychological status. | Detects early signs and symptoms of complications |
| 16. | Check chest dressing for drainage. | Assures occlusion of chest wound. |
| 17. | Record removal of tube, the amount of drainage in the collection bottle, appearance of wound and of dressing and patient's response. Patient's response also should include vital signs and respiratory assessment. | Documents procedure and status of wound and dressing. Documents patient's response |
| 18. | Obtain a chest X-ray if advised by physician. | |

## FOLLOW-UP ACTIVITIES

Notify physician immediately of respiratory distress, unstable vital signs, symptoms of subcutaneous emphysema, air leaks or psychological imbalances if observed.

## SPECIAL CONSIDERATION

When viewing chest X-ray immediately after tube removal, the chest tube tract may still be visible.

## 11.15: PERFORMING GASTRIC SUCTIONING

### DEFINITION

Removal of stomach contents through a nasogastric tub by aspiration using low suction.

### PURPOSES

1. To relieve abdominal distention
2. To maintain gastric decompression after surgery
3. To remove blood and secretions from the gastrointestinal tract
4. To remove contents of the stomach
5. To prepare the patient for general anaesthesia and gastric surgery
6. To aid in healing of the wound in case of surgery of the stomach and intestines.

### ARTICLES

1. Gastrointestinal tube (Ryle's tube) in place
2. Kidney tray for drainage from stomach
3. 20 cc syringe
4. Gauze pieces
5. Disposable gloves
6. Towel/non-absorbent pad
7. Pint measure
8. Basin with water

### PROCEDURE

| | Nursing action | Rationale |
|---|---|---|
| 1 | Explain procedure to patient. | Helps in obtaining co-operation of patient. |
| 2 | Position patient in semi fowler's position. | Prevents reflux of gastric contents and risk of aspiration. |
| 3 | Lower side rails on your side, spread non-absorbent pad near head end. | Provides easy access. Prevents soiling of bed linen. |
| 4 | Wash hands and don gloves. | Prevents transmission of microorganisms. |
| 5 | Remove cap from distal end of Ryle's tube and attach 20 cc syringe to the end by holding it with a gauze piece. | |
| 6 | Aspirate the stomach contents gently. | Facilitates removal of stomach contents using low suction. |
| 7 | As the syringe is filled with contents pinch the Ryle's tube disconnect the syringe from tube and empty contents into kidney tray. | Pinching the Ryle's tube prevents air entering into stomach. |
| 8 | Continue aspirating till all stomach contents are aspirated. | |
| 9 | Disconnect syringe and clamp the Ryle's tube. Rinse the syringe in a basin of water. | |
| 10 | Measure the amount of contents aspirated using a pint measure. | Amount of aspirate has to be included in 24 hrs output. |
| 11 | Discard the aspirated contents and wash the pint measure. Discard the non absorbent pad. | |
| 12 | Remove gloves and wash hands. | Prevents transmission of microorganisms. |

*Contd...*

*Contd...*

| | | |
|---|---|---|
| 13 | Assist patient for a mouth wash. | Provides a sense of well being for patient. |
| 14 | Document the colour, odour and quantity of contents aspirated. If necessary send sample to lab. | Helps communicating patient information with other health team members. |
| 15 | Include the amount of contents aspirated in Intake-output chart. | |

## SPECIAL CONSIDERATIONS

1. Only low pressure suction ( using 20 ml syringe) is used to aspirate stomach contents because an excessive negative pressure might cause the mucosa to be sucked in and can cause resultant damage to the stomach mucosa.
2. Adequate fluids should be administered by means of intravenous fluids for patient on gastric suction. This helps to prevent dehydration and maintain fluid and electrolyte balance.
3. Nasogastric tube should be irrigated frequently using normal saline to maintain its patency.
4. If continuous drainage of stomach contents is adviced by surgeon after GI surgeries, the Ryle's tube should be connected to an extension tube and the distal end of tube should be placed in a receptable which is kept at a level lower than the stomach. This achieves drainage of stomach contents by gravity.

# 11.16: ASSISTING WITH UPPER GASTROINTESTINAL FIBEROSCOPY (UPPER G.I SERIES/OGD SCOPY)

## DEFINITION

Visualization of esophagus, stomach and duodenum by a flexible endoscope that permits biopsy, cytology, pictures and video documentation (Figure 11.16(a)).

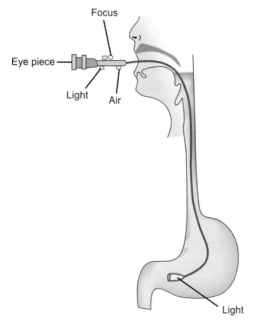

**Figure 11.16(a):** Fiberoptic scope *in situ*

## PURPOSES

1. To perform biopsy/cytologic study
2. To remove polyps and foreign bodies
3. To control bleeding
4. To open strictures.

## INDICATIONS

1. Chronic GI bleeding
2. Pernicious anemia
3. Esophageal injury
4. Masses in GI tract
5. Strictures
6. Dysphagia
7. Substernal pain
8. Epigastric discomfort
9. Neoplasms
10. Ulcer in upper GI tract
11. Esophageal and gastric varices
12. Gastroesophageal reflux disease.

## ARTICLES

1. Endoscopy tray/trolley
2. Suction equipment
3. Resuscitation equipment
4. Mouth guard
5. Drugs as prescribed, syringes and needles
6. Adhesive tape
7. Lubricant jelly
8. Gloves, gown and mask
9. Specimen containers
10. Slides.

## PROCEDURES

| | Nursing action | Rationale |
|---|---|---|
| 1 | Explain procedure to the patient. | Allays anxiety and helps in obtaining cooperation. |
| 2 | Get informed consent from patient. | Avoids medical legalities. |
| 3 | Keep patient NPO for 8–12 hours. | Prevents aspiration of stomach contents into lungs and allows for complete visualization of stomach. |
| 4 | Assess the oral cavity and report any lesions or loose tooth. If dentures are present, remove it. | Dentures may cause obstruction during procedure and removal of dentures facilitates passing the scope and preventing injury. |
| 5 | Spray the throat with local anaesthetic. | Suppresses gag reflex. |
| 6 | Intravenous sedative may be given. | Provides sedation and relieves anxiety during procedure. |
| 7 | Give injection atropine if ordered. | Reduces secretions. |
| 8 | Position patient in left lateral during procedure. | Left lateral position facilitates drainage of saliva and provides easy access for endoscope. |
| 9 | Lubricate the endoscope with water soluble jelly | Makes insertion easy and avoids friction. |
| 10 | Explain that room will be cool and dark and the patient will not be able to speak when the scope is in place. | Allows patient to have realistic anticipation and reduces anxiety. |
| 11 | Place mackintosh below head and neck of patient. | Protects bed linen from soiling. |
| 12 | Place mouth guard in place. | Prevents patient from biting on scope. |
| 13 | Instruct patient to swallow while endoscope is being advanced. Once inserted, instruct patient that he will not be able to swallow, talk or move the tongue. | |
| 14 | Suction out and examine secretions from oral cavity as necessary. | Prevents risk of aspiration. |
| 15 | Monitor vital signs and oxygen saturation throughout the procedure. | Helps in early identification of complication if any. |

## POSTPROCEDURAL CARE

| | | |
|---|---|---|
| 1 | Place the patient in Sim's position. | Prevents aspiration due to anesthetic effect. |
| 2 | After the procedure continue NPO status until gag reflex returns. | |
| 3 | Provide lozenges or normal saline gargles. | Eases throat irritation and hoarseness. |

*Contd...*

*Contd...*

| | | |
|---|---|---|
| 4 | Assess for signs of esophageal or gastric perforation. | Detects any complication if it occurs. |
| 5 | Provide complete bedrest for one hour. | Promotes comfort of patient. |
| 6 | Monitor patient for abdominal or chest pain, cervical pain, hemetemesis, malena, distended abdomen, fever, light headedness and firm distended abdomen. | Indicates complications |
| 7 | Monitor vital signs every 30 minutes for 3-4 hours and keep the patient in bed with side rails up. | |
| 8 | Record the procedure in nurse's record including timing of the procedure, tolerance and patient's reaction. | Gives information about the effectiveness of the procedure and any complications if it occurs. |

## COMPLICATIONS

1. Perforation of esophagus or stomach
2. Pulmonary aspiration
3. Hemorrhage
4. Respiratory depression
5. Infection
6. Cardiac arrhythmia.

## 11. 17: PREPARATION OF AND ASSISTING WITH COLONOSCOPY

### DEFINITION

Colonoscopy is the visual examination of the lining of rectum, colon and distal small bowel using a long flexible fibreoptic endoscope.

### PURPOSES

1. To evaluate active or occult lower intestinal bleeding.
2. To identify abnormalities found on radiographic examination.
3. To diagnose suspected caecal or ascending colonic diseases, anemia, cancer and inflammatory bowel diseases.

### ARTICLES

1. Light source
2. Endoscope
3. Suction apparatus
4. Lubricant
5. Topical anesthetic agent
6. Endoscopic accessories such as biopsy forceps, polypectomy snares, cytology brush
7. Dilatation devices.
8. Medications as prescribed by physician
9. Bicap Heater
10. Probe and hot biopsy forceps
11. Cardiac monitor
12. Oxygen source.

### GENERAL INSTRUCTION

Fluid and electrolyte status of elderly patients and those with renal or cardiac disease to be considered during bowel preparation.

### PROCEDURE

| | Nursing action | Rationale |
|---|---|---|
| 1 | Explain procedure to patient that carbon dioxide will be introduced into the colon and he may experience discomfort or abdominal cramps during procedure. | Allays anxiety and helps in obtaining co-operation of patient. |
| 2 | Get informed consent from the patient. | Prevents legal problems. |
| 3 | Keep patient on low residue diet for 3 days before procedure and NPO for 8 hours prior to the procedure. | |
| 4 | Administer laxatives 1-3 days before and cleansing enema the night before the procedure. | |
| 5 | Provide colonic wash using formula of salts like sodium sulphate and polyethelyne glycol that is dissolved in 5 liters of water and administer on the previous evening around 9PM. 2.5 litres of solution is to be administered on the morning of the day of the test between 5 am-8 am. | |

*Contd...*

*Contd...*

| | | |
|---|---|---|
| 6 | Advise patient to take clear fluids like glucose water or coconut water along with prepared solution on the day of procedure. | |
| 7 | Avoid premedication unless patient is apprehensive and anxious. Administer sedatives if ordered. | |
| 8 | Make patient to lie in left lateral position with lower limbs flexed at hip and knee and buttocks at table edge. | Helps in insertion of colonoscope into the rectum. |
| 9 | Lubricate the colonoscope and assist doctor in inserting the colonoscope. | Lubrication avoids friction and helps in easy insertion. |
| 10 | Instruct patient to take deep slow breaths while scope is being inserted. | |
| 11 | Apply pressure to areas of abdomen as directed by physician as he passes scope through splenic flexure, ascending colon and caecum. | |
| 12 | Monitor vital signs, color, warmth, dryness of skin, abdominal distention, level of consciousness and pain tolerance. | |
| 13 | Explain to patient that he may experience abdominal cramps during procedure | Abdominal cramps may be caused by stimulation of peristalsis and inflation with air. |
| 14 | Label and transport specimens to the lab that may be collected. | |
| 15 | Record the procedure in the nurses record. | |

## POSTPROCEDURE CARE

1. Monitor and document vital signs every 15 minutes for first hour and then every 30 minutes for 2 hours.
2. Observe signs of complications like rectal bleeding, vomiting severe and persistent abdominal pain, distention, rigidity, malaise, tenesmus, etc. which are indications of perforation.
3. Document time of procedure and patient's response.
4. Provide calm enviornment and make patient comfortable.

## SPECIAL CONSIDERATION

Patient may experience flatulence or gas pains because gas was used to distend the intenstine for better visibility.

# 11.18: ASSISTING WITH LIVER BIOPSY

## DEFINITION

Assisting in sampling of liver tissue by needle aspiration using aseptic technique.

## PURPOSE

To diagnose liver disease through histologic study.

## TYPES OF BIOPSY

A. Open biopsy.
B. Closed biopsy.

### OPEN BIOPSY

An open biopsy necessitates a general anesthetic and a major abdominal incision. It is not usually done unless abdomen is opened for a surgical reason.

*Advantages*

1. Direct observation of entire liver.
2. Identifies grossly altered tissue.
3. Removes the biopsy specimen for study.

### CLOSED BIOPSY (PERCUTANEOUS LIVER BIOPSY)

It is usual in current practice. It is performed under fluoroscopy and is a simpler procedure than open biopsy.

*Contraindications for Percutaneous Liver Biopsy*

1. Severe thrombocytopenia
2. Local infection of the lung base.
3. Prolonged prothrombin time or any other known bleeding disorder
4. Peritonitis
5. Massive ascites
6. Uncooperative client.
7. Extrahepatic obstructive jaundice, especially with an enlarged gallbladder.

## ARTICLES

A sterile tray containing:
1. Sponge holding forceps.
2. Syringe 5 ml with needles to give local anesthesia.
3. Liver biopsy needles with stiletts (Vim silverman or Menghini biopsy needle.)
4. Specimen bottles with cork.
5. Bowl to take cleaning lotion.
6. Aspiration syringe, if aspiration biopsy is to be done.
7. Dissecting forceps.
8. Dressing towels or slit towel.
9. Cotton balls, gauzepieces and cotton pads.
10. Gown, gloves and masks.

Clean tray containing:
1. Mackintosh and towel
2. Kidney tray and paperbag
3. Spirit, iodine, tincture benzoin, etc.
4. Lignocaine 2%
5. Apron
6. Adhesive plaster and scissors.
7. Formalin 10% to preserve the biopsy specimen.

## PROCEDURE

| | Nursing action | Rationale |
|---|---|---|
| 1 | Explain the procedure to patient and family and inform him how he has to cooperate. | Helps in obtaining cooperation of patient and reduces anxiety. |
| 2 | Obtain informed consent from patient | Prevents litigation to the staff members. |
| 3 | Ensure that patient's coagulation profile are in normal limits. | Prevents bleeding complication during procedure. |
| 4 | Check baseline vital signs and record. | Helps in obtains baseline data. |
| 5 | Instruct patient to be NPO for 6-8 hours before procedure. | Prevents risk of aspiration during procedure. |
| 6 | Administer premedication (analgesia, sedation) as per physician's instruction. | |
| 7 | Instruct patient to refrain from ingesting aspirin, NSAID or anticoagulants 2 weeks before procedure. | Prevents bleeding tendencies. |
| 8 | Make the patient to lie down in supine position or in left lateral position with right arm elevated. | This position helps for easy insertion of needle. |
| 9 | Shave and clean the eigth and ninth intercostal space at the incision site. | |
| 10 | Instruct patient to take several deep breaths and to hold the breath while the needle is introduced through the intercostal or subcostal tissues into the liver. | Avoids puncturing of the diaphragm. |
| 11 | The special needle assembly is rotated to separate a fragment of tissue and then is withdrawn | |
| 12 | Assist physcian to seal puncture site with tincture benzoin and apply pressure dressing. | |
| 13 | Collect the specimen in a sterile container, label it and send to laboratory. | |
| 14 | Instruct patient to lie on his right side. | |
| 15 | Record the procedure with date, time-method used and complications if any. | Acts as a communication between staff members. |

## POSTPROCEDURE CARE

1. Monitor vital signs every 15 minutes for 2 hours, and every 60 minutes for 4 hours.
2. Assess for tachycardia and decreasing blood pressure which may indicate hemorrhage.
3. Check the puncture site by monitoring the dressing, palpating the surrounding area for crepitus and observing for hematoma formation.
4. Observe for pain in the right upper quadrant of the abdomen caused by a subscapular accumulation of blood or bile, or at the right shoulder as a result of blood on the undersurface of the diaphragm.

5. Maintain the client on bedrest in right lateral position for 24 hours following procedure to reduce the risk of hemorrhage and bile leakage.
6. Administer postprocedure medications on an individual basis, depending on the client's physical status.
7. Give vitamin K if prescribed.
8. Assess respiratory status for manifestations of dyspnea.
9. Check abdominal girth every hour for first 12 hours.

**Table 11.18.1:** Complications after liver biopsy

| Immediate complications | Late complications |
|---|---|
| Pallor | Hemorrhage |
| Sweating | Shock and collapse |
| Restlessness | Bile peritonitis |
| Rising pulse rate | |
| Abdominal pain | |
| Pneumothorax | |
| Injury to the stomach, pancreas, small and large intestines, kidney, inferior vena cava and diaphragm. | |

## 11.19: GIVING A GASTRIC LAVAGE OR STOMACH WASH

## DEFINITION

Washing out of stomach with a solution using a lavage set.

## PURPOSES

1. To obtain samples of gastric contents for laboratory studies.
2. To relieve nausea and vomiting in case of acute dilatation of stomach, pyloric stenosis and intestinal obstruction
3. To reduce gastric bleeding.
4. To cleanse the stomach as a preparation for surgery
5. To remove poisonous or irritating substances from stomach.

## ARTICLES

1. Ryle's tube of appropriate size (12 –14 fr)
2. Bowl of water/normal saline/or specific solution ordered
3. Pint measure
4. Water soluble lubricant/Vaseline
5. A funnel to attach to the NG tube
6. Stethoscope
7. Kidney tray
8. Towel
9. Small mackintosh
10. Clean gloves
11. Apron
12. Mask
13. Adhesive plaster and scissors
14. Bucket/container for return flow
15. Syringe
16. Mouth gag.

## SOLUTIONS USED

1. Plain water (plain water is particularly useful when the poison is unidentified)
2. Normal saline
3. Weak solution of sodium bicarbonate or boric acid in corrosive poisoning.
4. Specific antidotes: if ingested poison is identified.

## PROCEDURE

| | Nursing action | Rationale |
|---|---|---|
| 1. | Identify patient and check the chart for physician's order and any specific instruction. | Ensures performance of correct procedure for the right patient. |
| 2. | Explain procedure to the patient | Helps in gaining co-operation of the patient |
| 3. | Wash hands and don gloves | Reduces risk of contamination. |
| 4. | Remove dentures if present and insert a mouth gag | Dentures may cause obstruction, and mouth gag is inserted to prevent biting of the tube. |
| 5. | Place patient in left lateral position | Prevents aspiration of fluid into the lungs. |

*Contd...*

# Clinical Nursing Procedures: The Art of Nursing Practice

*Contd...*

| | | |
|---|---|---|
| 6. | Pass lubricated nasogastric tube slowly and gently to prevent trauma to the tissues. | Lubricating the tube makes insertion easy and prevents friction. |
| 7. | Ensure proper placement of tube. | |
| 8. | Secure the tube with adhesive tape. | Prevents displacement of the tube. |
| 9. | Attach the syringe to the tube and aspirate the gastric contents completely and save it for laboratory analysis | |
| 10. | Remove the syringe and attach a funnel to the tube and fill the funnel with irrigating fluid. Raise the funnel to allow fluid to run into the stomach. Allow 2-3 funnels of fluid (150 – 200 ml) to flow into the stomach. | Ice cold water is used for irrigation when bleeding is present. |
| 11 | When 2 – 3 funnels of fluid have run into the stomach and before the funnel is completely empty, pinch the tube, wait for one minute and invert the funnel over a receptacle and allow the fluid to siphon back/aspirate using 50 cc syringe. | 200 ml of fluid is to be introduced at a time to reach all parts of the stomach and inversion of funnel helps in return flow of fluid from stomach. |
| 12. | In case of GI bleeding, if blood increases in the outflow, stop the procedure and inform the physician. | Prevents further complications. |
| 13. | During, the procedure observe the patient's vital signs and degree of consciousness every 15 minutes. | Monitors any deterioration in condition of patient. |
| 14. | Lavaging usually requires a total volume of at least 2 liters. | Some clinicians advocate use of 5-10 liters of solution. |
| 15. | Discontinue the treatment, by pinching the tube and pulling it out quickly. | Prevents entry of air into the stomach. |
| 16. | Leave the stomach empty at the completion of lavage. | |
| 17. | Remove gloves and wash hands. | |
| 18. | Give a mouthwash and dry the face. | Patient feels comfortable. |
| 19. | Replace articles, record the treatment with date, time, amount of solution used, character of return flow and condition of patient before, during and after the procedure. | These give detailed information about the procedure and patient's response to the procedure. |
| 20. | Continue to monitor the patient every 25 to 30 minutes as dictated by his/her condition. Check vital sign, breathing pattern, nausea and abdominal distention. | Identifies complication at an early stage. |

# 11.20: ASSISTING WITH INSERTION OF SENGSTAKEN BLAKEMORE TUBE/BALLOON TAMPONADE

## DEFINITION

Assisting in insertion of Sengstaken Blakemore tube or minnesota balloon which exerts pressure directly on bleeding sites in esophagus stomach.

### TYPES OF TUBES USED FOR TAMPONADE AND THEIR PARTS

1. Sengstaken blakemore tube
   a. Esophageal balloon
   b. Gastric balloon
   c. Gastric aspiration port
2. Minnesota balloon
   a. Esophageal balloon
   b. Gastric balloon
   c. Gastric aspiration port
   d. Esophageal aspiration port.

## PURPOSE

To arrest acute bleeding from esophageal varices and stomach.

## ARTICLES

1. Sengstakenblakemore tube (Figure 11.20(a))
2. Curved artery forceps, tips protected with rubber tubing
3. Lubricant
4. Adhesive
5. Syringes
6. Gloves
7. Vaseline gauze
8. Basin with icechips
9. Towel and emesis basin
10. Device to apply traction (optional)
11. Large scissors (for emergency deflation)
12. Manometer (to measure balloon pressure)

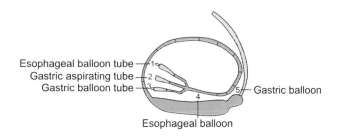

**Figure 11.20(a):** Sengstaken Blakemore tube

## PROCEDURE

| | Nursing action | Rationale |
|---|---|---|
| 1. | Explain procedure and give psychologial support to the patient. | Allays anxiety and helps in obtaining cooperation of the patient. |
| 2. | Elevate head of bed slightly unless the patient is in shock. | |
| 3. | Check balloon by trial inflation to detect leaks. | This is best done under water because it is easier to see escaping of air bubbles. |
| 4. | Chill the tube then lubricate it before the physician passes it via mouth or nose. | Chilling makes the tube more firm and lubrication lessens friction. |
| 5. | Provide the patient with a few sips of water. | This will help in passage of the tube more easily. |
| 6. | Verify placement of tube in stomach by irrigating the gastric tube with air while auscultating over the stomach. | It is imperative that the tube is in the stomach so that the gastric tube is not inflated in the esophagus. |
| 7 | Obtain an X-ray film of the lower chest and upper abdomen to verify placement of tube in the stomach. Inflate gastric balloon with air and gently pull tube back to seat balloon against gastroesophageal junction. | Exerts presence against cardiac sphincter. |
| 8 | Clamp gastric balloon tube and mark tube location at nares. | Prevents air leakage and tube migration. The mark on the tube allows easy visualization of movement of the tube |
| 9 | Apply gentle traction to the balloon tube and secure it with a foam rubber cube at the nares. | Prevents the tube from migrating with peristalsis and assists in exerting adequate pressure. |
| 10 | Attach Y-connector to esophageal balloon opening Attach syringe to one arm of the 'Y' connector and manometer to the other. Inflate esophageal balloon to 25-35 mmHg pressure (Figure 11.20(b)). Clamp esophageal balloon. | Maintains enough pressure to temponade bleeding while preventing esophageal necrosis |

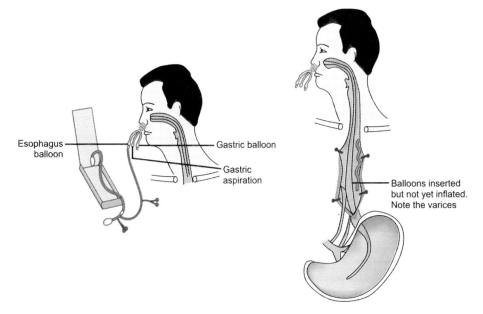

**Figure 11.20(b):** Sengstaken Blakemore tube *in situ*

*Contd...*

*Contd...*

| | | |
|---|---|---|
| 11 | Apply suction to gastric aspiration port and irrigate at least hourly. | Suctioning and irrigating the tube can remove old blood from the stomach and prevent hepatic encephalopathy and allows monitoring of bleeding status. |
| 12 | Insert a nasogastric tube, positioning it above the esophageal balloon and attach to suction . If using a Minnesota tube attach fourth port (esophageal suction port), to suction | Nasogastric tube serves to check for bleeding and suctions saliva accumulated above the esophageal balloon. |
| 13 | a. Label each port<br>b. Tape scissors at head of bed | Prevents accidental deflation or irrigation<br>Airway occlusion may occur if the esophageal balloon is pulled into the hypopharynx. If this occurs the esophageal balloon tube must be cut and removed immediately. |

## SPECIAL CONSIDERATIONS

1. Maintain constant vigilance while balloons are inflated in the patient.
2. Keep balloon pressures at required level to control bleeding.
3. Observe and record vital signs, monitor color and amount of nasogastric lavage fluid for evidence of bleeding.
4. Be alert for chest pain which may indicate injury or rupture of esophagus.
5. Irrigate suction tube as prescribed, observe and record nature and color of aspirated material.
6. Keep head of bed elevated to avoid gastric regurgitation and to diminish nausea and a sensation of gagging.
7. Maintain nutritional and electrolyte level parenterally.
8. Note nature of breathing, if counter weight pulls the tube into oropharynx, the patient may be asphyxiated.

# 11.21: ASSISTING WITH ENDOSCOPIC RETROGRADE CHOLANGIOPANCREATOGRAPHY(ERCP)

## DEFINITION

Endoscopic visualization of the common bile, pancreatic and hepatic ducts with a flexible fiberoptic endoscope inserted into esophagus passed through the stomach and duodenum and into common bile duct and pancreatic duct (Figure 11.21(a)).

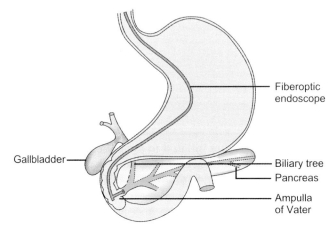

**Figure 11.21(a):** Fiberoptic endoscope inserted into duodenum

## PURPOSES

1. To diagnose obstruction in cholangiopancreatic tree.
2. To detect extrahepatic biliary obstruction.
3. To diagnose pancreatic disease.
4. To determine nature and level of pathology in biliary obstruction.
5. To evaluate pre- and post-operative conditions of obstructions.

## ARTICLES

1. Side viewing duodenoscope
2. ERCP catheters
3. X-ray compatible table
4. Contrast medium.

## PROCEDURE

| | Nursing action | Rationale |
|---|---|---|
| 1. | Explain procedure to the patient and confirm that an informed consent has been taken from the patient. Also explain to him how he has to cooperate. | Allays anxiety and helps in obtaining cooperation of patient. |
| 2. | Assess for any allergies to Iodine and seafood | Contrast medium usually contain iodine. |
| 3. | Explain to the patient that he will experience a flushing sensation during administration of contrast medium. | Prepares patient for the procedure. |
| 4. | Instruct patient to be NPO at least 4-6 hours before the procedure | Prevents aspiration during procedure. |

*Contd...*

*Contd...*

| | | |
|---|---|---|
| 5. | Ensure that artificial dentures are removed. | Prevents possibility of loose dentures obstructing airway. |
| 6. | Monitor vital signs and observe level of consciousness and tolerance to procedure. | Obtains baseline data for comparison in future. |
| 7. | Administer antibiotics as ordered. | Acts as a prophylaxis against postprocedural infection. |
| 8. | Administer sedatives, glucagon or anti-cholinergics as ordered. | Glucagon stops duodenal peristalsis. Anticholinergics reduce secretions. Sedatives reduce anxiety and help in relaxation of patient. |
| 9. | Spray throat with Xylocaine or instruct patient to gargle and swallow topical anesthetic agent. | Decreases gag reflex. |
| 10. | Place the patient in left semi propped position and multiple position changes are required during the procedure. | Enables easy passage of the endoscope and enables effective radiographic visualization. |
| 11 | Observe patient for any adverse effects of medication administered like respiratory depression, central nervous system depression, hypotension, vomiting, etc. Monitor IV fluids administered during procedure and help in changing position as required. | Sedatives may induce side effects like respiratory depression, central nervous depression, hypotension, vomiting, etc. Position changes may be required for radiographic visualization. |
| 12. | Record events of emesis, respiratory distress, vasovagal reaction or diaphoresis. | |
| 13. | Document all drugs administrated, stents placed and biopsies taken in nurses record. | Promotes communication among health care workers. |
| 14. | Record fluids administered, techniques used, and patient's condition at the end of the procedure. | Helps to identify patients tolerance to the procedure. |

## POSTPROCEDURAL CARE

1. Monitor vital signs and level of consciousness.
2. Position patient to prevent aspiration and transport to recovery area
3. Observe and report abdominal distention and signs of perforation, gastrointestinal bleeding or signs of possible pancreatitis including chills, fever, pain, vomiting, tachycardia and notify physician immediately.
4. Maintain NPO status until gag reflex returns. Check for gag reflex by applying gentle pressure using a tongue depressor placed on the back of the tongue.
5. Give verbal and written instructions to patient or relatives regarding diet, medications, activities and possible complications.
6. Instruct the patient to drink ample amount of fluid after administration of the dye.
7. Warn the patient that there may be some discomfort with urination while the dye is excreted.

## COMPLICATIONS

1. Pancreatitis.
2. Pleural effusion.
3. Gastrointestinal bleeding due to cervical perforation, esophageal perforation.

## SPECIAL CONSIDERATIONS

1. Cervical perforation would be exhibited by neck or throat pain, feeling of pressure, dysphagia or crepitus around the neck area
2. Epigastric or shoulder pain could be the result of esophageal perforation
3. Evaluate for cyanosis, dyspnea and pleural effusion-as a result of perforation affecting the respiratory system.

# 11: 22: ASSISTING IN ABDOMINAL PARACENTESIS

## PARACENTESIS

### DEFINITION

Paracentesis is the removal of fluid from peritoneal cavity through a small puncture made through the abdominal wall under sterile conditions (Figure 11.22(a)).

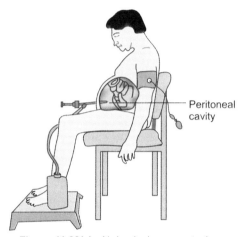

**Figure 11.22(a):** Abdominal paracentesis

## PURPOSES

1. To relieve pressure on the abdominal and chest organs due to ascites.
2. To study chemical, bacteriological and cellular composition of peritoneal fluid for diagnosis of disease.
3. To drain exudate in peritonitis.
4. To prepare for procedures like peritoneal dialysis.

## ARTICLES

A sterile tray containing (abdominal tapping set):
1. Sponge holding forceps.
2. 5 ml syringe with needle.
3. 20 ml syringe with Leur-Lock
4. Three-way adaptor and tubing
5. Trocar and cannula or aspiration needles.
6. BP handle with blade (optional)
7. Suturing needles (if incision is made)
8. Dissecting forceps.
9. Specimen bottles.
10. Sterile dressing articles.
11. Artery clamp
12. Surgical towel (4).

A clean tray containing:
1. Makintosh and towel.
2. Kidney tray and paper bag
3. Spirit, iodine, tincture benzoin.
4. Lignocaine 2%

5. Apron
6. Drainage receptacle
7. Pint measure
8. Measuring tape
9. IV set
10. IV bottle
11. Gloves, gown and mask.

## OTHER ARTICLES

1. Back rest
2. Low stool
3. Additional pillows.

## PROCEDURE

| | Nursing activity | Rationale |
|---|---|---|
| 1 | Identify the patient and explain the procedure to the patient and relatives. | Wins confidence and co-operation from patient. |
| 2 | Measure abdominal girth and weight of the patient. | Provides base line data. |
| 3 | Obtain informed consent. | Avoids legal problems. |
| 4 | Instruct the patient to void 5 min before the procedure. | Prevents risk of injury to bladder. |
| 5 | Bring the patient to the edge of bed. Place him in Fowler's position/Assist him to sitting position in a chair with legs supported. | Promotes good body mechanics and Fowler's position helps in shifting fluid down. |
| 6 | Place sphygmomanometer cuff around patient's arm to monitor BP during the procedure. | Hypotension. |
| 7 | Wash hands and put on gloves | Prevents transmission of infection. |
| 8 | Clean the area with antiseptic solution and assist the physician to administer local anesthesia. Drape patient with sterile towels | Reduces risk of infections. |
| 9 | Assist the physician in inserting trocar and cannula into the abdomen below the umbilicus. Remove the trocar and attach the cannula to the tubing which reaches the receptacle which is placed on a low stool. | The greater the vertical distance between the needle and receptacle the greater will be the pull on the fluid thus the cavity is drained more quickly and the patient may go into a state of shock. |
| 10 | Collect specimen in sterile bottles | |
| 11 | After enough fluid is withdrawn (1-2 liter )remove the cannula and place a tincture benzoin seal, sterile dressing and pressure bandage over puncture site. | Pressure dressing and bandage helps to prevent leakage of fluid. |
| 12 | Check the patient's general condition after procedure. Vital signs are checked every 15 min for 2 hrs: then 30 mins for 2 hrs. Examine the dressing for any leakage. | |
| 13 | Measure and describe the fluid collected and send the specimen to laboratory with labels and requisition form. | To rule out bacteriological and chemical composition of fluid and to diagnose the disease. |
| 14 | Record the procedure, date, time, amount of fluid collected, nature of fluid, color and general condition of patient during and after procedure. Include amount of fluid tapped in patients 24 hrs output. | |
| 15 | Clean all articles used. Wash with soapy water, rinse and dry it. Send for autoclaving. | Prevents cross infections. |

# 11.23: ASSISTING WITH ENDOSCOPIC SCLEROTHERAPY

## DEFINITION

Injection of a sclerosing agent through a fibreoptic endoscope into the bleeding esophageal varices to promote thrombosis.

## PURPOSES

1. To treat patient with acutely bleeding varices.
2. To treat patient who had bleeding from varices in the past and continues to have varices.
3. To treat patient with portal hypertension.

## CONTRAINDICATIONS

1. Hemoglobin less than 8 gm%
2. Uncooperative patient with severe coagulopathy
3. Acute myocardial infarction with arrhythmias
4. Encephalopathy
5. Acute respiratory distress
6. Shock.

## ARTICLES

1. Gastroscope with large biopsy channel
2. Sclerosing agent-Ethanolamine oleate, alcohol, sodium tetradecyl sulfate, methylene blue
3. Injector/needle
4. Emergency resuscitation equipments and drugs.

## PROCEDURE

| | Nursing action | Rationale |
|---|---|---|
| 1 | Identify the method of endoscopy to be performed. (involving upper gastrointestinal tract or lower intestinal tract) | |
| 2. | Explain procedure to the patient and obtain informed consent. Provide instruction to patient about preprocedural care depending on method of performing endoscopy. | Helps in obtaining cooperation of patient. |
| 3 | Identify any contraindication to the procedure and review physician's order for preprocedure medication. | |
| 4 | Instruct patient <br> • To remain NPO on the night before the procedure if sclerotherapy is done on upper gastro intestinal tract. | Prevents risk of aspiration. |
| 5 | Ensure that bowel preparation is done in case of patients posted for sclerotherapy for hemorrhoids in the lower gastrointestinal tract. | Ensures good visualization of varices. |
| 6. | Place the patient in left lateral position/Sim's position as per requirement. | Position helps in insertion of endoscope. |
| 7. | Place mouth guard if method involves upper gastrointestinal tract. | Ensures that patient does not bite on the scope. |

*Contd...*

*Contd...*

| | |
|---|---|
| 8. | Assist doctor to pass endoscope into the gastrointestinal tract to look for evidence of pathology. |
| 9. | Assist in introducing needle and injecting sclerosing agent. (Figure 11.23(a)) |

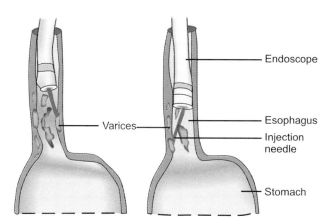

**Figure 11.23(a):** Injecting sclerosing agent in endoscopic sclerotherapy

| | | |
|---|---|---|
| 10. | Ensure patient's comfort and monitor for complication before shifting to day care unit. | Identifies complication that may occur during the early stage following procedure. |
| 11 | Record the procedure and care given in the nurse's record. | Documentation helps in continuity of care. |
| 12 | Transfer the patient to day care unit when stable. | |

## POSTPROCEDURAL CARE

1. Patient should be closely monitored in daycare area for at least 2 hours, till vital signs are stable.
2. Watch for signs and symptoms of bleeding.
3. Allow fluid after 1-2 hours.
4. Watch for complications like chest pain, dysphagia, fever, bleeding, stricture esophagus, and perforation.
5. Provide quiet environment and keep patient comfortable.
6. Record about starvation, time of sending patient to endoscopy room and time of receiving in recovery area.

## 11.24: PREPARATION OF PATIENT AND ASSISTING WITH CYSTOSCOPY

### DEFINITION

Cystoscopy is a method of direct visualization of the urethra and bladder by means of a cystoscope that is inserted through the urethra into the bladder (Figure 11.24(a)).

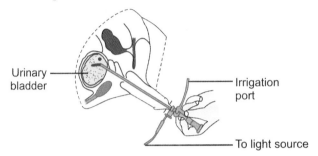

Urinary bladder

Irrigation port

To light source

**Figure 11.24(a):** Cystoscopic examination of the bladder

### PURPOSES

1. To inspect bladder wall directly for tumor, stone or ulcer.
2. To inspect urethra for abnormalities.
3. To allow insertion of urethral catheters for radiographic studies.
4. Prior to renal/genitourinary surgery.
5. To see configuration and position of ureteral orifices.
6. To remove calculi from ureter and bladder.
7. To diagnose and treat lesions of bladder, urethra and prostate.
8. To measure bladder capacity and look for evidence of vesicoureteral reflux.
9. To take biopsy from bladder and urethra.
10. To fulgurate bleeding areas in the bladder.
11. To implant radium seeds.
12. To dilate bladder in case of interstitial cystitis.

### ARTICLES

1. Sterile fiberoptic cystoscope
2. Irrigation solution –normal saline
3. Dressing pack
4. Cleaning solution
5. Draping set (leg draping)
6. Specimen container
7. Sterile gloves
8. Mask
9. Apron
10. Local anesthetic agent like lignocaine jelly
11. Syringes 20 ml (2).

### PREPROCEDURAL PREPARATION

1. Patient should be NPO for 6-8 hrs prior to the procedure if procedure is planned under general anesthesia or spinal anesthesia.

2. Encourage lots of fluids if procedure is planned under local anesthesia.
3. Perform bowel preparation on the evening before test.
4. Explain procedure and obtain informed consent.
5. Ask patient to empty bladder before sending to OT. Initiate IV access.
6. Administer prescribed pre-medications.
7. Send patient with records to OT.

## PROCEDURE

|   | Nursing action | Rationale |
|---|----------------|-----------|
| 1 | Receive patient with appropriate records. | Helps in confirming identity of patient and in obtaining information on the test to be done. |
| 2 | Position patient in lithotomy. | Helps in visualization of urethra. |
| 3 | Clean the genitalia with an antiseptic solution before procedure. | Prevents entry of infection. |
| 4 | Local anesthetic gel is instilled into urethra before insertion of cystoscope. | Reduces pain and discomfort. |
| 5 | Instruct patient to lie still and take deep breaths and relax. | Prevents trauma. |
| 6 | Ensure that the irrigation system is ready. | Saves time, energy and efforts. |
| 7 | Ensure that IV fluids are on flow. | Ensures that a good flow of urine is present at the time of procedure. |
| 8 | Reassure and comfort patient during insertion and examination with cystoscope as it is painful. Inform patient that he may experience an urge to void during insertion. | |
| 9 | Send specimens collected to laboratory with proper labels. | |
| 10 | Wash cystoscope with antiseptic solution and replace articles. | |
| 11 | Document time, findings, specimen collected and patient's response. | Helps in communication between staff members. |

## POSTPROCEDURAL CARE

1. Advise patient to be on bedrest for 4-6 hours.
2. Instruct patient to avoid standing immediately after procedure as it may cause syncope and dizziness.
3. Inform patient that pink colored urine is common, but report to the physician if bleeding and clots are present.
4. Instruct patient to expect back pain, bladder spasms and burning micturition during the initial period.
5. Administer or teach self-administration of antibiotics prophylactically as ordered to prevent urinary tract infection.
6. Advise warm sitzbath or analgesics to relieve discomfort after cystoscopy.
7. Provide routine catheter care if an indwelling catheter is present.
8. Encourage fluid intake and monitor intake and output.

## COMPLICATIONS

1. Bleeding due to trauma.
2. Perforation of the bladder.
3. Urinary tract infection.
4. Strictures (late complications).

# 11.25: ASSISTING WITH INTRAVENOUS PYELOGRAPHY

## DEFINITION

Intravenous pyleography is the roentgenographic visualization of the kidneys, ureters and bladder after injecting a dye into the vascular system.

## PURPOSES

1. To evaluate suspected cysts, tumors, tuberculosis, pyelonephritis, hydronephrosis, vesicoureteral reflux, hypertension and urinary tract calculi.
2. To evaluate the extent of renal injury.
3. To evaluate any renal condition in infants where cystoscopy may be unduly traumatic.
4. To assess congenital anomalies.
5. To assess renal function.

## CONTRAINDICATIONS

1. Hypersensitivity or allergy to iodine preparations.
2. Combined renal and hepatic disease.
3. Renal failure.
4. Patients receiving drug therapy for bronchiolitis and asthma.
5. Congestive cardiac failure.
6. Uncontrolled diabetes.
7. Multiple myeloma.

## PROCEDURE

| | Nursing action | Rationale |
|---|---|---|
| 1. | Explain procedure to the patient | Helps in reducing anxiety and obtaining cooperation of the patient. |
| 2. | Obtain informed consent from the patient | Prevents legalities to the medical staff. |
| 3. | Arrange for a preliminary X-ray (KUB) with the patient in supine position | Ensures that the bowel is empty. Visualizes the location of kidneys. |
| 4. | Assess the patient for allergic reactions to the dye | Prevents allergic reactions during procedure. |
| 5. | Instruct the patient to abstain from all food, liquid and medications for 12 hours before examination. | Dehydration is necessary for contrast material to concentrate in the urinary tract. |
| 6. | Ensure that bowel and bladder are emptied. | Provides clear visualization of the parts. |
| 7. | Explain to patient that there may be sensations of flushing warmth and salty taste in mouth, during dye injection. | Reassures the patient. |
| 8. | Emergency drugs and equipment should be kept ready during procedure. | Prepares to deal with possible complications. |
| 9. | Contrast medium is injected by physician and rapid films are taken at intervals of 6 minutes, 15 minutes, 1 hour, 2 hours and 6 hours after injecting dye. | |
| 10. | Arrange for postvoid film to be taken after 6 hours. | Checks clearance of dye. |
| 11. | Record the date, time and patients' response to procedure. | Helps in communication among health team members. |

## POSTPROCEDURE CARE

1. Advise patient to resume prescribed diet and activity after the examination.
2. Encourage patient to drink sufficient amount of water.
3. Instruct patient to take adequate rest.
4. Observe and document any mild reactions to the iodine material which may include fever, skin rashes, nausea and swelling of the parotid glands.

## 11.26: ASSISTING WITH RENAL BIOPSY

## DEFINITION

Assisting with insertion of a percutaneous needle under ultrasound guidance to obtain a biopsy specimen from kidney.

## PURPOSES

1.  To diagnose cause of glomerulonephritis.
2.  To diagnose renal malignancy.
3.  Prior to renal transplantation.
4.  To evaluate rejection response in renal transplant patient.
5.  To determine prognosis of renal disease.

## CONTRAINDICATIONS

1.  Single functioning kidney
2.  Malignant tumors
3.  Hydronephrosis
4.  Pregnancy
5.  Coagulation disorders.

## ARTICLES

### KIDNEY BIOPSY SET CONTAINING

1.  Artery clamp
2.  Surgical towels-2
3.  Gallipot with cotton balls
4.  Kidney tray
5.  Sterile trucut needle (biopsy needle)
6.  Scalpel blade 3/11 with holder
7.  Slit towel.

### A CLEAN TRAY CONTAINING

1.  5 cc syringe
2.  Disposable needles 22G (1), 20G (2)
3.  Iodine, spirit or other antiseptic solution
4.  2% Xylocaine
5.  Sandbag or firm pillow
6.  Broad adhesive
7.  Gloves (2 pairs)
8.  10% Formalin in small bottle
9.  0.9% Saline
10. Disposable plastic aprons
11. "Sharps" container
12. Urine specimen containers (3)

## OTHER ARTICLES

Portable USG machine.

# PROCEDURE

| | Nursing action | Rationale |
|---|---|---|
| 1 | Explain procedure and obtain consent. | Promotes patient co-operation and prevents legalities. |
| 2 | Ensure that X-ray films, IVP results and bleeding parameters are available before procedure. | Obtains baseline data to determine treatment guidelines. |
| 3 | Assemble equipment on trolley in treatment room. | Saves time, material and energy. |
| 4 | Assist patient to lie in prone position and place sandbag or firm pillow under abdomen. | Provides access to biopsy site. |
| 5 | Physician locates the position of kidney under USG guidance and the site is marked. | |
| 6 | Assist in administering local anesthetic to the patient. | |
| 7 | Assist in making small stab incision through skin and inserting biopsy needle. | |
| 8 | Ask patient to take a deep breath and to hold it while biopsy is being taken. | Avoids chances of injury to adjacent organs. |
| 9 | Reassure patient while physician removes needle and applies pressure bandages. | Pressure over incision site prevents bleeding. |
| 10 | Turn patient to supine position slowly and make him comfortable. | |
| 11 | Preserve biopsy specimen in formalin bottle, place label and send to laboratory. | |
| 12 | Replace equipment. | |
| 13 | Document time of biopsy, success of procedure, patient condition and vital signs. | |

# POSTPROCEDURAL CARE

1. After half an hour transfer patient from treatment room to bed or stretcher.
2. Explain to patient about strict bedrest for 24 hours and the need to avoid coughing or sneezing.
3. Check vital signs, BP, pulse and respiratory rate every 15 minutes for first hour; every ½ an hour for next two hours and every hour for next 3 hours.
4. Instruct patient to drink at least 2000-3000 ml of fluid in next few hours.
5. Give 3 small labelled bottles to collect first 3 urine specimens.
6. Inform doctor in case of hematuria, drop in blood pressure, rise in pulse rate, abdominal pain and any unusual symptoms.
7. Check biopsy site for bleeding. Assess for tightness of adhesive and do the needful.

# 11.27: ASSESSMENT OF CONSCIOUSNESS USING GLASGOW COMA SCALE (GCS)

## DEFINITION

Glasgow coma scale is a standardized scoring system used to assess level of consciousness in a patient with altered level of consiousness. GCS is a numeric expression of cognition, behavior and neurological function.

## PURPOSES

1. To monitor patient with suspected or confirmed head injury.
2. To monitor level of consciousness in any patient who has altered sensorium.

## ARTICLES

1. Glasgow coma scale proforma.
2. Knee hammer, pen and flashlight.

## PROCEDURE

| | Nursing action | Rationale |
|---|---|---|
| 1 | Explain procedure to the patient. | Unconscious patient may retain ability to hear. |
| 2 | Keep patient in comfortable position. | |
| 3 | Score responses in Glasgow coma scale sheets. | |
| 4 | Add total score at bottom of sheet during each assessment. | |
| 5 | Assess pupils, limb movements and vital signs for completion of procedure. | |
| 6 | Document accurately and report changes if any. | |

Table 11.27.1: Assessment guide to Glasgow Coma Scale

| | Category of response | Appropriate stimulus | Response | Score |
|---|---|---|---|---|
| I | Eye opening | • Approach to bedside<br>• Verbal command<br>• Pain | • Spontaneous response<br>• Opening of eyes to name or command.<br>• Lack of opening of eye to previous stimuli but opening to pain<br>• Lack of opening eyes to any stimulus<br>• Untestable | 4<br>3<br><br>2<br>1<br>U |
| II | Verbal response | • Verbal questioning with maximum arousal | • Appropriate orientation conversant, correct identification of self, place, year, and month<br>• Confusion, conversant but disorientation in one or more spheres.<br>• Inappropriate or disorganized use of words, lack of substained conversation.<br>• Incomprehensive words, sounds<br>• Lack of sound, even with painful stimuli<br>• Untestable | 5<br><br>4<br><br>3<br><br>2<br>1<br>U |
| III | Best motor response | • Verbal command<br>• Pain (pressure on (proximal nailbed) | • Obedience of command<br>• Localization of pain, lack of obedience but presence of attempts to remove offending stimulus<br>• Flexion withdrawal, flexion of arm in response to pain without abnormal flexion posture | 6<br>5<br><br>4 |

*Contd...*

*Contd...*

| | |
|---|---|
| • Abnormal flexion, flexing of arm at elbow and pronation, making a fist | 3 |
| • Abnormal extension, extension of arm at elbow usually with adduction and internal rotation of arm at shoulder | 2 |
| • Lack of response | 1 |
| • Untestable | U |

Minimum score ——3
Maximum score——15
Score less than 8 indicates coma

# 11: 28: PREPARATION OF PATIENT AND ASSISTING WITH ELECTROENCEPHALOGRAPHY (EEG)

## DEFINITION

Recording of electrical activity of the brain, using multiple electrodes on the scalp. Brain waves may be recorded at rest, after hyperventilation, with photic stimulation and during sleep.

## PURPOSES

To assess and diagnose
1. Seizures
2. Brain tumors
3. Brain abscess
4. Subdural hematomas
5. Cerebral infarcts
6. Intracranial hemorrhage
7. Alzheimer's disease
8. Brain death
9. Metabolic disorders
10. Mental retardation
11. Drug overdose.

## PROCEDURE: THE PROCEDURE IS PERFORMED IN A SPECIAL UNIT

| | Nursing action | Rationale |
|---|---|---|
| 1 | Explain procedure to the patient and instruct that no shock will be applied and it is a painless procedure. | Helps in obtaining cooperation of the patient. |
| 2 | Obtain an informed consent. | Protects staff and instituion from legalities. |
| 3 | Withhold medications such as anticonvulsants, stimulants, tranquilizers and depressants for 24-48 hours before the procedure. | This may alter the brainwave activity. |
| 4 | Withhold tea, cola and chocolates before procedure. Smoking should be restricted 24 hours before the procedure. | These products may stimulate brain activity. |
| 5 | Wash patient's hair thoroughly with shampoo and dry hair completely about 6 hours prior to procedure. Tell patient not to apply conditioners or oil after shampooing. | Oil interferes with the conduction of electrical activity. |
| 6 | If sleep study is ordered, the adult patient should sleep as little as possible the night before. | Induces sleep to the patient during the test. |
| 7 | Foods should not be withheld. | Decrease in blood glucose level interferes with brain activity. |
| 8 | Make the patient to lie in a recumbent position and fasten electrodes, contaning conduction gel to the scalp with a special glue or paste. | Conduction gel enhances effective electrical conduction. |
| 9 | Instruct patient to lie still during procedure. | Movement may affect the recording . |
| 10 | After the procedure is done, record the procedure in nurses record with date, time and patient's response to the procedure. | |

## POSTPROCEDURE CARE

1. Allow the patient to rest after the test. If a sedative was given during the test, raise bedside rails.
2. Tell patient that skin irritation from the electrodes usually disappears within few hours .
3. Wash hair after the test.
4. If a repeat testing is necessary, provide explanation and support to the patient.
5. Watch for seizures.
6. Obtain fresh order to resume drugs if they were withheld for procedure.

# 11: 29: PREPARATION OF A PATIENT FOR ELECTROMYOGRAPHY (EMG)

## DEFINITION

Electromyography is the recording of electrical potential of skeletal muscles and the nerves supplying them by inserting small needle electrodes into the muscles.

## INDICATIONS

1. To diagnose myasthenia gravis and myotonia.
2. To find out peripheral nerve injury or disease.
3. To differentiate among lesions of the anterior horn cell, root, plexus and specific nerves and muscles.
4. To measure conduction velocity of nerves.
5. To aid in differential diagnosis of primary and secondary muscle disorder such as motor neuron diseases and neurovascular junction disorders.
6. To localize the site of peripheral nerve disorders such as radiculopathy and axonopathy.

## INTERFERING FACTORS

1. Conduction can vary with age and normally decreases with increasing age.
2. Pain can yield false results.
3. Electrical activity from extraneous persons and objects can produce false results.
4. The test is ineffective in the presence of edema, hemorrhage or thick subcutaneous fat.

## PROCEDURE

The procedure is performed in a special unit.

| | Nursing action | Rationale |
|---|---|---|
| 1 | Explain procedure to the patient and instruct him how to cooperate. | Helps in obtaining cooperation of patient. |
| 2 | Tell the patient to lie down supine in the bed. | Promotes comfort of the patient. |
| 3 | Explain to patient that he may experience discomfort during insertion of needle electrode and there may be hematoma formation after removal of needle. | Reduces patient anxiety. |
| 4 | Obtain informed consent and ascertain whether patient is on anticoagulants. | Prevents risk for developing hematoma. |
| 5 | A needle is attached to an electrode and inserted into the muscle. A mild electric charge is delivered to stimulate the muscle at rest and during voluntary contraction. The response of muscle is measured on an oscilloscope screen. The electrode usually causes no pain unless the tip is near a terminal nerve. Ten or more needle insertions may be necessary. | The needle electrode detects electrical potential normally present in muscle. |
| 6 | The nurse and physician observe oscilloscope for normal waveform and listen for normal quiet sound at rest. A "machine gun popping" sound or a rattling sound like hail on a tin roof is normally heard when the patient contracts the muscle. | Identifies muscle activity. |
| 7 | Instruct patient that the test may take more than 3 hours. | The length of test depends upon the clinical problem. |
| 8 | Record the time and date of the procedure with patient's response. | Documentation helps in communication with other staff members. |

## OSTPROCEDURAL CARE

1. If the patient experiences pain, administer analgesics as per physician's order.
2. Promote rest and relaxation.
3. Interpret test results and monitor appropriately for nerve and muscle diseases.
4. Observe needle sites for hematoma formation.

## SPECIAL CONSIDERATIONS

1. Enzyme levels that reflect muscle activity (e.g. aspartate aminotransferase, lactate dehydrogenase, creatinine phosphokinase) must be determined before actual testing because the EMG causes elevation of these enzymes for up to 10 days postprocedure.
2. There may be hematoma formation at the needle site. Measures such as application of pressure at the site, controls bleeding.
3. During insertion of needle if patient complaints of pain, remove the needle because the pain stimulus yields false results.

# 11: 30: PREPARATION FOR SKULL AND SPINE X-RAYS

## DEFINITION

Preparing for radiological study taken at different planes and angles of skull, and various regions of spine (e.g. cervical, thoracic, lumbar, sacral).

## PURPOSES

### I. SKULL X-RAY

To furnish information about:
1. Presence of skull fracture
2. Position of pineal body
3. Unusual calcification
4. Size and shape of skull bones
5. Bone erosion
6. Abnormal vascularity.

### II SPINE X-RAY

To diagnose the following conditions:
1. Wedging of collapsed vertebra
2. Erosion of bone caused by neoplasm
3. Irregular calcification as a result of inflammatory process.
4. Narrowing of vertebral canal because of obstruction by neoplasm or protruding disk
5. Vertebral fractures and dislocations
6. Spondylosis
7. Spurs
8. Bony projections
9. Trauma to vertebral column.

## PROCEDURE

| | Nursing action | Rationale |
|---|---|---|
| 1 | Explain procedure to patient. | Helps in cooperation of patient. |
| 2 | Remove jewellery, dentures, hairclips, and glasses. | Presence of these articles interferes with procedure. |
| 3 | Send patient to X-ray department in wheelchair or stretcher with the case sheet and requisition form. | |
| 4 | Record in chart about the timing, patient was sent to X-ray department. | |
| 5 | After receiving patient back in ward, record time of arrival and X-ray taken. | |

# 11.31: ASSISTING WITH COMPUTERIZED AXIAL TOMOGRAPHY SCAN PROCEDURE

## DEFINITION

Obtaining a computerized image that reproduces the desired section of brain or spinal cord. The CAT scan becomes an invasive procedure when radiopaque dye is injected into peripheral vein to give a contrast scan.

## PURPOSES

To locate and diagnose various cranial lesions like:
a. Abscess
b. Cyst
c. Tumor
d. Infarction
e. Hematoma
f. Aneurysms
g. Contusion
h. Hydrocephalus.

## CONTRAINDICATIONS

1. Pregnancy
2. Renal failure.

## PROCEDURE

| | Nursing action | Rationale |
|---|---|---|
| 1. | Assess patient's knowledge and explain procedure to patient and instruct him how he has to cooperate. | Helps in obtaining cooperation of patient. |
| 2. | Determine if patient is allergic to dye. | Detects allergic reaction if contrast dye is used. |
| 3. | Get informed consent from patient. | Prevents risk of legalities. |
| 4. | Remove metal objects such as hair clips, dentures, etc. | Metal objects block body structures and will show upon X-ray film. |
| 5. | Keep the patient NPO for 4 hours before study. | Iodine dye may induce nausea. |
| 6. | Assist patient into desired position on examining table. | Proper position is necessary to obtain good films. |
| 7 | Instruct patient not to move, talk or sigh as the films are taken. | Movement causes computer generated artifacts on image produced. |
| 8 | X-ray beams pass through the body area from one side to other through 180 degree arc. | Multiple tomographic X-rays taken in successive layers provide three dimensional view of selected organ. |
| 9 | Iodinated dye is administered thorough peripheral IV line usually started in arm. | Dye enhances contrast and provides improved visualization. |
| 10 | Observe patient for signs of anaphylaxis. Signs include respiratory distress palpitation, itching and diaphoresis. | |
| 11 | X-ray procedure is repeated as necessary. | |
| 12 | Determine if patient feels back pain. | Results from lying on hard examining table. |
| 13 | Record in the nurse's note the time and part of the body where scan was performed. | Provides documentation of procedure in record. |
| 14 | Report duration of procedure and patient's tolerance to nurse in charge and to next shift staff. | Assures prompt follow-up. |

## FOLLOW UP ACTIVITIES

1. Assist patient in assuming comfortable position after scan
2. Provide meal for patient
3. Check with physician regarding test result.

## SPECIAL CONSIDERATIONS

1. Tell patient that " clicking" noise will be heard as scanner moves around and he will not be able to feel scanner rotating. Give cotton balls to plug the ears to avoid hearing sounds produced by scanner.
2. Encourage fluids for patient who received dye injection as dye is excreted through kidneys .

# 11.32: ASSISTING IN MAGNETIC RESONANCE IMAGING SCAN (MRI)

## DEFINITION

Magnetic resonance imaging is a non-invasive scanning technique that provides visualization of internal organs and structures by means of magnetic forces rather than by ionizing radiation.

## PURPOSES

1. To diagnose pathologic lesions in organs or tissues.
2. To provide contrast between normal and pathologic tissues.
3. To distinguish white from gray matter and to identify conditions such as
   - Necrotic tissue
   - Oxygen deprived tissue
   - Small malignancies
   - Degenerative disease of central nervous system
   - Cerebral and spinal cord edema
   - Hemorrhage
   - Congenital anomalies.

## CONTRAINDICATIONS

1. Implanted devices such as heart valves, surgical and aneurysm clips, plates, internal orthopedic screws and rods, pacemakers, etc.
2. Prosthetic devices
3. Respirators
4. Pregnancy
5. Patient with epilepsy.

## PROCEDURE

| | Nursing action | Rationale |
|---|---|---|
| 1. | Explain procedure to the patient and inform him what he has to expect during the course of procedure. | Helps in obtaining cooperation of patient. |
| 2. | Assess whether patient has signed informed consent form. | Minimizes institutions' legal risk. |
| 3. | Assess patient's weight. | Procedure is contraindicated in patients with over 300 pounds body weight. |
| 4. | Assess patient for any contraindication. | Procedure is contraindicated as the magnet may cause movement of metal or electric objects inside the body. |
| 5. | Assess patient for claustrophobia. | Sedation may be needed in case of these patients or if severe claustrophobia, procedure may be contra-indicated. |
| 6. | Assess patient's ability to remain still throughout the procedure. | Any movement may produce artifacts. Patients must remain still for 30-90 minutes. |
| 7 | Assess for allergies to dye and contrast medium. | Avoids anaphylactic reaction. |
| 8 | Tell the patient to empty bladder before procedure. | Helps in non-interruption of procedure. |
| 9 | Remove all metallic objects from patient such as watch, jewellery, coins, keys, hairpins, credit cards and dentures containing metals. | Metallic objects will create artifacts on the scan and some metal objects may be damaged by the magnetic field. |

*Contd...*

*Contd...*

| 10 | Assist patient onto padded table and position comfortably. | Provides for correct positioning and for patient's comfort. |
|----|---|---|
| 11 | Place special helmet around head if it is to be scanned and secure patient on table with velcro straps. | Allow for accurate imaging and helps to keep patient from moving during procedure. |
| 12 | Provide patient with ear plugs and intercom or ear phones. | Decreases sound of images and allows for communication between patient and technologist. |
| 13 | After examination, assist patient to sitting and then to standing positions slowly. | Decreases possibility of orthostatic hypotension. |
| 14 | Evaluate patients' status after procedure. | Verifies patient's comfort after procedure. |
| 15 | Record in patient's chart time and site where MRI was performed. If contrast medium was used record patient's tolerance of procedure. | Provides documentation of procedure in record. |
| 16 | Report duration of procedure and patient's response to nurse incharge. | Ensures follow-up. |

## SPECIAL CONSIDERATIONS

1. Certain types of eye make up and permanent eyeliners that contain metallic fragments cause discomfort during MRI
2. Common metallic equipment such as scissors, oxygen tanks and electronic devices can become lethal projectiles when exposed to strong magnetic fields. Therefore, a thorough screening of all visitors and staff is mandatory, before entering the room.

# 11.33: ASSISTING WITH LUMBAR PUNCTURE

## DEFINITION

Lumbar puncture is the insertion of a needle into the lumbar subarachnoid space to withdraw cerebrospinal fluid.

## PURPOSES

1. To administer spinal anesthesia before surgery.
2. To administer medication into spinal canal in case of meningitis.
3. To reduce intracranial pressure.
4. To perform diagnostic studies, e.g. Myelogram
5. To detect subarachnoid block.

## CONTRAINDICATIONS

1. Suspected epidural infection
2. Severe psychiatric/neurotic problems.
3. Chronic backache
4. Intracranial bleeding.

## ARTICLES

A sterile tray containing (LP set)
1. LP needle with stillette
2. Sponge holding forceps.
3. Small bowls
4. Specimen bottles
5. Cotton balls, gauze pieces, cotton pads, etc.
6. Dressing articles.

A clean tray containing:
1. Mackintosh and towel
2. Kidney tray/paper bag
3. Spirit, iodine, tincture benzoin
4. Lignocaine 2%
5. Sterile normal saline
6. Adhesive plaster and scissors
7. Sterile gloves, gown and mask.
8. 3 way adapter, manometer and tubing
9. Syringe and needle for local anesthesia.

## PROCEDURE

|   | Nursing action | Rationale |
|---|----------------|-----------|
| 1 | Identify the patient and explain the procedure to him. | Relieves anxiety and fear. |
| 2 | Instruct the patient to void before the procedure. | Ensures that patient is comfortable. |
| 3 | Instruct the patient not to make any movement during the procedure. | Movement during procedure causes injury to the spinal cord and its nerves. |
| 4 | Check BP pulse and respiration of patient. | Helps in obtaining a base line data. |

*Contd...*

*Contd...*

| | | |
|---|---|---|
| 5 | Position the patient on one side at the edge of the bed, with back towards the physician. Thighs and legs are flexed as much as possible (C-shaped position). The head and neck are flexed and brought towards chest. Keep hands between knees (Figure 11.33(a)). | Flexion of thighs and legs increases the space between vertebrae and facilitates easy entry of needle into sub arachnoid space. |

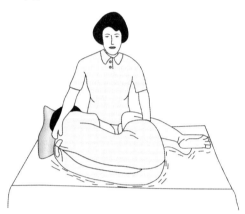

Figure 11.33(a): Positioning patient for lumbar puncture

| | | |
|---|---|---|
| 6 | Keep a pillow under the head and between the legs of patient | Pillow under the head maintains the spine in a horizontal position. Pillow under legs prevents the upper leg from rolling forward. |
| 7 | Encourage the patient to relax and breath normally during procedures. Remind patient that he should not talk. | Hyperventilation may cause an error in pressure reading. |
| 8 | Fold back the upper garments above the waist line and the lower garments below the hip exposing the site. | Avoids over exposure of the patient. |
| 9 | Assist the physician in cleaning the puncture site with antiseptic solution and injecting local anesthetic. | Prevents risk of infection. |
| 10 | Spinal needle is inserted into the subarachnoid space by physician through the 3rd, 4th and 5th lumbar intercostal space (Figure 11.33(b)). | |

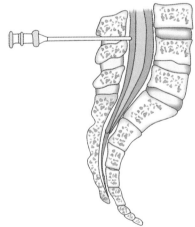

Figure 11.33(b): Spinal needle inserted into subarachnoid space

*Contd...*

*Contd...*

| | | |
|---|---|---|
| 11 | Physician removes the stilette and connects three-way adaptor with manometer filled with normal saline. | Obtains CSF pressure. Normal pressure is 6-13 mm of mercury or 80-180 cm of water |
| 12 | Collect CSF specimen into 3 specimen bottles after measuring pressure. | |
| 13 | Needle is withdrawn by physician. | |
| 14 | Assist physician in sealing the puncture site with tincture benzoin and apply sterile dressing. | Dressing protects and prevents leakage of CSF from puncture site. |
| 15 | Instruct the patient to be flat for 12-24 hours. | Decreases CSF pressure in the caudal area where the needle insertion occurred and decreases the risk of leakage. |
| 16 | Monitor for complications of lumbar puncture. Check vital signs every half an hour for 3-4 hrs till stable. | Postlumbar headache may appear a few hours to several days after procedure. |
| 17 | Check puncture site frequently for CSF leakage | |
| 18 | Encourage patient to take more fluids after the procedure. | Reduces the risk of postlumbar headache by re-establishing the CSF volume. |
| 19 | Record the procedure with date, time, CSF pressure, amount drawn, color, nature of cerebrospinal fluid and general condition of patient during and after the procedure. | |
| 20 | Send the specimen to the laboratory with proper labels and requisition forms. | Detects chemical, bacteriological and cellular composition of CSF and diagnose the disease. |
| 21 | If no complications are observed give upright position to the patient after 24 hours. | |

## SPECIAL CONSIDERATIONS

1. Monitor for neurological changes such as change in the level of consciousness, pupil size, numbness and tingling or pain in the legs or lower back, during and after the procedure.
2. If spinal headache is present, instruct patient to
   a. Increase fluid intake
   b. Avoid aspirin and caffeine
   c. Keep lights dim in the patient's room
   d. Avoid excessive stimulation
   e. Avoid Valsalva maneuver
   f. Administer pain medications
   g. Maintain flat position for 12-24 hours without pillows.
3. Once needle enters subarachnoid space, help patient to slowly straighten legs to reduce false recording of increased intracranial pressure, increased muscle tension and compression may elevate pressure recording.
4. If pressure reading is not required after introduction of the needle into the subarachnoid space, the CSF specimen is taken. In this case, the three-way adapter and manometer tubing is not required.

## COMPLICATIONS

1. CSF leakage
2. Infection
3. Postpuncture headache
4. Paralysis
5. Hematoma.

# 11.34: ASSISTING WITH BONE MARROW ASPIRATION AND BIOPSY

## DEFINITION

Assisting in obtaining a sample of bone marrow aspirated from sternum/ileum/ tibia using aseptic technique (Figure 11.34(a))

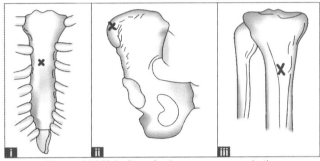

**Figure 11.34(a):** Sites for bone marrow aspiration

## PURPOSES

1. To diagnose hematological disorders.
2. To follow course of disease and patient's response to treatment.
3. To diagnose diseases such as primary metastatic tumors, infectious diseases and certain granulomas.
4. To isolate bacteria and other pathogens by culture.

## ARTICLES

Trolley with:
1. 5 cc syringe
2. Needles (no 22. 20)
3. Sterile gloves
4. Small bottle with FAA solution (Formalin, Alcohol, Actic acid)
5. Culture tubes
6. Slides
7. Mackintosh and draw sheet
8. Razor set
9. Adhesive tape and scissors
10. Tincture benzoin solution
11. Kidney tray.

Sterile pack containing:
1. Towels
2. Dissecting forceps
3. Cups with cotton balls and gauze pieces
4. Scalpel blade and handle
5. Artery forceps (2)
6. 20 cc glass syringe
7. Bone marrow aspiration needle
8. Sterile drapes.

## CONTRAINDICATION

1. Coagulation defect.

# PROCEDURE

| Nursing action | Rationale |
|---|---|
| 1 Check the physician's order and nursing care plan and investigation reports like coagulation studies. | Obtains specific information/instructions. |
| 2. Ascertain that consent has been duly signed and fully understood by the patient. | Fulfills legal requirements and hospital policies. |
| 3. Identify the patient. | Ensures performance of right procedure on right patient. |
| 4. Explain procedure to patient and ensure that pain medication is given. | Allays fear and gains patient's confidence and co-operation. |
| 5. Collect and assemble equipment. | |
| 6. Ensure privacy. | Avoids unnecessary embarrassment to the patient during the procedure. |
| 7. Help patient into correct position<br>  a. Supine for sternal puncture<br>  b. Lateral position with upper knee flexed for iliac crest puncture. | |
| 8. Open small dressing pack and put sterile slide, syringes, needle and scalpel blade into pack. | |
| 9. Assist physician to clean the site with solution and drape with sterile towels. | Reduces risk of infection. |
| 10. Inform patient, that anesthestic will be injected and the site infiltrated. | Prepares patient to anticipate what he will be experiencing. |
| 11. Continue to observe and reassure the patient as the physician punctures and aspirates the marrow (Figure 11.34(b)). | |

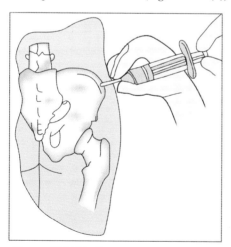

Figure 11.34(b): Bone marrow aspiration from the posterior iliac crest

| | |
|---|---|
| 12. Receive the syringe with bone marrow and collect specimen in various containers as indicated. | Bone marrow tissue is collected in containers with FAA (Formalin, Acetic acid and Alcohol). |
| 13. Once the physician removes the needle, apply pressure over puncture site for 5-10 minutes using a sterile topical swab until the bleeding stops. | Minimises bleeding and hematoma formation. Prolonged pressure i.e.5-10 minutes is required if the patient has low platelet count (thrombocytopenia). |

*Contd...*

*Contd...*

| | | |
|---|---|---|
| 14 | When bleeding stops, seal puncture site with tincture benzoin and apply small, firm dressing. | Avoids chances of oozing from puncture site. |
| 15 | Instruct patient not to wash or wet the area for 24 hours. | Provides an airtight seal over the puncture site and prevents entry of bacteria. |
| 16 | Make the patient comfortable. Instruct the patient that he or she may be mobile after 4-6 hours. | |
| 17 | Remove and dispose off waste, wash and replace reusable articles. | |
| 18 | Send specimen to laboratory with necessary data in the form and container, properly labelled. | |
| 19 | Record information in patient's chart including patient's tolerance and condition. | |

## POSTPROCEDURAL CARE

Keep patient in supine or lateral position
1. Administer analgesics if required
2. Monitor pulse and respiration every 30 minutes for 4-6 hours or until stable

## COMPLICATIONS

1. Bleeding
2. Infection

## SPECIAL CONSIDERATION

Aspirin containing analgesics should be avoided as these may cause bleeding.

# 11.35: PREPARING FOR AND ASSISTING WITH CEREBRAL ANGIOGRAPHY

## DEFINITION

Injecting radiopaque contrast medium into an artery for radiological visualization of intracranial and extracranial blood vessels.

## PURPOSES

1. To diagnose intracranial lesions.
2. To detect abnormalities of blood vessels
   a. Stenosis
   b. Aneurysms
   c. Arteriovenous malformation
3. To detect any displacement of cerebral vessels due to cysts, tumor or abscess.

## PROCEDURE

| | Nursing action | Rationale |
|---|---|---|
| 1 | Explain procedure to the patient and inform him that X-ray films will be taken from different angles during procedure. | Allays anxiety and helps in obtaining cooperation of the patient. |
| 2 | Remove any metal objects and jewellery from patient. | Presence of these may interfere with procedure results. |
| 3 | Assess the patient for allergic reactions to dye. | Prevents complications during dye injection. |
| 4 | Maintain NPO for six hours before procedure, and keep patient well hydrated with IV fluids. | Prevents vomiting and aspiration during procedure. |
| 5 | Perform skin preparation and remove hair from the sites of catheter insertion (femoral, carotid, brachial). | Prevents risk of iatrogenic infection. |
| 6 | Document baseline neurological signs | Helps in comparison after procedure. |
| 7 | Mark peripheral pulses with a pen, distal to the insertion site before procedure. | Helps in comparison after procedure. |
| 8 | Instruct patient about the effects of contrast medium to be expected such as feeling of warmth in face, behind the eyes, jaws, teeth, tongue, lips and a metallic taste in the mouth when it is injected. | Gives psychological support and reassurance to the patient. |
| 9 | Local anesthesia is administered before insertion of cathether | Reduces arterial spasm and prevents pain. |
| 10 | Catheter is introduced into the femoral artery or other sites chosen and contrast agent is injected. X-ray films are taken in different angles. | |
| 11 | Caution the patient to lie still during the procedure. | |

## POSTPROCEDURAL CARE

1. Maintain bedrest for 12-24 hours.
2. Apply direct pressure over puncture site for 15-20 minutes. Observe for bleeding, swelling, redness etc. After bleeding stops, apply a pressure dressing and place a sandbag over the dressing.
3. The extremity on which arterial puncture was performed should be kept straight for 12 hours.
4. Check the patient frequently for neurological symptoms such as motor or sensory alterations, reduced level of consciousness. Speech disturbances, dysrhythmias and blood pressure fluctuations.

5. Monitor for adverse reactions to contrast medium (e.g. restlessness, respiratory distress, tachycardia, facial flushing, nausea and vomiting).
6. Assess skin color, temperature and peripheral pulses of the extremity distal to the IV site. Change may indicate impaired circulation due to occlusion.

## COMPLICATIONS

1. Decreased hand grip on plantar pressure.
2. Facial weakness on the side opposite to the injection site.
3. Seizures
4. Aphasia
5. Stroke
6. Visual disturbances
7. Carotid sinus hypersensitivity
8. Infection
9. Hematoma (Bleeding from puncture site).
10. Air embolism.

# 11: 36: PREPARATION FOR AND ASSISTING WITH DIGITAL SUBTRACTION ANGIOGRAPHY

## DEFINITION

Digital subtraction angiography is a computer based imaging method for visualization of extracranial, intracranial and vascular system by passing a catheter to certain veins and arteries.

## INDICATIONS

1. To identify the cause of transient ischemic attacks.
2. Serial follow-up evaluations for known carotid stenosis.
3. Assessment of intracranial tumors.
4. Postoperative assessment of aneurysm.
5. Follow-up evaluation after extracranial or intracranial bypass procedures.
6. Assessment of dural venous sinuses.
7. Intravascular or extravascular tumors or other masses.
8. Total occlusion of arteries.
9. Preoperative and postoperative evaluation for vascular and tumor surgery.

## INTERFERING FACTORS

1. This examination is very sensitive and even slight physical movement may cause poor images.
2. Study should not be used for uncooperative or agitated patients.
3. The act of swallowing results in unsatisfactory images.

## PROCEDURES

| | Nursing action | Rationale |
|---|---|---|
| 1 | Explain to patient that he has to lie still during the procedure and what he will be experiencing during the procedure and how he has to cooperate. | Helps in obtaining cooperation of patient. |
| 2 | Ensure that patient is coherent and cooperative and able to hold his breath and remain absolutely still when instructed. | Even the act of swallowing may result in unsatisfactory images. |
| 3 | Obtain informed consent from patient. | Prevents litigations. |
| 4 | Determine whether the patient is allergic to iodine, contrast media or latex. | Reduces risks of hypersensitivity reactions. |
| 5 | In female patient check if patient is pregnant. | This procedure is contraindicated in pregnancy. |
| 6 | Obtain the following lab results before procedure<br>a. Prothrombin time drawn on day of procedure for patients on anticoagulation therapy.<br>b. Creatinine levels.<br>c. Recent prothrombin time and partial thromboplastin time.<br>d. Platelet count<br>(generally within 30 days of procedure) | |
| 7 | Administer glycogen intravenously just before procedure as ordered. | Reduces motion artifacts by stopping peristalsis. |
| 8 | Maintain NPO status before 2 hours of study. | Minimises risk of vomiting if an iodine contrast reaction occurs. |

*Contd...*

*Contd...*

| 9 | Assist the physician in cleansing, preparing and injecting the vascular access area with a local anesthetic using sterile techniques. | Prevents spread of microorganisms. |
|---|---|---|
| 10 | The physician advances the catheter containing a guide wire into the desired vessel and removes the guide wire and connects the catheter to a power injector that administers iodine under pressure in defined quantity at prescribed intervals. X-ray images are taken and stored. | |
| 11 | Remove the catheter after the procedure is terminated. | |
| 12 | Place a dressing over the insertion site and apply manual pressure to the puncture site for about 10-20 minutes. | Pressure application prevents bleeding. |
| 13 | Monitor the patient frequently for hemorrhage or hematoma formation. | Identifies early signs of complications. |
| 14 | Record the procedure in nurse's record. | Acts as a communication between staff members. |

## POSTPROCEDURAL CARE

1. Check vital signs frequently. Report unstable signs to physician.
2. Observe the catheter insertion site for signs of infection, hemorrhage or hematoma formation.
3. Monitor neurovascular status of the extremity. Report any problems to the physician immediately.
4. Observe for allergic reactions such as nausea, vomiting, dizziness and urticaria.
5. Instruct the patient to increase fluid intake during the first 24 hours following the procedure to facilitate excretion of the iodine contrast substance.

## SPECIAL CONSIDERATIONS

1. Check vital signs, observe puncture site and do neurovascular assessment every 15 min for few hours after the procedure. Neurovascular assessment includes color, motion, sensation, capillary refill time, pulse quality and temperature of the extremity.
2. If an arterial puncture was performed, the affected extremity should be kept straight for 12-24 hours and the patient must lie flat.
3. Do not raise the head of the bed because this can cause a strain on the femoral puncture site.
4. Sudden onset of pain, numbness or tingling, greater degree of coolness and absent pulse are signs of complication and should be informed to physician immediately.

# 11.37: PERFORMING AN EYE IRRIGATION

## DEFINITION

Washing of the eye externally using stream of water or other medicated fluids.

## PURPOSES

1. To clean the eye
2. To remove foreign particles, excessive secretion or discharge.
3. To apply heat or cold
4. To reduce inflammation
5. To relieve discomfort.

## ARTICLES NEEDED

1. Eye irrigator (undine)/syringe without needle
2. Large cotton swabs
3. Mackintosh
4. K-basin
5. Irrigating solution (sterile)
6. Paper bag
7. A squeezing plastic bottle/sterile irrigation set/ a large syringe

## PROCEDURE

| Nursing action | Rationale |
|---|---|
| 1. Identify the patient and provide explanation as to what will be done and how he may cooperate. | • Provides for performance of procedure on correct patient.<br>• Decreases patient's anxiety and promotes cooperation. |
| 2. Assemble articles at the bedside. | Facilitates orderly performance of procedure. |
| 3. Wash and dry hands. | |
| 4. Expose the lower conjunctival sac by separating the lids with the thumb and forefinger. Exert pressure on the bony prominence of the cheek bone and on the eyebrow when holding the eyelids (Figure 11.37(a)). | Prevents reflex blinking<br>Prevents pressure to the eyeball. |

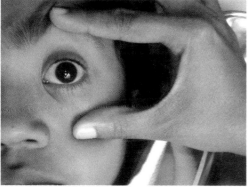

**Figure 11.37(a):** Exposing lower conjunctival sac

*Contd...*

*Contd...*

| | | |
|---|---|---|
| 5. | Hold the filled eye irrigator about 2.5 cm (1 inch) above the eye (Figure 11.37(b)). | Ensures an even, safe pressure of the solution and avoids possible injury to cornea. |

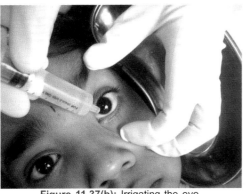

**Figure 11.37(b):** Irrigating the eye

| | | |
|---|---|---|
| 6. | Irrigate the eye directing the solution on the lower conjunctival sac, from inner canthus to the outer canthus. | Directing the solution in this way prevents fluid from flowing down the nasolacrimal duct. |
| 7. | Irrigate until the solution leaving the eye is clear (or) until all the solution has been used. | |
| 8. | Dry around the eye with cotton swabs. | Prevents infection. |
| 9. | Apply ointment if prescribed by physician. | Aids in healing and prevents infection. |
| 10. | Discard the irrigated fluid and swabs and sterilize and replace all the reusable articles. Wash hands. | Prevents transmission of microorganisms. |
| 11. | Record the treatment showing amount and color of discharge, consistency of discharge, presence of redness and swelling, treatment given. | Serves as a legal document. |
| 12. | Refer the patient to the physician if the eyes show evidence of ulceration. | Prevents complication. |

# 11. 38: PERFORMING AN EAR IRRIGATION

## DEFINITION

An ear irrigation is the washing of the external auditory canal with a stream of liquid.

## PURPOSES

1. To remove the earwax.
2. To remove foreign bodies (except hygroscopic substances)
3. To cleanse the ear in case of purulent discharge caused by middle ear infection.
4. For antiseptic effect.
5. To apply heat.
6. To evaluate vestibular functions (e.g. bithermal caloric test).

## SOLUTIONS USED

1. Boric acid 2-4%
2. Sodium bicarbonate solution 1%
3. Normal saline
4. Hydrogen peroxide 2%
5. Sterile water.

## ARTICLES

1. Prescribed sterile irrigating solution (w armed to 37 degree centigrade).
2. Irrigation set (Container and irrigating bulb syringe).
3. Waterproof pad.
4. Emesis basin.
5. Cotton tipped applicators.
6. Disposable gloves.
7. Cotton balls.
8. Spot light and head mirror.
9. Sterile gauzepiece.
10. Sterile jug with extra fluid.

## PROCEDURE

| | Nursing action | Rationale |
|---|---|---|
| 1 | Explain the procedure to the patient and inform him how he has to cooperate. | Explanation facilitates cooperation and provides reassurance. |
| 2 | Bring equipment to the patient's bedside. Check the physician's order, protect the patient and bedlinen with a moisture proof-pad. | Provides for an organised approach to the task. |
| 3 | Wash hands | Prevents spread of microorganisms. |
| 4 | Have the patient sit up or lie with the head tilted toward the side of the affected ear. Have the patient support the basin under the ear to receive the irrigating solution. | Gravity causes the irrigating solution to flow from the ear to the basin. |
| 5 | Clean the pinna and meatus at the auditory canal as necessary with moistened cotton-tipped applicators dipped in warm tap water or the irrigating solution. | Materials lodged on the pinna and at the meatus may be washed into the ear. |

*Contd...*

*Contd...*

| 6 | Ascertain whether impaction is due to foreign hygroscopic (attracts or absorbs moisture) body before proceeding. | If water contacts such a substance it may cause it to swell and produce intense pain. |
|---|---|---|
| 7 | Fill the bulb syringe with warm solution, if an irrigating container is used, allow air to escape from the tubing. | Air forced into the ear canal is noisy and therefore unpleasant for the patient. |
| 8 | Straighten the auditory canal by pulling the pinna up and back for an adult, upward and back for a child over 3 years of age and down and back for an infant or child upto 3 years of age. | Straigtening the ear canal helps to allow the solution to reach all areas of the ear canal. |
| 9 | Direct a steady, slow stream of solution against the roof of the auditory canal, using only sufficient force to remove secretions (Figure 11.38(a)). Do not occlude the auditory canal with the irrigating nozzle. Allow the solution to flow out unimpeded. | Directing solution at the roof of the canal helps prevent injury to the tympanic membrane. Continuous in and out flow of the irrigating solution helps to prevent pressure in the canal. |

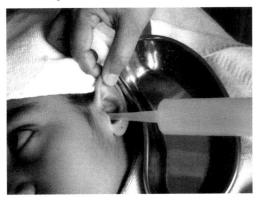

Figure 11.38(a): Irrigating the ear

| 10 | When the irrigation is completed, place a cottonball loosely in the auditory meatus and have the patient lie on the side of the affected ear on a towel or absorbent pad. | The cottonball absorbs excess fluid and gravity allows the remaining solution in the canal to escape from the ear. |
|---|---|---|
| 11. | Discard the irrigated fluid and swabs. Clean and replace reusable articles. | |
| 12 | Wash hands. | Prevents spread of microorganisms. |
| 13 | Record the irrigation, appearance of the drainage and the patient's response. | Acts as a communication between staff members. |
| 14 | Remove the cottonball and assess drainage after 15 minutes. | Drainage or pain may indicate injury to the tympanic membrane. |

## SPECIAL CONSIDERATIONS

1. Irrigation solution should be at least at room temperature.
2. An irrigating container with tubing and an eartip may be used if the purpose of the irrigation is to apply heat to the area.
3. If irrigation does not disloge the wax, instill several drops of prescribed glycerin, Carbonide peroxide or other solutions as directed, two or three times daily for 2-3 days which helps to soften and loosen impaction.
4. Take special care not to irrigate an older adult's ears with cool water because dizziness may occur.

# 11.39(A): ADMISSION AND INITIAL MANAGEMENT OF PATIENT IN BURNS UNIT

## DEFINITION

Admitting a burns patient directly to the unit to resolve the immediate problems resulting from burn injury.

## PURPOSES

1. To correct fluid and electrolyte imbalances.
2. To initiate life saving measures without delay.
3. To prevent infection.
4. To manage pain.

## ARTICLES

1. Sterile bed linen
2. Articles for:
    a. , Starting intravenous infusion
    b. Urinary catheterization
    c. Monitoring vital signs
    d. Monitoring ECG
    e. Nasogastric intubation
    f. Maintaining aseptic precautions and isolation technique.
    g. Obtaining blood for initial investigations.

## PROCEDURE

| | Nursing action | Rationale |
|---|---|---|
| 1 | Receive patient in the unit specially prepared for the purpose. | |
| 2 | Avoid air conditioning as far as possible for at least 48 hours. | Prevents evaporative loss of fluid from burned skin surfaces. |
| 3 | Assess airway, breathing and circulation. | Swelling of the upper airway interferes with patency of airway and breathing. |
| 4 | Establish airway and ensure adequate breathing by providing 100% oxygen if indicated as in suspected inhalation injury. | Clients with head and neck burn injury need immediate endotracheal intubation |
| 5 | Check vital signs | Provides baseline data |
| 6 | Assess for associated trauma | Helps in identifying risk for complications. |
| 7 | Meet patient's needs based on priority<br>a. Remove saturated clothing (chemical or scald burns)<br>b. Cool the tar burn<br>c. Copiously irrigate a chemical burn<br>d. Remove any jewellery present on patient. | |
| 8 | Collect history about the incident such as the cause of burns that is chemical, thermal, electrical or radiation. | Helps to know about the cause of burns and plan management during intial period. |
| 9 | Collect data about the time of occurrence of burns, level of consciousness at the scene, whether injury occurred in an enclosed or open space, presence of associated trauma etc. | Helps in planning management during initial period. |
| 10 | Assess the patient for depth, size and location of the burns. | Helps to identify type, extent and depth of burns. |

*Contd...*

*Contd...*

| 11 | Assess the duration of exposure in case of electrical, chemical or radiation burns. | |
|---|---|---|
| 12 | Assess percentage of burns by "Rule of 9".<br><br>Head and neck —9%<br>Anterior thorax—18%<br>Posterior thorax—18%<br>Right arm –9%<br>Left arm—9%<br>Perineum—1%<br>Right leg—18%<br>Left leg—18% | Helps in planning treatment and calculating fluid to be administered. |
| 13 | Cover the patient with a sterile sheet. | Conserves body heat. |
| 14 | Estimate the age of patient. | Infants and older adults tolerate burns poorly. |
| 15 | Assess general health of the patient with debilitating illnesses such as cardiac, pulmonary, endocrine and renal disease. | Influences patient's response to injury and treatment. Mortality is high in patients with such illnesses due to risk of development of cardiopulmonary complications and impaired immune function. |
| 16 | In chemical burns assess for<br>• Knowledge of offending agent<br>• Concentration<br>• Duration of exposure. | Determines the extend of injury |
| 17 | Incase of electrical injuries assess for<br>• Electrical source<br>• Type of current<br>• Current voltage | Determines the extent of injury |
| 18 | Initiate IV infusion through peripheral line. Assist for cut down if indicated. Fluid calculation depends upon patient's weight, extent of injury, presence of inhalation injury, any delay in initiation of resuscitation and deep tissue damage.(Refer to fluid resuscitation formula given at the end of procedure) (Figure 11.39(b)). | Maintains circulatory blood volume. |
| 19 | Catheterize the patient. Measure the amount of urine and record hourly. | Determines the adequacy of fluid therapy for the first 48 hours. |
| 20 | Initiate nasogastric feeding (Withhold feed if paralytic ileus is present). | Maintains nutritional status. Prevents and reduces the risk of aspiration. |
| 21 | Maintain strict isolation and follow aseptic technique in caring for patient. | Prevents spread of infection. |
| 22 | Check vital signs frequently. | Helps to identify deviation from normal. |
| 23 | Assess for baseline laboratory studies such as<br>• Blood glucose<br>• BUN<br>• Serum creatinine<br>• Serum electrolytes<br>• Hematocrit level<br>• Chest X-ray<br>• ABG (inhalation injury) | Identifies development of complications at an early stage. |

*Contd...*

*Contd...*

| | | |
|---|---|---|
| 24 | Monitor ECG continuously especially in high voltage electrical injury and major burns. | Patients are at risk of developing dysrhythmias in high voltage electrical injury and in major burns. |
| 25 | Administer narcotic agents through IV line as prescribed by physician | Reduces pain. Oral method of drug administration is not used due to gastrointestinal dysfunction. |
| 26 | Administer tetanus toxoid for patients who have not been immunized. If immunized, Tetanus booster dose should be given according to physician's order. | |
| 27 | Record the time of admission and document procedures done in nurses records. | Acts as a communication between staff members. |

## SPECIAL CONSIDERATIONS

1. Inform police in medicolegal case.
2. Use caution when patient is biohazard with hepatitis B and HIV infection.
3. Inform family by giving periodical information about patient's condition and progress.
4. Assess patient for known allergies.

# 11.39(B): FLUID RESUSCITATION IN ACUTE BURNS

## DEFINITION

Initiating and maintaining fluid resuscitation as per burns protocol.

## PURPOSES

1. To prevent hypovolemic shock
2. To prevent further complications.

## ARTICLES

1. Sterile pack-1
2. Antiseptic solution
3. Injection Xylocaine
4. Disposable needle 23
5. Cavafix
6. Cut down set
7. IV fluids as required
8. Blood administration set (for 2nd day's colloids transfusion)
9. Three-way with extension
10. Scalpel blade No 11.

## GENERAL INSTRUCTIONS

1. If patient does not tolerate feeds, keep nil orally with 4 hourly aspiration and dependent drainage.
2. Initiate fluid therapy within an hour following a severe burn.
3. Consider three types of fluids in calculating the needs of the patient:
   • Colloids-including plasma and plasma expanders such as dextran.
   • Electrolytes such as physiologic solution of sodium chloride, Ringer's solution.
   • Non-electrolyte fluids such as distilled water with 5% dextrose.
4. The amount of fluid replacement required during first 48 hours is determined by assessment of factors such as
   • Urinary output
   • Serum electrolyte levels
   • Blood gas findings
   • Central venous pressure
   • Body weight
   • Hematocrit level
   • Level of consciousness
   • Vital signs
5. Observe urine for color and volume. An urine outflow of 30-50 ml per hour for adults and 15 ml/hr for infants is considered adequate. If the urinary output falls below these figures notify physician immediately.

## PROCEDURE

| | Nursing action | Rationale |
|---|---|---|
| 1 | Explain procedure to patient | Helps in obtaining cooperation of patient. |
| 2 | Initiate IV access or assist for cut-down and connect IV fluids as per fluid resuscitation formula | Maintains homeostasis. |

*Contd...*

*Contd...*

| 3 | Assist in collecting blood samples while starting cut down. | Helps in investigation of blood for hematocrit, electrolytes bicarbonate, creatinine, HIV, HbsAg, grouping and cross-matching. |
|---|---|---|
| 4 | Enquire date and time of burns accident. | Helps in planning fluid calculation. |
| 5 | Check the weight of the patient. | Aids in determining the amount of the fluid to be infused. |
| 6 | Monitor urinary output. | Adequacy of fluid resuscitation can be judged by urine output. |
| 7 | Check vital signs frequently. | Determines adequacy of fluid resuscitation. |
| 8 | Monitor ECG continuously. | Identifies arrhythmias in patients with high voltage electrical injury. |

**Table 11.39.1:** Guidelines formulas for fluid replacement in burns patient

| Sl.No. | Fluid resuscitation formula | Crystalloids | First 24 hours Colloid containing solution | First 24 hours Dextrose in water | Crystalloids | Second 24 hours Colloid containing solution | Second 24 hours Dextrose in water |
|---|---|---|---|---|---|---|---|
| 1 | Evans | Normal saline 1 ml /kg/% BSA ½ given in first 8 hrs remaining ½ in next 16 hours | 1 ml /kg/ % BSA | 2000 ml | ½ of first 24 hours requirement | ½ of first 24 hours requirement | 2000 ml |
| 2 | Brooke | Lactated Ringer's Solution 1.5 ml/kg /% BSA ½ given in first 8 hrs remaining ½ in next 16 hours | 0.5 ml/kg % BSA | 2000 ml | Half to three fourth of first 24 hours requirement | Half to three fourth of first 24 hours requirement | 2000 ml |
| 3 | Modified Brooke | Lactated Ringer's 2 ml/kg/% BSA ½ given during first 8 hrs and remaining ½ given during next 16 hours | None | None | None | 0.3-0.5 ml/ Kg /% BSA | Titrate to maintain urine output |
| 4 | Parkland/ Baxter | Lactated Ringer's 4 ml/kg/% BSA ½ given first 8 hrs; 1/4th given in each next 8 hrs. | None | None | None | 0.3-0.5 ml/ Kg /%BSA | Titrate maintain urine output |
| 5 | Hypertonic saline solution | Fluid containing 250 mEq of sodium /L to maintain hourly urine output of 70 ml/in adults ½ given in first 8 hrs remaining ½ in next 16 hrs | None | None | Same solution to maintain hourly urine output of 30 ml in adults | None | None |

**Table showing fluid resuscitation**

## SPECIAL CONSIDERATIONS

1. If a burned patient is delayed for 2 hours in reaching emergency department, those 2 hours must be considered in calculation of needed fluid.
2. With the exception of Evans and Brooke formulas, for the first 24 hours colloid containing solutions are not given because of the changes in capillary integrity that allows leakage of protein rich fluid into the interstitial space resulting in formation of additional edema fluid
3. It is important to remember that all resuscitation formulas are only guides and that fluid resuscitation volumes should be adjusted according to the patient's physiologic response
4. Assessment of adequacy of fluid replacement is best made by use of more than one parameter
5. Modified Brook and Parkland formula for fluid resuscitation are widely used clinically.

## ASSESSMENT OF PARAMETERS FOR FLUID RESUSCITATION

1. Urine output-30-50 ml/hr in adult, 75-100 ml/hr for electrical burn in adult.
2. Cardiopulmonary factors: blood pressure (systolic greater than 90-100 mmHg) pulse rate (less than 120b/min) Respiration(16-20 breaths/min).
3. Blood pressure is most appropriately measured by a continuous arterial monitoring. Peripheral measurement is often invalid because of vasoconstriction and edema.
4. Sensorium: Alert and oriented to time, place and person.

# 11.40: PROVIDING EXERCISES FOR POST BURN PATIENTS

## DEFINITION

Physical therapy offered to burns patient from the time of admission to be continued at home in order to prevent post burn complications like contractures and deformities.

## PROCEDURE

|   | Area of burn | Common deformity | Procedure |
|---|---|---|---|
| 1 | Anterior neck | Flexion | Use sand bags on both sides of head. Position neck in extension with head kept straight. Hyperextend neck by placing a pillow beneath shoulders. |
| 2 | Shoulder | Adduction and internal rotation | Position with shoulder flexed and abducted using aeroplane splint. Give wall climbing exercise, range of motion exercises like flexion, extension, abduction, adduction, clockwise and anticlockwise shoulder rotation etc. |
| 3 | Elbow | Flexion and pronation | Position elbow in fully extended and supinated position. Provide range of motion to elbow joint like flexion, extension, pronation and supination exercises. |
| 4 | Hand | Claw hand | Dress fingers separately. Elevate to decrease edema. Position wrist in extension- metacarpophalangeal joints in extension and thumb in palmar abduction. |
| 5 | Hip | Flexion and extension | Provide range of motion exercises to hip joint. |
| 6 | Knee | Flexion | Position knee in full extension. Splint posterior part of knee. Give prone lying position and exercises like extension and flexion. |
| 7 | Ankle | Plantar flexion | Position ankle in zero degree dorsiflexion: splint with plaster of Paris or ankle-foot-orthosis. Give exercise to fully move ankle up, down, in and out. |

## 11.41(A): PERFORMING A HEIMLICH MANEUVER (ADULT)

### DEFINITION

An emergency procedure for dislodging a bolus of food or other obstruction from the trachea to prevent asphyxiation. It is a series of 5 abdominal thrusts just above a victim's navel and below the sternum to relieve a foreign body airway obstruction.

### PURPOSES

1 To prevent airway obstruction.
2 To remove foreign body from trachea.

### PROCEDURE

| | Nursing action | Rationale |
|---|---|---|
| 1 | Assess airway for complete or partial blockage. (partial airway obstruction will have some air exchange. Complete airway obstruction will have weak, ineffective cough and signs of respiratory distress) (Figure 11.41(a)). | If there is good air exchange and the patient is able to forcefully cough, do not interfere with the patient's attempts to expel the foreign body. Encourage attempts to cough. If complete airway obstruction is apparent, the Heimlich maneuver or alternative method of subdiaphragmatic thrust should be performed immediately. |

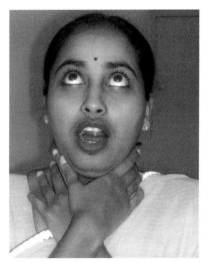

Figure 11.41(a): Signs of respiratory distress in foreign body obstruction

| | Nursing action | Rationale |
|---|---|---|
| 2 | Conscious adult patient (sitting or standing) <br> • Stand behind the patient (Figure 11.41(b)). <br><br><br> • Wrap your arms around the patient's waist <br> • Make a fist with one hand and grasp the fist with your other hand, placing the thumb side of the fist against | Proper positioning is necessary to provide an effective sub-diaphragmatic thrust. Correct hand placement is important to prevent internal organ damage. Produces artificial cough by forcing air from the lungs. Attempts to dislodge food or a foreign body to relieve airway obstruction should be continued as long as |

*Contd...*

*Contd...*

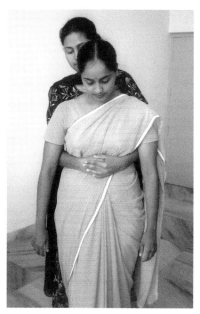

**Figure 11.41(b):** Position of rescuer

the patient's abdomen. The fist should be placed midline, below the xiphoid process and lower margins of the ribcage and above the navel (Figure 11.41(c)).
- Perform a quick upward thrust into the patient's abdomen: each thrust should be separate and distinct.
- Repeat this process six to ten times until the patient either expels the foreign body or loses consciousness.

necessary because of the serious consequences of hypoxia.

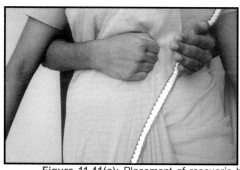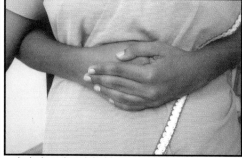

**Figure 11.41(c):** Placement of rescuer's hands below the xiphoid process

3  Unconscious adult patient or patient who becomes unconscious:
- Position the patient supine. Kneel astride the patient's thighs.

- Place the heel of one hand midline, below the xiphoid process and lower margin of the ribcage and above the navel. Place the second hand directly on top of the first hand.
- Perform a quick upward thrust into the diaphragm, repeating six to ten times.

Proper positioning is necessary to provide an effective subdiaphragmatic thrust.
Proper positioning is necessary to provide an effective subdiaphragmatic thrust.

Patient who is unconscious may become more relaxed so that the previously unsuccessful Heimlich maneuver may be successful.

*Contd...*

*Contd...*

| | | |
|---|---|---|
| 4 | Perform a finger sweep:<br>a. Use one hand to grasp the lower jaw and tongue between your thumb and fingers and lift. This will open the mouth and pull the tongue away from the back of the throat.<br>b. Insert the index finger of the other hand into the patient's mouth next to the cheek and using a hooking motion dislodge any foreign body.<br>Caution must be used to prevent pushing the foreign body farther down into the airway. | Should be used only in the unconscious patient who will not fight with the action. |
| 5 | Open the patient's airway and attempt ventilation. | The brain can suffer irreversible damage if it is without oxygen for over 4 to 6 minutes. |
| 6 | Continue sequence of Heimlich maneuver, finger sweep and rescue breathing as long as necessary. | Life saving efforts must continue until they are successful or until the rescuer becomes exhausted and cannot go on. |
| 7 | Record in nurses record the procedure performed, patient's condition and effectiveness of treatment. | Acts as a communication between staff members. |

## SPECIAL CONSIDERATIONS

1. If a choking victim is pregnant or extremely obese place your fist on the chest instead of the abdomen for the thrusts.
2. It is important to wrap your fingers around your thumb when performing the Heimlich maneuver so as not to perforate the spleen with an extended thumb.
3. The universal sign of airway obstruction is clutching the neck with hands. In addition, the inability to talk or breathe as well as cyanosis and progression to an unconscious state.

## 11. 41(B): PERFORMING HEIMLICH MANEUVER/PEDIATRICS

### DEFINITION

An emergency procedure for dislodging a bolus of food or other obstruction from the trachea to prevent asphyxiation in a child.

It is a series of 5 abdominal thrusts just above a victim's navel and below the sternum to relieve a foreign body airway obstruction.

### PROCEDURE

| | Nursing action | Rationale |
|---|---|---|
| 1 | Assess airway for complete or partial blockage. In children the signs of blockage can be similar to that of adults. In infants the signs are turning blue, crying without sound and flailing arms and legs. (partial airway obstruction will have some air exchange. Complete airway obstruction will have weak, ineffective cough and signs of respiratory distress). | If there is good air exchange and the patient is able to forcefully cough, do not interfere with the child's attempts to expel the foreign body. Encourage attempts to cough. If complete airway obstruction is apparent the Heimlich maneuver needs to be performed. |
| 2 | Differentiate between infection and airway obstruction. | Complication of infection that lead to airway obstruction require immediate medical attention, establishment of patent airway and treatment of underlying infection. |
| 3 | **I. Infant airway obstruction:** | |
| | a. Straddle infant over forearm in prone position on your lap with the head lower than trunk. Support the infant's head, positioning a hand around the jaws and chest. | Proper positioning is essential for success of the maneuver and to prevent other organ damages. |
| | b. Keeping the infants head down, deliver five back blows between the infant's shoulder blades. | Helps in dislodging the obstruction. |
| | c. Holding the infant's head, place the free hand on the infant's back and turn the infant over, supporting the back of the child with your forearm and thigh. | Safely rotates the infants position to continue life saving procedures. |
| | d. With your free hand, deliver five chest thrusts using two fingers. | Helps in dislodging the obstruction. |
| | e. Alternate chest thrusts and back blows till the child is relieved of the obstruction. | |
| | f. Assess for a foreign body in the mouth of an unconscious infant and utilise the finger sweep only if a foreign body is visualized. | A blind finger sweep is avoided in infants and children as a foreign object can be pushed back farther into the airway increasing obstruction. |
| | g. Open airway and assess for respiration. If respirations are absent, attempt rescue breathing. Assess for the rise and fall of the chest. If not seen, reposition infant and attempt resuce breathing again. | Irreversible brain damage can occur within 4 – 6 minutes |
| | h. Repeat the entire sequence again: five backblows, five chest thrusts, assessment for foreign body in oral cavity and rescue breathing as long as necessary. | Life saving efforts must continue until they are successful or until the rescuer becomes exhausted and cannot go on. |
| | **II. Small child-Airway obstruction** (Conscious, standing or sitting) | |
| | a. Assess air exchange and encourage coughing and breathing. Provide re-assurance to the child. | Provides psychological support |

*Contd...*

*Contd...*

| | |
|---|---|
| b. Ask the child if he or she is choking, and initiate the steps. | Proper positioning prevents organ damage and life saving efforts must continue until they are successful. |
| i. Stand behind the child with your arms positioned in the same way as in adults and administer six to ten subdiaphragmatic abdominal thrusts with lesser force. | |
| ii. Continue until foreign object is expelled or the child becomes unconscious. | |
| **III. Small child unconscious:** | |
| a. Position the child supine and kneel at the child's feet and gently deliver five sub-diaphragmatic abdominal thrusts using one hand by placing the heel of one hand at the umbilicus and pressing downward and upward. | Proper positioning prevents organ damage |
| b. Open airway by lifting the lowerjaw and tongue forward. Perform a finger sweep only if a foreign body is visualized. | Opening the airway allows visualization of the oral cavity. |
| c. If breathing is absent, begin rescue breathing. If the chest does not rise, reposition the child, check if airway is open and attempt rescue breathing again. | Irreversible brain damage occurs. |
| d. Repeat this sequence as long as necessary | Life-saving efforts must continue until they are successful. |
| e. Wash hands. | Reduces transmission of microorganisms. |

# Chapter 12

# Operating Room and Related Procedures

# 12.1: PERFORMING A SURGICAL SCRUB

## DEFINITION

Surgical handwashing is a procedure by which dirt and microorganisms are destroyed and removed from hands and fingers by chemical action and mechanical friction.

## PURPOSES

1. To remove dirt and transient micro-organisms from hands.
2. To reduce the risk of transmission of microorganisms to patients.
3. To reduce the risk of cross infection among patients.
4. To reduce the risk of transmission of infectious agents to oneself.
5. To prevent iatrogenic infections.

## ARTICLES

1. Soap/antiseptic detergent
2. Running warm water
3. Nail brush in antiseptic lotion
4. Towels (sterile)
5. Mask and cap.

## PROCEDURE

| | Nursing action | Rationale |
|---|---|---|
| 1 | Ensure that the nails are short. Remove artificial nails if any. | Short nails are less likely to harbor organisms, scratch the patient or puncture gloves. |
| 2 | Remove nail polish | Nail polish harbors microorganisms. |
| 3 | Inspect hands for abrasions, cuts, or open lesions. | These conditions increase likelihood of more micro-organisms residing on skin surfaces. |
| 4 | Remove jewellery of any type. | Microorganisms accumulate in jewellery. |
| 5 | After medical handwash, wear cap and mask. | |
| 6 | Turn on water using knee/foot/elbow (Figure 12.1(a)) | |

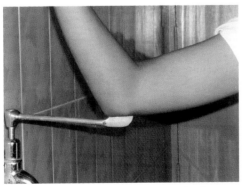

**Figure 12.1(a):** Turning on water with elbow

*Contd...*

*Contd...*

| | | |
|---|---|---|
| 7 | Wet hands and arms under running lukewarm water and lather with soap/detergent to 5 cm above the elbows (Hands need to be raised/held above elbows at all times). Use firm circular movements to wash palms, back of hands, wrists, forearms and interdigital spaces for 20-25 seconds. (Figure 12.1(b)) | Water flows from fingertips to elbows. Fingertips are considered to be cleaner than the elbows. |

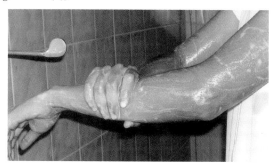

**Figure 12.1(b):** Lathering hands with soap

| | | |
|---|---|---|
| 8 | Rinse hands and arms thoroughly under running water (remember to keep hands above elbows). | Rinsing removes transient bacteria from hands. |
| 9 | Clean under nails of both hands with nail pick/nail brush (Figure 12.1(c)) | Removes dirt and microorganisms. |

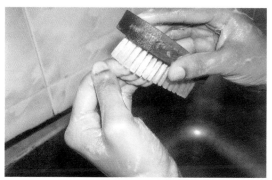

**Figure 12.1(c):** Cleaning under nails with brush

| | | |
|---|---|---|
| 10 | Scrub nails of each hand with 15 strokes using antimicrobial agent | |
| 11 | Holding the brush perpendicular scrub palm, each side of thumb and fingers and posterior side of hand with 10 strokes each. | Scrubbing loosens resident bacteria that adhere to skin surfaces. |
| 12 | Scrub from wrist to 5 cm above each elbow that is lower arm, upper forearm and antecubital fossa to marginal area above elbows. | Scrubbing is performed from cleaner area to less clean area (upper arms). |
| 13 | Entire scrub should last for 5 to 10 minutes. | Scrubbing time can be lengthened according to agency policy/according to the degree of contamination of hands. |
| 14 | Discard brush and rinse hands from fingertips to elbows (Figure 12.1(d)). | |

*Contd...*

*Contd...*

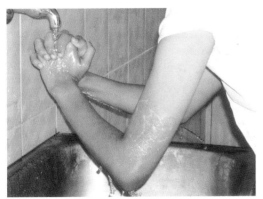

**Figure 12.1(d):** Rinsing hands from fingertips to elbow

| | | |
|---|---|---|
| 15 | Take care not to touch the tap or sides of the sink during the procedure. | Tap and sides of sink are considered to be contaminated. |
| 16 | Use a sterile towel to dry one hand moving from fingers to elbow. Dry from cleanest to least clean area (Figure 12.1(e)). | Drying prevents chapping and facilitates donning of gloves |

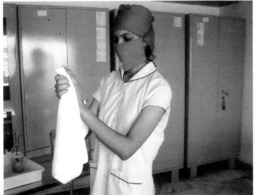

**Figure 12.1(e):** Drying hands from fingers to elbow

| | |
|---|---|
| 17 | Repeat drying of the other hand using a different towel. Use one side to dry one hand and reverse side for other hand, if only one towel is available. |
| 18 | Discard towel |
| 19 | Proceed with sterile gowning |

## SEPCIAL CONSIDERATION

Report any dermatitis to employee health or infection control as per agency policy.

# 12.2: CONDUCTING A GENERAL PREOPERATIVE ASSESSMENT AND CHECKLIST

## IDENTIFICATION DATA

Name        : _____

Age         : _____

Sex         : _____

IP No       : _____

Ward       : _____

Bed No     : _____

Diagnosis   : _____

Surgery proposed    : _____

Date of surgery      : _____

Type of anesthesia      : _____

## a) Day prior to surgery:

1. Weight                              : _____ kg
2. Height                              : _____ cm
3. Known allergy             : _____
4. Medications consumed (specify)    : _____
   (Place tick mark (✔) for items carried out)
1. Consent for surgery is obtained in specified format    : _____
2. Teaching about postoperative exercise given    : _____
3. Explanation about anesthesia and surgery given    : _____
4. Local skin preparation done    : _____
5. Nails cut and bath given    : _____
6. Enema/bowel wash given    : _____
7. Recording done about any cough/alteration in vital
   signs/loose teeth/skin infection/menstruation/any others    : _____
8. X- rays, scan, ECG, lab reports etc collected and
   attached to patient record    : _____
9. Instructions given about fasting    : _____
10. Nail polish and make-up removed    : _____
11. Old chart requested and obtained    : _____
12. Type and cross-match for blood done    : _____
13. Consent for receiving blood transfusion obtained    : _____
14. Notified surgeon for any abnormal lab report    : _____

...................................................................................................

**Signatures:**                                       **Date and time:**

a. Nursing student    : _____

b. Staff nurse    : _____

c. Ward sister/supervisor    : _____

## b. Day of surgery

1. Confirm PO status.    : _____
2. Enema/bowel wash given (if indicated)    : _____
3. Bath given    : _____

4. Final skin preparation done : _____
5. Ryle's tube passed (if indicated) : _____
6. Intravenous line in place : _____
7. Clean gown given, hair groomed : _____
8. Jewellery, dentures, glasses, contact lenses, : _____
   hairpins, nail polish, hearing aids removed
9. Vital signs checked and recorded : _____
10. Bladder emptied (catheterization if indicated) : _____
11. Pre-medication given : _____
12. Identification band and blood band checked for accuracy : _____
13. Siderails put up and bed brought down to lowest level : _____
14. Patient instructed not to get out of bed without nursing assistance : _____
15. Lab reports, X- rays, scan reports, ECG reports, blank
    prescription form, fresh doctor's order sheet and : _____
    operation record attached to patient's chart
16. Specify materials, such as drugs, articles to be sent with
    patient (Ryle's tube, Foley's catheter, urosac, : _____
    medications, asepto syringe)
17. Time when patient left the ward : _____

..................................................................................................................

**Signature:**                                    **Date and time:**
a. Nursing student                                : _____
b. Staff nurse                                    : _____
c. Ward sister/supervisor                         : _____

## 12.3: PERFORMING SKIN PREPARATION FOR SURGERY

### DEFINITION

Skin preparation is a preoperative procedure performed to decontaminate and reduce the number of organisms on skin to eliminate the transference of such organisms into the incision site.

### PURPOSES

1. To remove hair from well defined skin area.
2. To prevent wound infection postoperatively.

### METHODS OF HAIR REMOVAL

1. Wet shaving
2. Clipping
3. Use of depilatory cream.

### ARTICLES

1. Razor set
2. New blade
3. Soap
4. Bowl with water
5. Rag pieces/Paper tissues
6. Kidney basin
7. Mackintosh
8. Basin with water
9. Sponge towel
10. Bath towel
11. Duster
12. Depilatory cream -optional
13. Electric clippers if clipping is to be done
14. Clean gloves
15. Scissors.

### PROCEDURE

| | Nursing action | Rationale |
|---|---|---|
| 1. | Inspect general condition of skin | If lesions, irritation or signs of infection are present, shaving should not be done. These conditions increase chances of postoperative wound infections. |
| 2. | Review physician's order or the agency procedure book for specific area to be shaved. | Extent of area for hair removal depends upon site of incision, nature of surgery and physician's preference. |
| 3. | Assess patient's understanding and acceptance of the purpose of hair removal. | Patient may be anxious regarding removal of hair and implications regarding change in appearance. |
| 4. | Wash hands. | Reduces risk of transmission of microorganisms. |
| 5. | Close room doors or bedside curtains and raise bed to working level. | Provides privacy and promotes good body mechanics. |

*Contd...*

*Contd...*

| | |
|---|---|
| 6. Position patient comfortably with surgical site accessible. | Shaving and skin preparation can take several minutes. Nurse should have easy access to hard to reach areas |
| 7. Don disposable gloves | Use of disposable gloves safeguards the patient and the nurse, minimizing nurse's exposure to blood-borne pathogens |
| 8 Remove hair<br>**I. Wet shave**<br>a. Place towel or waterproof pad under body part to be shaved | Prevents soiling of bed linen |
| b. Drape patient with bath blanket, leaving only the area to be shaved at one time, exposed | Prevents unnecessary exposure of body parts and reduces patient's anxiety |
| c. Cut long hair short with scissors. Lather skin with gauze sponges dipped in antiseptic soap | Lathering with antiseptic soap softens hair and reduces friction from razor |
| d. Shave small area at a time. With non-dominant hand hold gauze sponge to stabilize skin. Hold razor at 45-degree angle in dominant hand and shave in the direction of hair growth. Use short gentle strokes (Figure 12.3(a)). | Shaving small area minimizes chances of cutting skin. Shaving in direction of hair growth prevents pulling of hair. |

**Figure 12.3(a):** Preoperative skin preparation—shaving

| | |
|---|---|
| e. Rinse razor in basin of water as soap and hair accumulate on the blade. Change and discard blades as they become dull | Maintains clean sharp razor edge to promote patients comfort |
| f. Rearrange bath blanket as each portion of shave is completed | Maintains patient comfort and privacy |
| g. Use wash cloth and warm water to rinse away remaining hair and soap solution. Change water as needed | Reduces skin irritation and allows good visualization of the skin |
| h. If shaved area is over body crevices, for example, umbilicus or groin, cleanse with cotton tipped applicators or cotton balls dipped in antiseptic solution | Removes secretions, dirt and other remaining hair clippings which harbour microorganisms |
| i. Dry crevices with cotton balls or applicators | Reduces maceration of skin from retained moisture |
| j. Discard waterproof towel or pad. | Reduces spread of microorganisms |
| k. Observe skin closely for any nicks or cuts | Any break in skin integrity increases risk of wound infection |
| **II Hair clipping**<br>a. Lightly dry area to be clipped with towel | Removes moisture which interferes with clean cut of clippers |
| b. Hold clippers in dominant hand, about one cm above skin, and cut hair in direction it grows. Clip small area at a time | Prevents pulling on hair and abrasion of skin |
| c. Rearrange drape as necessary | Prevents unnecessary exposure of body parts |

*Contd...*

*Contd...*

| | |
|---|---|
| d. Lightly brush off cut hair with towel | Removes contaminated hair and promotes comfort. Improves visibility of area being clipped |
| e. When clipped area is over body crevices, clean crevices with cotton tipped applicators or cotton balls dipped in antiseptic solution, then dry | Removes secretions dirt and hair clippings which harbour microrganisms |
| **III. Depilatory hair removal** | |
| a. Apply depilatory cream to the area (before application of cream sensitivity test to be done by applying a small amount of cream on skin on inner aspect of forearm or wrist. Check for any sensitivity reaction like redness, rashes, itching of skin after 15 to 20 minutes | Hair removal by depilation offers the primary advantage of leaving skin intact and free from cuts. If the patient is not sensitive to the depilatory preparation, it is a safer method of hair removal than shaving |
| b. Wait for the required number of minutes and wipe off the cream with rag pieces or paper towel. | Hair is removed simultaneously with wiping off the depilatory cream |
| c. Wash skin and rinse thoroughly | Removes microrganisms from the skin |
| 9. Inform patient that procedure is completed | |
| 10. Clean and dispose of article according to policy, do not re-cover razor blade. Dispose of gloves | Reduces spread of infection and reduces risk of injury from razor blades |
| 11. Wash hands | Reduces risk of spread of microorganisms |
| 12. Record procedure, area clipped or shaved and condition of skin before and after shaving in nurse's notes | Documents status of surgical site for comparison over time |
| 13 Inspect/check patient to be sure that sheets are dry, bath blanket is removed, hospital clothing is being worn and patient is placed in comfortable position | |
| 14. Report any skin alterations or nicks or cuts in skin to surgeon | Skin problems may pose a serious risk for postoperative infections. |

## SITES FOR SURGICAL PREPARATION VARY DEPENDING ON TYPE OF SURGERY TO BE PERFORMED

### HEAD AND NECK

The site extends from above the eyebrows over the top of the head and includes the ears and both anterior and posterior areas of the neck and face. In females, face and eyebrows are not shaved.

### LATERAL NECK

Clean the external auditory canal with a cotton swab. Anteriorly, prepare the side of the face from above the ear to the upper thorax to just below the clavicle. Posteriorly prepare from neck to the spine including the area above the scapula.

### CHEST SURGERY

The site extends from the neck to the umbilicus and to the lateral midline.

### ABDOMINAL SURGERY

The preparation site extends from axilla to the mid thighs extending bilaterally to the lateral midline. All visible pubic hair should be shaved.

### PERINEAL SURGERY

Shave all pubic hair and the inner thighs to the mid thigh. The area starts above the pubic bone anteriorly and extends beyond the anus posteriorly.

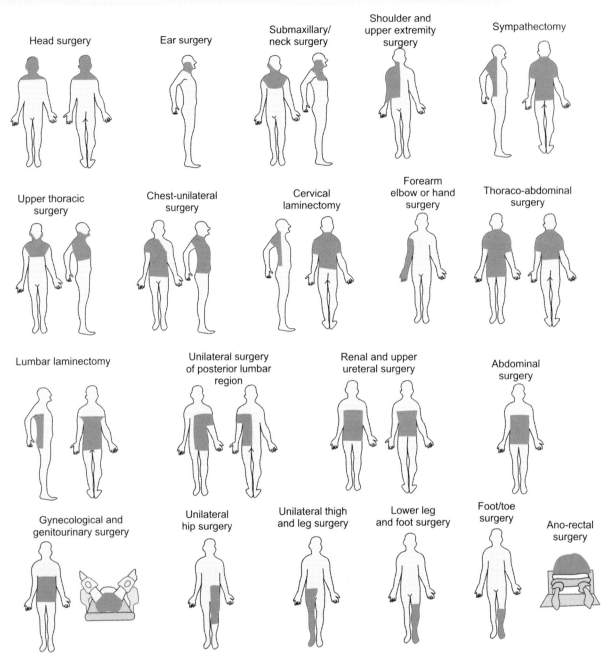

**Figure 12.3(b):** Skin areas to be prepared for surgery

## LUMBAR SPINE SURGERY

Shave entire back including shoulders and neck to hairline and down to knees including both axilla.

## RECTAL SURGERY

Shave the buttocks from iliac crest down to the upper third of the thighs including the anal region. The area extends to the mid line on each side.

**FLANK SURGERY**

Extends anteriorly from the axilla down to the upper thigh including external genital area. Posteriorly the area extends from mid scapular to the mid gluteal regions.

**HAND AND FOREARM SURGERY**

The area includes the full circumference of the affected hand from axilla to the fingertips.

**LOWER EXTREMITY SURGERY**

The area includes the area from umbilicus anteriorly including the entire leg, toes and foot of the affected leg and posteriorly
from top of buttocks to the heel.

**LOWER LEG SURGERY**

The area to be prepared includes the circumference of the entire leg from mid thigh to the distal toes of the affected leg.

**SPECIAL CONSIDERATION**

The site for preparation may vary according to the surgeon's preference.

# 12: 4: PREPARING AN OPERATION THEATER, TROLLEY AND PATIENT BEFORE SURGERY

## DEFINITION

Keeping the operating room ready and available for carrying out surgical procedures.

## PURPOSES

1. To ensure that appropriate equipment and machinery are available in working condition.
2. To clean equipment and machines.
3. To disinfect room, and work surfaces.
4. To collect necessary supplies of sterile and other items.

## ARTICLES

1. Operating room table and accessories like lights, cautery, sponge rack, etc.
2. Instrument trolleys
3. Articles required for positioning patient.
4. Sterile linen
5. Instrument sets
6. Cleaning solutions
7. Waste disposal containers.

## PROCEDURE

| | Nursing action | Rationale |
|---|---|---|
| 1 | Acquire information about the surgery to be carried out. | Helps in accurate, easy and quick preparation of operating room. |
| 2 | Assemble necessary equipment and machines. Minimise equipment as far as possible. | To save time and energy in preparation. Provides an organised approach to task. |
| 3 | Disinfect room, work surfaces, walls and floor including equipment and machines. Carbolise the surfaces and equipments after wet washing. | Ensures a sterile area and maintains sterile field. |
| 4 | Collect sterile linen and instrument sets. | |
| 5 | Account and collect other supplies. | |
| 6 | Ensure that scrub room is ready with soap, running water and sterile brush. | Ensures that articles are ready for scrubbing. |
| 7 | Ensure that airconditioning, lighting and power supply are adequate. | Preparation provides for an organised approach to task. |
| 8 | Check table and accessories, lights and cautery machine for proper functioning. | |
| 9 | Connect suction apparatus to electric source check central suction equipment. | |
| 10 | Receive patient from control desk/reception to operating room. | |

## SPECIAL POINTS

1. All personnel working in the operation theater use special dresses and shoes which are kept for use only for the time of theater work.
2. Anyone entering inside the theater after carbolising, should wear cap and mask along with the theater gown.

# STERILE TECHNIQUE OF DRAPING TROLLEY

## DEFINITION

Arranging appropriate sterile linen, instruments and supplies on designated trolleys for carrying out surgical operation, using aseptic technique.

## PURPOSES

1. To create a sterile field for carrying out surgical operation.
2. To ensure successful barrier against bacterial invasion of surgical wound.

## ARTICLES

1. Instrument trolleys
2. Mayo stand
3. Basin stand
4. Square trolley.

## PROCEDURE

| | Nursing action | Rationale |
|---|---|---|
| 1 | Scrub nurse after scrubbing her hands to put on sterile cap, mask, gown and gloves. | Interrupts chain of infection. Protects patient and nurse. |
| 2 | Check outer labels of all sterile linen bundles and instrument sets. | Ensures that correct instrument sets are opened. |
| 3 | Follow strict principles of asepsis while sterile packs are opened. | Maintains sterile field. |
| 4 | Ensure that whole trolley is dry by using waterproofing beneath sterile packs. | Moisture contaminates sterile field. |
| 5 | Circulating nurse, opens the sterile drum and hands over the sterile towel with the transfer forceps to the scrubbed nurse. | |
| 6 | Scrubbed nurse spreads the towel very carefully on the trolley without touching unsterile area. | Maintains sterile field. |
| 7 | Drape distal end of trolley first, then proximal. | Moving from distal to proximal prevents need to reach across the sterile field. |
| 8 | The circulating nurse opens the sterile pack using transfer forceps and scrub nurse removes the instrument tray and instruments from the sterile pack and gently places on instrument trolley. | Preparation provides for an organised approach to task. |
| 9 | Arrange instruments neatly according to the order of use. | |
| 10 | Circulating nurse pours sterile saline in sterile basin which is placed in basin stand. | Maintains sterile field. |
| 11 | Discard unnecessary wrappers and foils from sterile field. | Maintains sterile field. |
| 12 | Discard any contaminated drapes/instruments and substitute with sterile ones. | A sterile work area promotes proper aseptic technique. |
| 13 | After arranging, cover the trolley with a sterile towel till it is taken over to the surgeon. | Maintains sterile field. |

## STERILE TECHNIQUE OF DRAPING PATIENT

### DEFINITION

Receiving the preoperative patient on the theater table, and replacing patient's linen with sterile, theater linen, exposing operative site for preoperative skin cleaning and placing sterile mackintosh and towels for barricading operative site from surrounding areas.

### PURPOSES

1. To create a sterile field for carrying out surgical operation.
2. To ensure successful barrier against bacterial invasion of surgical wound.
3. To prevent contamination of operative site with unprepared skin surfaces.

### EQUIPMENT

1. Sterile bed linen
2. Big and small mackintosh
3. Surgical towels
4. Towel clips.

### PROCEDURE

|   | Nursing action | Rationale |
|---|---|---|
| 1 | Transfer the patient to theater table. | |
| 2 | Replace patient's linen with sterile linen | Sterile field is maintained. |
| 3 | Expose operative site while adequately covering other areas. | A neat work area promotes proper techniques |
| 4 | Assist surgeon to clean the site with bacteriocidal solution | |
| 5 | Offer sterile mackintosh, towels and towel clips to surgeon and assist in draping operative site. | Sterile field is maintained. |
| 6 | Drape patient according to nature, type of surgery and incision. | |
| 7 | Secure towel clips at each corner, viz above, below and sides of operative site. | Ensures that the sterile towels remain in place. |
| 8 | Assist surgeon to apply "Opsite" evenly without air pockets, soon after cleaning and drying operative site. | Sterile field is maintained. |
| | | Preparation provides for an organised approach to task. |

# 12.5: PERFORMING MASKING AND STERILE GOWNING

## DEFINITION

This procedure is the wearing of a mask and a specially stitched gown in the operation theater to maintain asepsis and to protect the nurse from contaminating herself and others around her.

## PURPOSES

1. To prevent dispersal of droplets from wearer to environment and patient.
2. To prevent contamination of sterile field.
3. To enhance easy handling of sterile equipment.

## ARTICLES REQUIRED

1. Articles for surgical handwashing.
2. Sterile cheattle forceps in a container of disinfectant solution.
3. Sterile drums containing sterile masks and sterile gowns.

## PROCEDURES

### MASKING

| | Nursing action | Rationale |
|---|---|---|
| 1 | After performing surgical handwashing take the sterile mask handed to you by the circulating nurse. Hold it by top two strings, keeping top edge above bridge of nose. | |
| 2 | Tie both top strings at back of head above ears (Figure 12.5(a) (i)) | |

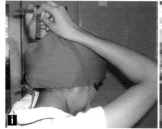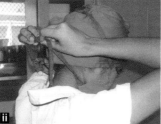

**Figure 12.5(a):** Sterile masking technique

| | | |
|---|---|---|
| 3 | Tie the two lower strings snugly around neck well under the chin (Figure 12.5(a) (ii)). | |
| 4 | Gently pinch upper portion of mask around bridge of nose. | Ensures proper fitting. |

### GOWNING

| | Nursing action | Rationale |
|---|---|---|
| 1 | Grasp the sterile gown at the crease near the neck, hold it away from yourself and permit it to unfold freely without touching anything including the uniform. | Prevents gown from becoming unsterile. |

*Contd...*

*Contd...*

| | | |
|---|---|---|
| 2 | Hold the gown at the shoulder level from inside and put each hand directly into the armhole (Figure 12.5(b) (i)). | Protects the outer portion of gown from contamination. |

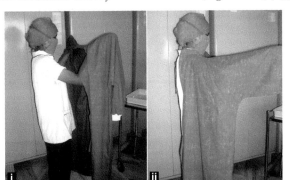

**Figure 12.5(b)** Sterile gowning technique

| | | |
|---|---|---|
| 3 | Extend the arms and hold hand upward at shoulder level while putting through the arm hole (Figure 12.5(b) (ii). | |
| 4 | The circulating nurse pulls back the gown from inside. So that the upper limbs go into the sleeves. The circulating nurse ties the gown from the back. | Prevents contamination of the outer portion of gown. |
| 5 | The waist ties are loosened by the scrub nurse and flap is brought around the waist by the use of cheatle forceps held by the circulating nurse and it is tied. | The waist flap cover the back, preventing contamination of the area when turning around. |

## REMOVAL OF GOWN AND MASK

| | | |
|---|---|---|
| | **GOWN:** | |
| 1 | Untie strings at the back of the gown. Remove gown, folding inside out to cover outside of gown. | Prevents contact with contaminated portion of gown. |
| 2 | Dispose gown into designated receptacle. | |
| | **MASK:** | |
| 1 | Wash hands. Untie lower strings first, then the top strings and pull mask away from face. | Avoids contact of the contaminated portion of mask to our body. |
| 2 | Hold mask by strings and discard into appropriate receptacle. | |

# 12.6: PERFORMING STERILE GLOVING

## DEFINITION

Gloving is defined as the donning of a pair of sterile gloves to protect one's own hands from pathogenic micro-organisms and to avoid contamination of a sterile area by hand.

## PURPOSES

1. To protect the nurse from pathogenic microorganisms.
2. To handle sterile articles without contaminating.

## ARTICLES REQUIRED

Soap/Antiseptic detergent, running warm water, nail brush in antiseptic lotion, towels (sterile) mask and cap.
A pair of sterile surgical gloves.

## PROCEDURE (DONNING OF GLOVES)

| | Nursing action | Rationale |
|---|---|---|
| 1 | Perform thorough surgical handwashing and dry hands using sterile towel. | Handwashing deters the spread of microorganisms. Gloves are easier to don when hands are dry. |
| 2 | The circulating nurse removes the outer glove package by carefully separating and peeling apart the sides. Scrubbed nurse pulls out the inner glove pack taking care not to touch the outer one. | Prevents inner glove package from accidentally opening and touching contaminated objects. |
| 3 | Grasp inner package and lay it on clean, flat surface just above waist level. Open package, keeping gloves on wrapper's inside surface (Figure 12.6(a)). | Sterile object held below waist is contaminated. Inner surface of glove package is sterile. |

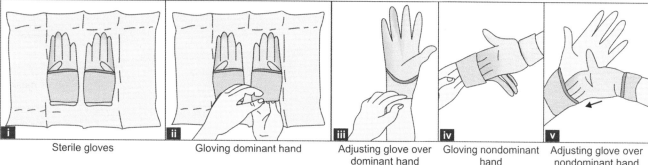

| i | ii | iii | iv | v |
|---|---|---|---|---|
| Sterile gloves | Gloving dominant hand | Adjusting glove over dominant hand | Gloving nondominant hand | Adjusting glove over nondominant hand |

**Figure 12.6(a):** Sterile gloving technique (illustrated)

| | | |
|---|---|---|
| 4 | If gloves are not pre-powdered, take packet of powder and apply lightly to hands over sink or waste basket. | |
| 5 | Identify right and left glove. Each glove has a cuff of approximately 5 cm (2 inches) wide. Glove dominant hand first. | Proper identification of gloves prevents contamination by improper fit. Gloving of dominant hand first improves dexterity. |
| 6 | With thumb and first two fingers of non-dominant hand, grasp edge of cuff of glove for dominant hand. Touch only the inside surface of gloves. | Inner edge of cuff will lie against skin and thus it is not sterile. |
| 7 | Carefully pull glove over dominant hand making sure the thumb and fingers fit into the proper spaces of the glove. | Prevents tearing the glove material, guiding the fingers into proper places facilitates gloving. |

*Condt...*

*Condt...*

| | | |
|---|---|---|
| 8 | With the gloved dominant hand, slip in fingers under the cuff of the other glove. Keep thumb of gloved dominant hand abducted back to avoid touching of exposed non-gloved hand. | If glove's outer surface touches hand/wrist, then it is contaminated. Cuff protects gloved fingers maintaining sterility. |
| 9 | Carefully slip the glove onto your non-dominant hand making sure that the fingers slip into the proper spaces. | |
| 10 | With gloved hands, interlock fingers to fit the gloves onto each fingers. | Promotes proper fit over the fingers. |

## REMOVAL OF GLOVES

| | | |
|---|---|---|
| 1 | Remove the first glove by grasping it on its palmar surface taking care to avoid touching wrist. | This keeps the soiled parts of the used gloves from touching the skin of the wrist/hand. |
| 2 | Pull the first glove completely off by inverting or rolling the glove inside out. | |
| 3 | Continue to hold the inverted removed glove by the fingers of the remaining gloved hand. Place the first two fingers of the bare hand inside the cuff of the second glove. | |
| 4 | Pull the second glove off to the fingers by turning it inside out. This pulls the first glove inside the second glove. | The soiled part of glove is folded to the inside to reduce the chance of transferring any microorganisms by direct contact. |
| 5 | Using the bare hand continue to remove the second glove, which is now inside out and dispose off the gloves in the waste receptacle. | |
| 6 | Wash hands. | |

# 12.7: POSITIONS USED IN SURGERY

## DEFINITION

Providing specific positions for patients undergoing surgery, which promote best visualization, and accessibility to operative site and promote safety and comfort.

## PURPOSES

1. To provide necessary accessibility and exposure for the site to be operated.
2. To facilitate administration of anesthesia and efficient monitoring.
3. To ensure safety for the patient and prevent injury.
4. To promote normal circulatory and respiratory functions.
5. To provide correct skeletal alignment.
6. To prevent undue pressure on muscles, nerves, skin over bony prominances and eyes.

## FACTORS THAT DETERMINE POSITION

1. The surgery to be performed.
2. Type of anesthesia used.
3. Age, size and physical condition of the patient
4. Surgical approach access.

## GUIDELINES FOR POSITIONING A PATIENT ON THE OPERATION TABLE

1. Explain to the patient in simple understandable terms why the positions and restraints are necessary and how he will be placed for surgery.
2. The patient should be in a comfortable and safe position as far as possible, whether asleep or awake.
3. Respiration and circulation should not be impeded by any kind of pressure.
4. Nerves must be protected from undue pressure, as improper positioning can cause serious nerve injury and paralysis.
5. Do not allow the extremities to dangle over the sides of table because this may impair circulation or cause nerve and muscle damage.
6. Avoid excessive stress on muscles, bones and soft body organs such as female breast, penis and eye.
7. Be certain that patient's body does not rest on hands or fingers, as circulation may be occluded.
8. Secure the patient to the table with well padded safety straps, usually placed 2 inches above knees.
9. Nerves, muscles and body prominences must be adequately padded to prevent nerve and tissue damage.
10. The physical condition (e.g. Arthritis) of the patient may place limitations on the desired position and should be taken into account.
11. Obtain sufficient physical or mechanical help to avoid unnecessary straining of self or patient.
12. Anesthetized patient is never moved without the anesthetist's permission.
13. Position changes (e.g. Lowering leg from lithotomy should be made slowly to allow the circulatory system to adjust thereby preventing a drop in blood pressure.
14. When using an armboard, do not abduct the upper extremity more than 90 degrees as this could crush the brachial plexus between the first rib and scapula.
15. Avoid contact between patient's skin and any metallic parts of operating room equipment.
16. Make sure that any apparatus which is to support patient's body is fully secure before body is brought to rest upon it.
17. Always ensure that head and cervical spine are adequately supported.
18. Position patient in correct alignment and protect patient from pressure and other injuries.
19. Consider normal joint movements while positioning the patient.

20. When positioning, lift the patient rather than slide, to prevent sheering forces on the skin.
21. Position the patient correctly before operation starts because it is much more difficult to do so afterwards.
22. The operative site must be adequately exposed. Preserve patient's dignity and avoid undue exposure.

## ARTICLES

1. Head rest
2. Arm board
3. Sand bags
4. Pillows
5. Towel roll
6. Mackintosh
7. Straps
8. Stirrups
9. Drapes

| Commonly used positions | Indications | Pressure points |
|---|---|---|
| **A  Supine position:**<br>1. Position the patient flat on back.<br>2. Position one arm at the side of table with hand placed palm down.<br>3. Position the other arm carefully on an arm board to facilitate infusion of fluids, blood or medications.<br>4. Position head and legs straight.<br>5. Check that legs are uncrossed.<br>6. Apply well padded safety straps 2 inches above knees.<br>7. For surgery on face or neck stabilize head on head rest.<br>8. For shoulder operation place a small sand bag or rolled sheet under shoulder.<br>9. For operations on upper extremity, radical mastectomy or axillary dissection, arm of affected side is placed on an arm board at right angle to body.<br>10. For saphenous ligations and groin operations, knees are slightly flexed over a pillow with thighs externally rotated. | • Abdominal operations<br>• Thoracic operations<br>• Abdomino-thoracic operations<br>• Operations on hip<br>• Operations on upper and lower extremities | • Heels<br>• Buttocks<br>• Elbows<br>• Shoulders<br>• Occiput |
| **B  Prone position:**<br>1. Carefully roll over the patient to prone position after the placement of intravenous line and the administration of general anesthesia.<br>2. Support fore-head on a horse-shoe.<br>3. Support arms on an arm board (angled towards the head end of table) | Thoracic/lumbar<br>Laminectomy | • Forehead<br>• Eyes<br>• Chest<br>• Abdomen<br>• Elbows<br>• Knees<br>• Breast (in case of female)<br>• Genitalia (in case of male) |
| **C  Lithotomy position:**<br>1. Lower the foot section of table and attach stirrups to table on either side to place patient's leg.<br>2. Place a mackintosh over the lower end of table before patient is transferred on to it. | Cystoscopy, operations on vagina, perineum and rectum. | • Forearm<br>• Buttocks<br>• Inner aspects of thighs<br>• Occiput |

*Contd...*

*Contd...*

3. Position the patient flat on back
4. Gently bring the patient towards foot end of table so that buttocks extend slightly past the lower edge of table.
5. Move both lower extremities simultaneously and put them up in stirrups, so that hips are not dislocated or muscles strained.
6. Position one arm on an arm board and secure the other arm across patient's abdomen.
7. Protect pressure points.
8. Secure patient safely using safety straps.

| | | |
|---|---|---|
| **Trendelenburg position:**<br>1. Place the patient flat on back.<br>2. Lower the foot end of the table so that patient's knees are flexed slightly.<br>3. Tilt the table in such a way that the head end of table is slightly lower than the foot end (usually operating table at an angle of 45 degree to the floor).<br>4. Pad the pressure points.<br>5. Secure the patient in position | Operations on lower abdomen and pelvis | • Occiput<br>• Shoulders<br>• Elbows<br>• Knees. |
| **E  Lateral position:**<br>1. Position the patient on the non-operative side with an air pillow 12.5 to 15 cm thick under the loin or on a table with a kidney or back lift.<br>2. Position the legs in such a way that the underneath leg is fully flexed at the knees with foot placed under upper leg.<br>3. Support the upper most arm on a padded rest and the underneath arm is pulled little away from the body.<br>4. Pad the pressure points.<br>5. Secure the patient safely. | Renal surgery | • Head<br>• Ear<br>• Shoulder<br>• Elbow<br>• Hip<br>• Knee |
| **F  Rose position/Neck position**<br>1. Place the patient flat on the back.<br>2. Place a rolled sheet or small sand bag between the scapulae to extend the neck.<br>3. Lower shoulders for better exposure of the operative site.<br>4. Stabilize head on a head ring.<br>5. Arms may be extended on an arm board. | Thyroidectomy<br>Tracheostomy<br>Parathyroidectomy | • Occiput<br>• Shoulders<br>• Elbows<br>• Buttocks<br>• Heels. |

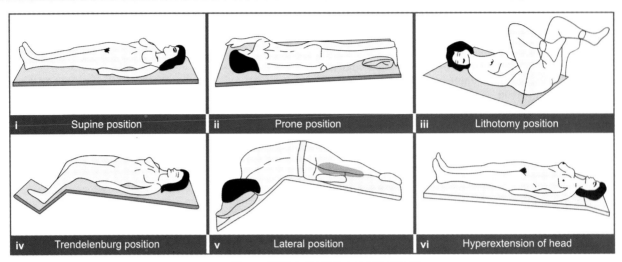

Figure 12.7(a): Position used in surgery

## SPECIAL CONSIDERATIONS

Even after careful positioning most patients feel stiff and sore after a long surgical procedure. Therefore, observe the patient throughout the surgery. Protect any unprotected bony prominence or pressure points.

# 12.8: ASSISTING WITH POSTOPERATIVE EXERCISES

## DEFINITION

Exercises done by patient independently or with assistance, to enhance a speedy recovery after surgery.

## EXERCISES INCLUDE

1. Ambulation
2. Diaphragmatic breathing
3. Turning in bed
4. Leg exercises.

## AMBULATION EXERCISE

Assisting a patient to walk after a period of being immobile following surgery.

*Purposes*

1. To exercise muscles and joints for regaining strength.
2. To increase patient's sense of independence
3. To increase mobility
4. To prevent postoperative complications.

*Procedure*

| | Nursing action | Rationale |
|---|---|---|
| 1 | Assess patient's condition, vital signs and any contraindications. | Predicts the patient's tolerance for ambulation. |
| 2 | Check the time when patient received last dose of sedative drug | |
| 3 | Assess patient's ability to walk | |
| 4 | Keep a foot stool beside bed if required | Assists in getting out of bed safely. |
| 5 | Keep a chair with backrest and extra pillows ready near the bed | |
| 6 | Make sure that the floor is clean and dry. Ensure that slippers or chappals worn by patient are made of non-skid material | Clutter free and well-lighted area prevents falls during ambulation. |
| 7 | Explain procedure and purpose of ambulation | Promotes patient cooperation for ambulation. |
| 8 | Ensure that patient is adequately dressed and well groomed | |
| 9 | Free all drains attached to bedside. Empty urobag. Ensure that the drainage bag is held below hip level. | Urine bag held below hip level prevents back flow of urine. |
| 10 | Raise head end of bed 40 to 60 degrees and assist patient to sit up. Bring patient's legs to edge of bed and allow feet to dangle. | Prevents orthostatic hypotension. |
| 11 | Check for dizziness, drowsiness, pain, etc. Administer pain medication half an hour before ambulation if ordered | Ensures that patient is able to tolerate ambulation. |
| 12 | Assist patient to get out of bed slowly and to stand with head erect and back straight. | |
| 13 | Support patient on either side by holding at inferior aspect of upper arms and assist him to walk with even gait. | Provides confidence for patient and prevents accidental fall. |
| 14 | After walking, allow patient to rest in chair for some time and then assist back to bed. Check vital signs and note untoward changes if any. | |

*Contd...*

| | | |
|---|---|---|
| 15 | Connect the drains back in position and make patient comfortable and leave the unit neat. | |
| 16 | Record in patient's chart the distance walked, duration of ambulation and patient's response. | Gives information about the patient's response to the exercise. |

### Special Considerations

1. Have chair/wheel chair readily available in case patient cannot tolerate the exercise.
2. Use safety-walking belt if available.

## DIAPHRAGMATIC (DEEP BREATHING) EXERCISE

### Definition

Lung expansion exercise to be performed by patient to reduce postoperative respiratory complications.

### Purposes

1. To enhance lung expansion and gas exchange
2. To prevent complications such as respiratory infections and atelectasis.

### Procedure

| | Nursing action | Rationale |
|---|---|---|
| 1 | Assess patient's risk for postoperative respiratory complications. Identify presence of chronic pulmonary condition or any condition that affects chest wall movement, history of smoking and presence of reduced hemoglobin. | General anesthesia predisposes patient to respiratory problems because lungs are not fully inflated during surgery. Cough reflex is suppressed and mucus collects within air passages postoperatively. Patient may have reduced lung volume and require greater efforts to cough and deep breath. Inadequate lung expansion can lead to atelectasis and pneumonia. |
| 2 | Explain procedure to patient including the advantages of diaphragmatic breathing. | Helps in obtaining cooperation of patient. |
| 3 | Assess patient's ability to cough and deep breath by instructing patient to take deep breaths. Observe movements of shoulders and chest wall. Measure chest expansion during deep breath. Ask patient to cough after taking a deep breath. | Reveals maximum potential for chest expansion and ability to cough forcefully. Serves as baseline to measure patient's ability to perform exercises postoperatively. |
| 4 | Assess patient's willingness and capability to learn exercise, note factors such as attention span, anxiety, level of consciousness and language known. | Ability to learn depends on readiness, ability and learning environment. |
| 5 | Assess family member's willingness to learn and support patient postoperatively. | Presence of families postoperatively can be a potential motivating factor for patient's recovery. Family members can coach patients on exercise performance. |
| 6 | Assess patient's medical orders– both preoperative and postoperative. | Determines if patient requires adaptations in the way exercises are performed. |
| 7 | Assist patient to comfortable sitting or standing position. If patient chooses to sit, assist to side of bed or to upright position in chair. | Upright position facilitates diaphragmatic excursion |
| 8 | Stand or sit facing patient for demonstrating breathing exercise to patient (Figure 12.8(a)). | Patient will be able to observe breathing exercise performed by nurse. |

*Contd...*

*Contd...*

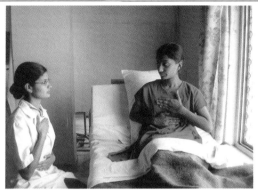

**Figure 12.8(a):** Demonstrating deep breathing exercises

| | | |
|---|---|---|
| 9 | Instruct patient to place palm of one hand on chest and another on abdomen and concentrate on filling up the abdomen by inhaling slowly through the nose. On exhalation the patient uses pursed lip breathing. | |
| 10 | Demonstrate for patient the exercise and instruct to perform every 2 hours while awake during postoperative period until mobile. Explain that abdominal organs descend and chest wall expands during inspiration. | Slow deep breaths prevent panting or hyperventilation. Inhaling through nose warms, humidifies and filters air. Explanation and demonstration focus on normal ventilatory movement of chest-wall. |
| 11 | Repeat breathing exercise 3 to 5 times. | Allows patient to observe slow, rhythmical breathing pattern. |
| 12 | Have patient practice the exercise. Patient is instructed to take 10 slow deep breaths every 2 hours while awake during postoperative period until mobile. | Repetition of exercise reinforces learning. Regular deep breathing will prevent postoperative complications. |
| 13 | Record the procedure. | Gives information about patient's response to the exercise. |

## CONTROLLED COUGHING

Lung exercise to be performed by patient including voluntary coughing.

*Purposes*

1. To promote lung expansion and gas exchange
2. To prevent complications like infection and atelectasis
3. To loosen and bring out secretions.

*Procedure*

| | **Nursing action** | **Rationale** |
|---|---|---|
| 1 | Explain procedure to patient | Helps in obtaining cooperation of the patient. |
| 2 | Explain importance of maintaining upright position | Position facilitates diaphragmatic excursion and enhances thoracic expansion. |

*Contd...*

*Contd...*

| 3 | Demonstrate coughing, taking two slow deep breaths inhaling through nose and exhaling through mouth. | Deep breath expands lungs fully so that air moves behind mucus, and facilitates effect of coughing. |
|---|---|---|
| 4 | Breath deeply a third time and hold breath to count of 3, perform 2 to 3 consecutive coughs without inhaling between coughs. | Consecutive coughs help remove mucus more effectively and completely than one forceful cough. |
| 5 | Caution patient against just clearing throat instead of coughing. | Clearing throat does not remove mucus from deep airways. |
| 6 | If surgical incision is either abdominal or thoracic, teach patient to place a small pillow or folded sheet over incisional area and splint incision. During breathing and coughing exercise, press gently against incisional area holding a small pillow or folded sheat over it (Figure 12.8(b)). | Surgical incision cuts through muscle tissues and nerve endings. Deep breathing and coughing exercises place additional stress on suture line and causes discomfort. Splinting incision with hands or pillows provides firm support and reduces incisional pulling. |

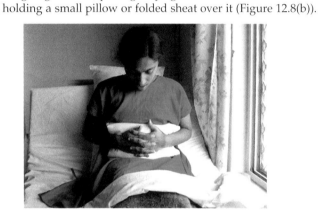

**Figure 12.8(b):** Splinting incisional area

| 7 | Instruct. the patient to cough two or three times every 2 hours while awake. | Value of deep coughing with splinting is stressed to effectively expectorate mucus with minimal discomfort. |
|---|---|---|
| 8 | Instruct patient to examine sputum for consistency, odour, amount and color changes. | Change in consistency odour, amount and colour of sputum may indicate the presence of pulmonary complications such as infection. |
| 9 | Record the procedure observations made and patient's response. | |

## TURNING EXERCISE

Assisting patient to change position while in bed.

*Purposes*

1. To improve circulation
2. To relieve pain and discomfort
3. To increase GI peristalsis
4. To avoid unrelieved pressure

# PROCEDURE

| | Nursing action | Rationale |
|---|---|---|
| 1 | Explain procedure to the patient | Helps in obtaining cooperation of the patient. |
| 2 | Instruct patient to assume supine position on right side of the bed. | Positioning begins on right side of bed so that turning to left side will not cause patient to roll towards edge of bed. |
| 3 | Assist patient to place the left hand over incisional area to splint it. | Splinting incision supports and minimizes pulling on suture line during turning. |
| 4 | Instruct patient to keep left leg straight and flex right knee up and over left leg. | Straight leg stabilizes patient's position. Flexed right leg shifts weight for easier turning. |
| 5 | Instruct patient to turn every two hours while awake. | Reduces risk of vascular complications. |
| 6 | Record the procedure in nurse's record. | |

## LEG EXERCISE

*Definition*

Assisting patient to move lower limbs.

*Purposes*

1. To improve circulation and prevent thrombophlebitis and thrombus formation.
2. To relieve pain/discomfort.

*Procedure*

| | Nursing action | Rationale |
|---|---|---|
| 1 | Explain procedure to the patient | Helps in obtaining cooperation of the patient. |
| 2 | Help patient assume supine position in bed. Demonstrate leg exercises by performing passive range of motion exercises and explaining each exercise. | Supine position provides normal anatomical position of lower extremities |
| 3 | Rotate each ankle in complete circle. Instruct patient to draw an imaginary circle with big toe. Repeat five times. (Figure 12.8(c)) | Leg exercises maintain joint mobility and venous return. |

**Figure 12.8(c):** Ankle exercises

| | Nursing action | Rationale |
|---|---|---|
| 4 | Alternate dorsiflexion and plantar flexion by moving both feet up and down. Direct patient to feel calf muscles contract and relax alternately (Figure 12.8(c)). | Stretches and contracts gastrocnemius muscles. |
| 5 | Instruct patient to continue leg exercise by alternately flexing and extending knees. Repeat five times (Figure 12.8(d)). | Contracts muscles of upper legs and maintains knee mobility. |

*Contd...*

*Contd...*

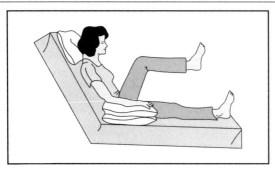

**Figure 12.8(d):** Flexion and extension of knees

| 6 | Instruct patient to alternately raise each leg straight up from bed surface, keeping legs straight. Repeat five times (Figure 12.8(e)). | Promotes contraction and relaxation of quadriceps muscles. |

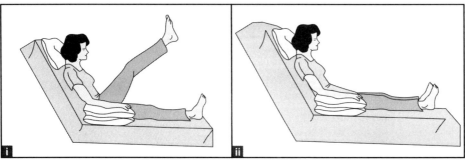

**Figure 12.8(e):** Leg exercises

| 7 | Have patient continue to practice exercises at least every 2 hours, while awake. Patient is instructed to coordinate turning and leg exercises with diaphragmatic and coughing exercises. | Repetition of sequence of exercises reinforces learning. |
| 8 | Record exercises that have been demonstrated to patient and whether patient performs exercises independently. | Ensures continuity of exercises. |
| 9 | Record physical assessment findings in nurse's notes or flowsheets. | Documents baseline for later comparison. |
| 10 | Report any problem patient has in practicing exercises. | Informs staffs so that reinforcement can be provided. |

## SPECIAL CONSIDERATIONS

1. The patient can benefit more from the use of incentive spirometry instead of diaphragmatic exercises.
2. Increase frequency of exercises if patient has difficulty practicing exercise.

# Chapter 13

# Mental Health Nursing

## 13.1: PERFORMING MENTAL STATUS EXAMINATION (MSE)

### DEFINITION

Mental status examination (MSE) is an assessment of general motor behavior, thought and emotional functioning, along with evaluation of insight and judgement of the patient's current status.

### PURPOSES

1. Mental status examination serves as a basis for comparison, to track the progress of patient.
2. It is used to detect changes or abnormalities in a person's psychological functioning.

### GENERAL INSTRUCTIONS

1. Collect identification data before doing mental status examination.
2. Perform a physical assessment from head to toe including vital signs.
3. Provide a comfortable environment for mental status examination.
4. Prepare some questions under each aspect of mental status examination.

### FORMAT FOR MENTAL STATUS EXAMINATION (MSE)

#### INSTRUCTIONS

1. Write observation findings obtained from patient in the space given.
2. Give details wherever required.

1. **Identification data**
   a. Name                  :
   b. Age                   :        Date of admission          :
   c. Sex                   :        Diagnosis                  :
   d. Bed No                :
   e. Date of MSE           :
   f. Time of MSE           :

2. **General appearance**
   a. Consciousness         :
   b. Body built            :        Well built/Moderately built/emaciated
   c. Personal hygiene      :
   d. Grooming              :
   e. Facial expression     :
   f. Eye contact           :

3. **Speech**
   a. Language              :
   b. Reaction time         :
   c. Unusual words         :
   d. Volume                :
   e. Rate                  :
   f. Characteristics       :

4. **Motor activity**
   a. Level of activity     :

   b.  Mannerisms             :
   c.  Type of activity     :

**5. Mood or Affect**
   a.  Mood – Sad/Happy/Irritable/Angry/Suspicious/Fearful/Restless/Worried/Any other (specify)
   b.  Affect – Appropriate/Inappropriate/Flat/Labile/Blunt/ Any other (specify)

**6. Perception**
   a.  Hallucination        :          Present/Absent
       if present specify        _____
                                _____

   b.  Type                 :          Visual/Auditory/Tactile/ Olfactory
   c.  Illusion             :          Present/Absent
       if present specify        _____
                                  _____

**7.  Thought**
   a.  Stream of thought   :          Normal/Increased/Reduced/Blocked/Any other
       if present specify        _____
                                _____

   b.  Content            :          Neologism/clang association
       if present specify        _____
                                _____

   c.  Form               :          Circumstantiality/Tangentiality/Flight of ideas
       if present specify        _____
                                _____

**8.  Orientation**
   a.  Oriented to time, Place, Person  :     Present/Absent
                                  _____

   b.   Confusion          :          Present/Absent

**9. Memory**
   a.  Remote             :          Intact/Impaired
   b.  Recent             :          Intact/Impaired
   c.  Immediate         :          Intact/Impaired

**10. Judgement**
   a.  Logical/Illogical (specify)

_____
_____

**11. Attention and Concentration**    :      Good/Distracted/Pre-occupied/Any other
                                  _____
                                  _____

**12. Intelligence**
   a.  Educational status
   b.  Learning disability     :          Present/Absent
       if present specify        _____
                                  _____

    c.  I.Q Level             :

    d.  General knowledge   :       Good/Poor/Moderate

**13. Insight**                :       Present/Absent

**14. Psychological factors**

    a.  Stressor             :       Present/Absent

       If present specify            _____

                                    _____

    b.  Coping skills(specify)  :       _____

                                    _____

    c.  Social relation       :       Good/Poor

    d.  Occupation           :

**15. Physiological factors**

    a.  Bowel and bladder habits  :

    b.  Appetite             :

    c.  Sleep               :

    d.  Libido              :

**16. Summary**

    • List of problems

# 13.2: CONDUCTING PROCESS RECORDING

## DEFINITION

Process recording is the interaction or interview conducted and recorded by the nurse by using various communication techniques.

## PURPOSES

1. To study the patient's psychological, social and emotional behavior
2. To evaluate the condition of patient during admission, hospital stay and at the time of termination of hospital stay.
3. To improve therapeutic communication skills of the nurse.
4. To establish a therapeutic relationship.

## GENERAL GUIDELINES

1. Record the conversation verbatim.
2. Use a recording device and obtain patient's permission for using it. This will help in reviewing the session if needed.
3. Note the non-verbal responses of patient and nurse when recording the session.

## FORMAT FOR PROCESS RECORDING

### IDENTIFICATION DATA

- Name                               :
- Age                                :
- Sex                                :
- Address                            :
- Ward & Bed No                      :
- Marital status                     :
- Language                           :
- Religion                           :
- Education                          :
- Occupation                         :
- Income                             :
- Diagnosis                          :
- Date of admission                  :
- Date of interview                  :
- Brief history of patient's illness :
- Objectives of interaction          :
- Time and duration of interaction   :

**DETAILS OF CONVERSATION**

### Nurse – Patient Interaction

| Nurse | | Patient | |
|---|---|---|---|
| Verbal | Nonverbal | Verbal | Nonverbal |
| | | | |

**INFERENCES**

# 13.3: PREPARATION OF PATIENT AND ASSISTING WITH ELECTROCONVULSIVE THERAPY (ECT)

## DEFINITION

Electroconvulsive therapy is a physical therapy, in which there is an application of electrical current to the temporal region of the brain to produce a grand mal type of seizure, for bringing about therapeutic effects.

## INDICATIONS

1. Major depression
2. Involutional melancholia
3. Schizophrenia
4. Mania
5. Postpartum depression.

## CONTRAINDICATIONS

1. Increased intracranial pressure
2. Recent myocardial infarction
3. Cerebral hemorrhage
4. Glaucoma
5. History of cardiovascular diseases
6. Pregnancy.

## ARTICLES

1. ECT machine, electrodes
2. ECG monitor
3. Pulse oximeter
4. Defibrillator
5. Suction apparatus
6. Oxygen cylinder and AMBU bag
7. Mouth gag and Tongue depressor
8. Sterile syringe and needles
9. IV stand
10. Emergency drugs
11. K-basin
12. Jelly

## PROCEDURE

| | Nursing action | Rationale |
|---|---|---|
| | **Preparation for ECT** | |
| 1. | Identify the patient and explain about procedure to the family and patient. | Helps in obtaining cooperation from patient. |
| 2 | Check if a thorough physical examination is completed which includes assessment of the cardiac, respiratory, skeletal system, etc. and investigation like routine blood and urine tests such as Hb% TC, DC, urine for glucose, albumin and X-ray. | These findings help rule out contraindication or risk of the patient for ECT |

*Contd...*

*Contd...*

| 3 | Get a written consent from the nearest relative after explaining the purposes, method of treatment and risks involved. | Prevents legal problems. Explanation to the relatives will help them to overcome fear of therapy. |
|---|---|---|
| 4 | Patient should be kept nil per orally from midnight, of the previous day . | Helps to prevent risk of vomiting and aspiration during and after the procedure. |
| 5 | Instruct the patient not to apply oil to head, on the day of ECT, wash hair using shampoo. | Oil is a bad conductor of electricity. |
| 6 | Remove all the metallic articles from his/ her body, e.g. watch, bangles, ring, safety pin, etc. | Prevents the electric current passing on unwanted areas, and causing burns since metal is a good conductor of electricity. |
| 7 | Remove artificial dentures | Prevents dislodging and blocking of the respiratory passage. |
| 8 | Remove lipstick, nail polish or any other makeup. | These colors may mask any changes, if present, e.g. cyanosis. |
| 9 | Provide a loose gown | |
| 10 | Administer medication as per physician's order. | Enhances the effectiveness of ECT |
| 11 | Encourage patient to empty the bladder before entering treatment room. | Prevents soiling of bed due to a relaxant effect of the drugs administered. |
| 12 | Give injection atropine 0.65 mg IM or S.C half to one hour prior to ECT as per order. | Blocks the vagal nerve thus decreases oropharyngeal secretions. |
| 13 | Check vital signs | Helps to evaluate the condition of patient. |
| 14 | Administer Tab. Lorazepam or calmpose if ordered. | Relieves anxiety of patient. |
| 15 | Transfer the patient to the waiting room. | |
| | **Assisting with administration of ECT** | |
| 16. | Shift the patient to ECT room. | |
| 17. | Provide a well padded bed with a pillow under lumbar curve. Patient can be placed in a supine position. | Well padded bed helps to prevent injury. |
| 18 | Administer short acting anesthetic agents like thiopental as prescribed by physician. | Muscle relaxant and anesthetic are used to reduce violent convulsive attacks. |
| 19 | Place well padded mouth gag or tongue depressor between the teeth. | Prevents tongue bite, injury to lips, and obstruction of airway caused by falling back of tongue. |
| 20 | Support the shoulder and arms lightly and restrain the knee joints firmly but gently. | Prevents fracture. Tight pressure may lead to fracture of femur or humerus. |
| 21 | Hyperextend the head with support to the chin | Prevents jaw dislocation or fracture and facilitates patent airway. |
| 22 | Administer 100% oxygen by using face mask. | Helps the patient to overcome a phase of apnea after convulsions. |
| 23 | Provide electrodes dipped in jelly for placement. (Electrodes may be placed as bilateral, unilateral or bifrontal) (Figure 13.3(a)) | Jelly is a good conductor of electricity, thereby facilitates passing of current and production of convulsions. |
| 24 | Observe grand mal seizures. Initial tonic stage lasts for 10-15 seconds, followed by convulsions lasting for 25-30 seconds. Then there is a phase of muscular relaxation. | Ensures that treatment is successful and there are no subshocks. |

*Contd...*

*Contd...*

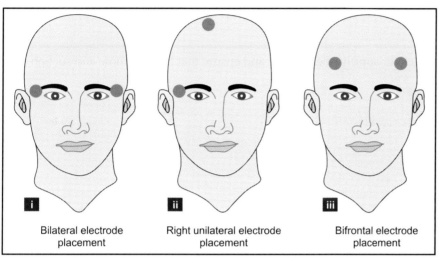

|  | i | ii | iii |
|---|---|---|---|
|  | Bilateral electrode placement | Right unilateral electrode placement | Bifrontal electrode placement |

**Figure 13.3(a):** Electrode placement in electroconvulsive therapy

| 25 | Do suction of mouth immediately. | Keeps airway patent and prevents from aspiration pneumonia. |
|---|---|---|
| 26 | Restore respiration by giving oxygen by mask if required. | Prevents the patient from respiratory and cardiac complications. |
|  | **Care after ECT** |  |
| 27 | Check and record vital signs. | Evaluates any respiratory or cardiac complications. |
| 28 | Put the side rails of bed up and place the patient on side lying position. Wipe the secretions. | Prevents falling of patient due to restlessness. Side lying position avoids aspiration. |
| 29 | Transfer the patient to the recovery room when he can answer simple questions. | Ensures that patient has come out of the phase of unconsciousness. |
| 30 | Check vitals every 15 minutes till stable and record. | Helps to evaluate signs and symptoms of complications if any. |
| 31 | Encourage the patient to sleep for some time. | Helps the patient to overcome physical exhaustion. |
| 32 | Shift the patient to ward. |  |
| 33 | Reorient the patient to the ward, toilet, nurse's station etc. | Reorientation helps to overcome the state of confusion. |
| 34 | Check for any injury pain, headache etc. | Helps to detect any complications, specially fracture. |
| 35 | Encourage the patient to drink clear tea followed by soft solids. | Meets the nutritional needs as they are kept nil per oral from previous midnight. |
| 36 | Record any change observed after ECT. | Evaluates the behavioral pattern after receiving ECT. |

## COMPLICATIONS

1. Impairment of memory
2. Fracture and dislocations
3. Aspiration pneumonia
4. Headache, backache
5. Painful mastication
6. Injury to mouth and tongue.

7. Subshocks
8. Confusion

## SPECIAL CONSIDERATION

Before starting the procedure, check for supply of electricity and ensure that ECT machine and suction apparatus are in working condition.

## 13.4: ASSISTING WITH NARCO ANALYSIS/ABREACTIVE THERAPY

### DEFINITION

Therapy in which a heightened psychological reaction is produced with an intention of ventilating the pent up emotions present in the unconscious mind of the individual.

### PURPOSES

1. To ventilate the traumatic, painful experiences in therapeutic situations.
2. To release the emotional conflicts and disturbances.
3. To give positive suggestions and improve tolerance.
4. To elicit suicidal or paranoid ideas from patient's mind.

### INDICATIONS

1. Hysterical stupor
2. Catatonic stupor
3. Personality disorders
4. Post-traumatic stress disorders
5. Hysterical convulsions
6. Dissociative disorders
7. Acute anxiety
8. Phobias.

### CONTRAINDICATIONS

1. Cardiac/renal/liver diseases
2. General disability
3. Severe anemia
4. Mental retardation
5. Schizophrenia.

### ARTICLES

1. Injection sodium pentathol – 250 - 500 mg
2. Distilled water
3. Syringe and needles
4. Oxygen cylinder
5. AMBU bag
6. IV stand, IV fluid
7. K. basin
8. Suction apparatus
9. Emergency drugs.

### PROCEDURE

| | Nursing action | Rationale |
|---|---|---|
| 1. | Explain procedure to the patient/relatives and obtain informed consent. | Legal implications are met and proper explanation helps to win patient's confidence and trust. |
| 2. | Perform thorough physical examination. | Identifies any medical illness or contraindication. |

*Contd...*

# Clinical Nursing Procedures: The Art of Nursing Practice

*Contd...*

| | | |
|---|---|---|
| 3. | Ensure that all laboratory investigations are done and reports collected. | Helps to rule out any physical pathology. |
| 4. | Instruct the patient to be nil per oral, (NPO) 4-6 hours prior to procedure. | Prevents complication due to anesthetic effect. |
| 5. | Keep ready all emergency drugs, suction apparatus, oxygen, etc. | Helps to meet the emergency situation if it occurs. |
| 6. | Transfer the patient to treatment room. Ensure that he/she is comfortable in a bed. | Since patient goes to hypnotic state, it is preferable that the patient lies in a bed. |
| 7. | Administer injection pentothal sodium mixed with 20–40 ml of distilled water, intravenously till it produces a state of trance between wakefulness and sleep where patient is able to answer questions. (Requires physician's prescription) | |
| 8. | Ensure that patient has gone to 'trance' state. | Trance state is ideal so that patient will release his emotional conflicts and receives suggestions when given |
| 9. | The therapist will ask questions, that will encourage the patient to ventilate deep seated conflicts. | Helps to release patient's pent up emotions. |
| 10. | Encourage expression of emotions like crying, anger, fear etc. | Helps to release patient's pent up emotions. |
| 11. | Record patient's conversations. | Helps to be legally safe. |
| 12. | Monitor and record vital signs during procedure | Evaluates patient's condition. |
| 13. | Once the patient has fully verbalized emotional conflicts the therapist can give positive suggestions. | Patient can take up suggestions easily in the 'trance' state. |
| 14. | Administer the remaining medications as per order | Ensures rest and sleep after an emotionally charged situation. |
| 15. | Check vital signs every 30 minutes after procedure for 2 hours | Helps to identify complications early. |
| 16. | Transfer the patient to his/her room. | |
| 17. | Monitor the patient | Identifies post anesthetic complications. |
| 18. | Give fluids or food when fully conscious and after gag reflex has returned. | Reduces risk of aspiration. |
| 19. | Record procedure and other findings in nurses record. | Recording enables communication between staff members. |

## COMPLICATIONS

1. Aggression
2. Depression
3. Disorientation
4. Suicidal tendency
5. Anxiety.

# Chapter 14

# Maternal and Child Nursing

# 14.1: PERFORMING AN ANTENATAL ABDOMINAL EXAMINATION AND PALPATION

## DEFINITION

Examination of a pregnant woman to determine the normalcy of fetal growth in relation to the gestational age, position of the fetus in uterus and its relationship to the maternal pelvis.

## PURPOSES

1. To measure the abdominal girth and fundal height.
2. To determine the abdominal muscle tone.
3. To determine the fetal lie, presentation, position, variety (anterior or posterior) and engagement.
4. To determine the possible location of the fetal heart tones.
5. To observe the signs of pregnancy.
6. To detect any deviation from normal.

## ARTICLES

1. Fetoscope/stethoscope/Doppler machine.
2. Measuring tape/Pelvimeter.

## PROCEDURE

| | Nursing action | Rationale |
|---|---|---|
| 1. | Explain to the woman what will be done and how she may cooperate | Reduces anxiety and promotes relaxation during the procedure. |
| 2. | Instruct the woman to empty her bladder. | Avoids discomfort during palpation . |
| 3. | Draw curtains around the bed. | Provides privacy. |
| | **INSPECTION** | |
| 4. | Position the woman for examination <br> • Place a pillow under her head and upper shoulders <br> • Have her arms by her sides <br> • Expose her abdomen from below the breasts to the symphysis pubis. | Promotes relaxation of abdominal muscles. <br><br> Enables visualization of the whole abdomen. |
| 5. | Inspect abdomen for the following: <br> Scars, Diastasis recti, Hernia, <br> Linea nigra, Striae gravidarum, Contour of the abdomen, <br> State of umbilicus, Skin condition. | |
| 6. | Determine the fundal height using the ulnar side of the palm (Figure 14.1(a)). | Provides an estimate whether fetal growth corresponds to gestational period. |

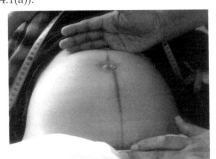

**Figure 14.1(a):** Identifying fundus

*Contd...*

*Contd...*

- 12 weeks – level of symphisis pubis
- 16 weeks – midway between symphisis pubis and umbilicus
- 20 weeks – 1-2 finger breadths below umbilicus
- 24 weeks – level of umbilicus
- 32 weeks – halfway between umbilicus and xiphoid process
- 36 weeks – at level of xiphoid process
- 40 weeks – 2-3 finger breadths below the xiphoid process
  if lightening occurs (Figure 14.1(b))

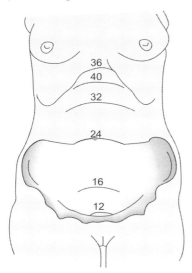

**Figure 14.1(b):** Fundal height at various weeks of pregnancy

7. Measure fundal height using any
   one of the following methods.
   a. Using measuring tape (Figure 14.1(c))
   - Place zero line of the tape measure on the superior
     border of the symphysis pubis
   - Stretch the tape across the contour of the abdomen to the
     top of the fundus along the midline.

The number of centimeters measured should be approximately equal to the weeks of gestation after about 22 to 24 weeks.

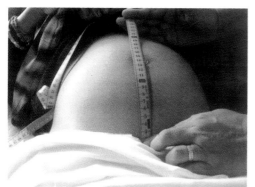

**Figure 14.1(c):** Measuring fundal height

*Contd...*

*Contd...*

| | |
|---|---|
| b. Caliper method (Pelvimeter)<br>• Place one tip of the caliper on the superior border of the symphysis pubis and the other tip at the top of the fundus. Both placements are in the midline.<br>• Read the measurement on the centimeter scale located on the arc, close to the joint. The number of centimeters should be equal approximately to the weeks of gestation after about 22 to 24 weeks. | This method is more accurate. |
| 8. Measure the abdominal girth by encircling the woman's body with a tape measure at the level of the umbilicus (Figure 14.1(d)) | Normally the measurement is 2 inches (5 cm) less than the weeks of gestation.<br>e. g. 32 inches at 34 weeks gestation. Measurements more than 100 cm (39 ½ inches) is abnormal at any week of gestation. |

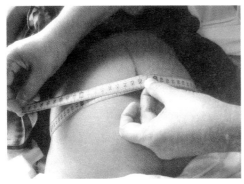

**Figure 14.1(d):** Measuring abdominal girth

### ABDOMINAL PALPATION OR LEOPOLD'S MANEUVERS

| | |
|---|---|
| 9. Instruct the woman to relax her abdominal muscles by bending her knees slightly and doing relaxation breathing. | These steps reduce the stretching and tension of abdominal muscles |
| 10. Be sure your hands are warm before beginning to palpate, rest your hand on the mother's abdomen lightly while giving explanation about the procedure. | Cold hands may cause muscle contraction and discomfort. Resting hands on mother's abdomen would help her to become accustomed to your touch and dissipate muscle tightening. |
| 11. For the technique of palpation,<br>• Use the flat palmar surface of fingers and not fingertips. Keep fingers of hands together and apply smooth deep pressure as firm as is necessary to obtain accurate findings. | These measures would aid in gathering greatest amount of information with least discomfort to the woman. |
| 12. Perform the first maneuver (Fundal palpation) (Figure 14.1(e))<br>• Face the woman's head<br>• Place your hands on the sides of the fundus and curve the fingers around the top of the uterus<br>• Palpate for size, shape, consistency and mobility of the fetal part in the fundus | Round, hard, readily, movable part, ballotable between the fingers of both hands is indicative of head. Irregular, bulkier, less firm and not well-defined or movable part is indicative of breech<br>Neither of the above is indicative of transverse lie |

*Contd...*

*Contd...*

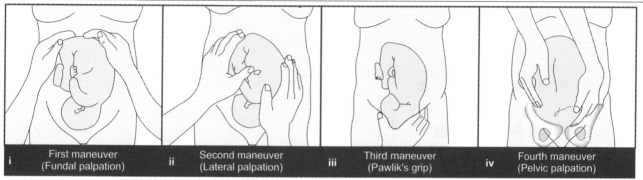

| i First maneuver (Fundal palpation) | ii Second maneuver (Lateral palpation) | iii Third maneuver (Pawlik's grip) | iv Fourth maneuver (Pelvic palpation) |

**Figure 14.1(e):** Abdominal palpation Leopold maneuver

13. Do the second maneuver (lateral palpation)
    • Continue to face the woman's head
    • Place your hands on both sides of the uterus about midway between the symphysis pubis and the fundus.
    • Apply pressure with one hand against the side of the uterus pushing the fetus to the other side and stabilizing it there.

    A firm convex, continuously smooth and resistant mass extending from breech to neck is indicative of fetal back. Small knobby, irregular mass, which move when pressed or may kick or hit your examining hand is indicative of the fetal small parts small parts all over the abdomen are indicative of a posterior position.

    • Palpate the other side of the abdomen with the examining finger from the midline to the lateral side and from the fundus using smooth pressure and rotatory movements.

    • Repeat the procedure for examination of opposite side of the abdomen.

14. Third maneuver (Pawlik's grip)
    • Continue to face the woman's head make sure the woman has her knees bent)

    Avoids discomfort

    • Grasp the portion of the lower abdomen immediately above the symphysis pubis between the thumb and middle finger of one of your hands.

    If the fetal head is above the brim, it will be readily movable and ballotable. If not readily movable, it is indicative of an engaged head.

15. Fourth maneuver (pelvic palpation)
    • Turn and face the woman's feet (make sure the woman's knees are bent)

    Avoids pain with the maneuver.

    • Place your hands on the sides of the uterus, with the palm of your hands just below the level of umbilicus and your fingers directed towards the symphysis pubis
    • Press deeply with your fingertips into the lower abdomen and move them toward the pelvic inlet

    This maneuver determines level of engagement.

    • The hands converge around the presenting part when head is not engaged
    • The hands will diverge away from the presenting part and there will be no give or mobility if the presenting part is engaged or dipping.

**AUSCULTATION**

16. Place fetoscope or stethoscope over the convex portion of the fetus closest to the anterior uterine wall (Figure 14.1(f)).

    Fetal heart sounds are heard over fetal back (scapula region) in vertex and breech presentation. Over chest in face presentation.

*Contd...*

*Contd...*

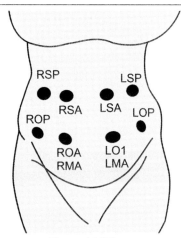

**Figure 14.1(f)**

| | |
|---|---|
| 17. | Inform the mother of your findings. Make her comfortable. |
| 18. | Replace articles and wash hands |
| 19. | Record in the patient's chart the time, findings and remarks if any. |

**Table 14.1.1:** Location of the maximum intensity of the fetal heart tones

| | Presentation and positional varieties | Location |
|---|---|---|
| 1. | Cephalic | Midway between umbilicus and level of anterior superior iliac spine |
| 2. | Breech | Level with or above umbilicus |
| 3. | Anterior | Close to the abdominal midline |
| 4. | Transverse | In lateral abdominal area |
| 5. | Posterior | In flank area |

# 14.2: TEACHING ANTENATAL EXERCISES

## DEFINITION

Systematic exercises to help the pregnant woman adapt to the physical changes in her body during pregnancy and to tone up the muscles that will be stretched or stressed during delivery.

## PURPOSES

1. To lessen the problem of backache in pregnancy.
2. To speed up return of muscle strength after delivery.
3. To prepare for effective pushing in labor.
4. To reduce problems related to sluggish circulation such as leg cramps, varicose veins and edema.

## PROCEDURE

| Nursing action | Rationale |
| --- | --- |
| 1. **Abdominal Breathing**<br>Teach mother to:<br>• Sit comfortably or kneel on all fours (hands and legs).<br>• Breath in and out normally.<br>• Pull on the lower part of the lower abdomen below the umbilicus while continuing to breath normally.<br>• Hold the muscles in the drawn- in position for ten seconds.<br>• Repeat up to 10 times. | This exercise strengthens the deep transverse abdominal muscles, which are the main support of the spine.<br>Prevents backache in future. |
| 2. **Pelvic floor exercises:**<br>Instruct mother to:<br>• Sit, stand or half lie with legs slightly apart.<br>• Close and draw up around the anal passage as though preventing a bowel action<br>• Then draw up around the vagina and urethra as if to stop the flow of urine in mid stream.<br>• Hold for as long as possible up to 10 seconds, breathing normally, then relax<br>• Repeat upto 10 times | This exercise will prepare the pelvic floor muscles for the stretching during delivery. |
| 3. **Foot and leg exercises:**<br>Instruct mother to:<br>• Sit or half lie with legs supported.<br>• Bend and stretch the ankle at least 12 times<br>• Circle both feet at the ankles at least 20 times in each direction<br>• Hold tight (brace) both knees for a count of four and then relax<br>• Repeat 12 times<br>• Perform this exercise before getting up from resting, last thing at night and several times during the day | Helps to improve venous circulation. |
| 4. **Breathing exercise:**<br>Teach mother to:<br>• Take a few deeper breaths now and again during the day<br>• At one time 3-4 breaths to be taken<br>• Avoid more number of deep breaths at one time | Aids oxygen supply to mother and fetus.<br><br>Prevents hyperventilation. |

*Contd...*

*Contd...*

| | | |
|---|---|---|
| 5. | **Posture for relief of aches and pains during pregnancy**<br>Instruct those who get sciatica like pain to:<br>• Lie on the side away from the discomfort so that the affected leg is uppermost<br>• Place pillows to support the whole limb | |
| 6. | **Exercise for relief of cramps:**<br>• Practice foot and leg exercises<br>• If in sitting position, hold the knees straight and stretch the calf muscles by pulling the foot upwards (dorsiflexing) at the same time<br>• Alternatively stand firmly on the affected leg and stride forwards with the other leg. | Dorsiflexion of the foot<br>Stretches the calf muscles |

## SPECIAL CONSIDERATIONS

1. Discourage pregnant women from standing for longer periods.
2. Encourage pregnant women to put their feet up whenever possible.
3. Teach them to avoid crossing legs at the knee or ankles as it may impede circulation.
4. Support stockings may be worn if varicose veins are present.
5. Practice exercises regularly.
6. Exercise should never be carried to the point of fatigue.
7. Walking outdoors at a good, brisk speed is recommended.
8. Exercise of any kind is more beneficial if combined with fresh air and sunlight.
9. It is important to take fluids frequently during excerise to prevent dehydration.
10. Women with pregnancy induced hypertension and heart disease must seek physician's advice to know the exercises they can safely practice.

## 14.3: PERFORMING A NONSTRESS TEST (NST)

### DEFINITION

A test that monitors the fetal heart rate in response to fetal movements in order to assess the integrity of fetal central nervous system and cardio-vascular system.

### PURPOSES

1. To assess the fetal ability to cope with continuation of a high-risk pregnancy.
2. To determine the projected ability of a fetus to withstand the stress of labor.
3. To assess the fetal status in women for whom contraction stress test is contraindicated such as previous cesarean section, placenta previa or preterm labor.

### INDICATIONS (MATERNAL)

1. Post dated pregnancy
2. Rh sensitization.
3. Maternal age 35 or more
4. Chronic renal disease
5. Hypertension
6. Collagen diseases
7. Sickle cell disease
8. Diabetes
9. Premature rupture of membranes
10. History of still birth
11. Trauma
12. Vaginal bleeding in 2nd and 3rd trimester.

### INDICATIONS (FETAL)

1. Decreased fetal movement
2. Intrauterine growth retardation (IUGR)
3. Fetal evaluation after amniocentesis
4. Oligohydramnios/polyhydramnios.

### ARTICLES

1. Electronic fetal heart monitor (Figure 14.3(a)).

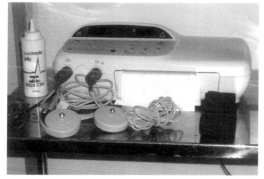

Figure 14.3(a): Fetal monitor

*Contd...*

*Contd...*

2. Ultrasound transducer
3. Tocotransducer (Tocodynamometer)
4. Monitor strip
5. Ultrasound gel
6. Belts to hold the transducers in place.

## PROCEDURE

| | Nursing action | Rationale |
|---|---|---|
| 1. | Explain to mother about the procedure and its purpose and how she has to cooperate. | Reduces anxiety and promotes full cooperation |
| 2. | Make sure that the woman had eaten food and ask her to empty her urinary bladder. | Promotes comfort during the procedure. |
| 3. | Turn on the monitor and press the TEST button to see that it is working and adjust the paper speed (set at 3 cm per minute). | Setting the paper speed at 3 cm per minute increase the accuracy of interpretation. |
| 4. | Perform an abdominal palpation (Leopold's maneuver). | Locates the fetal position and awakens the fetus. |
| 5. | Confirm the presence of fetal heart tones with a fetoscope or stethoscope and note the area of maximum intensity. | Ensures that the source of pulse detected by the electronic monitor is the fetal heart tones. |
| 6. | Position the woman in semi Fowler's or lateral tilt position and place the monitor belts under her back so that they are flat against her skin. | Supine position compresses maternal blood vessels and causes potential supine hypotension. |
| 7. | Connect the ultrasound transducer and the tocotransducer to the fetal monitor. Apply ultrasound gel to the ultrasound transducer. | Ultrasound gel improves sound conduction. |
| 8. | Place the ultrasound transducer on the fetal back. Move the transducer until clear, audible fetal heart tones are heard and the signal light is flashing steadily. Secure the device in place with belt (Figure 14.3(b)). | |

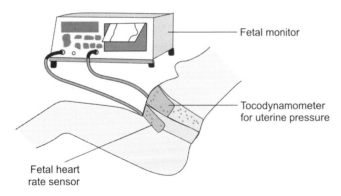

**Figure 14.3(b):** Nonstress test

| | | |
|---|---|---|
| 9. | Place the tocotransducer on the fundus of the uterus and secure in place with the belt. | |

*Contd...*

*Contd...*

| | | |
|---|---|---|
| 10. | Run the monitor and evaluate the quality of the tracing to determine if it is adequate for interpretation. If it is not, reposition the transducer until interpretable, data is obtained. | |
| 11. | Give the hand button to the woman and ask her to press the button every time she feels fetal movement. | Monitors the recorded mark at each point of fetal movement, which is used as a reference point to assess FHR response. |
| 12. | Run the monitor and obtain a tracing for at least 20 minutes | Observes fetal heart rate and uterine activity. |
| 13. | On completion, put off the monitor and take out the strip of paper. | |
| 14. | Remove the abdominal straps and wipe off the gel from the abdomen and transducer. | |
| 15 | Make the woman comfortable and give relevant instructions. | |

### Interpretation of the tracing for term fetus of more than 37 weeks

| | | |
|---|---|---|
| 1. | **Reactive or negative test** <br> At least two or more accelerations of fetal heart rate with an amplitude of at least 15 beats per minute and duration of at least 15 seconds during a 20 minutes period. | Healthy fetus <br> Less than 1% chance of fetal death within one week of NST. |
| 2. | **Nonreactive test** <br> No accelerations or accelerations less than 15 beats per minute or less than 15 seconds in duration, for a 40 minute period. | Fetus may be compromised and there needs to be furthre follow up with bio-physical profile, CST and OCT. |
| 3. | **Unsatisfactory or unequivocal test** <br> A tracing that cannot be interpreted because of poor quality of fetal heart rate tracing. | NST needs to be repeated in 2-3 hours or follow up with CST, OCT or BPP. |

Baseline FHR – 120 – 160 bpm
Baseline bradycardia – less than 120 bpm as in hypoxia due to cord compression
Baseline tachycardia – more than 160 bpm
Mild tachycardia <180 bpm
Severe tachycardia > 180 bpm as in cases of hypoxia and maternal or fetal fever

### Interpretation of tracing for preterm fetus <37 weeks

| | | |
|---|---|---|
| 1. | Reactive | At least a minimum of 2 accelerations within 60 to 90 minutes lasting at least 10 seconds with a fetal heart rate increased by 10 bpm above baseline in response to fetal activity. |
| 2. | Nonreactive | The above criteria is not met. |

# 14.4: PERFORMING AN OXYTOCIN CHALLENGE TEST (OCT)

## DEFINITION

A test in which the fetus is exposed to the stress of contractions to determine whether there is adequate placental perfusion under simulated labor conditions (Induced uterine contractions).

## PURPOSES

1. To assess the fetal ability to cope with the continuation of a high-risk pregnancy.
2. To determine the projected ability of the fetus to withstand the stress of labor.

## INDICATIONS

1. IUGR
2. Postmaturity
3. Hypertensive disorders of pregnancy
4. Diabetes mellitus
5. Women with nonreactive NST.

## CONTRAINDICATIONS

1. Third trimester bleeding
2. Incompetent cervix.
3. Multiple gestation
4. Previous classical uterine incision
5. Hydramnios
6. History of preterm labor
7. Premature rupture of membranes.

## ARTICLES

1. All the articles required for NST (Fetal monitor, monitor strip, transducers and monitor belts)
2. An IV line to administer a dilute dose of oxytocin (Pitocin).
3. An IV infusion pump to monitor the flow rate.
4. Medication and IV fluids.

## PROCEDURE

| | Nursing action | Rationale |
|---|---|---|
| 1. | Explain to mother the procedure and its purpose. | Reduces anxiety and promotes full co-operation. |
| 2. | Make sure that the woman had eaten food and ask her to empty her urinary bladder. | Promotes patient's comfort. |
| 3. | Turn on the monitor and press the "TEST" button to see that it is working and adjust the paper speed (set at 3 cm per minute). | Setting the paper speed at 3 cm per minute increases the accuracy of interpretation. |
| 4. | Perform an abdominal palpation (Leopold's maneuver). | Identifies the fetal position and awakens the fetus. |
| 5. | Position the woman in semiFowler's or lateral tilt position and place the monitor belts under her back so that they are flat against her skin. | Supine the position is avoided to prevent compression of maternal blood vessels and potential supine hypotension. |

*Contd...*

*Contd...*

| | | |
|---|---|---|
| 6. | Connect the ultrasound transducer and the tocotransducer to fetal monitor. Apply ultrasound gel to the ultrasound transducer. | Ultrasound gel improves sound conduction. |
| 7. | Confirm the presence of fetal heart tones with a fetoscope or stethoscope. | Ensures that the source of pulse detected by the electronic monitor is the fetal heart. |
| 8. | Place the ultrasound transducer on the maternal abdomen over the fetal back. Move the transducer until clear, audible fetal heart tones are heard and the signal light is flashing steadily. Secure the device in place with belt. | Aids monitoring of fetal heart tones. During the procedure. |
| 9. | Place the tocotransducer on the fundus of the uterus and secure in place with the belt. | Facilitates monitoring of uterine contractions. |
| 10. | Run the monitor and evaluate the quality of the tracing to determine if it is adequate for interpretation. If it is not, reposition the transducer until interpretable data is obtained. | |
| 11. | Start the oxytocin infusion at the rate of 1 mu/minute. | |
| 12. | Step up the infusion rate every 15 minutes at the prescribed rate until effective uterine contractions are established. | |
| 13. | Monitor the uterine contractions using hands to palpate the hardening of the uterus. | Abdominal palpation while observing the monitor tracing aids to confirm the uterine contractions. |
| 14. | Continue the infusion until the contractions are occurring at a frequency of at least one in a 10 minute period and lasting at least 30 seconds. | |
| 15. | The recorded strip is then taken out for interpretation and infusion of oxytocin discontinued. | |
| 16. | Monitoring and IV infusion without oxytocin are continued until contractions have diminished to their baseline activity. | |

## INTERPRETATIONS

1. **Negative:** No decelerations occur with contractions as frequent as three in a ten-minute period. Indicates fetal well being and predicts that the fetus will continue to be alright for another week without intervention of delivery.
2. **Positive:** Repeated late decelerations of fetal heart patterns occur during the test (more than 3 in a ten minute period). Further assessment is done to decide on the need for immediate termination of pregnancy.
3. **Hyperstimulation:** Contractions are more frequent than two minutes or for duration of more than 90 seconds. The test should be stopped and repeated within 24 to 48 hours with a more dilute solution.
4. **Suspicious:** Occasional late decelerations with continued contractions. The CST should be repeated within 24 to 48 hours.
5. **Unsatisfactory:** The recording is not of good quality to be interpreted. This may be due to problems inherent with monitoring.

## SPECIAL CONSIDERATIONS

Discontinue infusion when:
1. Criteria are met
2. Hyperstimulation occurs
3. Prolonged deceleration/bradycardia occurs

## 14.5: PREPARING A PRENATAL PATIENT FOR ULTRASOUND EXAMINATION

### DESCRIPTION

Ultrasound is the transmission of low energy, high frequency waves through a medium such as fluid or tissue. The echoes received by the transducer crystals are converted to electric signals and displayed on a monitor. The intensity and delay time for reflected echoes are recorded which are interpreted to arrive at data regarding the fetus and the intrauterine environment.

### PURPOSES

1. To diagnose pregnancy as early as 6 weeks of gestation.
2. To confirm the size and location of placenta and amount of amniotic fluid.
3. To identify the growth of the fetus and to detect any gross abnormality.
4. To diagnose presentation and position of the fetus.
5. To predict maturity of the fetus.
6. To confirm suspected ectopic pregnancy.
7. To locate an intrauterine contraceptive device.
8. To confirm suspected multiple gestation, placenta praevia and cord presentation.
9. As adjunct to cervical encirclage, amniocentesis and external version.
10. To estimate fetal growth and normalcy.
11. To establish gestational age.
12. To obtain biophysical profile for determining fetal wellbeing.

### ARTICLES

1. Ultrasound machine with transducer
2. Ultrasound gel/coupling gel
3. A gown for the patient.

### PROCEDURE

| | Nursing action | Rationale |
|---|---|---|
| a. | **Transabdominal ultrasound scan** | |
| 1. | Explain to the woman, the nature of examination, purpose and her role | Reduces anxiety and helps in obtaining cooperation |
| 2. | Instruct the women to drink eight glasses of water 2 hours prior to the examination if in the first trimester of pregnancy. (In second and third trimester, drinking water is not necessary) Instruct the woman not to void until examination is over. | Having the patient drink water will distend her bladder. Distended bladder displaces bowel out of the pelvis, lifts the uterus from behind the symphysis pubis, and produces an acoustic window enabling optimal imaging of the uterine contents. During the second and third trimester of pregnancy, amniotic fluid serves as an acoustic window while the gravid uterus displaces the bowel. |
| 3. | Assist the patient to wear a hospital gown. | |
| 4. | The patient is assisted to lie in supine position on the examining table and expose her abdomen from costal margin to symphysis pubis. | Exposure of abdomen from the costal margin to symphysis pubis will provide a complete area for visualization. |

*Contd...*

*Contd...*

| | | |
|---|---|---|
| 5. | Apply the ultrasound gel or coupling gel generously to the abdomen (A towel or disposable tissues should be provided to the patient to protect her clothing). | Ultrasound gel eliminates the air interface between ultrasound transducer and patient's skin, thereby providing better transmission and reflection of the ultrasound waves. |
| 6. | After completion of procedure remove gel from the women's abdomen and assist her to dress back into her clothes. | |
| **b.** | **Transvaginal ultrasound examination** | |
| 1. | No pre-examination preparation is required. | No acoustic window is required for a transvaginal scan because the transducer is in direct contact with pelvic organs. |
| 2. | Explain procedure to the patient. | Reduces anxiety and helps in obtaining cooperation |
| 3. | Instruct patient to remove any clothing below waist. | |
| 4. | Place the woman in lithotomy position and place a pillow under her buttocks to raise the pelvic area. | Elevating the patient's hips will provide better imaging of pelvic organs. |
| 5. | Place a transducer sheath or a condom, filled with ultrasound gel over the vaginal transducer. | Ultrasound gel will eliminate the air interface between the transducer and the patient's skin. Lubricant applied to the transducer reduces discomfort. Lubricant applied outside the sheath increases the ease of insertion. |
| 6. | The transducer is then inserted through the introitus into the mid vagina by radiologist. | |
| 7. | Remove the condom after the examination and clean the transducer with disinfectant (cidex) | |
| 8. | Assist the woman to clean herself and change to her clothes | |
| 9 | Forward the findings of the ultrasound scan to the unit or physician who has requested the test. | |
| 10 | Wash hands and record the procedure and findings. | |

# 14.6: ASSISTING WITH AN AMNIOCENTESIS

## DEFINITION

Amniocentesis is the deliberate puncture of the amniotic sac per abdomen for diagnostic and therapeutic purposes.

## DESCRIPTION

Amniocentesis is a procedure needing informed consent, in which amniotic fluid is removed from the uterine cavity by inserting a needle through the abdomen and uterine walls into the amniotic sac. The normal time for the procedure is between 16 to 18 weeks' gestation, when approximately 20 ml of amniotic fluid is removed and sent for analysis.

## INDICATIONS

A.  Diagnostic:
*   Early months (14 to 16 weeks)
    For diagnosis of chromosomal and genetic disorders
    1.  Sex-linked disorders
    2.  Karyotyping
    3.  Inborn errors of metabolism
    4.  Neural tube defects
*   Later months
    1.  Fetal maturity
    2.  Degree of fetal hemolysis in Rh sensitized mother
    3.  Meconium staining of liquor
    4.  Amniography or fetography
B.  Therapeutic
*   First half of pregnancy
    1.  Induction of abortion by instillation of chemicals, such as hypertonic saline, urea or prostaglandin.
    2.  Decompression of the uterus in acute hydramnios
*   Second half of pergnancy
    1.  Decompression of uterus in unresponsive cases of chronic hydramnios
    2.  To give intrauterine fetal transfusion in severe hemolysis following Rh – isoimmunization
    3.  Amnioinfusion- infusion of warm normal saline into the amniotic cavity, transabdominally or transcervically to increase the volume of amniotic fluid.

## PREPROCEDURAL PREPARATIONS

1.  Obtain informed consent.
2.  Ensure that ultrasonogram is done for sonographic localization of placenta to prevent bloody tap and fetomaternal bleeding.
3.  Prophylactic administration of 100 mg of anti-D immunoglobulin in Rh negative non-immunized mother.
4.  Ask patient to empty her bladder.
5.  Skin preparation is needed on the day of procedure.
6.  Obtain maternal vital signs and a 20 minutes fetal heart rate tracing to serve as baseline.

## ARTICLES AND EQUIPMENTS NEEDED

*   TPR tray
*   Stethoscope
*   Sterile gloves
*   Dressing tray

# Maternal and Child Nursing

- Sterile towels – 4
- 1% lignocaine
- Disposable syringes – 5 ml, 20 ml
- Cotton swabs
- Antiseptic solutions.
- Sterile bottles – to collect the specimen
- 20 – 22 gauge spinal needle of 4 inch length with stillette
- Adhesive plaster.

## PROCEDURE

| | Nursing action | Rationale |
|---|---|---|
| 1. | Explain to patient the need/ purpose of procedure and how it will be done. | Minimizes anxiety and facilitates patient cooperation |
| 2. | Ensure that informed consent is signed. | Ensures full awareness of procedure for patient and protects the health care professionals. |
| 3. | Have the woman empty her bladder if the fetus is more than 20 weeks gestation (If the fetus is less than 20 weeks gestation the woman's full bladder will hold the uterus steady and out of the pelvis) | Avoids injury to the woman's bladder |
| 4. | Assemble equipment. | Promotes organization and saves time and effort. |
| 5. | Provide privacy. | Reduces anxiety. |
| 6. | Assist patient to lie in dorsal position. | Exposes the area of puncture. |
| 7. | Check the maternal vital signs and fetal heart rate. | Obtains baseline data. |
| 8. | Wash hands and don sterile gloves. | Reduces risk of transmission of microorganisms and maintains surgical asepsis. |
| 9. | Start IV fluids in accordance with institutional policy. | |
| 10. | Administer terbutaline SC or IV or ritodrine IV per institutional policy. | Reduces chances of uterine contractions during and after the procedure. |
| 11. | An ultrasound examination is performed and the placenta localized and a pool of liquor found. | Reduces the possibility of bloody tap and abortive attempts and reduces risk of complications. |
| 12. | Drape the area with sterile towels. | Prevents unnecessary exposure. |
| 13. | Prepare abdominal wall aseptically. | Reduces the risk of pathogens entering the skin through the puncture site. |
| 14. | Assist the physician in infiltrating the proposed site of puncture with 2 ml of 1 % lignocaine. | Causes loss of painful sensation in the area. |
| 15. | Ensure adequate time between infiltration of local anesthetic and introduction of needle into the amniotic sac. | Reduces pain and discomfort related to the procedure. |
| 16. | Assist physician while inserting the needle and stillette (A 20 to 22 gauge spinal needle about 4 inch length) through the abdominal wall into the uterus, under direct ultrasound guidance. The stillette is then withdrawn and a few drops of liquor are discarded (Figure 14.6(a)). | A suitable pool of liquor is identified by ultrasound<br><br>First 2 ml may be contaminated by maternal cells or blood and should be discarded. |
| 17. | Physician withdraws 10 – 20 ml of amniotic fluid for analysis or a smaller amount if the amniocentesis is performed in the first trimester | |

*Contd...*

*Contd...*

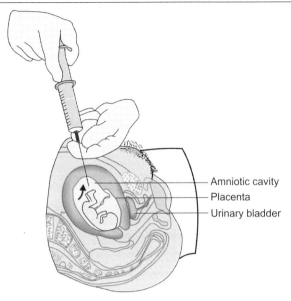

**Figure 14.6(a):** Amniocentesis

| | |
|---|---|
| 18. Physician withdraws the needle, keep a dressing gauze and place an adhesive bandage over the puncture site. | Minimizes tissue damage and discomfort to patient. |
| 19. Monitor the woman during the procedure for signs of premature labor, bleeding or fetal distress. | Facilitates early detection of maternal/fetal complications. |
| 20. Discard the used materials. | Prevents spread of microorganisms. |
| 21 Remove and discard the gloves. | Prevents spread of microorganisms. |
| 22. Wash hands. | Prevents cross infection. |
| 23. Replace articles in the utility room | Prevents spread of microorganisms. |
| 24. Obtain maternal vital signs and a 20 minute fetal heart tracing | Serves as a baseline to evaluate possible complications. |
| 25. Instruct the woman to report signs of bleeding, unusual fetal activity abdominal pain, cramping, or fever while at home after the procedure. | Identifies early signs of complications. |
| 27. Label the specimen container adequately, including the estimated weeks of gestation and EDD. Send the specimen to laboratory for investigation immediately. | Ensures proper identification of the specimen and reporting of the findings. |
| 28. Record the procedure done, date, time, name of physician who performed the test, maternal and fetal responses and details of specimen taken. | Provides for accurate documentation of procedure. |

## COMPLICATIONS

*Maternal*
- Infection
- Antepartum hemorrhage
- Rhesus–isoimmunization
- Fetal loss
- Abortion

- Preterm labor
- Amniotic fluid leakage.

*Fetal:*
- Hemorrhage
- Trauma to umbilical cord and vessels
- Fetal trauma resulting from needle puncture
- Death.

## SPECIAL CONSIDERATION

1. Color of amniotic fluid indicates condition of fetus
    a. Opaque with greenish brown discoloration—Meconium in the amniotic fluid
    b. Yellow with slight turbidity—Hemolytic diseases of the newborn
    c. Opaque with dark red—Blood in the amniotic fluid
    d. Opaque with yellow brown (tobacco juice)—Intrauterine death

# 14.7: ADMITTING A CLIENT TO LABOR ROOM

## DEFINITION

Admitting a woman to labor room for observation, treatment, care and safe delivery.

## PURPOSES

1. To prepare the woman for safe delivery
2. To induce labor
3. To monitor high risk mothers
4. To monitor maternal and fetal conditions.

## ARTICLES

Tray containing:
1. Soap solution
2. Rag pieces
3. Razor with blade
4. Enema can
5. Rectal tube
6. Kidney tray
7. Thermometer tray
8. Disposable gloves and patient records.

## GENERAL INSTRUCTIONS

1. Admit women with contractions, leaking or bleeding per vagina, reduced or absent fetal movements and woman less than 22 weeks gestation if they have pregnancy induced hypertension or heart disease.
2. Admit women with communicable disease, HIV positive, and HBSAg positive in separate room.
3. If patients are referred from elsewhere the reference letter should be pasted on patient's folder for physician's reference.
4. Contra-indications for giving enema are:
   - Severe pregnancy induced hypertension (PIH)
   - Cardiac disease
   - Pre-term labor
   - Leaking per vagina
   - Bleeding per vagina
   - Decreased fetal movements
   - Women in 2nd stage of labor
   - Grand multiparae
   - Malpresentations

## PROCEDURE

| | Nursing action | Rationale |
|---|---|---|
| 1. | Welcome patient to the unit | |
| 2. | Collect history and reason for admission | Helps in knowing about patient's condition and needs. |
| 3. | Explain admission procedure to patient and relatives. | Helps in obtaining co-operation of patient. |

*Contd...*

# Maternal and Child Nursing

*Contd...*

| No. | Action | Rationale |
|---|---|---|
| 4. | Help patient to change clothes to hospital gown and hand over valuables to the relatives. | Prevents chance of losing valuables. |
| 5. | Collect samples of blood and urine. | Helps in diagnosing any complications. |
| 6. | Check height and weight of patient. | Obtains baseline data. |
| 7. | Check vital signs. | Gives information about patient's general condition. |
| 8. | Assess maternal and fetal condition | Gives information about condition of mother and fetus condition. |
| 9. | Collect following information from patient<br>a. Booked or unbooked status<br>b. Obstetrical score<br>c. Gestational age<br>d. Any bleeding or leaking PV<br>e. Time of onset of labor contractions<br>f. Fetal movements<br>g. Any other complaints. | |
| 10. | Perform a careful abdominal examination which includes inspection, palpation, auscultation of fetal heart sounds and monitoring of contraction. | Aids in identification of any deviation from normal condition. |
| 11. | Check perineum for condition of membranes | Gives information about progress of labor. |
| 12. | Prepare pubic area using razor or depilatory cream (optional). | Prevents infection and gives clear visualization during delivery. |
| 13. | Administer an evacuant enema unless contraindicated. | Prevents contamination by fecal matter during bearing down. |
| 14. | Document time of admission, reason for admission, assessment findings and procedures done in admission room | Serves as a communication between hospital staff. |
| 15. | Instruct patient to lie on bed allotted to her in labor room and inform doctor about admission. | |

# 14.8: ASSISTING WITH INDUCTION OF LABOR

## DEFINITION

Assisting in initiation of labor or uterine contraction by artificial means before the onset of spontaneous labor.

## INDICATIONS

*Maternal*
1. Post-term pregnancy
2. Hypertension including pre-eclampsia and eclampsia
3. Medical problems—renal, respiratory and cardiac disease.
4. Previous stillbirth
5. Premature rupture of membranes
6. Chronic polyhydramnios and maternal distress.

*Fetal*
1. Placental insufficiency.
2. Rh-Isoimmunization.
3. Unstable lie, after correcting into longitudinal lie.
4. Intrauterine death.
5. Certain congenital anomalies.
6. Postmaturity.

## COMBINED INDICATIONS

1. Pre-eclampsia and eclampsia
2. Minor degree of placenta praevia
3. Abruptio Placenta
4. Chronic hypertension.
5. Premature rupture of membranes.

## CONTRAINDICATIONS

1. Contracted pelvis and cephalopelvic disproportion.
2. Persistent malpresentation—transverse or compound presentation.
3. Pregnancy with history of previous cesarean section.
4. Elderly primigravida
5. High risk pregnancy with compromised fetus.
6. Cord presentation or cord prolapse
7. Placenta praevia
8. Pelvic tumor.

## METHODS OF INDUCTION

1. Medical
2. Surgical
3. Combined.

## MEDICAL INDUCTION

Medical induction is done by administration of drugs such as:
1. Oxytocin/syntocinon
2. Prostaglandin.

# Maternal and Child Nursing

## Oxytocin Induction

*Equipments*
1. Foley's catheter No 16Fr
2. Distilled water.
3. Syringe 2cc or 5cc
4. Bowl
5. Bivalve speculum
6. Sterile gloves
7. Antiseptic solution
8. Spot light or flash light
9. Mask and apron
10. IV set
11. IV solution – normal saline or Ringer's lactate
12. IV pump if available to regulate the flow.
13. Medication – oxytocin/syntocinon/cerviprime.

## Procedure

| | Nursing action | Rationale |
|---|---|---|
| 1 | Explain to patient what will be done, the purpose of it and how she may cooperate. | Reduces anxiety and promotes cooperation. |
| 2 | Wash hands. | Prevents transmission of infection. |
| 3 | Check the chart for doctors order. | |
| 4 | Instruct mother to empty bowel and bladder. | A full bladder interferes with contraction and descend of fetus. |
| 5 | Provide privacy. | Prevents embarrasment to the mother. |
| 6 | Prepare the perineal area as for labor. | |
| 7 | Check the fetal heart rate, uterine contraction rate, abdominal and vaginal findings. | Identifies presence of any contraindication. |
| 8 | Maintain labor progress chart every 15 min, and monitor BP every 2 hours. | Detects any abnormal findings. |
| 9 | Set up the IV tubings, IV pump and adjust the drops/min. | |
| 10 | Add the loaded syntocinon in the IV bottle after adjusting the drops/min. | Sudden increase or decrease in syntocinon concentration may lead to an abnormal uterine contraction. |
| 11 | Gradually increase the drops after ensuring that everything is normal. | |
| 12 | Indications for stopping:<br>• Strong contractions lasting over 60 seconds and occurring frequently with intervals less than 3 min.<br>• Tonic uterine contractions<br>• Fetal distress<br>• Deterioration in the woman's condition<br>• Occurrence of increased or decreased fetal movement. | Complications caused by increasing level of oxytocin may result in fetal distress.<br><br><br>Fetal movements will increase if fetal distress is present. |

*Prostaglandin Induction*

*Procedure*

|   | Nursing action | Rationale |
|---|----------------|-----------|
| 1 | Wash hands | Prevents transmission of infection |
| 2 | Check the chart for doctors order | |
| 3 | Instruct mother to empty bowel and bladder. | A full bladder interferes with contraction and descend of fetus. |
| 4 | Provide privacy | Prevents embarrassment to the mother. |
| 5 | Prepare the perineal area as for labor | |
| 6 | Perform vaginal examination | |
| 7 | Insert prostagandin E2 or E1 (misoprostal) gel into the posterior fornix close to cervix. | Absortion of the medication is facilitated from posterior fornix. |
| 8 | Instruct the woman to stay recombent as contractions begin. | Frequent, low intensity contractions begin as medication gets absorbed. |
| 9 | Monitor vaginal changes using Bishop score. | Assesses the need for readministration of prostaglandin. |
| 10 | Monitor uterine contractions and fetal heart rate continuously. | |
| 11 | Repeat the dose of E2 or E1 if required after 6-8 hours according to physician's order. | Labor will result in 30-50% of women. |

## SURGICAL INDUCTION

Surgical induction of labor is done by two methods:
1. Stripping of membranes:
   i. It is the digital separation of the chorioamniotic membranes from the wall of the cervix and lower uterine segment. It is thought to work by release of endogenous prostaglandins from the membranes and decidua.
   ii. Stripping the membranes off its attachment from the lower segment is an effective procedure for induction, provided cervical score is favorable. It is used as a preliminary step prior to rupture of membranes. It is also used to make the cervix ripe.
   iii. Manual exploration of the cervix triggers release of oxytocin from pituitary causing increased levels in plasma. Sweeping of the membranes is done prior to artificial rupture of membranes.
2. Artificial rupture of membrane.

## PROCEDURE

|   | Nursing action | Rationale |
|---|----------------|-----------|
| 1 | Wash hands using surgical asepsis. | Prevents risk of infection. |
| 2 | Help the mother to lie down in lithotomy position. | Ensures better visualization. |
| 3 | Follow strict aseptic technique. | Reduces chances of infection. |
| 4 | Wear sterile gloves, gown and mask. | |
| 5 | Clean the perineum using aseptic technique. | |
| 6 | Physician introduces two fingers of left hand inside the vagina, upto the cervical canal beyond the internal os. | Helps to guide the ARM forceps. |
| 7 | Physician assesses the membranes, and places palmar surface of the lefthand upwards. | Guiding hand will prevent injury to the cervix or vaginal tract. |

*Contd...*

*Contd...*

| 8 | Physician introduces long kocher's forceps with blades closed up to the membranes along the palmar aspect and ruptures the membranes. | |
|---|---|---|
| 9 | Assess fetal heart rate, note the color, amount of the aminiotic fluid, status of the cervix, station of head, presence or absence of cord prolapse. | Identifies any complications at the earliest. |
| 10 | administer prophylactic antibiotics as per order. | Acts as a prophylaxis against infection. |
| 11 | Record the date and time and the type of induction done. | Acts as a communication between staff members. |

*Hazards of ARM*
1. Intrauterine infection, particularly iatrogenic from digital or instrumental contamination.
2. Chance of umbilical cord prolapse.
3. Bleeding from the following sources:
   • Fetal vessels in the membranes in case of vasa previa
   • The friable vessels in the cervix
   • A low lying placental site.
4. Amniotic fluid embolism.

## COMBINED METHOD

The combined medical and surgical methods are commonly used to increase the efficacy of induction by reducing the induction - delivery interval.

## SPECIAL CONSIDERATIONS

1. Oxytocin should not be given as a bolus injection during labor because of the risk of hyperstimulation.
2. Prolonged use of oxytocin causes uterine atony during the postpartum period.
3. The rate of oxytocin administration should be closely monitored to ensure uterine activity that is adequate to maintain progress of labor.
4. The midwife should be vigilant for signs of fetal distress such as suspicious or abnormal tracing or signs of meconium stained liquor.
5. Instruct the mother to lie on her sides to prevent aortacaval compression and to increase placental blood flow.
6. Water retention and water intoxication can occur with prolonged use of oxytocin and care should be taken to identify the signs of water retention like hypotension, tachycardia, and cardiac dysrhythmias.

# 14.9: PERFORMING VAGINAL EXAMINATION FOR A PATIENT IN LABOR

## DEFINITION

It is the examination done per vagina to detect the status of the vagina and cervix, and to assess the progress of labor as the fetal presenting part descends through the birth canal.

## PURPOSES

1. To make a positive diagnosis of labor.
2. To monitor cervical dilatation and effacement.
3. To make a positive identification of the fetal presentation.
4. To ascertain whether forewater have ruptured.
5. To determine if cord prolapse is likely to occur.
6. To assess the progress or delay in labor.
7. To detect whether second stage has begun.
8. To assess status of head and degree of moulding.
9. To apply fetal scalp electrode.

## EQUIPMENTS

A sterile tray containing:
1. Sterile cottonballs to give perineal care.
2. Artery clamp.
3. Bowl with antiseptic solution.
4. Sim's vaginal speculum.
5. Sterile cream in a bowl for lubrication.
6. Sterile gloves (outside the tray).

## GENERAL INSTRUCTIONS

1. The bladder should be empty.
2. The fingers should not be withdrawn until the required information has been obtained.
3. Perineal care should be given before performing vaginal examination.
4. It should be restricted or limited after membranes have ruptured.
5. It should be avoided in case of antepartum hemorrhage.

## PROCEDURE

| | Nursing action | Rationale |
|---|---|---|
| 1 | Explain procedure to mother. | Promotes compliance. |
| 2 | Ask mother to void if the bladder is not empty. | Avoids discomfort during procedure. |
| 3 | Explain how she should relax during the examination. | For smooth and safe performance of the procedure. |
| 4 | Read the chart for previous findings. | Serves as a baseline data. |
| 5 | Position the women in dorsal recumbent position with knees flexed . | For good visualization. |
| 6 | Drape the patient. | Provides privacy. |
| 7 | Do a surgical handwashing. | Prevents spread of infection from hands to the mother and fetus. |

*Contd...*

*Contd...*

| | | |
|---|---|---|
| 8 | Don sterile gloves | |
| 9 | Observe the external genitalia for the following:<br>—Signs of varicosities, edema, vulval warts or sores<br>—Scar from previous episiotomy or laceration.<br>—Discharge or bleeding from vaginal orifice.<br>—Color and odour of aminiotic fluid, if membranes have ruptured. | The external genitalia must be observed before cleansing the vulva. |
| 10 | Cleanse the vulva and perineal area. | |
| 11 | Dip the first two fingers of the right hand into the antiseptic cream. | Lubricates the fingers. |
| 12 | Holding the labia apart with thumb and index fingers of left hand, insert the lubricated fingers into vagina, palm side down, pressing downwards. | |
| 13 | With the fingers inside, explore the vagina for required information taking care not to touch the clitoris or anus.<br>Note the following:<br>—The feel on touch of vaginal walls<br>—Consistency of vaginal walls<br>—Scar from previous perineal wound, cystocele or rectocele. | —Touching clitoris causes discomfort<br>—Touching anus causes contamination.<br>Normally vagina is warm and moist. Hot dry vagina is a sign of obstructed labor.<br>—Hot vagina is seen in maternal fever.<br>Firm and rigid walls suggest long labor.<br>Normal finding is soft vaginal walls. |
| 14 | Examine the cervix with the fingers in the vagina turned upwards. Locate the cervical os by sweeping the fingers from side to side (Figure 14.9(a)).<br>Assess the cervix for:<br>a) Effacement<br>b) Dilatation<br>c) Consistency<br>d) Forewaters | - Normally cervix is situated centrally.<br>- In early labor cervix is situated posteriorly.<br><br>Thinning of the cervix and shortening of the canal indicates effacement.<br>Enlargement of the external Os indicates dilatation.<br>Normal cervix is soft, elastic and well applied to the presenting part in normal labor.<br>Intact membranes, which become tense during contractions with well fitting presenting part indicates forewater.<br>- Protruding membranes are seen with ill fitting presenting part. Membrances will not be felt if they rupture early. |

**Figure 14.9(a):** Vaginal examination during labor

*Contd...*

*Contd...*

| 15 | Assess the level of presenting part in relation to maternal ischial spines (Figure 14.9(b)). | |
|---|---|---|

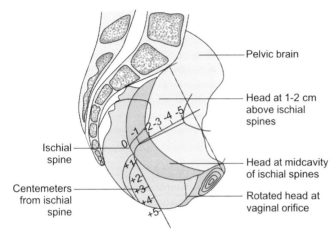

**Figure 14.9(b):** Station of fetal head in relation to ischial spine

| 16 | Identify the presentation by feeling the hard bones of the vault of the skull, the fontanalle and sutures. | The distance of the presenting part above and below the ischial spines is expressed as - and + station respectively. |
|---|---|---|
| 17 | Identify the position by feeling the features of the presenting part. | The sagittal suture may be felt in the right, left or transverse diameter of the pelvis in early labor. |
| 18 | With the fingers, follow the sagittal suture to feel the fontanalle | —posterior fontanalle will be felt in a well flexed head.<br>—location of the fontanalle in relation to the pelvis will give information about the position. |
| 19 | Assess the moulding, by feeling the amount of overlapping of skull bones. | The parietal bones override the occipital bone in case of moulding. |
| 20 | At the completion of the examination, withdraw fingers from vagina, take care to note the presence of any blood or aminiotic fluid. | For comparison with the earlier findings. |
| 21 | Remove gloves and wash hands | |
| 22 | Auscultate the fetal heart tones. | |
| 23 | Assist the woman to a comfortable position and inform her of the progress of labor | Encourages mother to relax and participate in labor. |
| 24 | Record the findings and observations in the patient's chart and inform the physician of the observations and progress of labor. | Acts as a communication between the staff members. |

# 14.10: CONDUCTING A NORMAL VAGINAL DELIVERY

## DEFINITION

Conducting or managing a normal vaginal delivery involves the hand maneuvers used to assist the baby's birth, immediate care of the newborn and the delivery of the placenta.

## PURPOSES

1. To have the child birth event take place in a prepared and safe environment.
2. To conduct delivery with least trauma to mother and baby.
3. To assist mother go through the process without undue stress, injury or complication.
4. To promote smooth and safe transition of newborn to the extrauterine life.
5. To avoid complications.

## ARTICLES

### FOR MOTHER

A Sterile delivery pack containing:
a. Articles for cutting and suturing an episiotomy.
   - Episiotomy scissors
   - Artery clamps 3
   - Tissue forceps—1
   - Needle holder—1
   - Syringe and needle for infiltration—10 ml
b. Scissors for cutting the cord.
c. Bowl for cleaning solution
d. Basin to receive placenta
e. Cottonballs
f. 4 × 4 gauze pieces.
g. Towel to cover the hand supporting the perineum
h. Sterile gown
i. Leggings for the mother.
j. Apron, gloves and mask for staff.

### FOR NEWBORN

1. Baby blanket or flannel cloth-2, one to receive and dry the baby of excess secretions and another to wrap the baby.
2. Neonatal resuscitation equipment checked and ready for use.
3. Oxygen source with tubing.
4. Suction apparatus and mucous extractor.
5. Cord clamp.
6. Bulb syringe for nasal and oropharyngeal suctioning of the baby.

### OTHER ARTICLES

- Antiseptic lotion-savlon or dettol
- Suture material
- Perineal pads for the mother
- Oxytocic drugs
- Sterile gloves

- Methergine
- Lignocaine 2%.

## POINTS TO REMEMBER

- Follow strict aseptic technique
- Never ask the mother to bear down before full dialatation
- Always give episiotomy at the peak of a uterine contraction
- Check that the resuscitation set, suction apparatus and other equipments are in good working condition.
- Record any alteration in uterine contraction or FHR. Record the time of rupture of membranes and color of amniotic fluid.
- Note FHR when the uterine contractions are not present.

## PREPARATION

1. Provide local preparation as per agency policy.
2. Administer enema.

## PROCEDURE

| | Nursing action | Rationale |
|---|---|---|
| 1 | Transfer mother to the delivery room | |
| 2 | Change her clothings into hospital gown | |
| 3 | Monitor uterine contraction and PV findings | Helps in assessing progress of labor |
| 4 | Assess the presentation, lie, position, attitude, station, cervical dilatation, effacement etc. | Helps in assessing progress of labor |
| 5 | Maintain labor progress chart (Partograph) | Helps in determining abnormalities. |
| 6 | Note the color of the liquor if the membranes rupture | Meconuim stained liquor indicates fetal distress. |
| 7 | Note the fetal heart rate every 10-15 mts, if not on continuous fetal monitoring. | Detects fetal distress at an early stage. |
| 8 | Avoid giving solid foods. | During labor emptying time of the stomach is delayed and may cause regurgitation. |
| 9 | Give her fluids in form of lemon juice or fruit juice (If an operative delivery is anticipated keep mother on NPO). | |
| 10 | Instruct her to follow breathing techniques | Ensures more oxygen supply to the fetus and promotes relaxation. |
| 11 | Instruct mother to lie down in left lateral position | Enhances more blood supply to the fetus as well as prevents supine hypotensive syndrome. |
| 12 | Give adequate explanation regarding breathing, relaxation and pushing (bearing down) to mother. | Obtains her co-operation and participation during the process. |
| 13 | Once the onset of second stage has been confirmed, place the woman in dorsal position with knees bent at lower end of the delivery bed. Ensure that bladder is empty. | Gives view to the perineum and to assess the progress clearly. |
| 14 | Open the delivery pack, arrange the articles and pour cleansing solution in the bowl. | For convenience and timely use. |
| 15 | Perform a surgical hand scrub and put on sterile gown and gloves. | |

*Contd..*

# Maternal and Child Nursing

| | | |
|---|---|---|
| 16 | Drape the mother's perineum and delivery area | Obtains a sterile field for delivery. |
| 17 | Clean the perineum in the following manner using one cotton ball separately for each stroke. | Proper cleansing makes the perineum free from microorganism. |
| a) | Monspubis in zig-zag manner from level of clitoris upward | |
| b) | Clotoris to fourchette-one downward stroke | |
| c) | Farther labia minora and then near side | |
| d) | Labia majora fartherside first and then near side | |
| e) | Thighs in long strokes away from the perineum | |
| f) | Anus in one circular stroke. | |
| 18 | Delivery of the head (Figure 14.10(a) (i))<br>As the head becomes visible at the introitus, place the pads of your fingertips on the portion of the vertex at vaginal introitus.<br>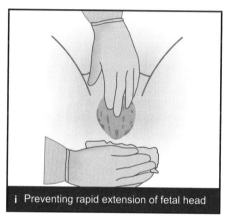<br>**Figure 14.10(a) (i):** Normal vaginal delivery (illustrated) | |
| 19 | As more of the head is visible, spread your fingers over the vertex of the baby's head, with fingertips pointing towards the unseen face of the fetus and the elbow pointing upwards, towards the mother (Figure 14.10(a) (ii)).<br>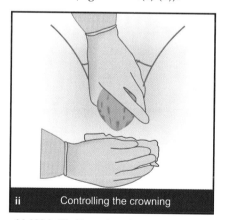<br>**Figure 14.10(a) (ii):** Normal vaginal delivery (illustrated) | Gives pressure against the fetal head to keep it well flexed. |

*Contd...*

*Contd...*

| 20 | Cover the hand not used on baby's head with a towel and place the thumb in the crease of the groin midway on one side of the perineum. Place the middle finger in the same way on the other side of perineum. | Prevent contamination from the anus. |
|---|---|---|
| 21 | As the head advances allow it to gradually extend beneath your hand by exerting control but not prohibitive pressure. | Control of the head in this manner will prevent explosive crowning and pressure on the perineum. |
| 22 | With the hand over the perineum, apply pressure downward and inward towards each other across the perineal body at the sametime. | This support will prevent rapid birth of head causing intracranial damage to baby and laceration to perineum. |
| 23 | Observe the perineum in the space between the thumb and middle finger while offering head control and perineal support. | Detects signs of impending tear such as stretch marks beneath the perineal skin. |
| 24 | Give an episiotomy if required when there is bulging thinned perineum during the peak of a contraction or just prior to crowning. | Avoids injury to the anal sphincter and spontaneous laceration of the perineum. |
| 25 | As soon as the head is born, during the resting phase, before the next contraction, place the fingertips of one hand on the occiput and slide them down to the level of shoulders. | |
| 26 | Sweep the fingers in both directions to feel for the umbilical cord. | Detects the presence of nuchal cord, which can prevent the descend of the fetus and the delivery of the body. |
| 27 | If the cord is felt and if it is loose, slip it over the baby's head. If the cord is tight apply clamps about 3 cm, apart and cut the cord at the middle of the neck (mother must be instructed to pant while clamping, cutting and unwinding the cord). | Prevents the cord from becoming tightened around the neck. |
| 28 | Wipe the baby's face and wipe off fluid from nose and mouth. | Facilitates breathing. |
| 29 | Suction the oral and nasal passage with a bulb syringe. | Prevents aspiration of the fluid. |
| 30 | Delivery of shoulders:<br>–Wait for a contraction and watch for restitution and external rotation of head. | Allows time for shoulders to rotate to the anteroposterior diameter of the outlet. |
| 31 | When the shoulders reach the anteroposterior diameter of the pelvic outlet, proceed to deliver one shoulder at a time in the following manner.<br>-Place a hand on each side of the head over the ears and apply downward traction to deliver the anterior shoulder.<br>(Figure 14.10(a) (iii)) | |

iii — Downward traction of fetal head

**Figure 14.10(a) (iii):** Normal vaginal delivery (illustrated)

# Maternal and Child Nursing

*Contd...*

| | | |
|---|---|---|
| | -When the axillary crease is seen, guide the head and trunk in an upward curve to allow the posterior shoulder to escape over the posterior vaginal wall (Figure 14.10(a) (iv)) | Avoids overstretching of the perineum |

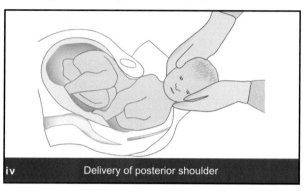

**Figure 14.10(a) (iv):** Normal vaginal delivery (illustrated)

| | | |
|---|---|---|
| 32 | Grasp the baby around the chest and lift the baby towards the mother's abdomen. | This allows the mother to have an immediate sighting of the baby and close contact. |
| 33 | Note the time of birth | |
| 34 | Place two clamps on the cord about 8-10 cm from the umbilicus and cut it while covering it with a gauze | Covering with a gauze while cutting prevents spraying the delivery field with blood. |
| 35 | Give the baby to the nursery nurse who will place him in the designated area, dry him and carry out the assessment and care. | |
| 36 | Place the placenta receiver against the perineum. | For receiving the placenta and membranes. |
| 37 | Place one hand over the fundus to feel the contraction of the uterus. | |
| 38 | Watch for signs of placental separation: lengthening of cord, gush of bleeding, fundus becoming round and placenta descending into the vagina. | Contraction and placental separation may occur in minutes. |
| 39 | When placental descend is confirmed ask the patient to beardown as the uterus contracts, as she did during the second stage of labor (controlled cord traction can be used to deliver placenta) (Figure 14.10(b)). | Bearing down simultaneously with a contraction aids expulsion of the placenta. |

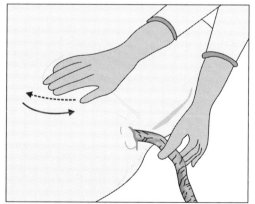

**Figure 14.10(b):** Controlled cord traction (Brandt-Andrew's method)

*Contd...*

*Contd...*

| | | |
|---|---|---|
| 40 | As soon as the placenta passes through the introitus, grasp it in cupped hands. | |
| 41 | Twist the placenta round and round with gentle traction so that the membranes are stripped off intact. If the length of the membranes make the movements difficult, catch the membranes with an artery forceps and give gentle traction till they are stripped off and expelled intact. | |
| 42 | If spontaneous expulsion fails to occur in 20-30 min, perform controlled cord traction or Brandt Andrew's maneuvers. | |
| 43 | Examine the patient's vulva, vagina and perineum for any laceration. | |
| 44 | Massage the uterus to make it contract for expulsion of any retained blood clots. | |
| 45 | Suture episiotomy layer by layer if one was made. | |
| 46 | Clean the vulva and surrounding area with antiseptic solution and place perineal pad. | |
| 47 | Straighten mother's legs, cross them and make her comfortable. | Reduces bleeding. |
| 48 | Clean and replace articles. | Prevents spread of microorganisms. |
| 49 | Remove gloves and wash hands. | |
| 50 | Record the details of delivery and condition of the mother and baby in the patient's chart. | |

## 14.11: PERFORMING AN EXAMINATION OF PLACENTA

### DEFINITION

A thorough inspection and examination of the placenta and membranes, soon after expulsion, for its completeness and normalcy.

### PURPOSES

1. To ensure that the entire placenta and membranes have been expelled and no part has been retained.
2. To make sure that placenta is of normal size, shape, consistency and weight.
3. To detect abnormalities such as infarctions, calcification or additional lobes.
4. To ascertain the length of the cord, number of blood vessels and site of insertion of the cord.
5. To prevent PPH and infection.
6. To check weight of placenta and measure length of cord.

### ARTICLES

1. Placenta in a bowl.
2. A washable surface to lay the placenta
3. A weighing machine.
4. Measuring tape
5. Kidney tray
6. Pair of gloves.

### PROCEDURE

| | Nursing action | Rationale |
|---|---|---|
| 1 | Don gloves | Protects nurse from contamination. |
| 2 | Using gloved hands hold the placenta by the cord allowing the membranes to hang (twisting the cord twice around the fingers will provide a firm grip). | Hanging membranes will provide a better view to check its completeness. |
| 3 | Identify the hole through which the baby was delivered. | If the membrances are not torn into pieces, a single round hole can be identified clearly. |
| 4 | Insert hand through the hole and spread out the fingers to view the membranes and the blood vessels (Figure 14.11(a)). | The position of cord insertion and the course of blood vessels can be noted in this position. |

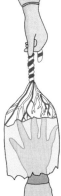

Figure 14.11(a): Examination of the membranes

*Contd...*

*Contd...*

| | | |
|---|---|---|
| 5 | Remove the hand from inside the membranes and lay the placenta on a flat surface with the fetal surface up. Identify the site of cord insertion (Figure 14.11(b)). | Normally the cord is inserted in the center of placenta. Lateral or velamentous insertion may be noted. |

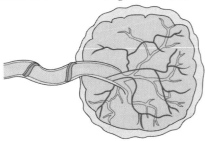

Figure 14.11(b): Fetal surface of placenta

| | | |
|---|---|---|
| 6 | Examine the two membranes, amnion and chorion for completeness and presence of abnormal vessels indicating succenturiate lobe. | Amnion is shiny and chorion is shaggy. Amnion can be peeled from the chorion upto the umbilical cord. |
| 7 | Invert the placenta, expose the maternal surface and remove any clots present (Figure 14.11(c)). | |

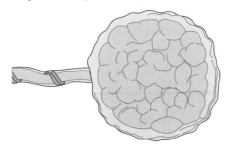

Figure 14.11(c): Maternal surface of placenta

| | | |
|---|---|---|
| 8 | Examine the maternal surface by spreading it in the palms of your two hands and placing the cotyledons in close approximation (any broken fragments must be replaced before accurate assessment is made). | Ensures that no part of the placenta or membranes is left inside the uterus. |
| 9 | Assess for presence of abnormalities such as infarctions, calcifications or succenturiate lobes. | |
| 10 | Inspect the cut end of the umblical cord for presence of three umbilical vessels (Figure 14.11(d)). | Two arteries and one vein should normally be seen. Absence of an artery may be associated with renal abnormalities. |

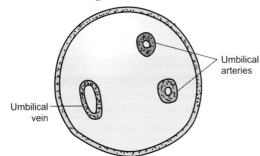

Umbilical arteries

Umbilical vein

Figure 14.11(d): Cross-section of umbilical cord

*Contd...*

*Contd...*

| | | |
|---|---|---|
| 11 | Measure the length of the umbilical cord by holding it extended against a graduated surface/side of the weighing scale. (The length of the cord on the baby may be added to get the total length where applicable) | Average length of the cord is 50 cm. |
| 12 | Weigh the placenta by placing it on the weighing scale meant for the purpose. | Normally the placenta weighs about 1/6 th of the baby's weight. |
| 13 | Place the placenta in the bin for proper disposal. | |
| 14 | Clean the area used for examination of the placenta and membranes, the weighing scale and the bowl. | |
| 15 | Remove gloves and wash hands. | |
| 16 | Record in the patient's chart, the findings of placental examination and weight of the placenta, length of the cord and any special observations made. | Acts as a communication between staff members. |

# 14.12: PERFORMING AND SUTURING AN EPISIOTOMY

## DEFINITION

A surgically planned incision on the perineum and posterior vaginal wall during the second stage of labor to facilitate delivery.

## PURPOSES

1. To substitute a straight surgical incision for the laceration that may otherwise occur.
2. To facilitate repair of laceration and promote healing.
3. To spare the newborn's head from prolonged pressure and to avoid pushing against rigid perineum.
4. To shorten the second stage of labor.
5. To speed delivery if there is fetal distress.
6. Prior to an assisted delivery such as forceps or ventouse extraction.
7. To minimise the risk of intracranial damage during preterm and breech delivery.
8. To prevent overstretching of the perineal muscles.

## TYPES OF EPISIOTOMIES

1. Median or midline: Incision is made in the middle of the perineum and directed toward the anus.
2. Mediolateral: Incision begins at the midline and is directed laterally.

## INDICATIONS

1. Inelastic rigid perineum
2. Primigravida
3. Anticipated perineal tear.
4. Operative delivery
5. Previous perineal surgery.

## EQUIPMENTS

A Sterile tray containing:
1. Sterile syringe with needle.
2. Needle holder-1
3. Scissors-1 and episiotomy scissors -1
4. Cutting needle-1 for skin
   Round body needle-1 for muscles.
5. Thumb forceps
6. Suture material-2-0 chromic catgut-1
7. Kidney tray
8. Plain Lignocaine 2%
9. Antiseptic solution
10. Sterile gloves
11. 4 × 4 gauze pieces
12. Tampons.

## GENERAL INSTRUCTIONS

1. Ensure that
   a. The presenting part is directly applied to the perineal tissues, which will be evidenced as bulging perineum.
   b. Vaginal orifice is distended by approximately 3 cm diameter of presenting part between contractions.

2. The presenting part of the fetus should be protected from injury.
3. A single cut in any direction is preferable to repeated snipping, as the latter will have jagged ends.
4. The episiotomy should be large enough to meet the purpose
5. The timing of the cut should be such that lacerations are prevented and unnecessary blood loss avoided .

## PROCEDURE

| | Nursing action | Rationale |
|---|---|---|
| 1 | Place the patient on the delivery table in dorsal recumbent position when the fetal head is distending the perineum. | Gives clear visualization. |
| 2 | Infilterate the perineum using 10 ml of local anesthetic. Wait for 3-5 min for the anesthetic to act (Figure 14.12(a)). | Minimizes pain during incision. |

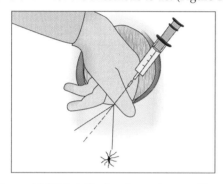

**Figure 14.12(a):** Infiltrating the perineum with anaesthetic

| | Nursing action | Rationale |
|---|---|---|
| 3 | Place your index and middle fingers in the vagina with palmar side down and facing you. Separate them slightly and exert outward pressure on the perineal body. | Provides protection to the presenting part in two ways. a) The fingers are against the presenting part and are thick enough so that the scissors properly placed will not hurt the baby. b) The outward pressure directs the perineal body away from the baby. The pressure also flattens the perineal body a bit more, making it easier to incise using a single cut. |
| 4 | Place the blades of the scissors in a straight up and down position, so that one blade is against the posterior vaginal wall and the other blade against the skin of the perineal body with the point where the blades cross at the middle of the posterior fourchette (Figure 14.12(b)). | |

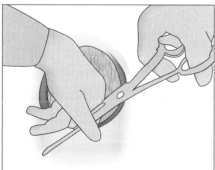

**Figure 14.12(b):** Performing an episiotomy.

*Contd...*

*Contd...*

| | | |
|---|---|---|
| 5 | Adjust the length of the blades of the scissors on the perineal body and predict the length of the incision accordingly. | The length of the incision should be adequate to meet the purpose. |
| 6 | a. A mediolateral episiotomy is cut at a slant starting at the midline of the fourchette with the points of the scissors directed toward the ischial tuberosity on the same side as the incision.<br>b. A midline episiotomy is cut in the middle of the central tendinous points of the perineum from the posterior fourchette down to the external anal sphincter. (The ideal timing of episiotomy is a bulging thin perineum at the peak of a contraction just prior to crowning). | |
| 7 | If a midline episiotomy was cut, palpate for the external anal sphincter. | |
| 8 | Cut again if needed, avoid snipping. Two cuts should accomplish the incision. | |
| 9 | Extend the vaginal side of the incision if needed by incising the vaginal band. For this, the scissors must come from above the backside of the hand to slide down the fingers and make the cut. | Protects the fetal presenting part. |
| 10 | Apply pressure with 4" × 4" sponges | Controls any slight bleeding present. |
| 11 | After completion of delivery assist for suturing of episiotomy incision. | |
| 12 | Wipe the wound area with sterile antiseptic cotton swabs. | Prevents spread of microorganisms. |
| 13 | Focus light on the perineal area | Gives clear visualization of the perineum. |
| 14 | Diagnose the degree of perineal tear if any. | |
| 15 | Pack the vagina with vaginal plug or tampon | Continuous bleeding may obscure the place of suturing. |
| 16 | Visualize the apex of the mucosa, start suturing little above the apex. Appose the vaginal tear by continuous suture using round body needle (Figure 14.12(c)). | |

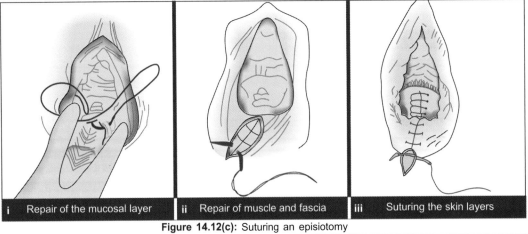

i    Repair of the mucosal layer     ii    Repair of muscle and fascia     iii    Suturing the skin layers

**Figure 14.12(c):** Suturing an episiotomy

*Contd...*

*Contd...*

| | | |
|---|---|---|
| 17 | Repair the perineal muscles by interrupted sutures, include the deeper tissue to enclose dead space. | |
| 18 | Perineal skin is apposed by mattress suture. | |
| 19 | Remove the vaginal pack which was inserted during suturing. | |
| 20 | Clean the perineum and apply perineal pads. | |
| 21 | Straighten patient's legs and assist her to supine position with legs crossed. | Makes the patient comfortable and reduces the chance of bleeding. |
| 22 | Wash and dry the instruments used for episiotomy along with those used for conduct of delivery and suturing. | |
| 23 | Record in the labor record, the time episiotomy was performed, type of episiotomy, suturing carried out, and patient's reaction. | Acts as a communication between staff members. |

## AFTER CARE

1. Check for any bleeding from inner areas or hematoma formation.
2. Check vital signs.
3. Check for any other tear or laceration.

## COMPLICATIONS

1. Hematoma
2. Infections
3. Wound dehiscence
4. Perineal laceration
5. Dyspareunia
6. Scar endometriosis.

## SPECIAL CONSIDERATIONS

1. Repair of the skin edges should begin at the fourchette so that vaginal opening is properly aligned.
2. A rectal examination is made when suturing is completed in order to ensure that no sutures have penetrated the rectal mucosa to prevent fistula formation
3. The thread should not be pulled too tightly to prevent edema formation.

# 14.13: ASSISTING WITH FORCEPS DELIVERY

## DEFINITION

Assisting with application of forceps to extract fetal head and thereby accomplish delivery of fetus.

## INDICATIONS

1. Maternal
   a. Maternal exhaustion (distress)
   b. Severe pre- eclampsia
   c. Heart disease.
2. Fetal
   a. Fetal distress
   b. Low birth weight baby
   c. Postmature baby
   d. Aftercoming head of breech.

## TYPES OF FORCEPS APPLICATION ACCORDING TO THE STATION OF FETAL HEAD

1. High forceps
   Application on a non-engaged fetal head. This method is not practiced in modern-day obstetrics.
2. Mid forceps
   Application on fetal head that is engaged in the pelvis, but presenting part is above + 2 station.
3. Low forceps
   Presenting part of the fetal head is at + 2 station or below but has not reached the pelvic floor.
4. Outlet forceps
   Forceps are applied on the fetal head lying on the perineum and is visible at the introitus between contractions. It is the widely practiced type of application (90%).

## CLASSIFICATION OF OBSTETRIC FORCEPS

1. Long curved forceps with or without axis traction device.
2. Short curved forceps (Wrigley's)
3. Kielland's forceps.

## CRITERIA FOR APPLICATION OF FORCEPS

1. Fetal criteria
   a. Fetal head must be engaged.
   b. The position and station of the head must be suitable to apply the blades correctly to the sides of the head.
2. Maternal criteria
   a. No major cephalopelvic disproportion
   b. Bladder must be empty.
   c. Adequate analgesia.
   d. Cervix must be fully dilated
   e. Membranes must be ruptured
   f. Presence of good uterine contractions.
3. Others
   a. Written consent.

- Mnemonic for FORCEPS
  - F  Favorable head position and cervix.
  - O  Open os
  - R  Ruptured membranes
  - C  Contractions present
  - E  Engaged head and empty bladder
  - P  Pelvimetry
  - S  Stirrups (Lithotomy position)

## ARTICLES

- All articles for conducting delivery plus forceps.

## PROCEDURE

| | Nursing action | Rationale |
|---|---|---|
| 1 | Explain to mother and family the need for forceps delivery | Helps in obtaining co-operation. |
| 2 | Obtain informed consent. | Prevents chances of legal problems. |
| 3 | Assess fetal heart rate | |
| 4 | Assess the state of cervix, membranes, presentation and position of head by an internal examination. | |
| 5 | Empty the bladder by catheterization | Full bladder interferes with contractions. |
| 6 | Infiltrate the perineum with local anesthetic (1% lignocaine) | |
| 7 | Give an episiotomy when the perineum becomes bulged and thinned out by the advancing head. | Helps in insertion of forceps blades. |
| 8 | Assess fetal heart rate frequently. (every 5-10 minutes) If not on continuous fetal monitoring. | |
| 9 | Physician identifies the forceps blades. | Helps to select the blade to be inserted first. |
| 10 | Inserts four fingers of the semisupined right hand along the left lateral vaginal wall, the palmar surface of the fingers rest against the side of the fetal head. | The fingers are to guide the blade during application and to protect the vaginal wall. |
| 11 | The handle of the left blade is taken in the left hand in a pen-holding manner and is held vertically. The fenestrated portion of the blade is then introduced between the internal fingers and fetal head, manipulated by the left thumb. (when correctly applied, the blade should be over the parietal eminence, the shank in contact with the perineum and the handle directed upwards) (Figure 14.13(a) (i)). | As the blade is pushed up, the handle is carried downwards and backwards. 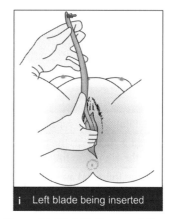 i  Left blade being inserted<br>**Figure 14.13(a) (i):** Forceps delivery |

*Contd...*

*Contd...*

| 12 | Introduction of the right blade is done after introducing two fingers of the left hand into the right lateral wall of the vagina along the side of baby's head.<br>Right blade is introduced in the same manner as with the left one but holding it with the right hand (Figure 14.13(a) (ii)). | Fingers in the vagina guide the blade inside preventing injury to vaginal wall. |
|---|---|---|

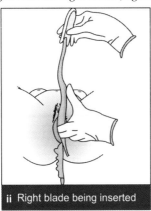

**ii** Right blade being inserted

**Figure 14.13(a) (ii): Forceps delivery**

| 13 | With the right blade over the left one the physician articulates and locks the blades. In case of difficulty in locking, the blades are removed and reapplied. With correct application, locking is easy. | |
|---|---|---|
| 14 | During the next uterine contraction the physician gives steady but intermittent traction (Figure 14.13(a) (iii)).<br>In outlet forceps, the traction may be continuous and contraction is not awaited as the head is already on the perineum. | The direction of the pull corresponds to the axis of the birth canal. |

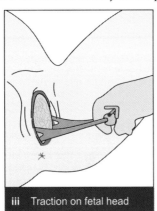

**iii** Traction on fetal head

**Figure 14.13(a) (iii): Forceps delivery**

| 15 | Once the baby's head is deliverd, the blades are removed one after the other, the right one first. | |
|---|---|---|
| 16 | Further steps are to be followed as in normal vaginal delivery. Intravenous methergine is to be administered with the delivery of the anterior shoulder. | Prevents chances of increased blood loss. |
| 17 | Episiotomy is repaired in the usual manner. | |

# COMPLICATIONS

## MATERNAL COMPLICATIONS

*Immediate*
1. Injury-Vaginal laceration, cervical tear, extension of episiotomy, complete vaginal tear.
2. Nerve injury-Femoral, lumbosacral trunk with midforceps delivery.
3. Postpartum hemorrhage
4. Anesthetic complications.
5. Puerperal sepsis and maternal morbidity.

*Remote complications:*
1. Painful perineal scars
2. Dyspareunia
3. Low backache
4. Genital prolapse
5. Stress urinary incontinence
6. Sphincter dysfunction.

## FETAL

*Immediate complication:*
1. Asphyxia
2. Facial bruising
3. Intracranial hemorrhage
4. Cephalhematoma
5. Facial palsy
6. Skull fractures
7. Cervical spine injury.

*Remote complications:*
1. Cerebral or spastic palsy due to residual cerebral injury.

# SPECIAL POINTS

1. The direction of the pull for extracting fetal head corresponds to the level at which the forceps is applied on fetal head.
   In low forceps, the direction of the pull is downwards and backwards until the head comes to the perineum.
2. The pull is then directed downwards till the head is almost crowned. (Horizontally straight towards the operator).
3. The direction of the pull is gradually changed to upwards and forwards towards the mother's abdomen to deliver the head by extension.

# 14.14: ASSISTING WITH VENTOUSE EXTRACTION

## DEFINITION

Assisting in the delivery of a fetus presenting by vertex using an instrument called ventouse or vacuum extractor.

## INDICATIONS

1. As an alternative to forceps delivery.
2. As an alternative to rotational forceps as in occipitotransverse or occipitoposterior position.
3. Delay in descent of the head in case of second baby of twins.
4. Delay in late first stage or second stage of labor.
5. Maternal exhaustion
6. Mild fetal distress.

## CONTRAINDICATIONS

1. Any presentation other than vertex (Face, brow, breech).
2. Preterm fetus (Less than 34 weeks).
3. Chance of scalp avulsion or sub-aponeurotic hemorrhage.
4. Suspected fetal coagulation disorder.
5. Suspected fetal macrosomia(more than 4 kg).

## CONDITIONS TO BE FULFILLED

1. There should not be any bony resistance below the level of head.
2. The head of a singleton baby should be engaged.
3. Cervix should be at least 6 cm dilated.

## EQUIPMENTS

1. Suction cups of varying sizes(30, 40, 50 and 60 mm)
2. A vacuum generator.
3. Traction tubing and handle
4. Delivery pack containing
   a. Artery forceps
   b. Dissecting forceps
   c. Cord clamp
   d. Episiotomy scissors
   e. Suture needle and suture material
   f. Vaginal tampon
   g. Mucous sucker.
5. Neonatal resuscitation equipments
6. Emergency drugs.

## PROCEDURE

| | Nursing action | Rationale |
|---|---|---|
| 1 | Explain procedure to mother and family. | Helps in obtaining co-operation of family and mother. |
| 2 | Obtain informed consent from mother. | Prevents litigation. |

*Contd...*

*Contd...*

| | | |
|---|---|---|
| 3 | Instruct mother to empty the bladder, if not possible catheterization should be done. | |
| 4 | Ensure that bowel is empty. | |
| 5 | Maintain lithotomy position and start good IV line. | |
| 6 | Assess FHR frequently. | |
| 7 | Assess for descent of fetal head with mother's uterine contraction. | |
| 8 | Infilterate perineum with 1% lignocaine | Acts as a local anesthetic. |
| 9 | Perform episiotomy when the contractions are strong. | Provides sufficient space for applying vacuum cup. |
| 10 | Assist obstetrician in applying suction cup and traction and maintenance of pressure (Figure 14.14(a)). | |

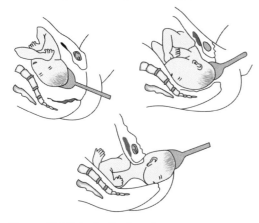

**Figure 14.14(a):** Application of vacuum extractor

| | | |
|---|---|---|
| 11 | As soon the head is delivered the vacuum is reduced by opening the screw-release valve. | Aids in release of the cup. |
| 12 | Complete the delivery of the fetus in the normal manner. | |
| 13 | Repair the episiotomy in the usual manner. | |
| 14 | Clean the perineum and check for bleeding or laceration. | |
| 15 | Record the date, time, pressure and traction applied and any complication in nurses record. | Acts as a communication between staff members. |

## COMPLICATIONS

### FETAL COMPLICATIONS

1. Superficial scalp abrasion
2. Sloughing of the scalp
3. Cephal hematoma
4. Subaponeurotic hemorrhage
5. Intracranial hemorrhage
6. Retinal hemorrhage.
7. "Chignon" formation.

### MATERNAL COMPLICATION

Injuries are uncommon but may be due to inclusion of the soft tissues such as the cervix or vaginal wall inside the cup.

## 14.15: ASSISTING WITH DILATATION AND CURETTAGE PROCEDURE

## DEFINITION

Assisting in expansion of cervical canal of uterus and scraping the surface lining of the uterine wall by a metal device called curette. This procedure is done during the premenstural phase.

## INDICATIONS

### DIAGNOSTIC

1. Infertility
2. Dysfunctional uterine bleeding
3. Pathologic amenorrhea
4. Endometrial tuberculosis
5. Endometrial carcinoma
6. Postmenopausal bleeding
7. Chorion epithelioma.

### THERAPEUTIC

1. Dysfunctional uterine bleeding
2. Endometrial polyp
3. Removal of IUD
4. Incomplete abortion
5. Evacuation of hydatidiform mole
6. Prior to insertion of intrauterine radium implants.
7. To prevent cervical stenosis in Manchester operation for uterine prolapse
8. To drain pyometra.

## CONTRAINDICATIONS

1. Vaginal and cervical infection
2. Pelvic infection
3. Suspected uterine pregnancy.

## ARTICLES

The procedure is carried out in the OT .

## SPECIAL INSTRUMENTS USED

1. Dilators (Different sizes of Hegar's dilators)
2. Vulsellum
3. Uterine sound
4. Curette.

## PROCEDURE

| | Nursing action | Rationale |
|---|---|---|
| 1 | Explain procedure to patient | Helps in allaying fear and anxiety. |
| 2 | Obtain, informed consent from patient. | Prevents legalities to staff members. |
| 3 | Instruct patient to empty the bladder prior to operation. | |
| 4 | Maintain NPO for six hours before procedure. | Prevents chances of aspiration during procedure. |

*Contd...*

*Contd...*

| | | |
|---|---|---|
| 5 | Administer premedication as per physician's order. | |
| 6 | Start IV line | |
| 7 | Maintain lithotomy position and clean the perineum with antiseptic solution. | Enhances good visualization. Prevents spread of micro-organisms. |
| 8 | Physician performs vaginal examination to note conditions of vulva, vagina and cervix, including the size, consistency position and mobility of the uterus. | Helps to know the position of uterus and to exclude possibility of pregnancy. |
| 9 | Assist the physician in administering anesthesia. | |
| 10 | Physician introduces Sim's vaginal speculum inside the vagina.<br>• In nulliparous women the blade of the speculum is lubricated with savlon solution and introduced from the side of the vaginal outlet after separating the labia minora with the otherhand till the entire blade is introduced inside the vagina.<br>• In parous women, the blade is introduced on separating labia minora. | Helps in visualization of cervix. |
| 11 | The anterior lip of the exposed cervix is grasped by the toothed vulsellum and pulled down near the vaginal introitus. | |
| 12 | An uterine sound is introduced with the tip directed forward into uterus. | Helps to measure the length of uterine cavity and position of the uterus. |
| 13 | Assist in dilatation of the cervix. The tip of the dilator should be directed anteriorly or posteriorly according to position of the uterus. | |
| 14 | After the desired dilatation, the uterine cavity is curretted by uterine curette either in clockwise or anti-clockwise direction in a smooth manner. | Vigorous curettage may damage the basal layer of the endometrium and uterine muscle. |
| 15 | Take out the vulsellum and curette. | |
| 16 | Clean the cervix with antiseptic solution and check for any unusual bleeding. | |
| 17 | The curetted material is preserved in 10% normal saline, labelled properly and sent for histological examination. | |
| 18 | Record the data and time of procedure with patient's reactions. | Acts as a communication between staff members. |

## POSTOPERATIVE CARE

1. Check the vital signs.
2. Instruct patient to rest in bed until the anesthtic effect is reversed.
3. Check the amount of bleeding.

## COMPLICATIONS

### IMMEDIATE COMPLICATIONS

1. Injury to the cervix.
2. Uterine perforation.
3. Bowel injury
4. Pelvic inflammation.

### REMOTE COMPLICATIONS

1. Cervical incompetence due to injury to internal os, resulting in midtrimester abortion.
2. Uterine synechiae due to injury to uterine muscle resulting in secondary amenorrhea.

# 14.16: GIVING A PERINEAL CARE

## DEFINITION

Cleansing the patient's external genitalia and surrounding skin using antiseptic solution.

## PURPOSES

1. To cleanse the perineal skin.
2. To reduce chances of infection of episiotomy wound.
3. To stimulate circulation.
4. To reduce body odour and improve self-image.
5. To promote the feeling of wellbeing.

## EQUIPMENT

a. A clean tray containing
   1. Sterile antiseptic lotion – 2% dettol or savlon.
   2. Sterile normal saline in a bottle.
   3. Cheatle forceps.
   4. Antiseptic or antibiotic medication if ordered.
   5. Sterile sanitary pad.
   6. Kidney tray.
   7. Sterile gloves.
   8. Mackintosh
b. Sterile pack or tray containing
   1. Artery forceps—2
   2. Dissecting forceps—1
   3. Cottonballs.
   4. Gauze pieces.
   5. Sterile towel to wipe hands after surgical scrub.
c. Additional items
   1. Infrared light.
   2. Bedpan (if procedure is done at bedside).

## PROCEDURE

| | Nursing action | Rationale |
|---|---|---|
| 1. | Explain the procedure to patient, the purpose and how she has to cooperate. | Gains confidence and cooperation of the patient. |
| 2. | Assemble articles at the bedside or in the treatment room. | Saves time and effort. |
| 3. | Ask the patient to empty her bowel and bladder and wash the perineal area before coming for perineal care. | Ensures cleanliness and reduces number of organisms in the perineal area. |
| 4. | Screen the bed or close the doors as appropriate. | Provides privacy reduces embarrassment. |
| 5. | Assist the patient to assume dorsal recumbent position with knees bend and drape the area using diamond draping method. | Dorsal position facilitates better viewing of the perineum. |
| 6. | Open sterile tray, arrange articles with cheatle forceps and pour antiseptic solution in the sterile gallipot in this tray. | |

*Contd...*

*Contd...*

| | | |
|---|---|---|
| 7. | Adjust the position of the infrared light so that it shines on the perineum at a distance of 45-50 cm. | |
| 8. | Scrub hands and dry with the sterile towel. | |
| 9. | Put on sterile gloves. | |
| 10. | Take the cotton swabs with artery forceps, dip in savlon and squeeze excess lotion with dissecting forceps into the kidney tray. | Maintains asepsis |
| 11. | With the swab clean from urethra towards anus. Clean the area from midline outward in the following order until clean and discard the swab after each stroke. Strokes are to be in the following order:<br>• Separate the vestibule with non-dominant hand and clean vestibule starting from clitoris to fourchette<br>• Inside of labia minora downward, farther side first then nearer side<br>• Take off the non-dominant hand<br>• Labia majora downward farthest side and then nearer side<br>• Discard the used forceps (if a second one is available)<br>• Using the second forceps clean the episiotomy wound from center outwards and outside of episiotomy both sides. | Cleaning from more cleaner area to least clean area prevents contamination |
| 12. | Wipe all traces of antiseptic away with sterile normal saline swabs in the same manner as described above using thumb forceps. | |
| 13. | Dry the episiotomy with gauze pieces. Do not use cotton balls for this purpose. | Cotton fibers are likely to get caught while drying if cotton balls are used. |
| 14. | Provide perineal light/infra red light for 10 mts if indicated. | Provides soothing effect from heat |
| 15. | Put prescribed medication on a gauze piece and apply to the episiotomy. | Prevents entry of pathogenic organisms. |
| 16. | Place sanitary pad from front to back. Do not shift position of the pad once it is applied. | Avoids chances of contamination. |
| 17. | Discard gloves and used items in the kidney tray, wash forceps and tray and keep ready for sterilization. | Reduces chances of contamination. |
| 18. | Replace other articles in designated places. | |
| 19. | Make the patient comfortable and leave the unit clean. | |
| 20. | Record procedure in the patient's chart including details regarding status of lochia and condition of episiotomy wound. | Documentation helps for communication between staff members and provides evidence of care given and observations made. |

## SPECIAL CONSIDERATIONS

1. If a sitz bath is prescribed, give it before perineal care.
2. If patient has urinary catheter, provide catheter care along with perineal care.

**Studies have shown that healing takes place effectively even when patient's practice perineal hygiene by themselves.**

## 14.17: MEASURING INVOLUTION OF UTERUS

## DEFINITION

Assessing the state of uterus in the post-delivery period as it returns to the pregravid state.

## PURPOSES

1. To rule out infection.
2. To estimate the rate at which involution is taking place.
3. To assess the puerperal condition of the woman with complicated labor.

## EQUIPMENTS

1. Screen
2. Inch-tape
3. Clean gloves.

## PROCEDURE

| | Nursing action | Rationale |
|---|---|---|
| 1. | Explain the procedure to patient and instruct her on how she has to cooperate. | Enhances cooperation. |
| 2. | Arrange the unit and assemble necessary articles at bedside. | Saves time and energy. |
| 3. | Ensure that patient's bladder is empty. | Full bladder may cause upward displacement of uterus. |
| 4. | Pull curtains/screen the bed | Provides privacy |
| 5. | Position the patient in supine and drape the patient exposing only the lower abdomen. | Enhances easy assessment. |
| 6. | Don gloves | |
| 7. | Locate fundus with the palm of one hand. | |
| 8. | Place lateral side of hands slightly above fundus. | |
| 9. | Place your other hand above the symphysis pubis. | Supports and stabilizes uterus during palpation. |
| 10. | Gently but firmly press into abdomen towards the spine and then slightly downwards towards the perineum until a mass is felt in the palm of the hand. | |
| 11. | Measure the number of finger breadth at which the fundus is felt below the umbilicus.<br>With the help of an inch-tape measure from the level of fundus to the upper border of symphysis pubis. | Finger breadth measurement should correspond to the number of days after delivery.<br>Or<br>On 1st postpartum day the fundus is felt about 10-12 cm above the symphysis pubis and from 2nd-11th day fundus descends at a rate of ½ inch (1.25 cm) per 24 hours.<br>By 11th day uterus sinks below the level symphysis pubis and becomes a pelvic a organ (Figure 14.17 (a)). |

*Contd...*

*Contd....*

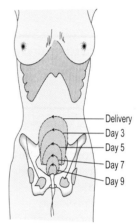

**Figure 14.17(a):** Involution of uterus

| | | |
|---|---|---|
| 12. | With gloved hand check perineal pad for color of lochia. | Allows for assessment of rate of involution. |
| 13. | Offer perineal care if needed and provide a clean pad. | Maintains hygiene and prevents infection. |
| 14. | Replace the articles and wash hands. | Prevents spread of microorganisms. |
| 15. | Mark the fundal height in nurses record. | Documentation helps in obtaining a clear picture about involution of uterus. |

# 14.18: TEACHING POSTNATAL EXCERCISES

## DEFINITION

A series of physical exercises that are performed by the postnatal mother to bring about optimal functioning of all systems and prevent complications.

## PURPOSES

1. To improve the tone of muscles which are stretched during pregnancy and labor specially the abdominal and perineal muscles
2. To educate about correct posture and body mechanics
3. To minimize the risk of puerperal venous thrombosis by promoting circulation and preventing venous stasis
4. To prevent backache
5. To prevent genital prolapse
6. To prevent stress incontinence of urine.

## PROCEDURE

Teach exercises in the early postpartum period to strengthen the abdominal muscles and firm the waist. The exercise can be started soon after childbirth and repeated upto five times twice a day, at first. The number of exercises is gradually increased as the mother gains strength.

| | Nursing action | Rationale |
|---|---|---|
| 1. | Explain the procedure to patient. | Minimizes anxiety and facilitates patient cooperation. |
| 2. | Provide privacy | |
| I. | **Abdominal exercises** | |
| | a. *Abdominal breathing:* | |
| | • Instruct the woman to assume a supine position with knees bent. | |
| | • Instruct her to inhale through the nose, keep the rib cage as stationary as possible, and allow the abdomen to expand and then contract the abdominal muscles as she exhales slowly through the mouth (Figure 14.18 (a)). | Strengthens the diaphragm. |
| | • Instruct her to place one hand on the chest and one on the abdomen when inhaling. The hand on the abdomen should rise and the hand on the chest should remain stationary | Ensures that the exercise is being done correctly and ensures adequate intake of air while inhaling. |
| | • Repeat the excerise five times. | |

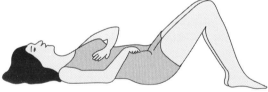

**Figure 14.18(a):** Abdominal breathing

| | | |
|---|---|---|
| | b. *Head lift* | |
| | This exercise can be started within a few days after childbirth | |
| | • Instruct the mother to lie supine with knees bent and arms out stretched at her side. | Strengthens abdominal muscles. |
| | • Instruct her to inhale deeply at first and then exhale while lifting the head slowly, to holds the position for a few seconds and relax (Figure 14.18 (b)). | |

*Contd...*

*Contd...*

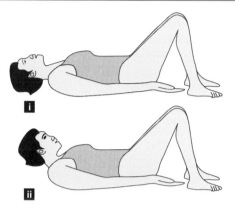

**Figure 14.18(b):** Head lift exercises

c. *Head and shoulder raising*
   On the second postpartum day instruct woman to:
- Lie flat without pillow and raise head until the chin touches the chest.
   On the 3rd postpartum day instruct her to:
- Raise both head and shoulder off the bed and lower them slowly (Figure 14.18 (c)).
- Gradually increase the number of repetitions until she is able to do this for 10 times.

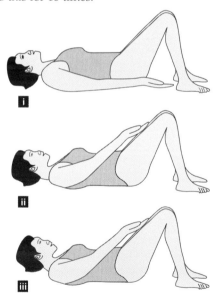

**Figure 14.18(c):** Head and shoulder raising exercises

d. *Leg raising*
This exercise may begin on the 7th postpartum
day. Instruct woman to:
- Lie down on the floor with no pillows under the head, point toe and slowly raise one leg keeping the knee straight.

*Contd...*

*Contd...*

- Lower the leg slowly.
- Gradually increase to ten times each leg.

e. *Pelvic tilting or rocking*

Instruct woman to:
- Lie flat on the floor with knees bent and feet flat, inhale and while exhaling flatten the back hard against the floor so that there is no space between the back and the floor
- Inhale normally hold breath for upto 10 seconds and then relax
- Repeat upto 10 times

f. *Knee and leg rolling* (Figure 14.18 (d))

Instruct woman to:
- Lie flat on her back with knees bent and feet flat on the floor or bed.
- Keep the shoulders and feet stationary and roll the knees to side to touch first one side of the bed, then the other.
- Maintain a smooth motion as the exercise is repeated five times.
- Later, as flexibility increases, the exercise can be varied by the rolling of one knee only (the mother rolls her left knee to touch the right side of the bed, returns to center and rolls the right knee to touch the left side of the bed).

Tightens abdominal muscles and muscles of the buttocks

This exercise will strengthen the oblique abdominal muscles.

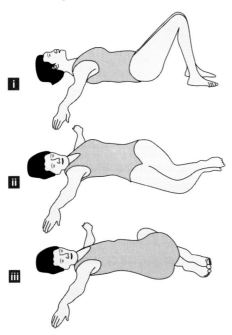

i

ii

iii

**Figure 14.18(d):** Knee and leg rolling

g. *Hip hitching*

Instruct mother to:
- Lie on her back with one knee bent and the other knee straight.
- Slide the heel of the straight leg downwards, thus lengthening the leg.

*Contd...*

*Contd...*

| | |
|---|---|
| • Shorten the same leg by drawing the hip up towards the ribs on the same side.<br>• Repeat upto 10 times keeping the abdomen pulled in.<br>• Change to the opposite side and repeat.<br>h. *Abdominal tightening*<br>Instruct woman to:<br>• Sit comfortably or kneel on all fours.<br>• Breath in and out, then pull in the lower part of the abdomen below the umbilicus while continuing to breath normally.<br>• Hold for upto 10 seconds.<br>• Repeat upto 10 times. | This very easy exercise will strengthen the the deep transverse muscles which are the main support for the spine and play a large part in prevention of long-term back problems. |
| **II   Circulatory exercises**<br> a. *Foot and leg exercises*<br>Instruct mother to:<br>• Sit or half lie with legs supported.<br>• Bend and stretch the ankles at least 12 times.<br>• Circle both feet at the ankle at least 20 times in each direction.<br>• Brace both knees, hold for a count of four, then relax.<br>• Repeat 12 times. | This exercise must be performed very frequently in the immediate postnatal period to improve circulation, to reduce edema and to prevent deep vein thrombosis. |
| **III  Pelvic floor exercise**<br> (Kegel exercise)<br>Instruct woman to:<br>• Sit, stand or half -lie with legs slightly apart, close and draw up around the anal passage as though preventing a bowel action, then repeat for front passages (Vagina and urethra) as if to stop the flow of urine in midstream.<br>• Hold the contraction for ten seconds (to a count of six)<br>• This is repeated upto ten times.<br>• Continue to do this exercise for 2 to 3 months.<br>• After three months if the mother is able to cough deeply with a full bladder without leaking urine, she may stop the exercise.<br>• If leaking occurs, she may continue the exercise for the rest of her life. | This exercise helps to regain full bladder control, prevents uterine prolapse and ensures normal sexual satisfaction in future. |
| **IV  Chest exercise (Figure 14.18 (e))**<br>Instruct mother to:<br>• Lie flat with arms extended straight out to the side, bring both hands together above the chest, while keeping the arms straight, hold for a few seconds and return to the starting position.<br>• Repeat the exercise five times initially and follow the advice of the health care provider for increasing the number of repetitions. | |

*Contd...*

*Contd...*

• Instruct the mother to bend her elbows, clasp her hands together above her chest, and press her hands together for a few seconds. Repeat this at least five times.

This exercise increases strength and tone of the chest muscles.

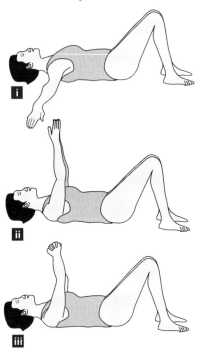

**Figure 14.18(e):** Chest exercises

## 14.19: PROVIDING IMMEDIATE NEWBORN CARE

### DEFINITION

Care provided to baby soon after birth.

### PURPOSES

1. To clear air passage and facilitate breathing.
2. To observe for any external anomalies.
3. To provide adequate warmth.
4. To help the newborn to adapt to the extrauterine environment.
5. To prevent injury and infections.
6. To keep the baby clean.

### EQUIPMENTS

1. Suction machine
2. Mucous sucker
3. Radiant warmer
4. Cord clamp
5. Sterile cotton balls
6. Sterile cord cutting scissors
7. Measuring tape
8. Rectal thermometer
9. Baby cloth (frock)
10. Baby sheet
11. Identification tag
12. Acriflavin solution/chlorhexidine powder.

### GENERAL INSTRUCTIONS

1. The emergency equipment for neonatal resuscitation is to be always kept ready in neonatal area.
2. Inj. Naloxane to be kept ready in case mother was sedated prior to delivery.
3. Do not stimulate baby (rubbing the back or suctioning nose and avoid bagging) if amniotic fluid is meconium stained.
4. If there is any deviation from normal, a neonatologist is to be informed. If mother has diabetes mellitus and is on insulin, and if the baby's weight is less than 2 kg or more than 3.8 kg transfer to nursery.

### PROCEDURE

| | Nursing action | Rationale |
|---|---|---|
| | **Immediate care:** | |
| 1 | Place the baby soon after delivery in a tray covered with sterile linen with the head slightly downward (15°) | Facilitates drainage of the mucus accumulated in the tracheo-bronchial tree by gravity. |
| 2 | Place the tray between the legs of the mother at a lower level than the uterus. | Facilitates gravitational flow of blood from the placenta to the fetus. |
| 3 | Clear the air passage off mucus using a mucus extractor or bulb syringe. | Maintains patent airway. |
| 4 | Check Apgar rating at 1 minute and 5 min and record. | Assesses the health status of newborn. |

*Contd...*

# Clinical Nursing Procedures: The Art of Nursing Practice

*Contd...*

| 5 | Clamp and cut the cord. Cord is to be clamped and divided as soon as convenient following birth of the baby. | Identifies abnormality. Separates the baby from mother for extrauterine life. |
|---|---|---|
| 6 | Dry the baby thoroughly, remove the linen and wrap the baby in dry, warm blanket / sheet | Prevent loss of heat by evaporation and chilling. |
| 7 | Tie identification tags which has mother's name and hospital number on wrists of both mother and baby and on leg of baby | Avoids confusion between staff and chances of wrong identification |
| 8 | Apply cord clamp or ligature and cut the cord shorter to desirable length. | |
| 9 | Place the baby under a radiant warmer (if one is available) until temperature is stable. | Maintains body temperature of the baby. |
| 10 | Clean the eyes with sterile cotton balls soaked in normal saline | |
| 11 | Instill soframycin eyedrops /erythromycin eye ointment to each eye. Acts as a prophylaxis against opthalmia neonatorum and Chlamydia trachomatis | |
| 12 | Clothe the baby using a dress that is appropriate for the climate. Extremities should be free for movement. Apply a napkin which should be changed periodically. | Moisture increases chances of microorganisms colonizing in the skin and crevices. |
| 13 | Check patency of rectum by introducing lubricated rubber catheter. Identifies imperforated anus. | |
| 14 | Check the weight and length of the baby, the baby should be weighed naked.<br>- Weight- Indian baby 2.5-3.0 kg<br>- Length – 50 cm | Normal measurements |
| 15 | Check vital signs | Identifies any deviation from normal. |
| 16 | Administer vitamin-K, 1 mg intra muscularly | Minimizes risk of hemorrhage |
| 17 | Administer prophylactic antibiotic therapy if ordered in conditions like<br>- Delivery following premature rupture of membranes<br>- Instrumental delivery. | Prevents secondary infection |
| 18 | Observe the baby frequently atleast for 4-8 hours. | Identifies any abnormal signs developing in newborn |
| 19 | Fill baby card and antenatal folder and document any abnormality | Acts as a communication between staff members. |

# 14.20: PERFORMING A NEWBORN ASSESSMENT

## DEFINITION

A detailed and systematic whole body examination of a stabilized newborn during the early hours of life.

## PURPOSES

1. To determine the normalcy of different body systems for healthy adaptation to extrauterine life.
2. To detect significant medical problems for immediate management.
3. To detect any congenital problems present for early management and parent education.

## ARTICLES

1. Measuring tape
2. Soft rubber catheter/rectal thermometer
3. Stethoscope
4. Flash light
5. Clean gloves.

## GENERAL INSTRUCTIONS

1. The newborn must be stabilized before starting the assessment procedure, i.e. normal body temperature and color.
2. The examination can be conducted without awakening the baby, although he will need to be exposed at intervals for a complete and accurate examination.
3. Nurse's hands must be washed thoroughly before touching the baby
4. The newborn should be protected from harmful processes such as chilling or nosocomial infection.
5. Examination should be done systematically.
6. A head to toe and systems approach to be followed for complete examination.
7. The examination may be carried out with the baby in a warmed crib or on an examination table.

## PROCEDURE

| | Nursing action | Rationale |
|---|---|---|
| 1 | Wash hands thoroughly and dry them and don gloves. | Avoids any chance of introducing infection to the baby. |
| 2 | General appearance:<br>• Uncover the baby and note general appearance. | For a normal baby the findings include:<br>• Body symmetrical and cylindrical in contour.<br>• Head large in proportion to the body.<br>• Narrow chest<br>• Protruding abdomen<br>• Small hips. |
| 3 | Take the head and body measurements (Figure 14.20 (a)).<br><br><br>Figure 14.20(a): Measuring crown to heel length | Normal measurements are:<br>• Head circumference 33-35 cm<br>• Chest circumference 30-33 cm<br>• Crown rump length 34-35 cm<br>• Crown heel length 48-52 cm |

*Contd...*

*Contd...*

| | | |
|---|---|---|
| 4 | Assess skin:<br>Note the color of skin especially around mouth and finger nailbeds. | Normal skin is smooth, soft, elastic, warm and moist. The skin is pink, nail beds are blue. Color of palms and soles will improve with activity. |
| 5 | Note any vascular nevi, milia, mongolian spots, or trauma marks on the head, neck or body. | Trauma marks may be present on babies born by instrument delivery or those who had tight nuchal cord. |
| 6 | Assess head:<br>Examine the head for symmetry, caput, cephalhematoma and the status of fontanelle (Figure 14.20 (b)).<br><br><br>**Figure 14.20 (b):** Examination of head | Asymmetry indicates moulding.<br>• Swelling on the scalp from pressure of the cervix indicates caput succedaneum.<br>• Subperiosteal bleeding, which does not cross suture line indicates cephalhematoma.<br>• Depressed fontanelle indicates dehydration.<br>• Bulging fontanelle indicates increased intracranial pressure. |
| 7 | Assess face:<br>Observe symmetry of infant's face<br>Note any characteristic feature like flattened nose, folds below eyes, upturned nose, etc. | Asymmetry is usually related to damage to the facial nerve and becomes obvious when the infant cries. These are seen in babies with fetal alcohol syndrome, chromosomal abnormality or due to oligohydramnios. |
| 8 | Assess eyes:<br>Examine the baby's eyes for response to light, puffiness, discharge, opacity or conjunctival hemorrhage. | Normally the eyes are gray, blue or brown in color.<br>• Infants will close their eyes in response to light.<br>• Puffiness is common after forceps delivery.<br>• Subconjunctival hemorrhage occurs due to pressure on the fetal head during delivery.<br>• Opacity suggest cataract formation.<br>• Ptosis of the eyelids suggest nerve damage.<br>• Minor drainage may occur after prophylactic eye medication. |
| 9 | Assess nose:<br>Observe the nose for appearance, breathing and any flaring of nostrils. | Newborns breath through the nose flaring of nostrils indicates respiratory distress. |
| 10 | Assess ears:<br>Examine the ears for the following:<br>• Firm and cartilaginous<br><br>• Presence of ear canal<br><br>• Location on the head<br><br><br>• Hearing | <br><br>• Ear lobes are firm and cartilaginous in mature or term babies.<br>• Startle reflex to sudden noise indicates that the newborn can hear.<br>• Deformed ear lobes with the upper margin of the pinna rolled down and thickened are seen in Down's syndrome.<br>• Low set ears are seen in Trisomy 15 and 18. |

*Contd...*

*Contd...*

| | | |
|---|---|---|
| 11 | Assess mouth:<br>• Examine the mouth and note the presence of any of the following:<br>• Cleft lip or palate<br>• Epstein pearls<br>• Asymmetry when crying<br>• Natal teeth<br>• Macroglossia<br>• Pooling of saliva | • Asymmetry of the mouth when open indicates facial nerve paralysis.<br>• Pooling of saliva is a sign of tracheooesophageal fistula/atresia.<br>• Macroglossia is seen in Down's syndrome. |
| 12 | Assess neck:<br>Examine the neck for the following:<br>• Head freely movable<br>• Neck webbed on shoulders<br>• Extended arms on one side (shoulder dystocia)<br>• Tightness of muscles on one side | • Short neck with flexible movement of head to each side is normal.<br>• Neck webbed on shoulder is seen in Down's syndrome and Turner's syndrome.<br>• Extension of one arm indicates clavicle fracture or damage to brachial nerve.<br>• Tightness of neck muscle is a sign of torticollis. |
| 13 | Assess chest:<br>Examine the chest for the following:<br>• Shape and movement with breathing<br>• Respiration pattern<br>• Grunting sound on expiration<br>• Retractions on inspiration<br>• Heart rate<br>• Clavicles palpable on both sides<br>• Presence of breast engorgement and secretion of milk. | Diaphragmatic breathing with symmetric movement of chest and abdomen is normal.<br>• Quiet and free respiration at the rate of 40-60/min is normal after initial activity.<br>• Grunting indicates respiratory distress.<br>• Clavicles clearly palpable if fracture is present.<br>• Milk secretion is present in response to maternal hormones. |
| 14 | Assess abdomen:<br>Observe the abdomen and note:<br>• Shape<br><br>• Umbilical cord stump for presence of three vessels<br><br>• Any mass<br><br>• Bowel sounds<br>• Passage of meconium | • Normal abdomen should be round and protruding<br>• Small scaphoid abdomen may indicate diaphragmatic hernia.<br>• If three vessels are not found congenital malformations should be investigated.<br>• Mass may indicate umbilical or inguinal hernia or abdominal mass<br>• Bowel sounds are normally active.<br>• Passage of meconium indicates a patent anus. |
| 15 | Assess genitalia:<br>Male:<br>Examine if:<br>• Foreskin covers the glans penis.<br>• Urethral meatus opens at the tip of the penis.<br>• Testicles are palpable in the scrotum bilaterally.<br><br>Female:<br>• Labia minora is prominent and is not covered by labia majora<br>• Edematous genitalia.<br>• Vaginal discharge and pseudomenstruation. | • Normally foreskin covers glans penis.<br>• Deviations indicate hypospadiasis or epispadiasis.<br>• If not palpable, undescended testicles should be investigated.<br><br><br>• Edema is normal in breech born babies.<br>• Vaginal discharge is a normal response to maternal hormones. |

*Contd...*

*Contd...*

| | |
|---|---|
| 16 Assess back:<br>Hold the newborn prone and examine the back to evaluate the spine<br>Note the presence of any<br>• Dimple in the coccygeal or sacrococcygeal region.<br>• Sinus opening or spina-bifida.<br>• Tufts of hair. | • Normally no abnormal curvatures and lesions are seen.<br><br>• May denote pilonidal cyst.<br>• May indicate fistula. |
| 17. Assess anus:<br>Verify the presence of a perforate anus by inserting a soft rubber catheter gently into the rectum.<br>(if the newborn passes meconium earlier, patency need not be checked). | Presence of meconium on the catheter on withdrawal indicates patency of anus. |
| 18 Assess upper extremities:<br>Note the proportions to the rest of the body, symmetry and spontaneous movements of arms and hands.<br>• Check if the baby holds hands in fists<br>• If fingers show webbing, polydactylism or syndactylism<br>• If fingernails are developed and extend beyond fingertips.<br>• If any skin tags are present. | Arms should be of equal length when extended.<br><br>Infant should normally resist having arm extended.<br><br>Long nails are present in post-term babies. |
| 19 Assess lower extremities:<br>Check the legs for the following:<br>• Symmetry and length.<br>• Range of motion<br>• Proportion to the rest of the body.<br>• Symmetry of creases of legs and buttocks (Figure 14.20 (c))<br>With knees flexed, abduct legs to the table in frog-like position (Figure 14.20 (d)). | Should be of equal length when extended.<br><br><br><br>If abduction is asymmetrical or hip click is present, dislocated hip to be suspected. |

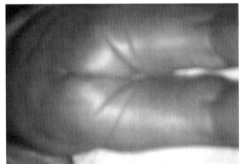

**Figure 14.20(c):** Symmetry of gluteal folds

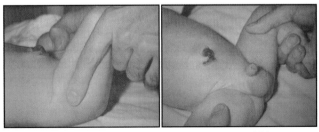

**Figure 14.20(d):** Assessing for dislocation of hip

| | |
|---|---|
| • Assess if the legs are persistently limp. | Persistent limpness, indicates spinal cord lesion |

*Contd...*

*Contd...*

| | | |
|---|---|---|
| 20 | Assess feet:<br>Examine the soles for presence of wrinkles, acrocyanosis and conditions such as Talipes equinovarus, Talipes calcaneovalgus, bow leg, webbing, polydactylism or syndactylism. | Wrinkles are normally present in full term babies.<br>Wrinkles are absent in pre-term babies.<br>The first and second toes are widely separated in Down's syndrome.<br>Acrocyanosis is common immediately after birth. |
| 21 | Assess CVS:<br>After making the baby quiet, auscultate the heart sounds and feel for pulses in the upper and lower extremities. | The normal heart rate is 120-160 bpm.<br>If cardiac murmurs are heard these should be documented and informed to the pediatrician.<br>— Murmurs are common in newborns during the transition from intrauterine to extrauterine life.<br>Congenital heart defects must be excluded. |
| 22 | Perform neurologic examination:<br>Elicit the following reflexes to assess the nervous system:<br>a. Moro or embracing reflex: (Figure 14.20 (e))<br>   —Hold infant at an angle of 45 degree and then permit the head to drop one or two centimeters or<br>   —Strike the examining table near the head of the baby. | The infant should respond by abducting and extending his arms and fanning of fingers. Sometimes there may be an accompanying tremor. The arms then flex and embrace the chest. |

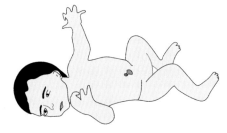

Figure 14.20(e): Moro reflex

| | | |
|---|---|---|
| | b. Rooting reflex:<br>Stroke side of cheek, lips or mouth with the finger. | Baby's head turns towards the stimulated side, the mouth opens and begins to suck on the stimulating object.<br>Rhythmical sucking movements will be felt. |
| | c. Sucking and swallowing reflex.<br>Place finger in baby's mouth | |
| | d. Palmar grasp reflex: (Figure 14.20(F))<br>With the baby in supine position and the head in midline, place your fingers in both the infant's hands. | Infant will grasp and hold the finger. |

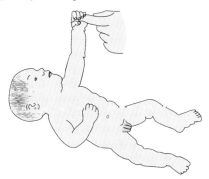

Figure 14.20(f): Palmar grasp reflex

*Contd...*

*Contd...*

---

e. Plantar grasp reflex (Figure 14.20 (g)):
Place a finger or a thin object like pen or pencil at the base of toes or phase the examiner's thumb against ball of the infant's feet.

Baby will curl toes for a short period.

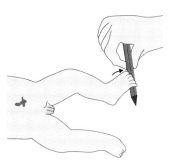

**Figure 14.20(g):** Plantar grasp reflex

f. Tonic neck reflex or fencing (Figure 14.20 (h)):
Place infant in supine position and turn head to one side.

The arm and leg on the same side will extend and the arm and leg on the opposite side will flex assuming a fencing position.

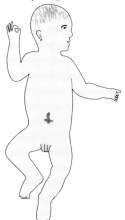

**Figure 14.20(h):** Tonic neck reflex

g. Stepping or walking reflex (dancing reflex). Hold infant upright with feet on a flat surface (Figure 14.20(i))

Stepping movement with alternating flexion and extension will be seen.

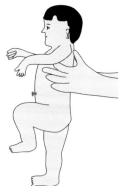

**Figure 14.20 (i):** Stepping reflex

---

*Contd...*

*Contd...*

h.  Babinski reflex:
    Stroke the lateral aspect of the sole of the foot going from heel to the greater toe with fingernail (Figure 14.20(j)).

Toes will fan out temporarily

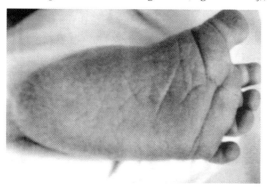

**Figure 14.20(j):** Babinski reflex

i.  Head lag:
    Grasp the infant's hands and arms and gently pull the infant to a sitting position. Note the degree of head lag and alignment of head with the body when in sitting position (Figure 14.20(k)).

If head lag persist beyond 3 months of age it signifies neurological complication.

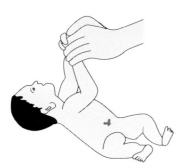

**Figure 14.20(k):** Head lag

j.  Ventral suspension:
    Hold the baby prone and suspended over examiners arm, the baby temporarily holds the head level with the body and flexes the limbs (Figure 14.20(l)).

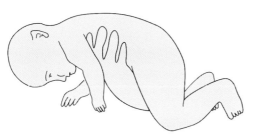

**Figure 14.20(l):** Ventral suspension

*Contd....*

*Contd....*

| | | |
|---|---|---|
| k. | Blink reflex:<br>Shine a sudden bright light at the baby's eyes. A quick closure of the eyes and a slight dorsal flexion of the head are elicited. | This response shows normal light perception. |
| l. | Corneal reflex:<br>When the eyes are open touch the cornea lightly with the piece of cotton. Normally the eyes close (avoid touching the eyelids and lashes). | Absence of this response denotes lesions of the 5th cranial nerve. |
| m. | Doll's eye response:<br>Move the head slowly to left or right. Eyes lag behind and do not immediately adjust to new position of head. | This disappears as fixation develops. |
| n. | Extrusion:<br>Touch or depress the tongue with finger, infant responds by forcing it outward. | This reflex usually lasts for about 4 months. |
| o. | Gallant reflex: Stroke the back of the infant lightly lateral to the vertebral column. The infant responde by flexing the entire trunk to the side stimulated. Lack of response indicates neurological deficit. | The reflex lasts for about one month. |
| p. | Perez reflex (Incurvation of the trunk reflex): Support the baby in prone position over the examiners hand and stroke with one finger along the infant's back parallel to the spine from sacrum to neck. Normally movement of the pelvis towards the stimulated tide occurs. | The examiner detects presence or absence of movement of the pelvis towards the stimulated side. This reflex is seen up to six months. Persistence beyond six months indicates brain damage. |
| 24 | Inform the mother about the baby's condition and wellbeing. | |
| 25 | Record the findings in the newborn assessment record. | |

## 14.21: PERFORMING NEONATAL RESUSCITATION

## DEFINITION

Measures taken to revive newborns who have difficulty in establishing respiration at birth and includes suctioning, positive pressure ventilation, external cardiac massage, intubation and medications as necessitated by the neonate's condition at one minute of age.

## PURPOSES

1. To establish and maintain a clear airway
2. To ensure effective circulation.
3. To correct any acidosis present.
4. To prevent hypothermia, hypoglycemia and hemorrhage.

## ARTICLES

1. Suctioning articles:
   - Bulb syringe
   - De lee mucous trap with no. 10 Fr catheter or mechanical suction.
   - Suction catheters no 6, 8, 10
   - Feeding tube no 8 Fr and 20 ml syringe.
2. Bag and mask articles:
   - Infant resuscitation bag with pressure release valve or pressure gauge with reservoir, capable of delivering 90-100% oxygen
   - Face masks with cushioned rims (Newborn and premature sizes)
   - Oral airways (newborn and premature sizes)
   - Oxygen with flowmeter and tubing.
3. Intubation articles:
   - Laryngoscope with straight blades No "O"(premature), No "1"(Newborn)
   - Extra bulbs and batteries for laryngoscope
   - Endotracheal tubes. Sizes – 2.5, 3.0, 3.5 and 4.0 mm internal diameter.
   - Styllet
   - Scissors
4. Medications:
   - Epinephrine 1:10, 000 ampoules (1ml ampoule of 1:1, 000 available in India)
   - Nalaxone hydrochloride (Neonatal narcan 0.02 mg/ml)
   - Volume expander
     a. 5% albumin solution
     b. Normal saline
     c. Ringer's Lactate
   - Sodium bicarbonate 4.2% (1 mEq/2 ml)
   - 7.5% strength available in India approximately 0.9 mEq/ml)
   - Dextrose 10% concentration 250 ml
   - Sterile water 30 ml
   - Normal saline 30 ml
5. Miscellaneous:
   - Radiant warmer
   - Stethoscope
   - Adhesive tape and bandage scissors
   - Syringe 1 ml, 2 ml, 5 ml and 20 ml sizes.

- Needles Nos 21, 22 and 26 G
- Umbilical cord clamp
- Gloves
- Warm dry towels.

## PROCEDURE

| | Nursing action | Rationale |
|---|---|---|
| 1 | Assess the Apgar score. | Helps to know if resuscitation measures are to be instituted. |
| 2 | Place infant under warmer, quickly dry off aminiotic fluid, replace wet sheets with a dry one. | Prevents heat loss. |
| 3 | Place the baby on his back with slightly head down 15 degree tilt, neck slightly extended. | Straightens the trachea and opens the airway. Hyperextension may cause airway obstruction. |
| 4 | Suction the mouth first and then nose. | Clears the airway passage. Infants often gasp when the nose is suctioned and may aspirate secretion from the mouth into lungs. |
| 5 | Give tactile stimulation if infant does not breathe (Flick or tap the sole of foot twice or rub the back). Do not slap | Tactile stimulation of drying may bring spontaneous respiration. |
| 6 | Check the vital signs, and color of the newborn. | Helps in determining further need for resuscitation. |

Note: Evaluation should be done on respiration, heart rate and color. If the baby is apnoeic, heart rate is less than 100 bpm and central cyanosis is present, proceed for bag and mask ventilation or positive pressure ventilation.

## BAG AND MASK VENTILATION/POSITIVE PRESSURE VENTILATION

### INDICATIONS

- Apnea
- Heart rate less than 100 bpm

### PROCEDURE

| | Nursing action | Rationale |
|---|---|---|
| 1 | Place the newborn on his back with head slightly extended. | Helps in opening airway. Hyperextension may cause airway obstruction. |
| 2 | A tight seal is to be formed over the infant's mouth and nose with the face mask. | Prevents leakage of air from the sides of the mask. |
| 3 | Ventilate at a rate of 40-50 per minute . | |
| 4 | Ventilate for 15-30 seconds and evaluate | Spontaneous respiration may be initiated with initial attempts to ventilate. |
| 5 | Have an assistant to evaluate, listen to the heart rate for 6 seconds and multiply by 10. | |

## EVALUATION

- If heart rate is above 100b pm and spontaneous respirations are present, discontinue bagging.
- If heart rate is 60-100 bpm and increasing, continue ventilation, check whether chest is moving adequately.
- If heart rate is below 80 bpm, start chest compression.
- If heart rate is below 60 bpm, in addition to bagging and chest compressions, consider intubation and initiate medications.

- Signs of improvement:
- Increasing heart rate
- Spontaneous respirations
- Improving color.

Continue to provide free flow oxygen by face mask after respirations are established. If the baby deteriorates, check the following:
- Placement of face mask for tight seal.
- Head position and presence of secretions.
- Pressure being used.
- Presence of air in the stomach preventing chest expansion.
- Oxygen being delivered (100% or not).

For bagging lasting for more than two minutes insert an orogastric tube to vent the stomach.

## CHEST COMPRESSIONS

Chest compressions consist of rhythmic compressions of the sternum that compresses the heart against the spine, increases the intrathoracic pressure and circulates blood to the vital organs.

Chest compressions must always be accompanied by ventilation with 100% oxygen to assure that the circulating blood is well oxygenated.

## INDICATIONS

1.  Heart rate less than 60 bpm after bagging with 100% oxygen for 15-30 seconds.
2.  Heart rate 60-80 bpm and not increasing after bagging with 100% oxygen for 15-30 seconds.

## PROCEDURE

| | Nursing action | Rationale |
|---|---|---|
| 1 | Compress the chest by placing the hands around the newborn's chest with the fingers under the back to provide support and the thumbs over the lower third of the sternum (just above the xiphoid process). <br> Or <br> Use two fingers of one hand to compress the chest and place the other hand under the back to provide support. (Figure 14.21(a)) | Correct hand position compresses the heart and avoids injury to the liver, spleen, fracture of the ribs and pneumothorax. |

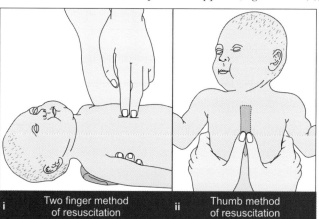

**Figure 14.21(a):** Chest compression for neonatal CPR

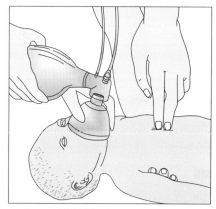

**Figure 14.21(b):** Chest compressions accompanied by bag and mask ventilation

*Contd...*

*Contd...*

| | | |
|---|---|---|
| 2 | Compress the sternum to a depth of approximately one third of the anteroposterior diameter of the chest and with sufficient force to cause a palpable pulse. The fingers should remain in contact with the chest between compressions. | The size of the newborn determines the depth of compressions to avoid injury. |
| 3 | Use three compressions followed by one ventilation for a combined rate of compressions and ventilations of 120 each minute. This provides 90 compressions and 30 ventilations each minute. Pause for ½ second after every third compression for ventilation (Figure 14.21(b)). | Simultaneous compression and ventilation may interfere with adequate ventilation. The short pause allows air to enter the lungs. |
| 4 | Check the heart rate after 30 seconds. If it is 60 bpm or more, discontinue compressions but continue ventilation until the heart rate is more than 100 bpm and spontaneous breathing begins. | Periodic evaluation is necessary to ensure that treatment is appropriate to the infant's status. |

Note: If cardiac compression fails, endotracheal intubation should be initiated.

## ENDOTRACHEAL INTUBATION

### INDICATIONS

1. Heart rate below 60 per min inspite of bagging and chest compressions.
2. Presence of meconium in the amniotic fluid.

### PROCEDURE

| | Nursing action | Rationale |
|---|---|---|
| 1 | Place infant with head slightly extended with a rolled towel under the shoulder. | Position makes the airway open. |
| 2 | Introduce laryngoscope over the baby's tongue at the right corner of the mouth. | |
| 3 | Advance 2-3 cm while rotating it to midline, until the epiglottis is seen. Elevation of the epiglottis with the tip of the laryngoscope reveals the vocal cords. | |
| 4 | Suction secretions if needed. | Clears the airway. |
| 5 | Pass the endotracheal tube a distance of 1.5-2 cm into the trachea, hold it firmly but gently in place and withdraw the laryngoscope slowly. | Ensures adequate air entry into both lungs. |
| 6 | Attach the endotracheal tube to the adapter on the bag. | |
| 7 | Ventilate with oxygen by bag. An assistant should check for adequate ventilation of both lungs with stethoscope. | |

### MEDICATIONS

Medications should be administered if despite adequate ventilation with 100% oxygen and chest compressions the heart rate remains at 80 bpm.

### RECORDING

Record the procedure in nurses record. Document the baby's condition before and after procedure.

# Maternal and Child Nursing

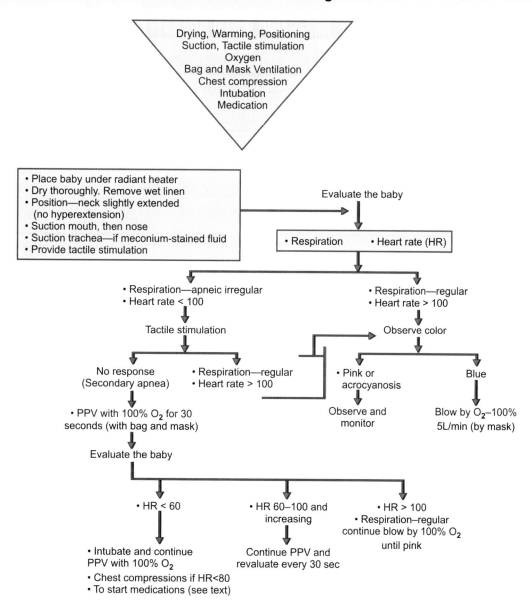

Figure 14.21(c): Resuscitation of the newborn in the delivery room

Chest compression—After every third chest compression ventilation should be continued.

In one minute, 90 chest compressions and 30 PPVs should be carried out (3:1 ratio).

Medications: Epinephrine: 0.1-0.3 ml/kg in 1: 10, 000 dilution is given I.V. when there is persistent bradycardia. Intratracheal adminsitration can also be given. It may be repeated every 5 minutes. Sodium bicarbonate to combat metabolic acidosis (PH<7.2) I.V. (4 ml/kg of 0.5 mEq/ml, 4.2% solution) is given. Reversal of narcotic drug is needed when mother has been given pethidine or morphine within three hours of delivery. Naloxone 100 mg/kg is given to the baby by IV, IM or endotracheal. Volume expansion is needed when blood pressure is low and tissue perfusion is poor. Whole blood, 5% albumin or packed red blood cells(10 ml/kg) I.V. is given. Dopamine infusion may be given for hypotension. PPV = Positive pressure ventilation.

*Resuscitation protocol following American Heart Association and the American Academy of Pediatrics.*
*Recommended by the National Neonatology Forum (NNF), India.*

# 14: 22: ASSISTING WITH BREASTFEEDING

## DEFINITION

Assisting new mothers with positioning and technique of breastfeeding during the early postpartum days.

## PURPOSES

1. To enable mothers to feed their babies adequately without discomfort.
2. To enable the newborn meet his/her nutritional needs adequately.
3. To promote mother – baby bonding.
4. To minimise chances of developing breast problems due to stasis of milk.

## EQUIPMENTS

1. Bowl with lukewarm water
2. Tray lined with towel
3. Kidney tray
4. Few rag pieces or sponge towel
5. Bath towel
6. Pillows (1 –2)
7. Soap (if mother has not taken bath or feeding baby for first time after delivery).

## CONTRAINDICATIONS

1. Maternal disease such as tuberculosis cardiac disease, acute illness or contagious disease, severe grade of anemia, severe puerperal sepsis, puerperal psychosis.
2. Local conditions preventing breastfeeding:
   - Fissures of the nipple
   - Acute mastitis
   - Abscess of the breast

3

|  | Temporary | Permanent |
|---|---|---|
| Maternal | 1. Acute puerperal illness<br>2. Acute breast complications such as cracked nipples, mastitis or breast abscess<br>3. Following exhaustive and complicated labour and delivery | Chronic medical illness such as decompensated organic heart lesion, active pulmonary tuberculosis, Puerperal psychosis.<br>Patient having high doses of antiepileptic and antithyroid drugs. |
| Neonatal | 1. Very low birth weight baby<br>2. Asphyxia and intracranial stress<br>3. Acute illness | Severe degree of cleft palate<br>Galactosaemia |

## PROCEDURE

| | Nursing action | Rationale |
|---|---|---|
| 1 | Explain to the mother about breastfeeding and how you can assist with the procedure. | Prepares mother for the act of breastfeeding. |
| 2 | Instruct the mother to expose her breasts | |

*Contd...*

*Contd...*

| | | |
|---|---|---|
| 3 | Clean the nipples and areolar region with a wet wash cloth and dry them. With a rag piece first clean nipple area then clean breast with soap and water. Clean one breast at a time. | Use of soap on nipples is not recommended as it is a drying agent and can lead to cracking. |
| 4 | Postoperative mothers<br>a) Assist the mother to a sidelying position<br>b) Tuck a pillow under her ribs if feeding from the lower breast. | Facilitates feeding without strain to the incisional area. Placing a pillow under the ribs brings baby and breasts closer and provides a shirls over the incision. |
| 5 | Post vaginal delivery mother who wishes to feed in sitting position. Instruct the mother to use one of the following positions:<br>i) Cradle hold<br>ii) Football hold<br>iii) Cross-cradle or modified cradle hold.<br><br>i. For cradle hold:<br>Position the infants head at or near the antecubital space and level with her nipple, with her arm supporting the infants body and with her other hand to hold the breast (Figure 14.22 (a)). | Sitting in a chair with back and feet supported is comfortable for feeding.<br><br>This would adjust the height so that she need not bend forward. |

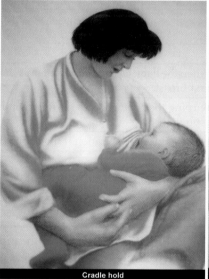 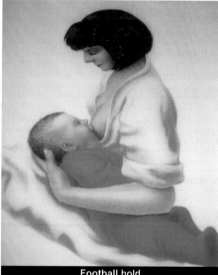

Cradle hold          Football hold

**Figure 14.22 (a):** Breastfeeding – techniques

ii. For football hold:
• Instruct mother to support the infants head in her hand with the infant's body resting on pillows alongside her hip.
iii. For cross-cradle or modified cradle hold:
• Assist the mother to sit with her back upright and at right angles to her lap.
• Place a pillow on her lap.
• Let the mother hold the baby supporting his head with her extended arms.

**Feeding techniques:**

| | |
|---|---|
| 6 | Move the baby near the breast, turned towards the mother's body with neck slightly extended and the mouth near the nipple. |
| 7 | Let the mother move the baby's mouth against her nipple. |

*Contd...*

*Contd...*

| 8 | As the baby opens his mouth dropping his lower jaw and darting his tongue, insert the nipple and breast tissue inside his mouth, so that the baby latches on to the nipple and areola correctly (Figure 14.22 (b)). | Having the bottom lip about 1.5 cm away from the base of the nipple allows the baby to latch on the breast.<br>With this position the lactiferous sinuses will be inside the baby's mouth. |

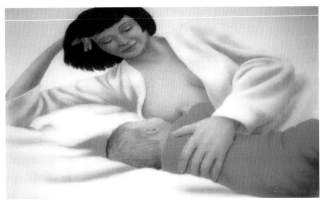

Figure 14.22 (b): Technique of breastfeeding – good attachment

| 9 | Provide assistance as needed to help for correct attachment of the baby to the breast and to start sucking | |
| 10 | When the baby releases the breast, burp him | |
| 11 | Encourage the mother to feed the baby from the second breast in the same manner. | When the baby has had sufficient milk, he releases the first breast. |
| 12 | Burp the baby as he comes off the second breast | Burping the baby reduces risk of vomiting and aspiration. |
| 13 | Wrap the baby and lay him on his side in the crib | Prevents risk of aspiration if the baby vomits. |
| 14 | Replace the articles | |
| 15 | Record in the chart the time and duration of feeding and any observations made. | |

## HEALTH TEACHING TO MOTHER

1. Placement of the baby on the breast should enable him to feed from the breast rather than from the nipple.
2. The finishing breast at one feed should be the starting breast for the next feeding so that both breasts get emptied.
3. Baby led feeding/demand feeding generally will be long feeding with longer intervals (6-8 hours) in between for the first one or two days and shorter and frequent after two days (that is every 3- 4 hours).
4. Daily bathing and change of dress are important for breast hygiene for nursing mothers.
5. Breastfeeding mothers need to wear proper fitting brassieres to provide comfortable support to breasts.
6. Arouse baby in between feeds by stroking the sole of this feet or earlobe.

## 14.23: CARE OF BABY UNDERGOING PHOTOTHERAPY

### DEFINITION

Caring for a baby being exposed to light source for prescribed period of time.

### PURPOSE

To bring down serum bilirubin level to normal.

### ARTICLES

1. Fluorescent lamps and fiberoptic pads (if available).
2. Eye pads or eye shields.
3. Napkin to cover the genitalia of male babies.
4. Baby blankets/sheets – 2 nos.

### INDICATIONS

Elevated serum bilirubin levels
- Healthy term babies > 17 mg/dl
- Pre-term babies (weighing more than 1500 gm >8 mg/dl
- Pre-term babies (weighing less than 1500 mg >5 mg/dl

Phototherapy can be delivered in several ways. The most common methods are:
1. Fluorescent lamps or "bililights" placed over the infant who is usually in an incubator or under a radiant warmer.
2. Halogen lamps.
3. Fiberoptic phototherapy blankets or pads.

### PROCEDURE

| | Nursing action | Rationale |
|---|---|---|
| 1. | Provide explanation to mother that her baby will be kept in an isolette and exposed to a blue- green light for bringing down the bilirubin levels. | Allays anxiety and convinces her about the need for phototherapy. |
| 2. | Instruct mother to feed the baby. | Prevents dehydration when exposed to phototherapy. |
| 3. | Check machine for electrical safety and proper insulation of wires | Prevents electrical hazards. |
| 4. | Check whether all bulbs are burning in machine. | |
| 5. | Transfer the baby to nursery where phototherapy equipment is present and place the baby in the isolette over which phototherapy lights are placed. | Heat loss is minimized and temperature is controlled when an incubator is used. |
| 6. | Adjust height between baby and lamp to 45 cm. | Lights that are too close increases the risk of burning the skin. Lights too far away from the infant will not be effective. |
| 7. | Place baby naked under light in the isolette (Figure 14.23 (a)) | Exposes the skin as much as possible for maximum exposure to light. |
| 8. | Cover the baby's eyes with eyepads. | Protects eyes from the effect of high intensity lights on retina and avoids abrasions to cornea. |
| 9. | Cover the genitals of male babies with the napkin | Protects testicles from the high intensity lights. |

*Contd...*

# Clinical Nursing Procedures: The Art of Nursing Practice

*Contd...*

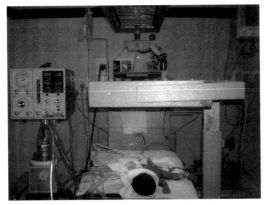

**Figure 14.23(a):** Baby undergoing phototherapy

| 10. a. If fiberoptic pad is used, place it under the baby in contact with the baby's skin | Aids in maximum exposure of skin surface. |
| b. Keep the baby on his side with a rolled baby sheet on the side. | Maintains the position |
| 11. Switch on bili lights and /or machine for the fiberoptic pad. | |
| 12. Change position every 2 hours. | Ensures that light reaches all areas of the body |
| 13. Record in baby's chart, all details about starting the procedure, observations made and precautions taken. | Acts as a communication between staff members |

## CARE AND OBSERVATION DURING PHOTOTHERAPY

1. Provide feeding at regular intervals to maintain adequate hydration. If breastfeeding, mother should be encouraged to give demand feeding.
2. If baby is hyperthermic, discontinue phototherapy and keep baby exposed under fan. When temperature reaches normal, restart phototherapy.
3. Monitor bilirubin level and other hematologic assessments at regular intervals.
4. Check baby at least every hour and see that the eyeshields remain in place. The eyeshields should not press against the eyes.
5. The infant may be removed from the lights for feeding, diaper changes and other general care but should receive phototherapy for 18 hours every day.
6. If fiberoptic blanket is used, it should be kept next to baby's skin at all times. Be sure that the baby does not roll off the blanket. It is not necessary to cover the eyes if blanket alone is used.
7. Monitor body temperature at regular intervals.
8. Observe the skin for rashes, dryness and excoriation.
9. Feed the baby every 2-3 hours because phototherapy causes the baby to loose fluid from the skin and have loose stools . This may cause dehydration.
10. Count your baby's wet diapers and stools. Increase feeding if the baby has less than six wet diapers a day or if urine appears dark.
11. Do not apply oil to the skin of the baby.
12. Observe for side effects like:
   - Loose green stool resulting from increased bile flow and peristalsis. Stool may damage the skin and cause fluid loss.
   - Tanning effect from the light
   - Bronze baby syndrome – a grayish brown discoloration of skin and urine
   - Skin rash
   - Temporary lactose intolerance.

# 14.24: CARE OF NEWBORN IN INCUBATOR (ISOLETTE)

## DEFINITION

Providing care to prematurely born or sick infants in a device called incubator which keep them warm.

## PURPOSES

1. To maintain a baby's core temperature stable at 37 degree celsius.
2. To provide humidified air.
3. To administer oxygen.
4. To observe the baby without disturbing him.
5. To conserve the energy of premature canopy.

## PARTS OF INCUBATOR

1. Deck
2. Mattress which is enclosed by a clear plastic canopy
3. Air intake pipe
4. Micro filter assembly
5. Oxygen inlet
6. Thermostat
7. Caliberated dial
8. Arm ports
9. **Hood**: Single walled rectangular hood. The hood has a large door to aid in placing or removing baby from incubator. There are four elbow operated parts for better access during small procedures, inlet for IV tubes, probes, endotracheal tubes etc. Canopy can be lifted for cleaning and access
10. **Control panel**: Heater, blower and electronics
11. **Lower unit**: This consists of control box, touch sensor, front panel with display, humidifier, airducts and filter
    The following are displayed on the front of the panel
    a. Air temperature
    b. Patient temperature
    c. Control temperature
12. **Cabinet:** This provides support for hood, canopy and lower unit. It houses main switch, fuse and power cord connector. The cabinet has three drawers for storage space.
13. **Humidity percentage**: Air is circulated by configural blower. Fresh air enters through air filters located at the end of incubator. Fresh air is mixed with circulating air from incubator conopy and passed over heater and humidifier. Temperature inside incubator is maintained by sensor placed on hood. Thus, heated air flow maintains surroundings of infant at desired temperature.

## PROCEDURE

| | Nursing action | Rationale |
|---|---|---|
| 1 | Identify the premature, weak or ill baby who needs to be nursed in an isolette. | Promotes chances of survival for premature baby who needs thermoregulation. |
| 2 | Verify physician's orders for management of baby in the incubator. | Facilitates adequacy of required unit assembly for care. |
| 3 | Explain procedure to mother/parents | Promotes understanding and acceptance of parents. |

*Contd...*

*Contd...*

| 4 | Prepare the incubator for placing the baby by cleaning it with soap and water and disinfecting. | Use of clean disinfected incubator prevents growth of microorganisms. |
|---|---|---|
| 5 | Switch on the incubator and adjust the temperature at 36 degree centigrade on " servo control mode" (Figure 14.24 (a)). | 36 degree centigrade set on servo-control mode maintains the baby's skin temperature at 36 degree centigrade. |

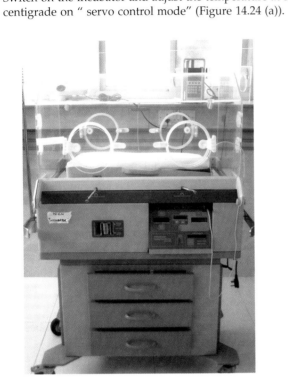

**Figure 14.24(a):** Incubator

| 6 | Prewarm the incubator for 15 minutes. | Pre warming facilitates flow of warm air on body surface. |
|---|---|---|
| 7 | Transfer the baby to the prepared isolette. | Facilitates provision of required care to baby without causing stress. |
| 8 | Undress the baby except for diapers. | Facilitates observation of the baby through the clear plastic canopy. |
| 9 | Check temperature of newborn and the incubator every hour until the temperature of the baby is stabilized. | Prevents over exposure to heat |
| 10 | Maintain flow chart to record, temperature, heart rate, respiration and oxygen saturation. | |
| 11 | Change humidifier water everyday. | Prevents growth of microorganisms. |
| 12 | Give care for baby by introducing hand through arm ports. | |
| 13 | Permit mothers/parents to see and bond with the baby according to hospital policy. | Reduces the chances of sensory deprivation. |
| 14 | Weaning a baby is important and has to be taken care of. This is done by gradually decreasing the temperature of incubator and monitoring the infants' body temperature. Keep port holes open for some time. Then take baby out and keep warm by dressing and wrapping. | |
| 15 | Do not tap incubator | Avoids disturbance to the baby. |

# 14.25: ASSISTING IN EXCHANGE TRANSFUSION

## DEFINITION

Assisting in withdrawing a baby's blood which has high bilirubin content and replacing with fresh blood through umbilical vein.

## AIMS

1. To correct anemia by replacing the Rh positive sensitized red cells.
2. To remove the circulatory antibodies.
3. To eliminate circulatory bilirubin.

## INDICATIONS

1. Non-obstructive jaundice with serum bilirubin level of 20 mg/dl or more in fullterm and 15 mg/dl in preterm infants, e.g. Rh or ABO incompatability
2. Kernicterus irrespective of serum bilirubin level.
3. Hemolytic disease of the newborn under following situations:
   - Cord Hb 10% or less.
   - Cord bilirubin 5 mg/dl or more.
   - Rise of serum bilirubin of more than 1mg/dl/hour.
   - Maternal antibody titer of 1:64 or more, positive direct Coombs' test and previous history of a severely affected baby.

## ARTICLES

1. Exchange transfusion set containing:
   - Kidney tray-1
   - Bowl-2
   - Metal scale-1
   - Suture scissors-1
   - Fine scissors-1
   - Vein dilator-1
   - Fine toothed forceps-1
   - Fine non-toothed forceps-1
   - Curved mosquito forceps-1
   - Straight mosquito forceps-1
   - Dressing forceps-1
   - Surgical towel-2
   - 20 cc syringe 2, 10 cc syringe 2
   - Cross splint, pads and bandages
2. Injection tray with antiseptic
3. Small dressing pack
4. Sterile scalpel blade 3 /11
5. Sterile feeding tray with pacifier.
6. I.V. stand
7. Injection normal saline 500ml
8. Injection heparin
9. 3-way stopcock.
10. Resuscitation equipment and oxygen source

11. Heat source
12. Suction apparatus with mucus sucker
13. Umbilical vein catheter
14. NG tube no 5, 6, 8
15. Sterile linen bundle with 2 sheets and 1 biopsy towel
16. Mask and gloves
17. Cord tie
18. Specimen containers
19. Specimen tubes
20. Adhesive plaster, scissors and extra syringes.
21. Emergency drugs like
    1. Inj. Adrenalin
    2. Inj. Calcium gluconate
    3. Inj. Soda bicarbonate
    4. Inj. Aminophylline
22. Blood giving set
23. Cross splint.

## CHOICE OF DONOR BLOOD

1. The donor blood should be fresh (less than 3 days old).
2. The amount needed for an adequate exchange is about 160 ml/kg (double the blood volume of baby).
3. The blood should be crossmatched against mother's blood.
4. It should be made sure that the blood is slowly warmed to infant's temperature.
5. Fresh heparinized blood or blood preserved with acid citrate dextrose is used.
6. In Rh incompatability the transfusions are performed with group O, Rh negative blood whereas in case of ABO incompatability and G-6-PD deficiency the procedure has to be performed with the same ABO and Rh groups of the baby.
7. 20-30 ml of blood is withdrawn and about 10-20 ml are replaced each time.

## PROCEDURE

| | Nursing action | Rationale |
|---|---|---|
| 1 | Explain procedure to the parents. | Helps in reassuring the parents. |
| 2 | Get informed consent from the parent. | Prevents legalities. |
| 3 | The procedure is best carried out in an airconditioned room. | |
| 4 | Collect the blood from blood bank and place in tepid water and check the blood type and group against the neonate's blood before administering. | Prevents hemolytic reaction caused by mismatched donor blood. |
| 5 | Procedure should be carried out in an incubator maintaining the temperature at 27-30 degree centigrade. | |
| 6 | NPO should be maintained for 4 hrs before procedure. The stomach should be aspirated before the exchange. | Minimises the risk of vomiting and aspiration into lungs. |
| 7 | Expose and immobilise baby on cross splint. | Prevents movements during procedure. |
| 8 | Open dressing pack and assist in cleaning of umbilical stump. | Removes microorganisms. |
| 9 | Assist in cleaning umbilical cord and draping with sterile linen. | |

*Contd...*

*Contd...*

| | | |
|---|---|---|
| 10 | Pour 500 ml of I.V. normal saline into a sterile bowl and add 1 ml inj. heparin into it. | Before beginning the exchange the whole apparatus should be primed with the saline as it prevents syringes becoming sticky. |
| 11 | Umbilical cord is cut to less than 2.5 cm from the skin surface. | Helps in location of vein. |
| 12 | Attach ligature loosely round the base of the cord. Insert umbilical catheter into the vein. | |
| 13 | The catheter should be filled with a flushing solution, or donor blood before insertion. | Minimises the risk of air embolism. |
| 14 | When free flow of blood is obtained, ligature is tightened and the catheter should be deep enough to reach the inferior vena cava. | |
| 15 | Make sure that heat source is available throughout the procedure. | Hypothermia may lead to metabolic acidosis. |
| 16 | Measure CVP after insertion of catheter into the umbilical vein. | |
| 17 | Take sample of pre-exchanged blood as well as after exchange for investigation. | Helps in estimation of bilirubin and hemoglobin. |
| 18 | Monitor heart rate, respiratory rate and condition of baby hourly during procedure. | |
| 19 | The physician removes 10 ml of umbilical blood and replaces with 10 ml of freshblood immediately, until calculated volume has been exchanged. | |
| 20 | Apply cord tie at umbilicus, seal umbilicus with tincture benzoin apply small gauze and secure with adhesive. | Prevents risk of hemorrhage and infection. |
| 21 | Replace equipments and start phototherapy. | |
| 22 | Document time of starting, duration, completion time, amount and type of blood exchanged, condition of baby during and after procedure, drugs given during procedure and samples sent to lab. | Gives information to the staff members. |

## POST TRANSFUSION CARE

1. Place the baby in a radiant warmer.
2. Inspect umbilicus for evidence of bleeding.
3. Repeat serum bilirubin as required.
4. Check infant's blood glucose level hourly.

## COMPLICATIONS

1. Bacterial sepsis
2. Thrombocytopenia
3. Portal vein thrombosis
4. Umbilical vein perforation
5. Dysrhythmia
6. Cardiac arrest
7. Hypocalcemia
8. Hypoglycemia
9. Hypomagnesemia
10. Metabolic acidosis

11. Alkalosis
12. HIV, Hepatitis B infections
13. Graft versus host disease.

## SPECIAL CONSIDERATIONS

1. If citrated or heparinized donor blood is used, one should be prepared for hypocalcemia, hypoglycemia, hyperkalemia and metabolic acidosis. Further, citrated blood leaves the infant with low Hb level. So, as a precaution calcium gluconate at regular intervals should be given when using citrated blood for exchange.
2. For every 100 ml of blood transfused one milli equivalent of sodium bicarbonate is given to combat metabolic acidosis.

## 14.26: BATHING A NEWBORN

### DEFINITION

Baby bath is a cleansing bath given to a newborn by immersing the baby's body in a tub of water.

### PURPOSES

1. To keep the baby's skin clean
2. To refresh the baby
3. To maintain normal temperature of the skin
4. To stimulate circulation.

### ARTICLES

1. A bath basin or tub
2. Jugs with hot and cold water
3. Buckets—2
4. Mackintosh and towel
5. Bath blanket/towel
6. Small towel
7. Mild, non-perfumed soap in a dish
8. Cotton balls in a container
9. Clean gloves
10. Sterile water
11. Kidney tray
12. Dress for the baby (baby frock and napkin)
13. Apron for the midwife
14. Alcohol swabs
15. TPR tray.

### PROCEDURE

| | Nursing action | Rationale |
|---|---|---|
| 1 | Check the physician's order to note the special precautions to be taken, if any | |
| 2 | Check the baby's temprature, respiration and color. | Ensures safety and readiness of the baby for bath. |
| 3 | Ensure that the baby was not fed within the previous one hour. | |
| 4 | Provide explanation to mother | |
| 5 | Ensure that the bathing room is not cold | |
| 6 | Close the windows and put off fan | Prevents draughts |
| 7 | Prepare the bathing area<br>- keep the table against wall<br>- place the tub or basin on one end and the toilet tray and clothing on the other end. | Prevents baby from falling |
| 8 | Place the mackintosh and towel on the table | |
| 9 | Assemble all articles before beginning the procedure | Avoids need of leaving the baby in the middle of bath. |
| 10 | Fill basin with warm water(100 degree F). Water should feel warm to the inside of wrist or elbow | |

*Contd...*

*Contd...*

| | | |
|---|---|---|
| 11 | Wash hands and wear apron. | |
| 12 | Bring baby for bath wrapped in bath blanket or towel. | |
| 13 | Check if the baby is wet with urine or stool, and if wet clean the baby. | |
| 14 | Undress the baby and wrap in a big towel. Wrap in such a manner that hands are restricted inside towel. | |
| 15 | Pick up cotton swabs dipped in sterile water and wipe the eyes from inner canthus to outer canthus using separate swab for each eye. Use one swab for each stroke | Cleans eyes and prevents infection. |
| 16 | If the eyes are not clean and crusts are not removed, repeat the procedure gently until eyes are clean. | Promotes hygiene. |
| 17 | If secretions are crusted in the nostrils take a rolled wisp of cotton, moisten it with normal saline or water and gently introdue it into the nostrils and rotate. The baby will sneeze and bring out secretions. Cotton-tipped applicators are contra-indicated. They can break when the baby moves causing injury to mucous membrane. | Cleaning nostrils with rolled wisp of cotton avoids chances of injury to baby's nostrils. |
| 18 | Clean the inside of ears with another rolled wisp of cotton | Cotton applicators can injure the eardrum |
| 19 | With the wet hand, clean face and behind ears. Do not apply soap on face. Dry face by patting and not by rubbing. | |
| 20 | Observe mouth for thrush as the baby cries. | |
| 21 | Reassure the baby before and during bath. Pick the baby up using the " football" hold and supporting the head in your palm. Hold the baby's head over the basin. Wet the scalp, apply soap, rinse with water and dry thoroughly. While washing the head, close ears using your thumb and middle fingers on either side of head. | "Football" hold provides for firm support to baby's body. Provides for washing the baby's head easily. |
| 22 | Discard the dirty water and take fresh water in basin. | |
| 23 | Unwrap the baby on the table, apply soap giving special attention to the neck, arms, axillae, groins and toes. | |
| 24 | The baby is held firmly and submerged gradually into water in the tub to rinse the soap completely The palm and fingers of the nurse are kept under the axilla of the baby for better support (Figure 14.26 (a)). Rinse him once again in clean water in the tub. | Helps in rinsing the body quickly. |

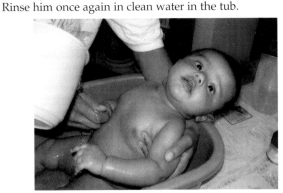

**Figure 14.26(a):** Proper technique of holding baby during bath

*Contd...*

*Contd...*

| | | |
|---|---|---|
| 25 | Turn the baby back in the same manner so that he lies over the forearm. | |
| 26 | To pick up the baby, slide the left hand under the baby's right shoulder and hold the infant at shoulders firmly. The head rests on the forearm and with the right hand, hold the baby at the ankles keeping the index fingers between two legs/feet. | A firm grip will prevent slipping of the baby. |
| 27 | Take the baby from water and place on spread towel. Dry him by patting gently. Special attention to be given to dry the body creases. | |
| 28 | Clean the cord stump with alcohol swabs. | Provides antiseptic and drying effects on the cord stump. |
| 29 | Dress the baby and swaddle wrap him in the blanket at the earliest. | Prevents chills |
| 30 | Arrange the hair. | |
| 31 | Handover the baby to his/her mother. | |
| 32 | Place the towel for washing and discard the waste water. | |
| 33 | Wash hands. | |
| 34 | Record the procedure in baby's chart. | |

## SPECIAL CONSIDERATIONS

1. Baby bath should be given prior to feeding or at least one hour after previous feeding.
2. Bath to be given about the same time every day to form a regular schedule.
3. Calm the baby before starting bath.
4. Use gloves for the first bath for preventing contact with body fluids.

## 14.27: WEIGHING A NEWBORN

### DEFINITION

Quantitative expression of body mass that indicates state of growth and health. It is measured in kilograms or pounds using infant weighing scale.

### PURPOSES

1. To check whether infant has adequate weight for age
2. To calculate food requirements
3. To calculate intravenous fluids and medications
4. To monitor whether infant is gaining or losing weight depending on disease condition

### ARTICLES

1. Infant weighing scale (Figure 14.27 (a))
2. Baby sheet
3. Duster.

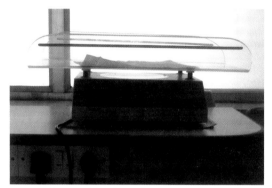

**Figure 14.27(a):** Infant weighing scale

### PROCEDURE

|   | Nursing action | Rational |
|---|----------------|----------|
| 1. | Explain procedure to parents. | Helps in obtaining cooperation. |
| 2. | Note infant's previous weight from record of last weighing. | Sudden loss in weight can indicate presence of serious disease or significant change in dietary habits. |
| 3. | Ensure that room temperature is warm. | Infants are weighed nude and are susceptible to temperature fluctuations because of immature thermo-regulation. |
| 4. | Clean the weighing pan with wet duster. | Wet dusting removes dust. |
| 5. | Calibrate scale by setting weight at zero and noting if balance beam registers in the middle of mark. Scale with digital display should read "zero" before use. | Calibrated scales ensure accurate measurements. |
| 6. | Place baby sheet on pan in which infant is to be placed. Note the weight. | Weight of the baby sheet to be subtracted from the combined weight of baby and sheet. |
| 7. | Place naked infant in basket or on platform. Hold hand lightly above infant during measurement. | Prevents accidental fall. |

*Contd...*

*Contd...*

| | |
|---|---|
| 8. Note weight in grams and kilograms or pounds and ounces. | |
| 9. Lift infant from pan and help mother to dress baby. | Maintains temperature of the infant. |
| 10. Check and compare with previous day's weight. | Gives information about change in weight. |
| 11. Difference of more than 100 grams need to be clarified by checking infants weight once again. | If weight is in pounds and ounces, it has to be converted using conversion table. |
| 12. If difference is still same it should be informed to head nurse or physician concerned. | |
| 13. Record weight in nurse's notes or flow sheet. | Repeated weight measurements are entered in flow sheet for comparison. |

## SPECIAL CONSIDERATIONS

1. Normally, weight can fluctuate daily because of fluid loss or retention (1 liter of water weighs 1 kg).
2. Infant should be weighed on same scale at same time, with same type of clothing each day.
3. Explain that it is best to weigh in the morning after voiding and before feed is taken.
4. Infants are weighed nude.
5. Assess if the infant is on any medication. Weight gain or loss can be a side effect of this medication.

# 14.28: FEEDING INFANTS WITH CLEFT LIP AND CLEFT PALATE

## DEFINITION

Feeding babies who have cleft lip and cleft palate using devices conducive for the baby to ingest feeds.

## PURPOSES

1. To meet nutritional needs of baby.
2. To prevent complications such as aspiration.

## GENERAL INSTRUCTIONS

1. Give frequent feeds to keep palate from drying
2. Administer gavage feeding if nipple feeding is to be delayed
3. If sucking is permitted, use a soft nipple with crosscut to facilitate feeding. Nipples can be softened by boiling them.
4. If sucking is ineffective due to inability to create a vacuum, try alternate oral feeding methods.
   a. Feeding devices include:
      • Preemie nipple
      • Crosscut nipple
      • Ross cleft palate nurser
      • Haberman feeder
      • Palatal obturator
   b. Avoid enlarging nipple holes as the infant's inability to control the flow of milk will result in choking. Crosscut nipples allow milk to flow only when infant squeezes the crosscut open.
   c. Using a squeezable bottle or plastic liner can be helpful by applying rhythmic pressure along with the infants normal sucking and swallowing.
   d. When using rubber tipped asepto syringe or dropper; the rubber extension should be long enough to extend into back of mouth to prevent regurgitation through the nose. Direct tip to side of mouth, and feed slowly.
   e. Teach the parents ESSR method of feeding
      E ….. Avoid enlarging nipple.
      S ….. Stimulate the suck reflex
      S ……Swallow
      R……Rest to allow baby to finish swallowing what has been placed in the mouth.

## PROCEDURE

|   | Nursing action | Rationale |
|---|----------------|-----------|
| 1. | Explain procedure to mother and encourage mother to clear her doubts. | Helps mother to acquire knowledge about feeding technique. |
| 2. | Assess for sucking and swallowing reflex of the baby. | Helps to choose the feeding method. |
| 3. | Make mother to sit in comfortable position with the baby held in upright position. | Decreases possibility of fluid being aspirated or returned through the nose or back to the auditory canal |
| 4. | Place the nipple (teat) angled to the side of mouth away from the cleft. | Prevents aspiration. |
| 5. | Feed slowly over approximately 15 to 30 minutes. | Feedings longer than 45 minutes expends too many calories and tires the infant. |
| 6. | Give small frequent feeds and burp after each feeding. | Decreases amount of air swallowed. |

*Contd...*

*Contd...*

| | | |
|---|---|---|
| 7. | Avoid repeated removal of nipple due to fear of choking. | Frustrates the infant causing crying which increases chances of aspiration |
| 8. | Feed infant before he becomes too hungry. | Infant gets agitated when hungry and feeding becomes a problem. |
| 9. | Give adequate amount of water after each feeding. | |
| 10. | Position the baby on side after feeding. | Prevents regurgitation. |
| 11. | Document time, feed, amount and baby's tolerance to given feed in nurses records. | Acts as a means of communication between staff members. |

## SPECIAL CONSIDERATIONS

Special methods of feeding include:
- Cup and spoon (Figure 14.28 (a))
- Paladai (Feeder with beaked tip) (Figure 14.28 (a))
- Feeder with compressible plastic sides which can be squeezed to help eject milk.

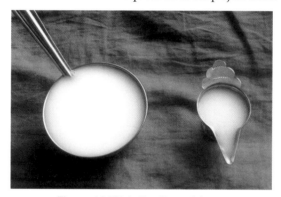

**Figure 14.28(a):** Feeding articles

# 14.29: ASSISTING IN INSERTION OF INTRAUTERINE CONTRACEPTIVE DEVICES

## DEFINITION

Introduction of a specially designed device into the uterine cavity of a fertile woman who desires to prevent conception/pregnancy for a specific period of time.

## PURPOSES

1. To avoid unwanted pregnancy.
2. To space pregnancies.

## CONTRAINDICATIONS

*Absolute:*
1. Suspected pregnancy.
2. Pelvic inflammatory disease.
3. Vaginal bleeding of undiagnosed etiology.
4. Cancer of cervix, uterus or adnexae and other pelvic tumors.
5. Previous ectopic pregnancy.

*Relative:*
1. Anemia
2. Menorrhagia.
3. History of pelvic inflammatory disease.
4. Purulent cervical discharge.
5. Distortions of the uterine cavity due to congenital malformations, fibroids.

## ADVANTAGES OF IUCD

1. Simplicity –No complex procedures are involved in insertion.
2. Hospitalization is not required.
3. IUCD stays in place as long as required (Different types of IUCDs have varying durations recommend for replacement depending on the amount of impregnated medication).
4. Inexpensive.
5. Contraceptive effect is reversible by removal of IUCD.
6. Free from systemic metabolic side effects associated with hormonal pills.
7. There is no need for continual motivation.

## ARTICLES

1. IUCD pre-sterilized insertion package
2. Sterile tray containing:
   - Vaginal speculum (cuscos)—1
   - Vulsellum—1
   - Uterine sound—1
   - Sponge holding forceps—2
   - Bowl containing cotton swab
   - Sterile gloves
   - Scissors
   - Disinfectant solution
   - Kidney tray

## PROCEDURE: (INSERTION OF COPPER T)

| | Nursing action | Rationale |
|---|---|---|
| 1 | Explain the procedure including advantages, disadvantages effectiveness and side effects of IUCD. | Helps in obtaining co-operation of patient and reduces anxiety. |
| 2 | Arrange the equipments on examination table. | |
| 3 | Instruct woman to empty her bladder. | |
| 4 | Position woman on her back with knees flexed and buttocks at the edge of the table. | |
| 5 | Provide privacy and drape patient appropriately. | Prevents embarassment. |
| 6 | Wash hands and don sterile gloves. | |
| 7 | Load IUCD inside applicator as per manufacturer's instruction. (Figure 14.29 (a)) | |

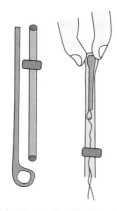

**Figure 14.29(a):** Placing the IUCD in the inserter

| | | |
|---|---|---|
| 8 | Inspect external genitalia, urethra and vagina for signs of infection, lesions or discharge. | |
| 9 | Explain to the woman that there will be slight discomfort during speculum insertion. | Helps in obtaining cooperation. |
| 10 | Insert the speculum gently and observe the cervix for signs of infection and erosion. | |
| 11 | Clean the external cervical os with an antiseptic soaked swab by using sponge holding forceps. | |
| 12 | Instruct the patient that there will be disocmfort (pinching pain) when applying the vulsellum. Apply vulsellum at the 12o' clock position on the cervix, grasp the lip of the cervix. | Applies traction to the cervix and straightens the cervical canal. |
| 13 | Pass the uterine sound into the cervical canal and insert carefully into the uterine cavity while pulling steadily downward and outward on the vulsellum. (A slight resistance indicates that the top of the uterine sound has reached the fundus), and remove the uterine sound. | Determines the length of the uterine cavity by noting the level of mucus or blood on the uterine sound. |
| 14 | Measure the length of the device to be inserted into the uterine cavity. The depth of gauge on the inserter- tube is used to mark the depth of the uterus. | |

*Contd...*

*Contd...*

|  | Pull the loaded inserter tube gently until the distance between the top of the folded "T" and edge of the depth gauge closest to the "T" is equal to the depth of the uterus as measured on uterine sound. |  |
|---|---|---|
| 15 | Carefully peel the clean plastic cover of the package away from the white packing. Lift the loaded inserter keeping it horizontal so that neither the " T" nor the white rod falls out. Be careful not to push the white rod towards the "T". |  |
| 16 | Grasp the vulsellum and pull firmly downwards and outwards to align the uterine cavity and cervical canal with the vaginal canal. |  |
| 17 | Gently introduce the loaded inserter assembly through the cervical canal. Keeping the depth gauge into a horizontal position (Figure 14.29 (b)). |  |

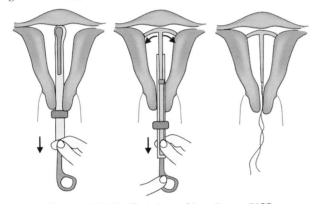

**Figure 14.29 (b):** Technique of inserting an IUCD

| 18 | According to the position and direction of the uterine cavity gently and carefully advance the loaded inserter assembly until the depth gauge comes in contact with the cervix or resistance of the uterine fundus is felt. | Places the loaded applicator in the uterine cavity. |
|---|---|---|
| 19 | Hold the vulsellum and the white rod in one hand. |  |
| 20 | Gently and carefully push the inserter tube upwards, towards resistance. | This action frees the IUCD into the uterine cavity. |
| 21 | Remove the white rod while holding the inserter tube stationary. |  |
| 22 | Gently and slowly withdraw the inserter tube from the cervical canal and check for the strings protruding from the uterus. Cut the strings shorter so that they protrude only 3 cm outside the cervix. | The strings can be seen and felt in the vagina. |
| 23 | Remove the vulsellum. If there is excessive bleeding from the vulsellum site, press a sterile cotton ball to the site using forceps until the bleeding stops. |  |
| 24 | Remove speculum and drapes. |  |
| 25 | Instruct patient to stay in bed for sometime. |  |
| 26 | Wash perineum with soap and water and dry it. |  |
| 27 | Remove gloves and discard. |  |

*Contd...*

*Contd...*

28  Instruct the woman on follow-up measures:
1. To confirm presence of IUCD periodically by feeling the presence of threads in vagina.
2. Instruct patient to visit clinic whenever she experiences the warning signs of problems related to IUCD such as:
   **P** -Delayed period, spotting, bleeding or missing period.
   **A**-Abnormal pain or pain during coitus.
   **I** -Infection, any vaginal discharge.
   **N**-Not feeling well, fever or pelvic pain.
   **S**- Strings in vagina (Feeling the device in vagina).

## SIDE EFFECTS AND COMPLICATIONS

1. Excessive bleeding
2. Low back pain during menstruation.
3. Pain during menstruation
4. Pelvic infection
5. Uterine perforation
6. Ectopic pregnancy
7. Expulsion of device.

## 14.30: GIVING A NEWBORN A SPONGE BATH

## DEFINITION

A sponge bath is a cleansing bath given to a newborn using a sponge and towel until the cord stump has fallen.

## PURPOSES

1. To keep the baby's skin clean.
2. To refresh the baby.
3. To stimulate circulation.

## ARTICLES

1. Big basin
2. A soft wash cloth or absorbent pad for sponging and drying
3. Mild non-perfumed soap in a container.
4. Cotton balls.
5. A towel to place under the baby during bath.
6. Bath blanket or towel to cover the infant during bath.
7. Baby comb for cleaning infants scalp.
8. Sterile water to clean the eyes of baby.
9. Diaper.
10. Baby cloth (shirt or gown).
11. Baby oil or mild lotion.
12. Tissue paper.

## PROCEDURE

| | Nursing action | Rationale |
|---|---|---|
| 1 | Explain the procedure to mother. | Helps in obtaining cooperation. |
| 2 | Ensure that the room is warm and free of draughts. This is particularly important when caring for newborns. | Temperature regulating mechanisms are not completely developed in newborn. |
| 3 | Remove the infant's diaper, and wipe away any faeces on the baby's perineum with the tissues. | |
| 4 | Reassure the infant before and during bath by holding the infant firmly but gently. | |
| 5 | Undress the infant and place him or her in supine position on a towel and cover him. | |
| 6 | Place small articles such as safety pins out of the infant's reach. | Prevents injury. |
| 7 | Ascertain the infant's weight and vital signs. | |
| 8 | Clean the baby's eyes with sterile water using clean cotton swabs. Use separate cotton ball for each eye wipe from inner to outer canthus. (In some agencies the infant's eyes and scalp are cleaned before the infant is undressed). | Using separate cotton balls prevent the transmission of microorganisms from one eye to the other. Wiping away from the inner canthus avoids entry debris into the nasolacrimal duct. |
| 9 | Wash and dry the baby's face using water only. Soap is used to clean the ears. | Soap can be irritating to the eyes, if used on face. |

*Contd....*

*Contd....*

| | | |
|---|---|---|
| 10 | Pick the baby up using the football hold (hold the baby against your side supporting the body with your forearm and the head with the palm of your hand) Position the baby's head over the wash basin and lather the scalp with a mild soap. Massage the lather over the scalp using fingertips. | Loosens any dry scales from the scalp and helps to prevent cradle cap. If cradle cap is present it may be treated with baby oil, a dandruff shampoo or ointment prescribed by physician. |
| 11 | Rinse and dry the scalp well. Place the baby supine again. | |
| 12 | Apply soap, wash rinse and dry each arm and hand paying particular attention to the axilla. Avoid using soap to the palmar surface and avoid excessive rubbing. Dry thoroughly. | Rubbing can cause irritation and moisture can cause excoriation of the skin. Avoiding soap on palms prevents baby putting soapy fingers in mouth. |
| 13 | Apply soap, wash rinse and dry the baby's chest and abdomen. Keep the baby covered with the bath blanket or towel between washing and rinsing. | Covering the infant prevents chilling. |
| 14 | Apply soap and rinse the legs and feet. Dry them. Expose only one leg and foot at a time. Give special attention to the area between toes. | Keeping exposure to a minimum maintains the baby's warmth. |
| 15 | Turn the baby on her or his stomach or side, wash, rinse and dry the back. | |
| 16 | Place the baby on his or her back. Clean and dry the genitals and anterior perineal area from front to back.<br>a. Clean the folds of the groin.<br>b. For females, separate the labia and clean them. Clean the genital area from front to back using moistened cotton balls. Use a clean swab for each stroke.<br>c. If a male infant is uncircumcised, retract the foreskin if possible and clean the glans penis using a moistened cotton ball.<br><br>If the foreskin is tight do not forcibly retract it. Gentle pressure on a tight foreskin over a period of days or weeks may accomplish eventual retraction. After swabbing, replace the foreskin to prevent edma of the glans penis. Clean the shaft of the penis and scrotum. (In some agencies foreskin is not retracted).<br>d. If a male infant has been recently circumcised, clean the glans penis by gently squeezing a cotton ball moistened with sterile water over the site. Note any signs of bleeding or infection. Petroleum jelly or bacteriocidal ointment is applied to the circumcision site. Avoid applying excessive quantities of ointment. | The rectal area is cleaned last since it is most contaminated.<br><br>The smegma that collects between the folds of the labia and under the foreskin in males, facilitates bacterial growth and must be removed. Lotions and powders, can also accumulate between the labia and need to be removed. Clean swabs are used to avoid spreading microorganisms from the rectal area to the urethra.<br><br><br><br>Excess ointment may obstruct the urinary meatus. |
| 17 | Clean the posterior perineum and buttocks, grasp both of the baby's ankles, raise the feet and elevate the buttocks. Wash and rinse the area with the wash cloth. Dry the area and apply ointment. Do not apply powder. | |
| 18 | Clean the base of the umbilical cord with a cotton ball dipped in 70% ethyl alcohol. (Some agencies use other antiseptics such as povidone-Iodine). | Alcohol promotes drying and prevents infection. |
| 19 | Check for dry, cracked or peeling skin and apply a mild baby oil or lotion. | |

*Contd...*

*Contd...*

| | | |
|---|---|---|
| 20 | Dress the baby in clean shirt and diaper. Diaper to be fixed below cord site lumbilicus. | Exposing the cordsite to air will promote healing. |
| 21 | Until the umbilicus and circumcision site are healed, position the baby on his side in the crib with a rolled towel or diaper behind the back for support. | This position allows more air to circulate around the cord site. |
| 22 | Swaddle wrap the baby. | Gives the baby a sense of security as well as keeps him warm. |
| 23 | Return the baby to mother and provide needed instructions. | Mother continues care and observation of the baby. |
| 24 | Clean and replace/discard used articles as appropriate | |
| 25 | Record any significant observation such as reddened area or skin rashes, the color and the consistency of the stool and the state of the cord stump. | Helps in planning treatment. |

# Chapter 15

# Community Health Nursing

## 15.1: PERFORMING HANDWASHING AT HOME

### DEFINITION

Hand washing is a vigorous, brief rubbing together of all surfaces of hands lathered in soap, followed by rinsing under a stream of water.

### PURPOSES

1. To remove dirt and transient micro-organisms from the hands.
2. To reduce total microbial counts over time
3. To prevent cross infection.

### ARTICLES

1. Soap in a soap dish
2. Water
3. Nail brush
4. Hand towel
5. Piece of paper/old newspaper

### PROCEDURE

| | Nursing action | Rationale |
|---|---|---|
| 1 | Place the bag on the newspaper, spread over a clean floor area or platform. | Prevents contamination of bag. |
| 2 | Remove wrist watch and keep in a safe place. | |
| 3 | Open the bag and take out, soap dish, hand towel, nail brush and a small piece of paper to "wash area", spread the paper and place articles on the paper. | Arranging all articles needed for the procedure saves time and effort. |
| 4 | Select a place where water will drain off. | Stagnation of water promotes breeding of flies and insects. |
| 5 | Moisten hands with water so that soap will lather well. Apply soap to the hands while holding hands down. | Prevents splashing and protects uniform |
| 6 | Rub together to work up a good lather. Rub palms, inter-digital areas, all sides of each finger then back of hands, wrist, nails and cuticles. | Friction of hands with action of soap cleans the hand and destroys microorganisms. |
| 7 | Scrub for 2-3 minutes with nail brush if any surgical procedure or delivery to be conducted. | For surgical procedure or delivery asepsis has to be maintained. |
| 8 | Wash soap off the hands and hold hands up to prevent water running from elbows to hands. | Water should flow from more clean to less clean area. |
| 9 | Dry hands using hand towel and place it on the clean area. | Moisture promotes growth of microbes. |
| 10 | After the procedure, wash hands again and dry with towel | Prevents infection |
| 11 | Replace soap in soap dish and hand towel in bag. Close the bag | |
| 12 | Discard the paper on which soap dish was placed, and any other used materials. | |

## 15.2: PERFORMING BAG TECHNIQUES AT HOME

### DEFINITION

The principles and methods of organizing and utilizing the community nurses' bag for carrying out nursing care procedures during a home visit.

### PRINCIPLES

1. Use supplies and equipment in the bag economically.
2. The bag and its contents must be kept clean and dry for use at all times.
3. Clean or sterilize contaminated instruments and equipment before returning to the bag.
4. Keep sterile equipment in the separate sterile area of the bag.
5. Standard nursing procedures need to be carried out by utilizing the material and equipment found in the home.
6. Teach and demonstrate to a responsible member of the family, about how nursing care can be provided at home.
7. Standing orders need to be followed while providing care at home.
8. Follow aseptic technique and thorough cleanliness at all times to prevent the spread of disease.
9. Respect the family's cultural and religious practices as far as possible.
10. Provide privacy, consider comfort and maintain professional relationship.

### SUPPLIES AND EQUIPMENT

1. Bag with removable plastic (or) cotton lining.
2. Outside pockets
   : Soaps in a soap dish
   : Hand towel
   : Nail brush
   : Newspaper pieces
   : Apron.
3. Side pockets
   : Pencil, nail cutter, scissors, measuring tape, paperbags, newspapers, specimen bottles.
4. Top compartment
   : Dressing pack
   : Scissors – 5 inch
   : Artery forceps – 5 inch
   : Dissecting forceps – 4 inch
   : Thermometer – oral
   : Slides-2
   : Cotton and gauze pack
   : Solution bowls
   : Ounce glass
5. Cover compartment
   : Solutions (Benedict's, Hydrogen peroxide, Alcohol, Betadine)
   : Acetic Acid, Dettole or savlon
   : Kidney tray
   : Test tube
   : Test tube holder
   : Filler
   : Spirit lamp
   : 5-cc syringe
   : Match box
   : Fetoscope

# PROCEDURE

| | Nursing action | Rationale |
|---|---|---|
| 1 | Upon reaching the home select a work area which is well lighted and dry where the bag can be set up away from children and domestic animals. | Prevents the danger of contamination of the bag. |
| 2 | Spread newspaper on a flat, clean surface and place the bag in one of the corners of the newspaper. | Remaining area on the newspaper can be used to place articles from inside the bag for procedure. |
| 3 | Unbutton the outer lining of the bag. Remove the handwashing articles and wash hands. | Hands are washed before opening the inside of the bag to prevent contamination |
| 4 | Remove apron from the bag to put it on if necessary. | Prevents contamination of the uniform. |
| 5 | Touch the inner part of the outer cover to open the inner lining of the bag and keep the folds aside on both sides. | Outer part of outer layer is contaminated. |
| 6 | Remove necessary supplies and equipment and place on the clean area on newspaper. | Prevents contamination of equipment and supplies. |
| 7 | Close the bag (half covered) | Prevents exposure of articles inside the bag and thus prevents contamination. |
| 8 | Prepare a disposal bag using newspaper | |
| 9 | Carry out the required nursing procedure. Place soiled swabs inside the newspaper bag for disposal. | |
| 10 | Give the newspaper bag with used cotton to family for disposal by burning. | Promotes safe disposal of contaminated waste. |
| 11 a. b. | Clean the used articles. Boil the used instruments for 5 minutes and keep inside the bag. Place articles which are contaminated with infected material in a plastic cover in the outer part of the bag for autoclaving before replacing into the bag. | Keeps articles ready for next use. |
| 12 | Wash hands, open the bag to return articles into the bag | Washing hands before opening the bag helps to prevent contamination of the bag. |
| 13 | Use a cotton swab moistened with spirit and wipe outside of used bottle and bowls and replace in the bag. | Ensures that all the articles are clean before replacing into the bag. |
| 14 | Close the bag | |
| 15 | Fold the newspaper with used side inside and place it in the side pocket and carry the bag. | Used side is considered to be contaminated. |
| 16 | Write a report of observations, the procedure done, instructions given and also plans for the next visit. | Evaluates the nursing care given and plans for future visits. |

# 15.3: TAKING ANTHROPOMETRIC MEASUREMENTS

## DEFINITION

A system of assessment of body build and nutritional status of children using measurements such as weight, height, wrist circumference, skinfold thickness, upper arm circumference, chest circumference and head circumference.

## PURPOSE

Anthropometric measurements recorded over a period of time reflect the patterns of growth and development and how individuals deviate from the average in body size, build and nutritional status at various ages.

## ARTICLES

1. Spring balance for infants
   Weighing scale for older children
2. A ruler
3. Measuring tape
4. Calipers
5. Growth chart

## PROCEDURE

| | Nursing action | Rationale |
|---|---|---|
| **A** | **Measuring weight** | |
| 1 | Explain the procedure and the purpose of it to the mother and family. | Accepts the purpose of assessing anthropometric measurements and ensures cooperation. |
| 2 | Dress the baby in strong canvas pants with straps and fix to the hooks of spring balance. | |
| 3 | Hold the balance up with the baby hanging or hook the balance to a nail fixed on the upper beam of a door. | Obtains accurate reading of weight.<br>A spring balance will weigh upto 20 kg |
| 4 | Instruct an older child to stand on the weighing machine with minimum clothing on and note the weight. | Less clothing while checking weight adds to accuracy of measurement. |
| **B** | **Measuring height** | |
| 5 | Instruct the child (above 2 years) to stand against a wall without footwear, feet parallel and heels, buttocks, shoulders and back of head touching the wall. | Standing straight against the wall, with the head comfortably errect aids accurate measurement of height. |
| 6 | Make a mark on the wall with the help of the ruler touching the top of the head horizontally. | |
| 7 | Instruct the child to move away and measure the length on the wall using the measuring tape. | |
| **C** | **Measuring circumference of head, chest, wrist and mid upper arm** | |
| 8 | Check the circumference by encircling the specific body part with a measuring tape and read the result in centimeters. | These measurements are used to assess growth pattern and identify deviations from normal growth and development. |

*Contd...*

*Contd...*

| D | Measuring skinfold thickness | |
|---|---|---|
| 9 | Pinch lengthwise a double fold of subcutaneous tissue about 1 cm above the mid upper arm with thumb and index finger. Place the teeth of calipers on either side of the tissue fold and note the reading.<br>Other sites used for measuring skin-fold thickness include biceps, scapula and abdominal wall. | Determines the fat content of subcutaneous tissue. Detects any muscle wasting present. |
| 10 | Record the measurements in the growth chart | Aids in comparison of measurements with earlier recordings and assessment. |

## SPECIAL POINTS

- For surveillance of growth and development compare the findings with standard reference values such as weight for age, weight for height and reference curves.
- For determining the degree (grade) of malnutrition, refer the growth chart recommended by the government of India.
- Anthropometric measurements are taken for adults in order to estimate body frame, muscle wasting and fat content of tissues.

## 15.4: PROCEDURE FOR CHECKING WEIGHT AND HEIGHT

### PRINCIPLES FOR CHECKING WEIGHT

1. The weighing scale must be accurate
2. The baby scale platform must be safe and secure to prevent the baby from falling.
3. The mother or nurse must stay with the baby when he/she is being weighed to prevent falling.
4. The baby being weighed must wear the same amount of clothing each time he is weighed.
5. Record the weight as soon as the scale is read. Adjust the scale each time.
6. Place separate newspaper on the platform after each infant has been weighed to prevent direct contact or a piece of plastic which can be swabbed and dried after each weighing.
7. Emphasize importance of weighing during the growth period.
8. Read the weight by standing in front of the scale.

### EQUIPMENTS

1. Weighing scale
2. Record form
3. Pen

### PROCEDURE

| | Nursing action | Rationale |
|---|---|---|
| | **To weigh infant:** | |
| 1 | Place a clean paper or clean plastic sheet on the scale and balance it. | Prevents direct contact and gives accurate reading. |
| 2 | Look at the record and note the last recorded weight | It gives a value for reference |
| 3 | Place the baby on the platform of weighing machine. | |
| 4 | Read the weight and record | |
| 5 | Instruct the mother to take the child | |
| 6 | Inform the mother the weight noted and also explain how much the child has gained or lost. | |
| | **To weigh children and adults:** | |
| 1 | Place the scale on a flat even surface | Gives an accurate reading |
| 2 | Check whether the needle is at zero. | Gives an accurate reading |
| 3 | Instruct the person to stand on the scale straight (Ensure that the person is wearing light clothing, removed shoes, coat or has emptied the pockets. | Extra clothing or full pockets may give false readings. |
| 4 | Read the scale. Record the weight immediately and inform the person how much he weighs. | |

### MEASURING HEIGHT

#### PURPOSE

To estimate the rate of growth of the individual and correlate the relation of height with general health.

#### ARTICLES

1. Measuring tape

2. Record form
3. Ruler
4. Blocks/books/bricks
5. Pencil
6. Height rod (if available).

## PROCEDURE

| Nursing action | Rationale |
|---|---|
| **To measure an Infant:** | |
| 1 Lay the child on a flat even surface like table. | Uneven surface may give false result. |
| 2 Hold the head and heel firmly. | |
| 3 Place two blocks/books/bricks one each at the head and heel level. | Gives accurate reading. |
| 4 Instruct the mother to remove the infant. | |
| 5 Place a measuring tape between the two blocks and measure the height. | |
| 6 Record the height and inform the mother. | |
| **To measure school children and adults:** | |
| 1 Instruct the child or adult to stand against a straight wall on a flat even surface or against the height rod with his feet together, arms and hands down, head erect and eyes straight. | Gives accurate reading |
| 2 Place the ruler on top of the head level and mark the area with pencil where the ruler touches the head. | Measures the height. |
| 3 Instruct the child or adult to move away from the area marked. | |
| 4 Measure from ground level to the marked area with a measuring tape or if a height rod is used, read the measurement that appears at the point where the ruler touches the head. | |
| 5 Record the height and inform the person. | |

## SPECIAL POINTS

1. If food is taken, the weight has to be measured after one hour.
2. Before weighing, the person has to empty his bowel and bladder.
3. The weight has to be checked with the same weighing scale each time.

## 15.5: URINE ANALYSIS

Testing of urine for diabetic patients and antenatal mothers at home.

### PRINCIPLES

1. All articles must be clean.
2. When in doubt regarding results, perform a repeat test.
3. Check the expiry of solutions used.

### PURPOSE

To test the urine for evidence of albumin, sugar and other abnormalities.

### ARTICLES

1. Container for specimen
2. Litmus paper
3. Test tube
4. Test tube holder
5. Benedict's solution
6. Syringe (5 ml)
7. Acetic acid
8. Spirit
9. Spirit lamp
10. Match box
11. Dropper

### PROCEDURE

| | Nursing action | Rationale |
|---|---|---|
| 1 | Instruct the person to clean the genitalia with soap and water. | The microbes around the urethra can be flushed or cleaned out. |
| 2 | Instruct the person to pass little amount of urine in the toilet first, and then collect urine in specimen container (Mid stream urine). | |
| | **Test for pH:** | |
| 1 | Place a small piece of litmus paper in the container with urine and note the reaction | If red litmus turns blue – alkaline<br>If blue litmus turns red- acidic<br>If litmus is unchanged – neutral |
| | **Test for albumin:** | |
| 1 | If urine is alkaline, add acetic acid. | It makes the urine acidic. |
| 2 | Pour urine into a test tube filling about 3/4th of the test tube. | |
| 3 | Boil the top 1/3rd of the contents. | |
| 4 | Check if cloudiness developes, if so add 5 drops of 5% acetic acid and reheat.<br>a) If a precipitate is formed and does not disappear when acid is added, then the test is positive for albumin. If precipitate is heavy, the test is heavily positive or ++++ | The cloudiness may be due to the presence of albumin or phosphate.<br>The precipitate is due to presence of albumin |

*Contd...*

*Contd...*

| | | |
|---|---|---|
| | b) If precipitate disappears after acid is added, test is negative for albumin. | Precipitate is due to presence of phosphate. |
| 5 | Record the test | Record is a legal document |
| | **Test for sugar:** | |
| 1 | Pour 5 ml of Benedict's solution into the test tube and heat. | If there is no color change then the solution is appropriate for the test. |
| 2 | Add 5 – 10 drops of urine to the sides of the test tube and bring to boil very slowly. | |
| 3 | Place aside and allow to cool. | Presence of glucose in urine changes the color of the solution. |
| 4 | Read the test<br>Blue – negative<br>Green – 0.5% or +<br>Yellow – 1% or ++<br>Orange – 1.5% or +++<br>Brick red – 2.0% and above or ++++ | |
| 5 | Record the test | Record is a legal document. |

# 15.6: COLLECTION OF SPECIMEN FOR LABORATORY INVESTIGATIONS

## PRINCIPLES

1. The specimen must be collected from the most likely source of the organisms or substance to be tested.
2. Specimen must be free of extraneous contamination or adulteration.
3. Specimen must be collected in clean or sterile container.
4. Specimen must be properly labelled with the person's full name, address or clinic number.
5. Specimen must be transferred to the laboratory promptly and in a container that will not contaminate things that may come in contact with it.
6. Laboratory reports are confidential.
7. Laboratory examinations are only one to diagnosis.

## ARTICLES

1. Clean gloves
2. Face mask
3. Specimen container/cult tube as applicable
4. Spatula
5. Handwashing articles
6. Family health record.

## PROCEDURE

| | Nursing action | Rationale |
|---|---|---|
| 1 | **Procedure for collecting stool specimen for special examination:** Stool specimens are collected by special techniques for each type of examination. Some have to be cultured and then examined, while others are examined directly from fresh specimen. | |
| | a. Collecting specimens for amoebiasis examination: | |
| | 1. Instruct the person to go to lab and collect specimen there. | For amoebiasis, the specimen should be fresh and warm. |
| | 2. Provide a sterile container and instruct how to use it | |
| | 3. Seal the container and label it and immediately send to lab for examination. | Helps in preventing contamination of specimen. Any delay will result in wrong results. |
| | b. Collecting specimen for examination for enteric bacterial pathogens: The stool culture study includes a search for all the enteric bacterial pathogens including typhoid, paratyphoid, dysentery and cholera. | |
| | 1. Collect the specimen in a sterile container. | |
| | 2. Instruct the patient to deposit stool in a clean pan. | Prevents errors in the findings. |
| | 3. Dip a sterile cotton applicator into the specimen and drop the applicator into the container and close the bottle. | Prevents contamination |
| | 4. Wash hands thoroughly | |
| | 5. Label the specimen and send to the laboratory. | |
| | c. Collecting specimen for intestinal helminth: Intestinal helminth include nematodes, hookworm, round worm, pinworm, whipworm and cestodes like tapeworm, guineaworm etc. | |

*Contd...*

*Contd...*

| | |
|---|---|
| 1. Instruct the person to deposit a small portion of moist stool into a container . | |
| 2. Label it completely and send to laboratory with a requisition form. | |
| 3. If the person finds round worms or segments of tapeworm in the stool he should collect and put it into a bottle of alcohol and take it to the laboratory. | |

| | |
|---|---|
| d. Collecting specimens of pinworm for examination:<br>The pinworm's eggs are not generally found in stools of infected persons because the mature worm anigrates to the anus and deposits eggs in peri-anal area after which the adult worm dies. The larvae that hatch out may reinfest the person.<br>  1. Use an applicator stick with cotton swab attached to the end of it. | |
|   2. Rub the tip of the swab around the anal orifice using firm motion directed outward from the anal opening and penetrating the folds. | The pinworm lays eggs in the peri-anal area. |
|   3. Place the swab in a covered bottle or test tube with a stopper and send to the laboratory. | Prevents contamination of the specimen |
|   4. Wash hands thoroughly. | Prevents cross infection. |

| | |
|---|---|
| 2  Collecting specimen for throat culture (diphtheria) | |
|   1. Wash hands thoroughly and wear a mask. | Prevents cross infection. |
|   2. Explain the procedure to the patient | Helps in gaining cooperation of the patient. |
|   3. Place the patient in good light so that you can see the throat. | |
|   4. Instruct the patient to open his mouth wide and to breath in long deep breaths. | Helps in obtaining specimen. |
|   5. Depress the tongue with the handle of a spoon or tongue depressor. | Helps in obtaining specimen. |
|   6. Observe the mucous membranes for evidence of white spots, redness, swelling. | |
|   7. Swab the infected area so as to get membrane or discharge. Touch only the throat and tonsil area. | Prevents contamination from other areas of oral cavity. |
|   8. Take the culture by rotating the swab lightly over the surface of the lesion, being careful not to break the surface. | Diphtheria patch may bleed if handled rashly. |
|   9. Burn the swab and boil the spoon. Wash hands. | Prevents cross infection. |
|   10. Fill in the label stating the request and send to the laboratory. | Helps in proper investigation. |
|   11. Wash hands thoroughly. | Prevents cross infection. |

| | |
|---|---|
| 3  Collecting specimen of sputum for examination: | |
|   1. Collect the container and give it to the patient with the following instructions; | |
|     a. Rinse the mouth with water just before coughing in the early morning (before brushing) | Helps in removing the bacteria that are formed during the night. |
|     b. Take deep breath, cough and deposit sputum in the container. | Sputum from the respiratory tract helps in accurate findings. |
|     c. Label the specimen and send to the laboratory. | |
|     d. Wash hands thoroughly. | Prevents cross infection. |

## SPECIAL CONSIDERATION

- While collecting specimen, nurse should wear mask and gloves to protect herself.

# 15.7: CHECKING TEMPERATURE AT HOME

## PRINCIPLES OF THE THERMOMETER TECHNIQUE

1. Meticulous cleansing of thermometer before and after use is essential to prevent the spread of infection.
2. Checking temperature by axillary method is preferred to avoid the risk of transferring infection.
3. For accuracy allow the thermometer to remain in the mouth for 3 minutes in the rectum for 3 minutes and in the axilla or groin for 5 minutes.
4. Shake the thermometer till the mercury level comes down to 95 degree fahrenheit before taking the temperature.
5. Accuracy in temperature recording helps in making accurate treatment and medical decision for providing effective treatment.

## EQUIPMENTS

1. Cotton swabs —3
2. Pledget—1
3. Thermometer
4. Kidney tray
5. Spirit
6. Paper bag
7. Soap

## PROCEDURE

| | Nursing action | Rationale |
|---|---|---|
| 1 | Follow the steps involved in bag technique and open the top compartment of the bag. | Only necessary part of the bag should be opened to prevent contamination. |
| 2 | Remove necessary articles. | |
| 3 | Prepare a pledget of cotton | Pledget is used to cleanse the thermometer after the procedure. |
| 4 | Rinse the thermometer under cold running water and dry with cotton swab. | The spirit on the thermometer is an irritant to the mucous membrane. |
| 5 | Place thermometer in axilla for 3-5 min. | For accurate recording. |
| 6 | Remove and wipe the thermometer with the same cotton from stem to bulb and read. | Cleaning from least to most contaminated area prevents spread of microorganisms. |
| 7 | Return to the work area. Wrap the thermometer in cotton pledget with soap until completion of care. | |
| 8 | After, providing treatment and care, wash hands again. | Prevents contamination. |
| 9 | Remove the thermometer from the pledget using spiral motion downward using friction to clean the thermometer. | Spiral motion and friction helps to remove the dirt and microorganisms from the thermometer. |
| 10 | Rinse under running water and dry. Wipe the thermometer with spirit from bulb to stem. | Wiping from more clean to less clean area prevents contamination. |
| 11 | Wipe the outer surface of spirit bottle and replace into the top compartment after washing hands. | Prevents contamination of the bag. |
| 12 | Close the bag. Record the temperature in the nurses dairy. | |

# 15.8A: ESTIMATION OF HEMOGLOBIN AT HOME USING HAEMOGLOBINOMETER

## DEFINITION

Estimating the amount of hemoglobin, a conjugated protein present inside the RBC by using a hemoglobinometer, expressed in gram percentage.

## ARTICLES

1. Hemoglobinometer
2. N/10 hydrochloric acid solution
3. Filler
4. Capillary pipette
5. Hemoglobin meter tube
6. Water pipette
7. Disposale lancet
8. Alcohol swabs

## PROCEDURE

| | Nursing action | Rationale |
|---|---|---|
| 1 | Identify the person in need of hemoglobin estimation at home and assess the situation. | Determines the appropriateness of the procedure. |
| 2 | Provide explanation about the need of procedure and how it will be performed. | Promotes acceptance of procedure and reduces anxiety. |
| 3 | Assemble articles on a clean surface | Facilitates safe performance of procedure. |
| 4 | Wash and dry hands following principles of bag technique | Avoids chances of contamination of articles. |
| 5 | Fill the graduated measuring tube up to bottom graduation line with N/10 hydrochloric acid | Accuracy in use of solutions ensures accuracy in results. |
| 6 | Clean fingertip with alcohol and and prick with a lancet. | Fingertip is highly vascular. Proper cleaning reduces risk of infection. |
| 7. | Wait for a drop of blood to form at the fingertip. | |
| 8 | Suck blood into the capillary pipette precisely up to the mark, wipe the pipette point and blow the blood into the measuring tube. | Accuracy in amount of blood taken ensures correct dilution and hence accurate results. |
| 9 | Achieve good mixture of the liquid by repeated suction and blowing or using a stirrer. The mixture will be dark brown and clear after about one minute | Ensures uniformity through out the mixture. |
| 10 | Add water by means of the water pipette and mix with the glass stirrer until the colour of the solution matches the color of the test rods. | |
| 11 | Read the result in diffused day light exactly 3 minutes after adding blood to the hydrochloric acid | |
| 12 | Record the result in the family folder Normal values: The value of Hb in blood is expressed in gm per 100 ml of blood, i.e. in gm% Male: 14 – 17 gm% Female: 12 - 16 gm% | |

# 15.8B: ESTIMATION OF HEMOGLOBIN LEVEL USING HEMOGLOBIN TESTING PAPER

## DEFINITION

Estimating the level hemoglobin in blood using hemoglobin testing paper.

## PURPOSE

1. To determine the amount of hemoglobin in blood
2. To monitor hemoglobin level for patients on treatment for anemia
3. To determine the level in clients prone to anemias, e.g. pregnant and lactating mothers.

## ARTICLES

1. Hemoglobin testing paper
2. Standardized tint color chart (Hemoglobin scale by Dr. Tallovist)
3. Disposable lancet
4. Alcohol swabs.

## PROCEDURE

| | Nursing action | Rationale |
|---|---|---|
| 1 | Identify the person in need of hemoglobin estimation at home and assess the situation. | Determines the appropriateness of the procedure. |
| 2 | Provide explanation about the need of procedure and how it will be performed. | Promotes acceptance of procedure and reduces anxiety. |
| 3 | Assemble articles on a clean surface. | Facilitates safe performane of procedure. |
| 4 | Wash and dry hands following principles of bag technique. Don gloves. | Avoids chances of contamination of articles |
| 5 | Clean thoroughly fingertip with alcohol and prick with a lancet. | Fingertip is highly vasular. Proper leaning reduces risk of infection. |
| 6 | Place a drop of blood on the testing paper and wait for few seconds. | Allows time for absorption of blood by the paper. |
| 7 | Apply pressure over puncture site with cotton ball untill bleeding stops. | |
| 8 | Compare the testing paper with standardized color chart. | Helps to ascertain the percentage of hemoglobin. |
| 9 | Inform the patient and record the result in the family folder | |
| 10 | Clean and replaec the articles, place the used lancent in a puncture proof container and carry it to health center for appropriate disposal. | |
| 11 | Remove gloves and wash hands. | |

## SPECIAL POINTS

Read the test results preferably in day light.

# 15.9: COLLECTING BLOOD FOR PERIPHERAL SMEAR

## DEFINITION

Obtaining a small sample of blood by skin puncture for peripheral smear.

## PURPOSES

1. To detect malarial parasites.
2. To detect blood cell abnormalities.

## ARTICLES

1. Disposable lancet.
2. Pipette and tubing.
3. Slides.
4. Cotton swabs/Alcohol prep pads.
5. Alcohol.
6. Disposable gloves.
7. Laboratory forms

## PROCEDURE

| | Nursing Action | Rationale |
|---|---|---|
| 1 | Identify the patient, who needs a peripheral smear done | |
| 2 | Give explanation to patient about the procedure | Obtains patient's co-operation and consent |
| 3 | Assemble articles on a clean surface | Facilitates safe performance of procedure |
| 4 | Wash and dry hands following principles of bag technique | Avoids contamination of articles |
| 5 | Don gloves | Offers protection from possible exposure to blood. |
| 6 | Cleanse site (ball of finger) with alcohol and dry with sterile cotton swab | If any alcohol remains, it will alter red cell morphology. Blood will not collect into a compact drop, but will run down the finger if it is not dry. |
| 7 | Prick the skin sharply and quickly with sterile, disposable lancet | Pricking the skin sharply and quickly minimizes pain during procedure and helps to obtain a flowing sample. |
| 8 | Release pressure on the finger, wipe off the first drop of blood | Epithelial and endothelial cells may be found in the first drop of blood and may render the count inadequate. |
| 9 | Allow the blood to flow freely with an adequate puncture. | Pressing out the blood dilutes it with tissue fluid. |
| 10 | Obtain the blood sample, fill the pipette and make blood smears on the slides<br>a. Thin smear<br>  • Put a drop of fresh blood on the middle of the slide.<br>  • Use another slide to spread the blood drop along the slide.<br>  • Leave the film to dry. Do not blow on it.<br>b. Thick smear<br>  • Put three drops of fresh blood on the left hand quarter of the slide | |

*Contd...*

*Contd...*

| | |
|---|---|
| | • With the corner of another slide mix the blood and smear it in a round form about 1 cm in diameter.<br>• Leave the film to dry. Do not blow on it or shake the slide. |
| 11. | Apply pressure over the puncture site with a dry cotton ball until bleeding stops. |
| 12 | When the film is dry, label the slide wrap it and dispatch to laboratory. |
| 13. | Remove gloves, wash hands. |

# 15.10: DRESSING A WOUND AT HOME

## DEFINITION

Cleansing a wound using aseptic technique for the purpose of promoting healing and preventing infections in the home setting.

## PURPOSES

1. To remove and dispose off soiled dressing to prevent spread of infection.
2. To cleanse area around the wound to prevent additional infection.
3. To apply sterile dressings to promote healing.
4. To support or splint the wound site.
5. To promote thermal insulation to the wound surface.
6. To provide for maintenance of high humidity between the wound and dressing.
7. To promote physical, psychological and aesthetic comfort.

## PRINCIPLES

1. Everything that comes in contact with a wound must be sterilized in the most effective way consistent with facilities in the home, school, industry or health center.
2. Hands must be thoroughly washed when handling equipment before dressing the wound.
3. When cleaning a wound, clean from the least contaminated area to the more contaminated area.
4. Boil instruments, cotton (or) gauze at the same time to save fuel. Boil instruments vigorously for 5 minutes in a closed vessel.

## ARTICLES

1. Sterile dressings
2. Scissors
3. Artery forcep
4. Dissecting forceps
5. Cotton swabs
6. A bowl/basin for boiling instruments and supplies
7. A small bowl for sterile cleansing solution
8. Kidney tray – for collecting soiled instruments
9. Paper bags – for soiled swabs and gauze
10. Antiseptic lotion
11. A plate which is boiled to use as a sterile field.

## PROCEDURE

| | Nursing action | Rationale |
|---|---|---|
| 1 | Identify the patient who requires wound dressing and the type of dressing to be performed. | Ensures that right procedure is done for right patient. |
| 2 | Explain to patient and family about the importance of the procedure, how it is performed and how they have to cooperate. | Obtains confidence of patient and family and ensures cooperation. |
| 3 | Spread the paper, place bag in a suitable area and take out soap and brush for handwashing. | |

*Contd...*

*Contd...*

| | | |
|---|---|---|
| 4 | Wash hands and dry | |
| 5. | Open the bag and assemble all the required articles at the bedside either on a box, chair (or) table. | Saves time and helps in continuing the procedure without any hassle. |
| 6. | The work area may be arranged while the instruments are boiling. | |
| 7. | Remove bandage and outer dressing with fingers (or) forceps and discard it in a proper receptacle. | Soiled dressing are contaminated. |
| 8. | Wash hands thoroughly with soap, water and nail brush. | Prevents risk of contamination of wound. |
| 9. | Create a sterile field by keeping sterile articles in the bowl/basin used for boiling or plate, which is sterilized. | Reduces risk of contamination of articles. |
| 10. | Pour the cleaning solution into the small bowl. | |
| 11. | Clean the wound with cotton swab dipped in cleaning solution (normal saline) using artery forceps<br>a. For surgical wounds clean from center to periphery.<br>b. For infected wounds clean from periphery to center.<br>Clean using circular strokes, use one swab for one stroke. | Moving from a more clean area to less clean area reduces risk of contamination. |
| 12. | Apply medication as directed in the standing order with a cotton applicator. | Promotes healing. |
| 13. | Apply sterile dressing and fasten it with bandage. | Prevents contamination and promotes healing. |
| 14. | Explain the condition of wound to the patient/relatives and also provide instructions regarding care, rest, exercise and diet. | Promotes good practices from patient and family. |
| 15. | Record the procedure, condition of wound and medication used. | Record is a legal document. |
| 16. | Wrap soiled dressing and burn. | |
| 17. | Wash used instruments and bowls with soap and water, rinse and boil for 5 minutes. | |
| 18. | Wash hands and return clean boiled instruments to the nurse's bag. | |

## 15.11(A): BABY BATH (TUB BATH)

## DEFINITION

Cleaning the skin of the baby for promoting hygiene and comfort in the home setting.

## ARTICLES

| | | |
|---|---|---|
| 1. | Tub | : 1 No (plastic/steel) |
| 2. | Jugs | : 2 No (hot and cold water) |
| 3. | Towel | |
| 4. | Cotton swabs | |
| 5. | Soap in soap dish | |
| 6. | Cotton buds | |
| 7. | Baby clothes | |

## PROCEDURE

| | Nursing action | Rationale |
|---|---|---|
| 1. | Explain procedure to the mother and encourage her participation. | |
| 2. | Pour water into the tub and adjust the temperature by checking with the elbow (or) dorsal side of palm. | Prevents chances of scalding or hypothermia. |
| 3. | Undress the baby. | |
| 4. | Place the head of the baby on your non-dominant palm and support the body with the forearm and elbow | Safe guards the baby from slipping. |
| 5. | Close ears with the thumb and middle finger of the non-dominant hand. | Prevents entry of water into the ear. |
| 6. | Wet hair and apply soap/shampoo and gently wash the scalp. Rinse with water and dry hair with towel. | Drying immediately prevents risk of hypothermia. |
| 7. | Wipe the eyes from inner to outer canthus with cotton swab. Wash the face with watch and pat dry. | Wiping eyes from inner canthus to outer canthus prevents entry of debris and microorganisms into the lacrimal duct. |
| 8. | Place the baby into the tub with shoulders, neck and head supported by the non-dominant hand and the trunk and legs in water, wet the baby's neck, chest, hands, abdomen, legs and perineum. For cleaning back and buttocks transfer the baby to the other hand in such a way that neck and chest are supported over the palm, holding the baby securely. | |
| 9. | Apply soap, concentrating on skin folds and rinse with water. | |
| 10. | Spread the towel over a flat surface. Place the baby on it and dry . | |
| 11. | With the swab stick wipe the inner and outer circle of cord at site of insertion | |
| 12. | Dress the baby | |
| 13. | Hand over baby to the mother for feeding. | |

## SPECIAL NOTE

Advise mother not to bathe the baby within one hour of feeding.

## 15.11(B): LAP/LEG BATH

### DEFINITION

Bathing a baby by placing him on the legs in a home setting which is the traditional method used in bathing a baby at home in rural communities.

### PURPOSES

1. To clean the body off dirt and bacteria.
2. To increase elimination through the skin
3. To stimulate circulation
4. To regulate body temperature
5. To induce sleep
6. To promote comfort to the baby

### ARTICLES REQUIRED

1. Hot water [ temperature 90 – 100 degree F (32 . 2 to 37.8 degree C)]
2. Tepid water
3. Buckets – 2
4. Mug
5. Towels – 2
6. Mild soap
7. Hair oil
8. Swab sticks – 4
9. Cotton balls
10. K-basin
11. Thermometer
12. Disinfectant
13. Clean clothes
14. Low stool
15. Apron

### PROCEDURE

| | Nursing action | Rationale |
|---|---|---|
| 1 | Wash hands | Prevents transmission of infection |
| 2 | Collect articles from the community bag that are needed for bath like<br>a. Thermometer<br>b. Cotton balls<br>c. Disinfectant<br>d. Swab sticks<br>e. K-basin<br>f. Apron | |
| 3 | Place the articles on a clean paper | Avoids contamination of articles |
| 4 | Collect articles from the mother as follows<br>a. Clean clothes<br>b. Baby soap | |

*Contd...*

*Contd...*

| | | |
|---|---|---|
| | c. Towels – 2 | |
| | d. Hair oil | |
| | e. Low stool | |
| 5 | Put on the apron | Protects the nurse's uniform from soiling |
| 6 | Wash hands and check the temperature of the baby (axillary temperature). | Alterations in body temperature indicates alteration in thermo-regulation |
| 7 | Mix hot and cold water in the bucket | Temperature is maintained between 90-100 degree F |
| 8 | Undress the baby | |
| 9 | Swaddle wrap the baby . | Prevents hypothermia |
| 10 | Remove bindi/kajal using hair oil | |
| 11 | Sit on the low stool with knees flexed | |
| 12 | Wipe both eyes from inner canthus to outer canthus using cotton balls. One cotton ball for each eye. | |
| 13 | Clean the nostrils and ears using cotton wisps. | Avoids chances of injury to mucous membrane. |
| 14 | Wet face with water and wipe off dirt | No soap is used on face. |
| 15 | Wipe face dry using towel. | |
| 16 | Hold the baby with the non-dominant hand and use the dominant hand to pour water on scalp and apply soap. | |
| 17 | Wet hair and apply soap gently. | |
| 18 | Pour water over scalp and rinse hair thoroughly | |
| 19 | Wipe and dry the hair immediately using another towel | Heat is lost by conduction, convection and radiation |
| 20 | Unwrap the baby and place him over your extended legs with baby facing upward (supine). | |
| 21 | Support the baby with your non-dominant hand and use your dominant hand to pour water and apply soap on the body. | |
| 22 | Apply soap over the dorsal surface of the baby, paying attention to the neck, axilla, groin and genitalia. | |
| 23 | Avoid applying soap over the palms and soles of the baby. | Avoids chances of the baby putting soapy fingers in mouth. |
| 24 | Pour water and wash off soap. | |
| 25 | Place the baby facing downward over your legs (prone). Ensure head is turned to one side. | |
| 26 | Apply soap over the back, buttocks and legs, paying attention to the gluteal folds. | |
| 27 | Pour water and wash off soap | |
| 28 | Dry the baby using dry towel. | |
| 29 | Put on clean clothes | |
| 30 | Swaddle wrap the baby | Promotes comfort for the baby. |
| 31 | Hand over the baby to the mother | |
| 32 | Wash hands and replace articles | |
| 33 | Record the time and type of bath given and any significant findings noted. | |

# 15.12: CONDUCTING A DOMICILIARY DELIVERY

## DEFINITION

Conducting a vaginal delivery in the home of a pregnant woman who has had a normal obstetrical history.

## CONTRAINDICATIONS

Mothers with the following characteristics are regarded as-"high-risks" and contraindicated for domiciliary delivery.
1. Elderly primi (30 years and over)
2. Malpresentations, such as breech, transverse lie
3. Antepartum hemorrhage, threatened abortion
4. Pre-eclampsia and eclampsia
5. Anemia
6. Twins, hydramnios
7. Previous stillbirth, intrauterine death
8. Elderly grand multiparas
9. History of previous caesarian section
10. Pregnancy associated with general diseases such as heart disease, renal disease, diabetes, tuberculosis, etc.

## ARTICLES NEEDED

*Requirements for baby:*
1. Adequate clothes
2. Cotton wool or small pieces of clean, soft, old rag
3. Cradle with firm bottom

*Preparation for confinement:*
1. Newspapers or jute sacks (washed and sun dried)
2. Chula (stove)
3. Large container to be used as sterilizer
4. Linen—properly prepared and in adequate quantity
5. For mothers—sanitary towels, clean rags that have been washed, and sundried
6. Bed covering
7. Specially scrubbed bed, floor canvas or clean mat
8. Glass of water
9. Midwifery bag containing
    i. Plastic bag, with plastic apron and sheet.
    ii. Soap, nail brush and towel in a waterproof bag.
    iii. Kidney tray—1
    iv. Bowls (lotion)— 2
    v. Artery forceps— 2
    vi. Dissecting forceps—2
    vii. Scissors—1 pair
    viii. Gloves—1 pair
    ix. Disposable syringe—1
    x. Complete set of enema can with connection-1
    xi. Urethral catheter (rubber)—1
    xii. Mucus extractor—1
    xiii. Spring balance—1
    xiv. Oral thermometer—1

 xv.  Rectal thermometer—1
 xvi.  Stock of cotton for making boiled swabs
 xvii.  Sterile gauze pieces for cord dressing, mouth wipes
xviii.  Dettol—1 bottle
 xix.  Spirit—1 bottle
 xx.  Methergine or ergometrine—1
 xxi.  Fetoscope—1
 xxii.  Measuring tape—1
xxiii.  Spigmomanometer
10. Mothers antenatal check up record.

## PROCEDURE

**First stage of labor**

| | | |
|---|---|---|
| 1 | Greet the family and ascertain details regarding duration of labor contractions. | Helps in promoting family compliance and obtains necessary data. |
| 2 | Place the midwifery bag on a sheet of paper or on an elevated surface (box or stool) in the confinement room | Prevents contamination. |
| 3 | Place your watch and other personal belongings in a convient safe place. | |
| 4 | Ask the family to prepare boiling water. | |
| 5 | Take out soap and towel from midwifery bag. | |
| 6 | Wash hands thoroughly under running water and pat dry. | Prevents infection. |
| 7 | Put on the apron. Prepare the mother for examination. | Protects the nurse from soiling by mother's body fluids. |
| 8 | Examine the mother–palpate abdomen and ascertain fetal lie, presentation and position, assess for fetal heart rate. Observe nature of contraction. Enquire about bowel movement, when urine was last passed etc. If the mother is in first stage and membranes are intact give enema, examine the urine and take blood pressure. | Provides data to plan for getting the necessary articles ready. Helps to screen for immediate complications Enema stimulates uterine contraction. |
| 9 | Wash hands and take out the necessary equipments from bag and put them in a covered container and boil for 20 min. a. Enamel bowls, 2 kidney trays, 2 covered basins. b. A pair of artery forceps, scissors, 1 teaspoon, cord tie. | Boiling disinfects the articles and thereby prevents chances of contamination. |
| 10 | Boil eye dropper and cotton swab (if required) separately. | |
| 11 | Boil catheter separately | |
| 12 | Take mother's temperature, pulse blood pressure etc. | An elevation of values obtained indicates infection. |
| 13 | Watch the progress of labor and give sufficient nourishment (clear fluids only). | Solid foods may induce vomiting and clear fluids provide energy for labor and prevents dehydration. |
| 14 | Prepare to receive baby. | |

**Second stage of labor**

| | | |
|---|---|---|
| 1 | Wash hands and put on mask | Protects the nurse from contamination by body fluids |
| 2 | Set up articles on newspapers for conducting delivery. | |
| 3 | Prepare about a pint of dettol lotion 2% | |

*Contd...*

*Contd...*

| 4 | Take a sterile bowl, artery forceps, sterile swabs and prepare for perineal care. | Prevents mother from acquiring ascending infections. |
|---|---|---|
| 5 | Place the mother in a comfortable position for delivery and bring mother down towards foot end of bed leaving enough space for delivering baby. | Lithotomy position is preferred for easy delivery of baby. |
| 6 | Scrub hands thoroughly for about three minutes using any germicide. Don gloves. | Scrubbing reduces the bacterial count on hands. |
| 7 | Swab the perineal area with dettol lotion. Swab away from vaginal orifice | |
| 8 | a. Give an episiotomy if required, when there is bulging, thinned perineum during uterine contraction or just prior to crowning.<br>b. Support perineum with a sterile pad and deliver the head allowing for descend of the fetus | Good support applied at the perineum prevents chances of perineal tear. |
| 9 | Soon after the baby's head is delivered, clean the eyes, mouth and nose to remove mucus and if needed suck out mucus using a mucus extractor. | Mucus can be aspirated by the baby leading to respiratory arrest. |
| 10 | Deliver the body of the fetus after restitution and external rotation of the head is completed. | |
| 11 | Clamp the cord and separate the baby from mother by cutting the cord with scissors between two clamps. | |

**Third stage of labor**

| 1 | Keep a kidney tray at the base of perineum to receive placenta | |
|---|---|---|
| 2 | Watch for signs of separation of placenta and deliver it using counter traction. | Forceful separation of placenta can lead to incomplete expulsion of placenta. |
| 3 | After the placenta and membranes are expelled examine them for normalcy and completeness. | Placental examination is important to rule out any abnormalities |
| 4 | Rinse hands and clean perineum. Examine the labia and perineum for lacerations or tears. | Any tear or laceration should be repaired at the earliest to prevent further complications. |
| 5 | Massage the uterus to make it contract and for expulsion of any retained blood clots. | |
| 6 | Suture episiotomy layer by layer if one was made. | |
| 7 | Clean the vulva and surrounding area with antiseptic solution and place perineal pad. Straighten mother's leg's, cross them and make her comfortable. Clean and replace articles. | Crossing legs reduces risk of bleeding. |
| 8 | Remove gloves and wash hands thoroughly | |
| 9 | Take the mother's temperature pulse and respiration | An alteration of TPR denotes infection, PPH or shock |
| 10 | Assemble all the articles wash them and boil and replace in the midwifery bag. | |
| 11 | Examine the mother carefully before leaving the home for signs and symptoms of postpartum bleeding. | |
| 12 | Clean the baby off any blood stains or vaginal secretions. | |
| 13 | Wrap the baby and keep the baby warm. | |
| 14 | Record the details of delivery, and condition of mother and baby. | |

# Appendices

## APPENDIX 1: NURSING HEALTH HISTORY FORMAT

Date of Health History_____

**I   Biographical data**

**Name :**_____**Age**:_____ **Sex:M/F**

Address:—_____
_____
_____
_____

Hospital No : _____Ward_____:_____Bed No._____

Date of Admission:_____Language spoken_____

Name of Family Member/Significant other :_____

Relationship with client:_____

Address ( If same as of client write same)_____
_____
_____
_____

Marital Status_____ Religion_____

Educational Status_____Occupation_____

Income:_____

Source of Health Care: _____
(Family physician, Private Hospital, PHC, Ayurveda,Homeo or other system of medicine)

Diagnosis_____

**II   Patient's reason for seeking admission**

_____
_____
_____

**III History of present illness**
a.   (Symptoms, Onset, Duration, Sudden/Gradual, Precipitating factors, Relief measures)
     write in narrative form in order of occurrence including the points given in bracket

_____
_____
_____

     Details of medications taken for present symptoms

_____
_____
_____

**IV Past health history**

a. Past illnesses and treatment:

_____
_____
_____

b. Previous hospitalization:

_____
_____
_____

c. Surgeries:

_____
_____
_____

d. Allergies:

_____
_____
_____

e. Menstruation: Regular/Irregular                          LMP:_____
              Age at Menarche:_____Menopause_____

f. Immunization:

_____
_____
_____

g. **Habits** (include if patient smokes, uses alcohol or drugs, chews betel leaves etc.)

_____
_____
_____

h. Current medications

_____
_____
_____

i. Sleeping pattern:

_____
_____

j. Exercise pattern:

_____
_____
_____

k. Nutritional pattern: Vegetarian/non-vegetarian/special diets/ other details (24 hours diet pattern)

_____
_____
_____

l. Work pattern:

_____
_____
_____

**V  Family history**

_____
_____
_____

a.  History of chronic illnesses (include diabetes mellitus, hypertension, coronary artery diseases, renal diseases, psychiatric illness, cancer etc.)

_____
_____
_____

b.  History of any recent death in the family

_____
_____
_____

c.  History of any communicable disease in the family

_____
_____
_____

d.  Any other significant data

_____
_____
_____

**VI Environmental history**
a.  Environmental hygiene_____
b.  Drinking water_____
c.  Environmental pollution_____
d.  Disposal of excreta_____
e.  Presence of flies/ Mosquitoes/Rodents:_____

**VII Psychosocial history**
a.  Languages spoken_____
b.  Social support systems present_____
c.  Developmental stage_____
d.  Any psychological stressors present_____

**VIII  REVIEW OF SYSTEMS**
a.  **Head**
   Headache _____   Dizziness _____
   Convulsions _____

b.  **Eyes**
   Glasses/contact lens: _____   Blurring of vision_____
   Diplopia _____   Pain: _____
   Inflammation: _____   Watering/Discharge _____

c.  **Ears**
   Hearing  impairment: _____   Hearing aid _____
   Pain _____   Discharge _____
   Tinnitus _____   Loss of balance _____

d.  **Nose**
   Discharge _____   Frequency of URI _____
   Allergies _____   Sinusitis _____
   Polyp _____   Bleeding_____

**Appendices**

**e. Throat & mouth**
Dysphagia _____  Inflammation _____
Dental caries _____  Lesions _____
Halitosis _____  Speech disorder _____
Pain _____  Brushing habits _____

**f. Respiratory**
Cough _____  Sputum _____
Dyspnea _____  Dyspnea on exertion _____
Activity intolerance _____  Pain related to breathing _____
Hemoptysis _____

**g. Circulation**
Pain _____  Palpitation _____
Edema _____  Numbness _____
Change in color _____  Syncope _____
Dizziness _____  Paroxysmal nocturnal dyspnea _____

**h. Nutritional**
Appetite _____  Nausea _____
Vomiting _____  Pain related to eating _____
Dysphagia _____

**i. Elimination:** Normal bowel pattern/bladder pattern
Constipation _____  Incontinence _____
Diarrhea _____  Infection _____
Melena _____  Hematuria _____
Any surgeries _____  Presence of catheters _____

**j. Reproductive**
No of pregnancy _____  No. of live children _____
Bleeding _____  Vaginal discharge _____
Infection _____  Pain _____

**k. Neurological**
Confusion _____  Convulsions _____
Weakness _____  Loss of strength _____
Paralysis _____  Changes in sensation _____
Incoordination _____  Headaches _____
Tingling/Pricking _____  Pain _____
Memory _____

**l. Musculoskeletal system:**
Pain _____  Stiffness _____
Joint movement _____  Muscle strength _____
Posture _____  Gait _____
Weakness _____  Changes in ADL _____

**m. Skin**
Rashes _____  Lesions _____
Pallor _____  Texture _____
Turgor _____  Color _____
Temperature _____

( Include any other symptoms reported by patient other than those mentioned)

# APPENDIX 2: LATIN TERMS USED IN MEDICATION ORDERS

## Time and frequency of medication administration

| | | |
|---|---|---|
| ac | = ante cibos | = before meals |
| pc | = post cibos | = after meals |
| b.d or bid | = bis in die | = twice a day |
| H.S | = hora somni | = at bed time |
| Noct | = nocte | = night |
| o.d | | = once a day |
| p.r.n | = proarenate | = when required |
| s.o.s | = sli opus sit | = if needed |
| stat | = statim | = at once |
| t.id/t d s | = ter in die | = three times a day |
| q.i.d | = quartuor die | = four times a day |
| q | = quoque | = each/every |
| q.4.h | | = every four hours |
| q. 6. H | | = every six hours |
| qh/q h | | = every hour |
| q. am | | = every morning |
| q.o.d | | = every other day |
| qs | | = sufficient quantity |
| ad.lib | | = freely as desired |
| dil | | = dilute, dissolve |

## Amount to be given

| | |
|---|---|
| gr | = Grain |
| Gm/g/gm | = Gram |
| gtt | = Drops |
| ss or s̄s̄ | = one half |

## Form of medication

| | | |
|---|---|---|
| Cap | = Capsule | |
| Tab | = Tablet | |
| Inj | = Injection | |
| Mist | = Mixture | |
| Syr | = Syrup | |
| Susp | = Suspension | |
| Tr/Tinct | = Tincture | |
| Ung | = Ointment | |
| Oc | = Occulentum | = eye ointment |
| Collyr | = Collyrium | = eye lotion |
| Comp | = Compound | |
| Elix | = Elixir | |
| Supp | = Suppository | |
| Pulv | = Powder | |
| aq | = aqueous | |

## Where to administer

| | | |
|---|---|---|
| Aur | = Qurist | = ear |
| O.D | = Oculam Dexter | = right eye |
| O.S | = Oculam Sinister | = left eye |
| P.O | = per os | = orally |
| OS | = Orifice | |
| OU | | = Both eyes |
| IM | | = intramuscular |
| IV | | = intravenous |
| ID | | = intradermal |
| SC | | = subcutaneous |

## APPENDIX 3: WEIGHTS AND MEASUREMENTS

**Weights**

| | |
|---|---|
| 8 drams | 1 ounce |
| 12 ounces | 1 pound |

**Fluid volume**

| | |
|---|---|
| 60 minims | 1 fluid dram |
| 8 fluid drams | 1 fluid ounce |
| 20 fluid ounces | 1 pint |
| 2 pints | 1 quart ( 1000 ml) |
| 8 pints | 1 gallon |

**Weights**

| | |
|---|---|
| 1000 micrograms ( Mcg) | 1 milligram ( mg) |
| 1000 milligrams (Mg) | 1 gram ( gm) |
| 1000 grams (g) | 1 kilogram (kg) |
| 1 kilogram (kg) | 2.2 pounds (lbs) |

**Approximate equivalents**
**Weights**

| | |
|---|---|
| 1 grain | 60 milligram (mg) |
| 1 dram | 4 gram ( g) |
| 1 ounce | 30 gram (g) |
| 1 pound | 375 gram ( g) |
| 1 milligram | 1/60 grains ( gr) |

**Volume**

| | |
|---|---|
| 1 milliliter (ml) | 15 or 16 minims |
| | 15 or 16 drops |
| 1 liter | 35 fluid ounces |
| 1 fluid ounce | 30 ml |
| 1 fluid dram | 4 ml |
| 1 gallon | 4.5 liter |
| 1 minim | 0.04 ml = 1 drop |
| 1 pint | 500 ml. |

**Household measurements:**

| | |
|---|---|
| 1 teaspoonfull | 4 or 5 ml |
| | 1 fluid dram |
| | 60 drops |
| 1 table spoonfull | 15 ml |
| | 4 drams |
| | 1/2 fluid ounce. |

## APPENDIX 4: DRUG CALCULATION FORMULAE

1. **Fried's formula : Infant's dosage ( < 1 year )**

$$\frac{\text{Infant's age in months}}{150 \text{ months}} \times \text{Average adult dose}$$

2. **Young's rule : child dosage ( 1 –12 years)**

$$\frac{\text{Child's age in years}}{\text{Child's age in years} + 12} \times \text{Average adult dose}$$

3. **Clark's rule :**

$$\frac{\text{Weight of the child in pounds}}{150 \text{ pounds}} \times \text{Average adult dose}$$

4. **Surface area rule :**

$$\frac{\text{Surface area of the child in (sq.m)}}{1.73} \times \text{Average adult dose}$$

5. **Parenteral dosage**

$$\frac{\text{Dose ordered}}{\text{Dose available}} \times \text{Quantity in hand(ml)} = \text{volume to be given}$$

6. **Intravenous fluid flow rate**

$$\frac{\text{Total volume to be infused (ml)}}{\text{Total time of infusion in minutes}} \times \text{drops factor} = \text{Flow rate/min}$$

7. **Insulin dosage =**

$$\frac{\text{What we want}}{\text{What we have}} \times \text{Number of divisions on the given syringe.}$$

8. **Ordered dose of medication in Microgram/min =**

$$\frac{\text{Vol to be infused}}{\text{Wt (kg)} \times 60 \text{ min}} \times \text{concentration}$$

9. **Concentration =**

$$\frac{\text{Dose of medication (mg)}}{\text{Volume to be infused}} \times 1000$$

# APPENDIX 5: ABBREVIATIONS

| S.No. | Description | Abbreviations/Symbols |
|---|---|---|
| 1 | Less than | < |
| 2 | Greater than | > |
| 3 | Liter | l |
| 4 | Milliequivalent | mEq |
| 5 | Milliliter | ml |
| 6 | Deciliter | dl |
| 7 | Millimeter of mercury | mmHg |
| 8 | Femtoliter | fl |
| 9 | Millimeter | mm |
| 10 | Gram | g |
| 11 | Microgram | μg |
| 12 | Nanogram | ng |
| 13 | Picogram | pg |
| 14 | Liter | l |
| 15 | International unit | IU |
| 16 | Milliosmole | m Osm |
| 17 | Unit | U |
| 18 | Millimole | mmol |
| 19 | nanomole | nmol |
| 20 | picomole | Pmol |
| 21 | kilopascal | kPa |
| 22 | microkatal | μkat |

## APPENDIX 6: URINE—CHEMISTRY NORMAL VALUES

| Sl. No. | Test | Specimen | Conventional units | Higher | Lower |
|---------|------|----------|--------------------|--------|-------|
| 1 | Acetone | Random | Negative | Diabetes mellitus, high fat and low carbohydrate diets, starvation states. | |
| 2 | Bence Jones protein | Random | Negative | Multiple myeloma, biliary duct obstruction. | |
| 3 | Bilirubin | Random | Negative | Hepatitis | |
| 4 | Calcium | 24 hr | 100-250 mg/day | Bone tumor, hyperparathyroidism | Hypoparathyroidism malabsorption of ca and vit D. |
| 5 | Chloride | 24 hr | 110 – 250 mEq/day | Addison's disease | Burns, excessive perspiration, vomiting, diarrhea, mensturation. |
| 6 | Creatine | 24 hr | < 100 mg/day | Carcinoma of liver, hyperthyroidism, diabetes, infections, burns. | Hypothyroidism |
| 7 | Creatinine | 24 hr | 0.8-2.0 gm/day | Anemia, leukemia, muscular atrophy | Renal disease |
| 8 | Creatinine clearance | 24 hr | 85 – 132 ml/min | | Renal disease |
| 9 | Glucose | Random | Negative | Diabetes mellitus, low renal threshold for glucose resorption, pituitary disorders. | |
| 10 | Hemoglobin (Hb) | Random | Negative | Extensive burns, hemolytic transfusion reaction, glomerulonephritis, hemolytic anemia | |
| 11 | Ketone bodies | 24 hr | 20 – 50 mg/day | Marked ketonuria | |
| 12 | Myoglobin | Random | Negative | Crushing injuries, electric injuries, extreme physical exertion. | |
| 13 | pH | Random | 4.0–8.0 | Chronic renal failure, compensatory phase of alkalosis, vegetarian diet | Compensatory phase of acidosis, dehydration, emphysema. |
| 14 | Phenyl pyruvic acid | Random | Negative | Phenylketonuria | |
| 15 | Protein | 24 hr | < 150 mg /day | Cardiac failure, inflammatory processes of urinary tract, nephritis, nephrosis, toxemia of pregnancy. | |
| 16 | Sodium | 24 hr | 40 – 250 mEq /day | Acute tubular necrosis | Hyponatremia |
| 17 | Specific gravity | Random | 1.003- 1.030 | Albuminuria, dehydration glycosuria | Diabetes insipidus. |
| 18 | Uric acid | 24 hr | 250 – 750 mg/day | Gout, leukemia | Nephritis |
| 19 | Urobilinogen | 24 hr | 0 .5 – 4.0 EU/day | Hemolytic disease, hepatic parenchymal cell damage, liver disease | Complete obstruction of bile duct. |

# APPENDIX 7: HEMATOLOGY—NORMAL VALUES

| Sl. No. | Test | Conventional units | Possible etiology | |
|---|---|---|---|---|
| | | | Higher | Lower |
| 1 | Bleeding time | 3. 0 – 9. 5 min | Defective platelet function, thrombocytopenia | |
| 2 | Activated partial Thromboplastin time (APTT) | 24 – 36 sec | Deficiency of factors I, II, V, VIII, IX and X, XI, XII, hemophilia, liver disease, heparin therapy | |
| 3 | Prothrombin time | 10 – 14 sec | Warfarin therapy, deficiency of factors I, II, V, VII and X. Vitamin K deficiency. Liver disease | |
| 4 | Fibrinogen | 200 – 400 mg/dl | Burns ( after first 36 hr) inflammatory disease | Burns ( during first 36 hr) DIC, severe liver disease |
| 5 | Erythrocyte count Male Female | $4.5 – 6. 0 \times 10^6/\mu l$ $4.0 – 5. 0 \times 10^6/\mu l$ | | |
| 6 | Mean corpuscular Volume (MCV) | 82 – 98 fl | Macrocytic anemia | Microcytic anemia |
| 7 | Mean corpuscular Hemoglobin (MCH) | 27 – 33 pg | Macrocytic anemia | Microcytic anemia |
| 8 | Mean corpuscular hemoglobin Concentration (MCHC) | 32 - 36% | Spherocytosis | Hypochromic anemia |
| 9 | Erythrocyte Sedimentation rate (ESR) Male < 50 yr > 50 yr Female < 50 yr > 50 yr | < 15 mm/hr < 20 mm/hr < 20 mm/hr < 30 mm/hr | <u>Moderate increase:</u> acute hepatitis, myocardial infarction, rheumatoid arthritis. <u>Marked increase:</u> acute and severe bacterial infections, malignancies -Pelvic inflammatory disease. -Dehydration, high altitudes, polycythemia | Malaria, severe liver disease, sickle cell anemia. Anemia hemorrhage, over hydration. |
| 10 | Hematocrit Male Female | 40 - 54% 38 - 47% | COPD, high altitudes, Polycythemia | Anemia, hemorrhage |
| 11 | Hemoglobin Male Female | 13.5 – 18.0 g/dl 12.0 – 16.0 g/dl | | |
| 12 | Glycosylated hemoglobin | 4. 0 - 6. 0 % | Poorly controlled diabetes mellitus | Sickle cell anemia, chronic renal failure, pregnancy. |
| 13 | Platelet count (thrombocytes) | $150 - 400 \times 10^3/\mu l$ | Acute infections, chronic granulocytic leukemia, chronic pancreatitis, cirrhosis, collagen disorders, polycythemia, postsplenectomy | Acute leukemia, DIC, thrombocytopenic purpura |

*Contd...*

*Contd...*

| 14 | White blood cell count (WBC) | $4.0–11.0 \times 10^3/\mu l$ | Inflammatory and infectious processes, leukemia | Aplastic anemia, side effects of chemotherapy and irradiation |
|----|------|------|------|------|
| 15 | Lymphocytes | 20 - 40% | Chronic infections, lymphocytic leukemia, mononucleosis, viral infections. | Corticosteroid therapy whole body irradiation |
| 16 | Monocytes | 4 – 8% | Chronic inflammatory disorders, malaria, monocytic leukemia, acute infections, Hodgkin's disease | |
| 17 | Eosinophils | 0 - 4% | Allergic reactions, eosinophilic and chronic granulocytic leukemia, parasitric disorders, Hodgkin's disease | Corticosteroid therapy |
| 18 | Basophils | 0 - 2 % | Hypothyroidism, ulcerative colitis, myeloproliferative diseases | Hyperthyroidism stress |

# APPENDIX 8: SERUM, PLASMA AND WHOLE BLOOD CHEMISTRIES

| S. No. | Test | Conventional units | Higher | Possible etiology — Lower |
|---|---|---|---|---|
| 1 | Acetone | 0.3–2 .0 mg/dl | Diabetic ketoacidosis, high fat diet, low carbohydrate diet, starvation. | |
| 2 | Albumin | 3.5–5.00 g/dl | Dehydration | Chromic liver disease, malabsorption, malnutrition, nephrotic syndrome, pregnancy. |
| 3 | $\alpha_1$-Fetoprotein | <15 ng/ml | Cancer of testes and ovaries, carcinoma of liver. | |
| 4 | Ammonia | 30–70 µg/dl | Severe liver disease | |
| 5 | Amylase | 0–130 U/ L (method dependent) | Acute and chronic pancreatitis, mumps, perforated ulcers. | Acute alcoholism, cirrhosis of liver, extensive destruction of pancreas. |
| 6 | Bicarbonate | 20–30 mEq/L | Compensated respiratory acidosis, metabolic alkalosis. | Compensated respiratory alkalosis, metabolic acidosis. |
| 7 | Bilurubin Total Indirect (unconjugated) Direct (conjugated) | 0.2–1. 3 mg/dl 0.1–1. 0 mg/dl 0.1–0.3 mg/dl | Biliary obstruction, impaired liver function, hemolytic anemia, pernicious anemia, prolonged fasting. | |
| 8 | Blood gases Arterial pH Venous pH Arterial $pCO_2$ Venous $pCO_2$ Arterial $pO_2$ Venous $pO_2$ | 7.35–7. 45 7.35–7.45 35–45 mmHg 45–52 mmHg 75–100 mmHg 30–50 mmHg | Alkalosis Compensated metabolic alkalosis Respiratory acidosis Administration of high concentration of oxygen | Acidosis Compensated metabolic acidosis Respiratory alkalosis Chronic lung disease decreased Cardiac output |
| 9 | Calcium | 9–11 mg/dl (4.5 –5.5 mEq/L) | Acute osteoporosis, hyperparathyroidism, vitamin-D intoxication, multiple myeloma. | Acute pancreatitis, hypoparathyroidism, liver disease, malabsorption syndrome, renal failure, vitamin D deficiency. |
| 10 | Chloride | 95–105 mEq/L | Metabolic acidosis, respiratory alkalosis, corticosteroid therapy, uremia. | Addison's disease, diarrhea, metabolic alkalosis, respiratory acidosis, vomiting |
| 11 | Cholesterol HDL (high density lipoproteins) Male Female LDL ( low density lipoproteins) | 140–200 mg /dl (Age dependent) > 45 mg/dl > 55 mg/dl < 130 mg/dl | Biliary obstruction, Hypothyroidism, idiopathic hypercholesterolemia, renal disease, uncontrolled diabetes. | Extensive liver disease, hyperthyroidism, malnutrition, corticosteroid therapy. |

*Contd...*

*Contd...*

| 12 | Cortisol | 8 Am : 5 –25 µg/dl<br>8 pm : < 10 µg/dl | Cushing syndrome, pancreatitis, stress | Adrenal insufficiency, panhypopituitary states. |
|----|----------|------------|------------|------------|
| 13 | Creatine | 0. 2–1.0 mg/dl | Active rheumatoid arthritis, biliary obstruction, hyperthyroidism, renal disorders, severe muscle disease. | Diabetes mellitus. |
| 14 | Creatine kinase (CK)<br>Male<br>Female | 15–105 U/L<br>10–80 U/L | Musculoskeletal injury or disease, myocardial infarction, severe myocarditis, exercises, myocarditis numerous intramuscular injections, brain damage. | |
| 15 | CK-MB(CK– 2) | 0 - 9 U/L | Acute myocardial infarction. | |
| 16 | Creatinine | 0.5–1. 5 mg/dl | Severe renal disease | |
| 17 | Glucose<br>Fasting | 70–120 mg/dl | Acute stress, cerebral lesions, Cushing's disease, diabetes mellitus, hyperthyroidism, pancreatic insufficiency. | Addison's disease, hepatic disease, hypothyroidism, insulin overdosage, pancreatic tumor, pituitary hypofunction. |
| 18 | Lactic acid | 5–20 µg/dl | Acidosis, congestive heart failure, shock. | |
| 19 | Lactic dehydrogenase (LDH) | 50–150 U/L | Congestive heart failure, hemolytic disorders, hepatitis, metastatic cancer of liver, myocardial infarction, pernicious anemia, pulmonary embolus, skeletal muscle damage. | |
| 20 | Lipase | 0–160 U/L | Acute pancreatitis, hepatic disorders, perforated peptic ulcer. | |
| 21 | Magnesium | 1.5–2. 5 mEq/L | Addison's disease, hypothyroidism, renal failure. | Chronic alcoholism, hyperparathyroidism, hypoparathyroidism, severe malabsorption, hyperthyroidism |
| 22 | Phosphatase acid | 0–0.6 U/L | Advanced Paget's disease, cancer of prostate, hyperparathyrodism | |
| 23 | Phosphatase alkaline | 30–120 U/L | Bone diseases marked hyperpara-thyroidism, obstruction of biliary system, rickets. | Excessive vitamin D ingestion, hypothyroidism, milk alkali syndrome. |
| 24 | Potassium | 3.5–5. 5 mEq/L | Addison's disease, diabetic ketosis, massive tissue distruction, renal failure. | Cushing syndrome, diarrhea, (severe) diuretic therapy, gastro-intestinal fistula, pyloric obstruction, starvation, vomiting. |
| 25 | Sodium | 135–145 mEq/L | Dehydration, impaired renal function, primary aldosteronism, corticosteroid therapy | Addison's disease, diabetic ketoacidosis, diuretic therapy, excessive loss from gastrointestinal tract, excessive perspiration, water intoxication. |

*Contd...*

*Contd...*

| 26 | Proteins Total | 6.0–8.0 g/dl | Burns, cirrhosis, dehydration | Congenital -agamma globulinemia, liver disease, malabsorption. |
|---|---|---|---|---|
| | Albumin | 3.5–5.0 g/dl | | |
| | Globulin | 2.0–3.5 g/dl | | |
| | Albumin-globulin ratio | 1.5 : 1-2.5 :1 | -Multiple myeloma (globulin fraction) shock and vomiting | Malnutrition, nephrotic syndrome, proteinuria, renal disease, severe burns. |
| 27 | T4 ( thyroxine ) total | 5–12 µg/dl | Hyperthyroidism, thyroiditis | Cretinism, hypothyroidism, myxedema |
| | T4 ( thyroxine) free | 0.8–2 .3 ng/dl | | |
| | T3 uptake | 25 - 35% | Hyperthyroidism, metastatic neoplasms | Hypothyroidism, pregnancy. |
| | T3 ( triodothyronine) | 110–230 ng/dl | Hyperthyroidism | Hypothyroidism. |
| | TSH (thyroid stimulating hormone) | 0.3–5 .4 µU/ml | Myxedema, primary hypothyroidism, Graves' disease. | Secondary hypothyroidism. |
| 28 | Serum glutamic oxaloacetic ( SGOT ) or aspartate aminotransferase (AST). | 7–40 U /L | Liver disease, myocardial infarction, pulmonary infarction, acute hepatitis. | |
| | Serum glutmate pyruvate SGPT or alanine aminotransferase (ALT) | 5–36 U /L | Liver disease, shock | |
| 29 | Triglycerides | 40–150 mg/dl | Diabetes mellitus, hyperlipidemia, hypothyroidism, liver disease | Malnutrition. |
| 30 | Blood urea nitrogen (BUN) | 10–30 mg/dl | Increase in protein catabolism, renal disease, urinary tract infection. | Malnutrition, severe liver damage. |
| 31 | Uric acid | | | |
| | Male | 4. 5–6.5 mg /dl | Gout, gross tissue destruction, high protein weight reduction diet, leukemia, renal failure, eclampsia. | Administration of uricosuric drugs. |
| | Female | 2.5-5.5 mg/dl | | |

## APPENDIX 9: CEREBROSPINAL FLUID ANALYSIS

| Sl. No. | Test | Conventional units | Higher | Lower |
|---|---|---|---|---|
| 1 | Pressure | 60 – 150 mm H$_2$O | Hemorrhage, intracranial tumor, meningitis. | Head injury, spinal tumor, subdural hematoma. |
| 2 | Blood | Negative | Intracranial hemorrhage | |
| 3 | Cell count<br>WBC<br>RBC | <br>0 – 5 cells/μl<br>0 | Inflammations or infections of CNS | |
| 4 | Chloride | 100 – 130 mEq /L | Uremia | Bacterial infections of CNS |
| 5 | Glucose | 40 – 75 mg/dl | Diabetes mellitus, viral infections of CNS. | Bacterial infections and TB of CNS |
| 6 | Protein<br>Lumbar<br>Cisternal<br>Ventricular | <br>15 – 45 mg/dl<br>15 – 25 mg/dl<br>5 – 15 mg/dl | Guillain – Barre syndrome, poliomyelitis, traumatic tap. Syphilis of CNS Acute meningitis, brain tumor, chronic CNS infections, multiple sclerosis. | |

## APPENDIX 10: FECAL ANALYSIS NORMAL VALUES

| Sl. No. | Test | Conventional units | Higher | Lower |
|---|---|---|---|---|
| 1 | Urobilinogen | 30 – 220 mg/100 g of stool | Hemolytic anemia | Complete biliary obstruction. |
| 2 | Mucus | Negative | Mucous colitis, spastic constipation. | ——————— |
| 3 | Pus | Negative | Chronic bacillary dysentery, chronic ulcerative colitis, localized abscessess. | ——————— |
| 4 | Blood | Negative | Anal fissures, hemorrhoids, malignant tumor, peptic ulcer, inflammatory bowel disease | ——————— |
| 5 | Color<br>Brown<br>Clay<br><br>Tarry<br>Red<br>Black | ——————— | <br>Various color depending on diet.<br>Biliary obstruction or presence of barium sulphate.<br>More than 100 ml of blood in GI tract.<br>Blood in large intestine<br>Blood in upper GI tract or iron medication. | ——————— |

## APPENDIX 11: ANTENATAL ASSESSMENT FORMAT

1. Demographic data:
   - Name : _____
   - Age : _____
   - Education : _____
   - Occupation : _____
   - Marital status : _____
   - Years married : _____ Consanguineous: _____
   - Husband's name : _____
   - Age : _____ Occupation: _____
   - Economic status (Family income)

2. Biologic and Environmental history : _____
   - Nutritional status : _____
   - Vegetarian/ Non-vegetarian : _____
   - Sleep and rest : _____
   - Hygiene : _____
   - Exercise : _____

3. Family health history:
   - Cardiovascular : _____
   - Renal : _____
   - Endocrine : _____
   - Neurological : _____
   - Genetic disorders : _____
   - Any other : _____

4. Personal health history:
   - Habits : _____
   - Sleep pattern : _____
   - Bowel pattern : _____
   - Hygiene : _____
   - Allergies : _____
   - Menstrual history: : _____
     Menarche: _____
     Cycles: _____
   - Past medical & surgical history : _____

5. Obstetrical history:
   - Pregnancy induced hypertension : _____
   - Multiple pregnancy : _____
   - Stillbirth/IUD/Abortion : _____
   - Gestational diabetes : _____
   - Previous pregnancies : _____
   - Previous deliveries : _____

6. Present pregnancy:
   - LMP:EDD : _____
   - Obstetric score : _____
   - Minor discomforts of pregnancy : _____
   - Booked/unbooked : _____

7.   Investigations:
- Blood group          : _____  Rh          : _____
- Hemoglobin           : _____  VDRL        : _____
- HIV                  : _____

8.   Examination (General):
- Heart                : _____  Lungs         : _____
- Breasts              : _____  Head and neck : _____
- General condition    : _____  Vulva/vagina  : _____
- Cardiovascular       : _____
- Gastrointestinal     : _____
- Urinary              : _____
- Musculo-skeletal     : _____
- Respiratory          : _____

9.   Obstetrical examination:
- Inspection- palpation and auscultation  : _____
- Fundal height                           : _____
- Presentation:                           : _____  Position:_____ Lie:_____
- Presenting part engaged/not engaged     : _____
- Fetal heart rate                        : _____
- Remarks                                 : _____

10.   Antenatal visit record:

| Date | B.P | Wt in kg | Fundal height in cm | Blood | | Urine | | Presentation | F.H.R | Immunization | Remarks |
|------|-----|----------|---------------------|-------|----|------|------|--------------|--------|--------------|---------|
| | | | | Hb% | Grp | Alb | Sugar | | | | |
| | | | | | | | | | | | |

11.   Treatment and Diet:

12.   Health teaching:

## APPENDIX 12: NEWBORN ASSESSMENT FORMAT

1. Demographic data:
   - Name of baby       : _____
   - Date of birth       : _____
   - Time of birth       : _____
   - Sex       : _____
   - Gestational age       : _____

2. Condition at birth:
   - Apgar score 1 min_____ 5 mins _____
   - Throat suction       : _____
   - Oxygen       : _____
   - Bag and mask ventilation       : _____
   - Endotracheal intubation       : _____
   - Medication (specify)       : _____

3. Physical assessment:
   a. General:
      - Birth weight (Kg)       : _____
      - Length (cm)       : _____
      - Head circumference (cm) : _____
      - Chest circumference (cm) : _____
      - Temperature (axilla)       : _____
      - Heart rate       : _____
      - Respiration       : _____
      - Position       : _____
      - Others       : _____
   b. Activity and skin:
      - Active/Lethargy       : _____
      - Color       : _____
      - Cry       : _____
      - Skin turgor       : _____
      - Rashes       : _____
      - Birth marks       : _____
      - Vernix       : _____
      - Others       : _____
   c. Reflexes:
      - Moro reflex/startle reflex : _____
      - Rooting reflex       : _____
      - Sucking reflex       : _____
      - Grasp reflex       : _____
      - Tonic neck reflex       : _____
      - Stepping/ walking       : _____
      - Blink reflex       : _____
      - Pupillary reflex       : _____

   d. Head and neck:
      - Fontanelles       : _____
      - Sutures       : _____
      - Moulding       : _____
      - Facial features       : _____
      - Eyes       : _____
      - Nose       : _____
      - Ears       : _____
      - Mouth       : _____
      - Others       : _____

4. Thorax:
   - Symmetry       : _____
   - Retractions       : _____
   - Clavicles       : _____
   - Heart sounds       : _____
   - Breath sounds       : _____
   - Respiration       : _____
   - Others       : _____

5. Abdomen:
   - Shape       : _____
   - Feel       : _____
   - Umbilicus       : _____
   - Others       : _____

6. Spine       : _____

7. Extremities:
   - Movement       : _____
   - Length       : _____
   - Digits       : _____
   - Deformities       : _____

8. Genitals       : _____

9. Anus       : _____

# APPENDIX 13: POSTNATAL ASSESSMENT FORMAT

1. Demographic data:
   - Name : _____
   - Age : _____
   - Education : _____
   - Occupation : _____
   - Marital status : _____
   - Years married : _____
                    Consanguinous :
   - Husband's name : _____
   - Age : _____
                    Occupation : _____
   - Economic status (Family income)

2. Biologic and Environmental history :
   - Nutritional status : _____
   - Vegetarian/ Non-vegetarian : _____
   - Sleep and rest : _____
   - Hygiene : _____
   - Exercise : _____

3. Family health history:
   - Cardiovascular : _____
   - Renal : _____
   - Endocrine : _____
   - Neurological : _____
   - Genetic disorders : _____
   - Any other : _____

4. Personal health history:
   - Habits : _____
   - Sleep pattern : _____
   - Bowel pattern : _____
   - Hygiene : _____
   - Allergies : _____
   - Menstrual history: : _____
                    Menarche : _____
                    Cycles : _____

5. Obstetrical history:
   - Pregnancy induced hypertension: _____
   - Multiple pregnancy : _____
   - Stillbirth/IUD/Abortion : _____
   - Gestational diabetes : _____
   - Previous pregnancies : _____
   - Previous deliveries : _____

6. Present pregnancy:
   - LMP:_____ EDD : _____
   - Obstetric score : _____
   - Minor disorders of pregnancy : _____

7. Investigations:
   - Blood group:_____ Rh : _____
   - Hemoglobin:_____ VDRL : _____
   - HIV : _____

8. Birth History:
   - Onset of labor : _____
   - Rupture of membranes : _____
   - Spontaneous : _____
   - Artificial : _____
   - Mode of delivery:
     - Normal vaginal : _____
     - Assisted vaginal : _____
     - Cesarean : _____
   - Date and time of birth : _____
   - Sex of baby : _____
   - Apgar score 1 min_____5 min : _____
   - Birth weight (kg) : _____
   - Duration of labor:
     - 1st stage : _____
     - 2nd stage : _____
     - 3rd stage : _____
   - Blood loss : _____
   - Placenta : _____
     - Weight : _____
     - Complete/incomplete : _____
     - Other abnormalities : _____
   - Perineum : _____
     - Intact : _____
     - Episiotomy : _____
     - Laceration : _____

9. General examination:
   A. Vital signs : _____
      B.P. : _____
      Temperature : _____
      Pulse : _____
      Respiration : _____

   B. General appearance:
      - Skin : _____
      - Head : _____
      - Neck : _____
      - Breasts : _____
      - Nipples : _____
      - Laceration : _____
      - Respiratory system : _____
      - Cardiovascular system : _____
      - Gastrointestinal system : _____
        - Constipation : _____
        - Discomfort : _____
        - Pain : _____

- Genito-urinary system:
  - Uterus:
    - Involution : _____
    - Fundal height : _____
    - Consistency : _____
    - After pains : _____
  - Lochia:
    - Color : _____
    - Amount : _____
    - Odour : _____
  - Perineum: Episiotomy/ Laceration : _____
    - Healing : _____
    - Gaping : _____
    - Hematoma : _____
    - Edema : _____

- Musculoskeletal system:
  - Legs mobility : _____
  - Edema : _____
  - Homan's sign : _____
- Neurological system:
  - Emotional status : _____
  - Reaction to childbirth : _____
  - Adaptation to parenting and care taking : _____

10. Investigations : _____

11. Treatment : _____

12. Breastfeeding : _____

13. Psychological status : _____

## APPENDIX 14: ASSESSMENT OF POSTOPERATIVE CESAREAN SECTION MOTHERS

I. **Demographic data**
   **Mother**
   - Name of mother : _____      Age : _____
   - Address : _____              Hosp No : _____
   - Education : _____            Occupation : _____
   - Duration of marriage : _____  No of living children : _____
   - Age of last child : _____
   - Date of admission : _____    Date of operation : _____
   - Indication for operation : _____
   - Type of anesthesia : _____
   - Operated by : _____          Performed by :
                                           Nurse : _____
                   _____          Assistant nurse : _____

II. **History:**
   a. Family history:
      - Type of family (Joint/Nuclear) : _____
      - Family composition : _____
      - Consanguinous marriage :
   b. Socio-economic history
      - Income per month : _____
      - House (own/rental) : _____
      - Type of house
      - Facilities present : _____
   c. Environmental history:
      - Source of water supply : _____
      - Disposal of waste : _____
      - Any other health hazards : _____
   d. Personal health——history:
      - Habits : _____
      - Sleep pattern : _____
      - Bowel pattern : _____
      - Hygiene : _____
      - Allergies : _____
      - Menstruation (menarche, cycle) : _____
   e. Obstetrical history:
      - Previous pregnancies : _____
      - Previous deliveries : _____
      - Pregnancy induced hypertension :

      - Stillbirth/IUD/Abortion : _____
      - Gestational diabetes : _____
      - Abortions : _____
      - Twins : _____
      - Use of contraceptives : _____
      - Previous cesarean section Indication : _____
      - Any other problems : _____
   f. Present Pregnancy:
      - LMP, EDD : _____
      - Obstetric score : _____
      - Antenatal history : _____
      - Minor disorders : _____

- Any illness associated with pregnancy:
  - Diabetes               : _____
  - Tuberculosis       : _____
  - Blood disorders    : _____
  - Asthma              : _____
  - Heart disease      : _____

g. Present admission details
  - Complaints on admission   : _____
    Contractions/discharge/bleeding/rupture of amniotic sac/fluid leak
  - Investigation findings:
    - *Blood*              : _____
    - Blood group     : _____
    - Rh                : _____
    - Hemoglobin      : _____
    - VDRL           : _____
    - HIV              : _____
    - WBC           : _____
    - RBC            : _____
    - Any other       : _____
    - Urine           : _____
    - Glucose        : _____
    - Albumin        : _____

## History of labor and delivery
  - Onset of labor       : _____
  - Rupture of membranes: spontaneous /  : _____
                             artificial  : _____
  - Type of cesarean section   : _____
  - Date and time of delivery   : _____
  - Sex of baby          : _____
  - Apgar score 1 – minute & 5 minutes  : _____
  - Birth weight (kg)      : _____
  - Duration of labor –
    - 1st stage         : _____
    - 2nd stage        : _____
    - 3rd stage        : _____
  - Blood loss (ml)      : _____
  - Placenta & membranes   : _____

Weight            : _____
Complete/incomplete: _____
Any abnormalities    : _____

## Physical Examination
a. General
  - Appearance: pain/pallor   : _____
  - Pain: Incision site/backache/headache/limbs _____
b. Vital signs
  - B.P.             : _____
  - Temperature      : _____
  - Pulse            : _____
  - Respiration       : _____
c. Respiratory system
  - Breath sounds – Normal   : _____
               Any abnormality   : _____

d.  Cardiovascular system:
    Heart sounds — Normal    : _____
                — Any abnormality   : _____
e.  Gastrointestinal system:
    —Nausea/vomiting    : _____
    — Peristalsis    : _____
    — Abdomen
f.  Urinary system:
    Urine output ( amount in 24 hr )  : _____
    Any abnormality    : _____
g.  Musculoskeletal system:
    Homan's sign    : _____
    Leg cramps    : _____
    Any other    : _____

**Obstetrical examination**
- Bleeding from operated site  : _____
- Uterine contractions  : _____
- Pain:- specify type  : _____
- Postpartum hemorrhage  : _____
- Wound infection  : _____

**Breasts**
Size: Normal  : _____
    Soft  : _____
Symmetry  : _____
Primary/secondary areola  : _____
Nipples: Prominent/depressed/retracted  : _____
    Flat/Cracked/Inverted/Sore  : _____
Milk:  Colostrum/Milk  : _____
    Any abnormality  : _____

**Genitalia**
Appearance
    Normal  : _____
    Edematous  : _____
    Infections  : _____
    Any other  : _____

**Medications**
Analgesics  : _____
Antibiotics  : _____
Laxatives  : _____
Any other  : _____

**Nursing care**  : _____

## APPENDIX 15: ASSESSMENT OF PATIENT WITH GYNECOLOGICAL PROBLEMS

I  **Demographic Data:**
- Name of the patient
- Age
- Education
- Occupation
- Income
- Religion
- Marital status – Duration of marriage/single/widow
- Hospital No
- Date of examination
- Address
- Diagnosis

II  **History:**

a. Family History
- Type of family: Joint/Nuclear
- Family composition
- Genetic/Hereditary disease

b. Socioeconomic history:
- Income/Month
- Type of house: Own/rented
- Social customs/beliefs

c. Environmental history
- Source of water supply
- Disposal of waste
- Any other health hazards

d. Personal health history
- Diet
- Sleep pattern
- Bowel/Bladder pattern
- Allergies
- Hygiene
- Addictions

e. Menstrual history
- Age of menarche
- Menstrual rhythm—Normal/Irregular
- Duration: in days
- Premenstrual discomfort – yes/No
- Dysmenorrhea — yes/No
- Menorrhagia – duration prolonged
- Metrorrhagia – yes/No
- Scanty menstruation –yes/No
- Last menstrual period
- Amenorrhea – primary/secondary

f. Marital history
- Age of marriage
- Sexual intercourse
- Dyspareunia –present/absent
- Contraceptives used
- Sexual disorders.

g. Past medical history
- Major illness — TB/DM/HT/ Hep B/Cancer

- Hormonal therapy
- Hospitalization
- Surgery
- Radiation therapy
- Infectious disease
- Blood transfusion
- Endocrine disorders
- Malaria
- Use of contraception
- Psychiatric problems

h. Obstetrical history
Each pregnancy should be recorded as follows:

| Sl. No. | Date | Duration of Pregnancy | Abnormalities in pregnancy | Home Delivery/ Hospital | Puerperium | Infant breast-feeding |
|---|---|---|---|---|---|---|
| | Year and Month | Weeks of gestation | Abortion/ APH/PIH | ——— | Normal/ PPH/other | Baby alive/still born |

- Gravida
- Para
- Number of living children
- Age of last child

i. Complications in present pregnancy
- Abortion
- APH
- Genital infections
- Rh incompatability
- Polyhydramnios
- Retained placenta
- Multiple pregnancy
- Breast complications
- Infertility
- CPD
- Instrumental delivery
- Vaginal discharge
  Leukorrhea – purulent/offensive/foul smelling
  Color— White/yellow/greenish
  Quantity
  Duration —hours/days
  Character — irritating/bloodstained

III a.  **Physical examination**
  Height in cm:
  Weight in kg:
  Gait:
  Body built:
  Appearance:
  Pallor:
  Lymphadenopathy:
  Edema
  Temperature
  Pulse

Respiration
Blood pressure

**b. Systemic examination**

- G.I. system
abdominal pain ————Severe/intermittent/colicky.
Swelling /Mass/Motility/distension/nausea/vomiting
- Cardiovascular system
Heart rate
Rhythm
Heart sound
- Respiratory system
Rate—
Rhythm——-
Breath sounds———
- Central nervous system
Lethargy
Irritability
Dizziness
Headache
Nausea
Vomiting
- Musculoskeletal system
Pain in the legs/calf muscles/weakness in leg
Cramps
Varicose veins
Swelling
Any other infection
- Genitourinary tract
Pain in the back
Pain on micturition
Burning micturition
Retention of urine

Incontinence of urine
Frequency of micturition
Urethral orifice
- Rectum
Rectal bleeding/discharge
Hemorrhoids
Any other infection
- Gynecological examination
Vulva—lesions/abrasions, redness of vaginal wall/
abnormalities/edema
- Pervaginal examination
Perineal body - soft/hard
Cervix - soft/abnormal
Signs of infection
Bleeding discharge
- Breast examination
Size of breast
Shape of breast
Primary areola – present/absent
Secondary areola—present/absent
Montgomery's tubercles —present/absent
Lymph nodes —palpable/not palpable
Secretion from the breast ——yellow/clear/white/
blood stained
Nipple—normal/no sore/flat/inverted
- Laboratory examination
Blood –Hb/group/type/culture
Urine –culture/sugar/albumin
Vaginal discharge—culture/color / consistency
Cervical swab –culture

**IV Nursing Diagnosis**

# BIBLIOGRAPHY

## BOOKS

1. Altman G, Delmar's. *Fundamental and Advanced Nursing Skills*, 2nd edition, Thomson publications, 2004.
2. Augustine A, Augustine J, Chacko A. *Clinical Nursing and Procedure Manual*, B. I publications, 2004.
3. Brunner and Suddharths. *Textbook of Medical- Surgical Nursing*, 10th edition, published by Lippincott Williams and Wilkins, 2004.
4. Black J M, Hawks JH, Keene AM. *Medical - Surgical Nursing, Clinical Management for Positive Outcomes* volume 1 , 6th edition, published by Harcourt private limited, 2001.
5. Black J M, Hawks JH, Keene AM. *Medical -Surgical Nursing, Clinical Management for Positive Outcomes* volume 2 , 6th edition, published by Harcourt private limited, 2001.
6. Bennett VR, Brown Lk. *Myles Textbook for Midwives*. 13th edition, Harcourt publishers, 2000.
7. Black JM, Jacobs Em. *Luckmann and Sorensen's Medical–Surgical Nursing*. Fourth edition, Publication by Saunders Company, 1993.
8. Basavanthappa B T. *Community Health Nursing*. Jaybee Brothers Publications (p) Ltd, 1998.
9. Bourne M. Shaw's *Textbook of Gynaecology*. 13th edition. Elsevier Publications, 2004.
10. Dutta DC. *Textbook of Obstetrics including Perinatology and Contraception,* sixth edition, New Central Book Agency Publication Ltd, 2004.
11. Dutta DC. *Textbook of Gynaecology including Contraception,* third edition, New Central Book Agency Publication (p) Ltd, 2001.
12. Fischbach FT, Dunning MB. *A Manual of Laboratory Diagnostic tests,* 7th edition, published by Lippincott Williams and Wilkins, 2004.
13. Fraser DM, Cooper MA, (Ed). *Myles Textbook for Midwives*, 14th edition, Churchil livingstone publications, 2003.
14. Ghaiop, Gupta P, Paul VK. *Essential Pediatrics*, fifth edition, Mehta publishers, 2001.
15. Gupte S. *The Short Textbook of Pediatrics*, 9th edition, Jaybee Brothers Publications, 2001.
16. Jacob A. *A Comprehensive Textbook of Midwifery*, Jaypee Brothers Publications , 2005.
17. Kozier B, Erbg, Berman A, Burke K. *Fundamentals of Nursing*, 6th edition, Pearson education publication, 2003.
18. Lewis SM, Heitkemper MM, Dirksen SR. *Medical - Surgical Nursing*, 6th edition Mosby publications, 2000.
19. Marlow DR, Redding BA. *Textbook of Pediatric Nursing*, Sixth edition, published by Harcourt India private Ltd, 1988.
20. MC Kinney ES, James SR, Murray SS, Ashwill JW. *Maternal Child Nursing*, Second edition, Elsevier publications, 2005.
21. Menon MK, Palniappan B. *Clinical Obstetrics*, ninth edition, published by orient longman pvt Ltd, 1990.
22. Natesan S, Jacob S. *Manual on Nursing Principles and Practice*, published by Omayal Achi college of Nursing, 1999
23. Potter PA, Perry AG. *Fundamentals of Nursing*, 3rd edition, Mosby Publications, 1993.
24. Potter PA, Perry AG. *Fundamentals of Nursing* , 6th edition, Elsevier Publications, 2005.
25. Potter PA, Perry AG. *Clinical Nursing Skills and Techniques* 3rd edition, Mosby Publications, 1994.
26. Phipps WJ, Long BC. *Woods NF. Shafer's Medical - Surgical Nursing*, 7th edition, B. I publications pvt Ltd, 1985.
27. Prema TP, Graicy KF. *Essentials of Neurological and Neurosurgical Nursing*, First edition, Jaypee Brothers Publications, 2002.
28. Park K. *Textbook of Preventive and Social Medicine*, Seventeeth edition, Banarsidas Bhanot Publishers, 2002.
29. Russell R, Williams N, Bulstrode C, Bailey and Love's. *Short Practice of Surgery*, 23rd edition Published by Arnold, 2000.
30. Rao KS. *An Introduction to Community Health Nursing*, 4th edition, B.I publications pvt Ltd, 2004.
31. Sr. Nancy, Stephenies. *Priniciples and Practice of Nursing*, volume 1 , 5th edition, N.R. publishing house, 1996.
32. Sr. Nancy, Stephenies. *Principles and Practice of Nursing*, volume 2, 3rd edition, N.R publishing house, 1995.
33. Sister Nancy M. *A reference Manual for Nurses on, Coronary Care Nursing*, 2nd edition Kumar publishing house, 1996.
34. Taylor C, Lillis e, Lemone P. *Fundamentals of Nursing*, 5th edition, Lippincott Williams and Wilkins publications, 2005.
35. The Lippincott. *Manual of Nursing Practice*, 7th edition, Lippincott William and Wilkins publications, 2001.
36. Thygerson AL. *First Aid Handbook,* Jones and Bartlett publishers, 1995.
37. Yalayyaswamy NN. *First Aid and Emergency Nursing*, 1st edition, Gajanana book publishers, 1997.
38. Lasaria and Stuart. " *Principles and Practice of Psychiatric Nursing* ", 7th edition, Mosby Publication, 2001.
39. Niraj Ahaja."*A Short Text Book of Psychiatry*", 5th edition, Jaypee Publication, 2002.

40. Bimla Kapoor."*Text book f Psychiatric Nursing*"No1 I & vol I, Kumar Publication, 2001.
41. Omayal Achi college of nursing *" Manual on Nursing Principles andPractice "*1997.

## PERIODICALS

1. Ayello A. Elizabeth, Baranoski Sharon and David S. Salati. "Wound care – Survey report", *Nursing 2005, June* 2005, P 36-44.
2. Barton Merryn Davies Clare, Graham Jane and Teonlett Jamie. "A new approach to training in intravenous drug therapy," *Nursing times,* 3 November 2003, P 26-27
3. Braden J. Barbara and Marklebust Joan. " Preventing pressure ulcers with Braden scale, *American Journal of Nursing,* June 2005, P 70-72.
4. Boyd Stevie. " Treatment of Physiological and Pathological Neonatal Jaundice", *Nursing Times,* 30 March 2003, P40-41.
5. Bower M Lisa. " Is your patient's metered dose inhaler technique up to snuff ? *Nursing 2005,* August, Vol 35, P 50-51.
6. Cooley Candy and Gabriel Janice. "Reducing the risks of sharps injuries in health care professionals," *Nursing Times,* 29 June 2004, P 28-29.
7. Crowley Angela, Bains M Ranbir and Pellico H. Linda. "A model preschool vision and hearing screening program", *American Journal of Nursing,* June 2005, Vol 105, No.6, P 52-55.
8. Davies Caroline. " The use of phosphate enemas in the treatment of constipation", *Nursing Times,* 4 May 2004, P 32-33
9. Duimel Peters Inge. " Preventing pressure ulcers with massage ? *Americal Journal of Nursing,* August 2005, Vol 105, P 30-31.
10. English Jaqueline." Importance of breast awareness in identification of breast cancer", *Nursing Times,* 7 October 2003, P 18-19.
11. Grosser Lisa. "Meeting the needs of younger women with breast cancer", *Nursing Times,* 11 May 2004 P 43.
12. Grace J Pamela and Mc Langhlin Moriah. " When consent isn't informed enough", *American Journal of Nursing,* April 2005, Vol 105, P 79.
13. Hoban Victoria. " Online learning tool for preoperative assessment", Nursing Times, 11 May 2004 P 43.
14. Hainsworth, Terry. " Guidelines for preventing errors in administering blood transfusion", *Nursing Times,* 6 july 2004, P 30-31.
15. Hubbard Julia. " Management of atrial fibrillation" *Nursing Times,* 10 February 2004.
16. Hoban Vitoria. "How to improve your record keeping", *Nursing Times,* October 2003, P 78-79.
17. Lindgren A. Vicki, Ames J Nancy. " Caring for patients on mechnical ventilation, *American Journal of Nursing,* May 2005, P 50-59.
18. Mendez-Eastman Susan. " Using negative pressure wound therapy wound therapy for positive results" *Nursing 2005,* vol 35, P 48-49
19. Marders Julia. " Sounding the alarm for I.V. infiltration ", *Nursing, 2005,* April 17, P 18.
20. Nandi Ganga, Biswas Doli. "Effect of cold compress and manual application of pressure on cardiac catheterization related hematoma", Asian Journal of cardiovascular *Nursing,* June 2005, vol 13, No 2 P 26-28.
21. Nirmala R. " Urinary investigations", *Health screen,* May 2005, P 10-11
22. Privet Susan. " Clean hands are a vital part of care ", *Nursing Times,* 29 June 2004, P – 47.
23. Pittet, D and Boyce J.M. " Organising an awareness week to target hand hygiene practice", *Nursing Times,* 27 April 2004
24. Pruitt Bill. " Clear the air with closed suctioning, *Nursing* 2005, vol 35 P 44-49
25. Reising Deanna L, Scott Ronald. " Enteral tube flushing, *American Journal of Nursing ,* March 2005, vol 105, P 58 – 63.
26. Stevenson Tracy. " Improving policy and practice in the prevention of pressure ulcers", *Nursing Times,* 2 March 2004.
27. Sangar Kanta. " Engorgement of Breast, Potential problem in lactation, *Nightingale Nursing Times,* August 2004, vol 1 P 12-16.
28. Webb Catherine. " The benefits and the pitfalls of preoperative fasting", *Nursing Times,* 16 December 2003, P 32-33.

# INDEX